Retain - local interest - Chapter 19

Core Topics in Paediatric Anaesthesia

Core Topics in Paediatric Anaesthesia

Edited by

Ian James
Consultant Anaesthetist, Great Ormond Street Hospital for Children NHS Foundation Trust;
Honorary Senior Lecturer, Institute of Child Health, London, UK

Isabeau Walker
Consultant Anaesthetist, Great Ormond Street Hospital for Children NHS Foundation Trust;
Honorary Senior Lecturer, Institute of Child Health, London, UK

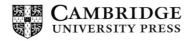
CAMBRIDGE
UNIVERSITY PRESS

CAMBRIDGE UNIVERSITY PRESS
Cambridge, New York, Melbourne, Madrid, Cape Town,
Singapore, São Paulo, Delhi, Mexico City

Cambridge University Press
The Edinburgh Building, Cambridge CB2 8RU, UK

Published in the United States of America
by Cambridge University Press, New York

www.cambridge.org
Information on this title: www.cambridge.org/9780521194174

© Cambridge University Press 2013

First published 2013

Printed and bound in the United Kingdom by Bell and Bain Ltd

*A catalogue record for this publication is available from the British
Library*

Library of Congress Cataloguing in Publication data
Core topics in paediatric anaesthesia / edited by Ian James,
consultant anaesthetist, Great Ormond Street Hospital for Children
NHS Trust, honorary senior lecturer, Institute of Child Health, London,
UK, Isabeau Walker, consultant anaesthetist, Great Ormond Street
Hospital for Children NHS Trust, honorary senior lecturer, Institute of
Child Health, London, UK.
    pages   cm
  Includes bibliographical references and index.
  ISBN 978-0-521-19417-4 (Hardback)
1. Pediatric anesthesia.   I. James, Ian (Ian Gordon) editor of
compilation.   II. Walker, Isabeau, editor of compilation.
  RD139.C67 2013
  617.9'6798–dc23
                                                              2012044102

ISBN 978-0-521-19417-4 Hardback

Contents

Preface

Children comprise almost a quarter of the population, and many will require general anaesthesia for surgery or an investigative procedure. It is important that the facilities and environment for such procedures are appropriate for a child, and it is crucial that those administering anaesthesia are knowledgeable, competent and safe. It is an oft-repeated adage that the child is not a miniature adult, and nowhere is this more true than in paediatric anaesthesia where there are significant differences, for instance in pharmacology, psychology, common clinical conditions and legal issues such as consent. Our intention with this book has been to provide the core knowledge, both theoretical and practical, necessary to assist all those regularly involved in anaesthetising children to do so safely and competently. We hope that this text will be particularly useful to trainees aspiring to become specialist paediatric anaesthetists.

We have tried to go further than just covering the core curriculum for training in paediatric anaesthesia. For the clinical chapters we asked our authors, who are all recognised experts in their specialist areas, to share their experience by outlining in a succinct manner how they manage their patients. It seems to us particularly helpful to read how those who are regularly anaesthetising patients with specific disorders have fine-tuned their practice to minimise problems and achieve good outcomes. We have included key references and additional reading for all chapters. Although we have discussed some of the more common syndromes affecting children, we have not provided a comprehensive list of all the congenital disorders that may be encountered. Many of these are rare, and their salient features can quickly and easily be obtained on the Internet.

We hope that our book will also be useful for those anaesthetists who work in the general hospital, especially those who only see children presenting as emergencies. Over the past 20 years or so a plethora of reports have espoused the benefits of centralisation of paediatric surgery. Subsequent organisational changes have resulted in the transfer of much of this work to specialised centres, particularly for children in the 0–4 year age range. For many anaesthetists working outside these specialist centres, this has resulted in reduced opportunity to maintain competence and, perhaps of equal importance, confidence in anaesthetising small children, even though over half of all procedures in children still take place in the District General Hospital. This book is no substitute for regular hands-on experience, but we hope that it will be helpful in providing core knowledge and tips from established experts that can be used to supplement refresher courses and clinical attachments to maintain skills.

We would like to thank those who have helped in developing this book, particularly family and friends who have been neglected during its long gestation. We are also grateful to Cambridge University Press for their patience as the book's post-conceptual age increased. Finally, we would like to thank Sally and Ash Suxena for allowing Joseph to grace our front cover.

Ian James
Isabeau Walker

Contributors

Lola Adewale
Consultant Anaesthetist, Birmingham Children's Hospital NHS Foundation Trust, Birmingham, UK

Nargis Ahmad
Consultant Anaesthetist, Great Ormond Street Hospital for Children NHS Foundation Trust, London, UK

James Bennett
Consultant Anaesthetist, Birmingham Children's Hospital NHS Foundation Trust, Birmingham, UK

Stephanie Bew
Consultant Anaesthetist, Leeds General Infirmary, Leeds, UK

Michael Broadhead
Consultant Anaesthetist, Great Ormond Street Hospital for Children NHS Foundation Trust, London, UK

Peter Bromley
Consultant Anaesthetist, Birmingham Children's Hospital NHS Foundation Trust, Birmingham, UK

Alison S. Carr
Consultant Paediatric Anaesthetist, Plymouth Hospitals NHS Trust, Plymouth, UK

David Chisholm
Consultant Anaesthetist, The Royal Marsden Hospital NHS Foundation Trust, London, UK

David de Beer
Consultant Anaesthetist, Great Ormond Street Hospital for Children NHS Foundation Trust, London, UK

Bruce Emerson
Consultant Anaesthetist, St Andrew's Centre for Plastic Surgery and Burns, Broomfield Hospital, Chelmsford, Essex, UK

Philippa Evans
Consultant Anaesthetist, Great Ormond Street Hospital for Children NHS Foundation Trust, London, UK

Lisa Flewin
Consultant Anaesthetist, Southampton University Hospital, Southampton, UK

Michael W. Frost
Consultant Anaesthetist, St Andrew's Centre for Plastic Surgery and Burns, Broomfield Hospital, Chelmsford, Essex, UK

Simon R. Haynes
Consultant Anaesthetist, Freeman Hospital, Newcastle-Upon-Tyne, UK

Jane Herod
Consultant Anaesthetist, Great Ormond Street Hospital for Children NHS Foundation Trust, London, UK

Alet Jacobs
Department of Anaesthesia, Birmingham Children's Hospital NHS Foundation Trust, Birmingham, UK

Ian James
Consultant Anaesthetist, Great Ormond Street Hospital for Children NHS Foundation Trust; Honorary Senior Lecturer, Institute of Child Health, London, UK

Ian A. Jenkins
Consultant in Paediatric Intensive Care & Anaesthesia, The Bristol Royal Hospital for Children, Bristol, UK

Adrian R. Lloyd-Thomas
Consultant Anaesthetist, Great Ormond Street Hospital for Children NHS Foundation Trust, London, UK

Daniel Lutman
Consultant Paediatric Anaesthetist, Children's Acute Transport Service, London, UK

Angus McEwan
Consultant Anaesthetist, Great Ormond Street Hospital for Children NHS Foundation Trust, London, UK

Su Mallory
Consultant Anaesthetist, Great Ormond Street Hospital for Children NHS Foundation Trust, London, UK

Vaithianadan Mani
Department of Anaesthesia, Royal Hospital for Sick Children, Glasgow, UK

George H. Meakin
Consultant Anaesthetist, Royal Manchester Children's Hospital, Manchester, UK

Anthony Moriarty
Consultant Anaesthetist, Birmingham Children's Hospital NHS Foundation Trust, Birmingham, UK

Neil Morton
Consultant in Paediatric Anaesthesia and Pain Management, Royal Hospital for Sick Children, Glasgow, UK

Reema Nandi
Consultant Anaesthetist, Great Ormond Street Hospital for Children NHS Foundation Trust, London, UK

Naveen Raj
Consultant Anaesthetist, Jackson Rees Department of Anaesthesia, Alder Hey Children's Hospital NHS Foundation Trust, Liverpool, UK

Steve Roberts
Consultant Anaesthetist, Jackson Rees Department of Anaesthesia, Alder Hey Children's Hospital NHS Foundation Trust, Liverpool, UK

Steven Scuplak
Consultant Anaesthetist, Great Ormond Street Hospital for Children NHS Foundation Trust, London, UK

Judith A. Short
Consultant Paediatric Anaesthetist, Sheffield Children's NHS Foundation Trust, Sheffield, UK

Jonathan Smith
Consultant Anaesthetist, Great Ormond Street Hospital for Children NHS Foundation Trust, London, UK

Ben Stanhope
Consultant in Paediatric Emergency Medicine, Birmingham Children's Hospital NHS Foundation Trust, Birmingham, UK

Peter A. Stoddart
Consultant Anaesthetist, The Bristol Royal Hospital for Children, Bristol, UK

Mike R. J. Sury
Consultant Anaesthetist, Great Ormond Street Hospital for Children NHS Foundation Trust; Portex Department of Anaesthesia, Institute of Child Health, University College London, UK

Dan Taylor
Consultant Paediatric Anaesthetist, Evelina Children's Hospital, St. Thomas' Hospital, London, UK

Karl C. Thies
Consultant Anaesthetist, Birmingham Children's Hospital NHS Foundation Trust, Birmingham, UK

Mark Thomas
Consultant Anaesthetist, Great Ormond Street Hospital for Children NHS Foundation Trust, London, UK

Isabeau Walker
Consultant Anaesthetist, Great Ormond Street Hospital for Children NHS Foundation Trust; Honorary Senior Lecturer, Institute of Child Health, London, UK

Agnes Watson
Consultant Anaesthetist, St Andrew's Centre for Plastic Surgery and Burns, Broomfield Hospital, Chelmsford, Essex, UK

Kathy A. Wilkinson
Consultant Paediatric Anaesthetist, Norfolk and
Norwich University Hospitals NHS Foundation
Trust, Norwich, UK

Glyn Williams
Consultant Anaesthetist, Great Ormond Street
Hospital for Children NHS Foundation Trust,
London, UK

Sally Wilmshurst
Consultant Anaesthetist, Great Ormond Street
Hospital for Children NHS Foundation Trust,
London, UK

Anatomical and physiological issues affecting anaesthesia in neonates and young children

Isabeau Walker

Introduction

Age is an important risk factor in anaesthesia, and the risks of anaesthesia are greater in neonates and infants, even in expert hands. There are important physiological and anatomical differences between neonates, young children and adults that influence anaesthesia techniques, and there are rapid changes that occur in the transition from fetal to neonatal life, and also during the first few months and years of life. This chapter will consider some of the differences in anatomy and physiology that affect neonates and young children during growth and development, and the clinical implications of these differences. The premature and ex-premature infant will be considered in more detail in Chapter 9.

The development of the respiratory system

The development of the lung starts early in the period of organogenesis; the lung buds with lobar structure are present by 6 weeks gestation and the structure of the bronchial tree is laid down by 16 weeks. The respiratory acinus consists of the respiratory bronchiole, alveolar ducts and alveolar sacs and starts to form by 24 weeks. The thin-walled terminal respiratory saccules appear by 24 weeks at the same time as complex pulmonary capillary networks start to develop. The respiratory saccules are lined by type I pneumocytes, which form the gas-exchanging surface, and type II pneumocytes, which produce pulmonary surfactant.

Surfactant is present in type II pneumocytes by 26 weeks and is secreted into the lumen of the airway by 30 weeks. Surfactant is important as it lines the airways and reduces surface tension to prevent the alveoli collapsing after birth. Fetal plasma cortisol levels rise from 24 weeks, which is important for lung maturation as cortisol stimulates surfactant release, alveolar cell differentiation and resorption of lung fluid. True alveoli start to develop at 32 weeks. Babies who are born at less than 30 weeks gestation benefit from antenatal steroids to facilitate lung maturation, and exogenous surfactant to assist in aeration of the lung. Babies born before 24 weeks gestation are unlikely to be viable owing to extreme immaturity of the respiratory system.

A baby born after 37 weeks gestation is considered as full term; the lung structure is mature with a large internal surface area and thin-walled alveoli in close proximity to the pulmonary capillaries. Alveolar development continues after birth and continues until the age of 18 months; in fact, 85% of alveolar development occurs in the post-natal period. Bronchial smooth muscle increases from birth to adulthood, with a rapid increase in the first few weeks after birth. Growth of the lungs occurs by increase in length and diameter of the airways, and continues until the long bones fuse.

Cardiorespiratory adaptation at birth

During fetal life, the placenta is the main site of respiratory gas exchange. Oxygenated blood returns from the placenta to the inferior vena cava via the ductus venosus, and is preferentially channelled across the foramen ovale to the left atrium, thence to the ascending aorta, coronary vessels and the brain (see Figure 1.1). Pulmonary arterioles are tightly constricted owing to low levels of oxygen, nitric oxide and prostacyclin (PGI_2), and pulmonary vascular resistance (PVR) is high. As a consequence, only about 10% of the right ventricular output enters

Core Topics in Paediatric Anaesthesia, ed. Ian James and Isabeau Walker. Published by Cambridge University Press. © 2013 Cambridge University Press.

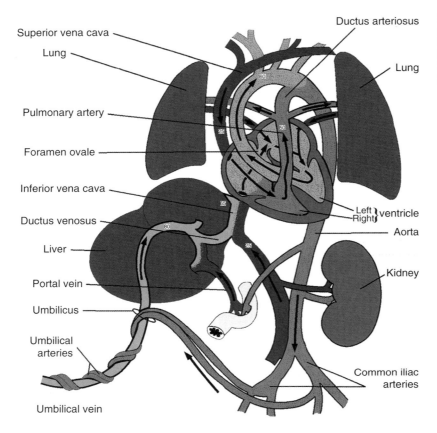

Figure 1.1 The fetal circulation. The numbers indicate oxygen saturation. From Murphy PJ. The fetal circulation. *Contin Educ Anaesth Crit Care Pain* 2005;5(4):107–112, with permission. See plate section for colour version.

the pulmonary circulation, and blood in the pulmonary artery is shunted across the ductus arteriosus to the descending aorta. Cardiorespiratory adaptation is the process whereby gas exchange is transferred from the placenta to the lungs and the fetal shunts close (foramen ovale, ductus arteriosus and ductus venosus).

In fetal life, the respiratory system is filled with liquid, and fetal breathing movements are present. Some lung fluid is squeezed out of the lungs during the second stage of labour, but most of the fluid is absorbed into the pulmonary lymphatics and capillaries when the first few breaths are taken. Sudden cooling and sensory inputs that increase central arousal act as the main stimuli for breathing. High negative pressures are generated initially, and active expiration during crying helps to distribute ventilation and facilitate clearance of lung fluid. Inflation breaths to clear lung fluid are an essential component of newborn resuscitation.

The foramen ovale

There is a marked fall in PVR associated with the mechanical changes that follow aeration of the lungs and the sudden increase in oxygen tension; pulmonary venous return is increased and the flap valve covering the foramen ovale closes, although the foramen ovale may remain 'probe patent' into adult life.

Ductus arteriosus

Patency of the ductus arteriosus is maintained *in utero* by low oxygen tension and the effect of prostaglandins. After birth, oxygen tension rises, and this causes the ductus arteriosus to constrict, a process that is usually complete by day 2 in healthy term infants, and by day 4 in most preterm babies. Anatomical closure of the ductus usually occurs by 2–3 weeks.

Patent ductus arteriosus (PDA) may be seen in up to 50% of babies with birth weight <800 g, with decreasing incidence as gestational age increases. PDA is due to persistently low oxygen tension or elevated prostaglandins, rather than abnormal ductal tissue per se. Pulmonary vascular resistance usually falls during the first few weeks of life, and the presence of a persisting PDA will lead to left to right shunting and increased pulmonary blood flow, with worsening respiratory distress and heart failure. Medical closure of the PDA may be attempted using prostaglandin synthetase inhibitors such as the NSAIDs ibuprofen or indomethacin. If unsuccessful, surgery may be required.

Continued ductal patency is essential in some congenital cardiac conditions, such as a duct dependent systemic circulation (e.g. hypoplastic left heart syndrome or critical coarctation) or duct dependent pulmonary circulation (e.g. pulmonary atresia with intact ventricular septum). Prostaglandin infusion may be required to keep the duct open until surgery can be performed.

Ductus venosus

The ductus venosus is a blood channel through the embryonic liver from the left umbilical vein to the inferior vena cava (IVC). It closes functionally within hours of birth, and anatomical closure starts after the first few days. It may be used immediately after birth to provide access to the right atrium via an umbilical venous catheter.

Pulmonary vascular resistance

Pulmonary blood flow increases eight-fold after birth owing to dilation of pulmonary arterioles in the first few minutes after birth, followed by a slow fall in PVR over the next few weeks and months (see Figure 1.2). The early fall in PVR is due to vasodilation of pulmonary arterioles mediated by increased lung volumes and increased oxygen tension, nitric oxide and PGI_2 levels, with later changes due to involution of smooth muscle in the arteriolar walls.

The PVR may remain high or increase during early neonatal life owing to asphyxia, hypoxia, sepsis, congenital diaphragmatic hernia and meconium aspiration. This results in shunting from right to left across the ductus arteriosus and severe hypoxaemia, so-called persistent pulmonary hypertension of the newborn (PPHN).

Infants who have congenital cardiac lesions associated with left to right shunting, such as unrestricted ventricular septal defect, usually become symptomatic during the first few weeks of life as PVR falls and pulmonary blood flow increases. If the child remains untreated and high pulmonary blood flow is sustained, pulmonary vascular remodelling occurs and the PVR rises. This reactive increase in PVR is the basis for subsequent flow reversal in Eisenmenger's syndrome.

Respiratory system in neonates and infants

Oxygen consumption in neonates is twice that in adults ($6-8\,ml\,kg^{-1}\,min^{-1}$ vs $3\,ml\,kg^{-1}\,min^{-1}$). The relatively high minute ventilation is achieved by increasing respiratory rate ($30-40\,min^{-1}$) as the tidal volume is relatively fixed ($7\,ml\,kg^{-1}$). Increased minute volume means that induction and emergence from inhalational anaesthesia is more rapid in infants compared with older children, and deep levels of anaesthesia may be obtained very quickly.

Neonates do not tolerate airway obstruction or pauses in ventilation and become hypoxic very quickly. Nasal resistance contributes one-third of pulmonary resistance, and a clear nasal airway is particularly important in small infants as they breathe predominantly through their noses. Hypoxia leads to profound bradycardia.

The airway is easily obstructed during anaesthesia. The tongue is relatively large, and the tongue and soft palate fall against the posterior pharyngeal wall. The occiput is prominent and encourages neck flexion. Airway patency is maintained by the action of pharyngeal dilators, but pharyngeal tone is lost on induction of anaesthesia. Airway obstruction may be improved by 'chin lift' and the use of an oropharyngeal airway.

The epiglottis is long and straight and tends to flop back over the laryngeal inlet, which is high and anterior, so intubation in neonates is best achieved with a straight blade laryngoscope, possibly with a roll placed under the shoulders to overcome the effect of the large occiput. The larynx is conical in shape with the narrowest portion at the level of the cricoid cartilage. Uncuffed tracheal tubes are commonly used in neonates to avoid airway oedema and potential subglottic stenosis. Cuffed tracheal tubes are increasingly used in older children, especially in children with pulmonary disease requiring ventilation in

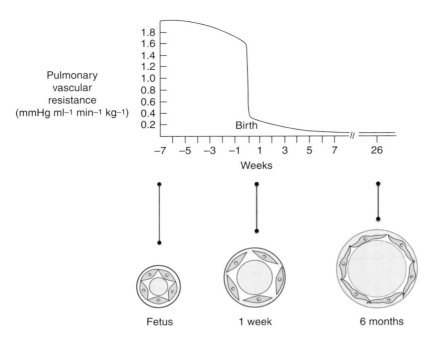

Figure 1.2 Structural changes in the pulmonary artery in the postnatal period and corresponding changes in pulmonary vascular resistance. Fetal pulmonary arteries have thick walls and a narrow lumen, with rounded densely packed smooth muscle cells (SMC). Within 1 week of life the SMC become thinner and spread around a larger lumen. By 6 months of age there is further decrease in the medial thickness of the vessel wall with reduced SMC density, and a larger lumen. (Adapted from Gao Y, Raj JU, *Physiol Rev* 2010;90:1291–1335, and Rudolph AM, *Congenital Diseases of the Heart*, Chicago: Year book, 1974.)

intensive care where a leak from an uncuffed tracheal tube may compromise ventilation. Care should be taken to avoid overinflation of the cuff, and the cuff pressure should be monitored (<20 cmH$_2$O).

The trachea is short in absolute terms, and it is easy to cause endobronchial intubation. The position of the tracheal tube should always be checked by auscultation. The airways are narrow and are easily blocked by oedema or secretions. According to Poiseuille's law, airway resistance is proportional to viscosity and inversely proportional to the fourth power of the radius of the airway:

$$R = 8\,nl/\pi r^4$$

where R = resistance
      n = viscosity
      l = the length of the airway
      r = the radius of the airway

Airway oedema that causes a small reduction in airway diameter in an infant results in a disproportionately large increase in airway resistance. Nebulised adrenaline (which reduces airway oedema) and heliox (which reduces airway resistance) may be useful in an emergency situation.

The thoracic cavity in neonates is round rather than dorso-ventrally flattened as in the adult. The cartilaginous ribs are soft and elastic and horizontally placed, so the 'bucket handle' action of the ribs that

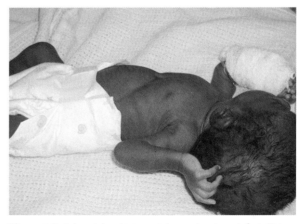

Figure 1.3 Subcostal and intercostal recession in an infant. Picture taken at Great Ormond Street Hospital (GOSH) with permission.

increases thoracic volume in adults does not occur. The lungs are very compliant, the chest wall is elastic and distending pressures on the lung are low. Closing volume occurs within tidal breathing in neonates and it is common to see intercostal and subcostal recession if lung compliance is reduced (e.g. infection or cardiac failure) (see Figure 1.3). Chest wall stability increases by about 1 year of age. Intercostal and subcostal recession in an older child is an ominous sign indicating severe lung disease.

The diaphragm is the predominant respiratory muscle in neonates, but it is less efficient than in adults as it is relatively horizontal rather than dome shaped. Neonates are prone to respiratory failure as they have a lower proportion of fatigue resistant type 1 muscle fibres in the diaphragm. Gastric insufflation is common after facemask ventilation and may result in abdominal distension and splinting of the diaphragm. A nasogastric tube should be passed to relieve abdominal distension as this will improve respiratory function and reduce the risk of aspiration.

Infants have little respiratory reserve, and apparatus dead space and resistance should be kept to a minimum to reduce the work of breathing. Infants should not be left to breathe spontaneously through a tracheal tube, and ventilation under anaesthesia should be assisted. Application of continuous positive airway pressure (CPAP) or positive end-expiratory pressure (PEEP) increases lung volumes, reduces the work of breathing and should be employed during anaesthesia to improve gas exchange and prevent atelectasis. Neonates should be intubated for all except the briefest of procedures and positive pressure ventilation should be used.

Control of ventilation

The control of ventilation is immature at birth. Neonates are at risk from post-operative apnoeas, especially if born prematurely, anaemic, cold or exposed to opioids.

Fetal breathing is detected from 14 weeks gestation, and increases with gestational age. The fetus responds to increased maternal hypercapnia by an increase in respiratory rate, and to hypoxia by a reduction in respiratory rate.

Neonates also respond to hypercapnia by increased respiratory rate, as in older children and adults. The response to hypoxia remains immature and results in a brief increase in ventilation followed by a fall in respiratory rate, or in premature neonates, by the baby becoming apnoeic. This apnoeic response to hypoxia may be due to persistence of the fetal response to hypoxia into neonatal life. In term infants this biphasic response disappears by 2 weeks of age, but maturation of respiratory control may be delayed in premature infants.

Anaesthetic agents depress ventilation in a dose dependent manner. Term neonates are probably at risk of post-operative apnoea after routine minor surgery (avoiding opioids) up to 1 month of age. Premature neonates are at low risk of post-operative apnoeas after 60 weeks postconceptional age; for a baby born at 28 weeks, this is when they are 8 months chronological age (5 months corrected age). Regional anaesthesia without sedation (e.g. spinal anaesthesia for hernia repair) may reduce the risk of post-operative apnoeas.

Cardiovascular system in neonates and infants

There is a period of ventricular remodelling after birth. *In utero*, the right ventricle dominates as it pumps 65% of the cardiac output and the left ventricle is relatively quiescent. After birth, the left ventricle becomes the dominant ventricle and supports the systemic circulation. The systemic vascular resistance increases after birth and the left ventricular wall thickness increases markedly during infancy, with a more modest increase in the right ventricular wall thickness. The newborn heart contains about half the myocytes present in the adult heart, and remodelling occurs by an increase in number, size and complexity of myocytes with age. The heart is relatively globular in the neonate, and the right ventricle is the same volume as the left. The right ventricle increases in volume relative to the left and reaches the adult volume ratio of 2:1 by 2 years of age. Left ventricular remodelling occurs as a consequence of increased systemic vascular resistance. Babies who have transposition of the great arteries and in whom the arterial switch operation is delayed beyond a few months may become inoperable, as the left ventricle is pumping into the pulmonary circulation where the PVR is low, and left ventricular remodelling does not occur.

Tissue oxygen delivery is achieved by a relatively high cardiac output ($300 \, \text{ml} \, \text{kg}^{-1} \, \text{min}^{-1}$ vs $60-80 \, \text{ml} \, \text{kg}^{-1} \, \text{min}^{-1}$ in adults) and high heart rate. There is limited cardiac reserve. The cardiac output is rate dependent, and the heart rate should be maintained in the normal range for age. The Frank–Starling relationship regulates cardiac output as in adults, but the ability to increase stroke volume is limited. Neonates can increase cardiac output with careful volume loading (bolus of $5-10 \, \text{ml} \, \text{kg}^{-1}$), but they do not tolerate volume overload. Afterload is a major determinant of cardiac output, and the neonatal heart is very sensitive to increases in systemic or pulmonary vascular resistance.

Innervation of the heart is functionally immature at birth, and sympathetic tone dominates, resulting in high contractility and high resting heart rate. Parasympathetic tone increases with age, but vagally mediated cardiac reflexes are well developed in infancy.

Neonates are sensitive to the negative inotropic effects of anaesthetic agents. Atropine may counteract the reduction in cardiac output seen with volatile agents and will protect against vagally mediated reflexes, especially those associated with intubation. It is useful as premedication, although no longer used routinely.

Oxygen transport to the tissues

Oxygen transport by haemoglobin is characterised by changes in the oxygen dissociation curve and described by the P_{50}, the partial pressure of oxygen at which haemoglobin is 50% saturated.

At birth, fetal haemoglobin (HbF) forms 70–80% of total haemoglobin – it is suited to the hypoxic conditions found during fetal life but provides relatively poor tissue oxygenation after birth (low P_{50}).

This is compensated for by a relatively high haemoglobin concentration.

Adult haemoglobin (HbA_2) production increases from birth, being the dominant haemoglobin by the first few months of life. It is very efficient at tissue oxygen delivery (high P_{50}), and tissue oxygen delivery increases during infancy to levels higher than found in adults, probably reflecting increased levels of 2,3-diphosphoglycerate (2,3 DPG) during a period of rapid growth (see Figure 1.4).

Coupled with a relatively high cardiac output, tissue oxygen delivery is extremely efficient in infants compared with adults. These factors affect the triggers for transfusion or the haemoglobin level at which a child should be considered significantly anaemic (see Table 1.1). A useful formula for transfusion is:

- $4 \, \text{ml} \, \text{kg}^{-1}$ packed cells raises the Hb by $1 \, \text{g} \, \text{dl}^{-1}$
- $8 \, \text{ml} \, \text{kg}^{-1}$ whole blood raises the Hb by $1 \, \text{g} \, \text{dl}^{-1}$

Table 1.1 Haemoglobin requirements for equivalent tissue oxygen delivery

	P_{50} (mm Hg)	Haemoglobin required for equivalent tissue oxygen delivery (g dl^{-1})		
Neonate <2 months	24	17.6	14.7	11.7
Infant >6 months	30	9.8	8.2	6.5
Adult	27	12	10	8

Adapted with permission from Motoyama EM, Finer JD. Respiratory physiology in infants and children. In Smith PJ, ed. *Smith's Anaesthesia for Infants and Children*, 8th edition. Elsevier Health Sciences. 2011, p. 63

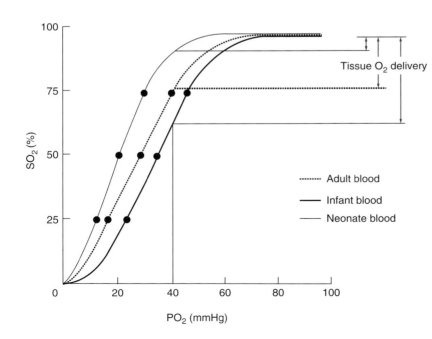

Figure 1.4 Oxygen–haemoglobin dissociation curves in infants and neonates. PO_2 = partial oxygen pressure; SO_2 = oxygen saturation. (Reproduced with permission from: Motoyama and Finer (2011) Respiratory physiology in infants and children. In Smith PJ, ed., *Smith's Anaesthesia for Infants and Children*. 8th edition. Elsevier Health Sciences. 2011, p. 62.)

Development of the kidney and changes with birth

Nephrogenesis begins at 5 weeks of gestation and is completed at 35 weeks. The main function of the fetal kidney is the production of amniotic fluid, which is in turn important for development of the fetal lung. Renal abnormalities *in utero* are associated with oligohydramnios and pulmonary hypoplasia. The full compliment of nephrons is present at birth, and maturation of the kidney is by increasing length and complexity of the tubules. The placenta performs the excretory functions of the fetus so at birth the urea and electrolytes in the neonate are similar to those of the mother, but fall within the first few days of life. Premature babies have impaired renal function in infancy, and may be hypertensive in later life. Glomerular filtration rate (GFR) is low after birth, but in normal children, reaches adult indexed values by 2 years of age.

The neonate does not take in very much fluid in the first few days of life during the time that lactation is established. Levels of antidiuretic hormone (ADH) are high so urine output is low and body water is conserved. A brisk diuresis occurs in the first few days of life as ADH levels fall and cardiorespiratory adaptation occurs, which results in increased pulmonary venous return and the release of atrial natriuretic hormone. Fluids should be restricted until the post-natal diuresis has occurred; excessive fluids may promote PDA, particularly in premature infants.

Sodium is retained in the first few days of life as the GFR is low, the mean arterial pressure is low, and the renin–angiotensin–aldosterone system is active and promotes the reabsorption of sodium in the collecting duct. Sodium is usually withheld in the first few days of life, but is added to maintenance fluids after the post-natal diuresis has occurred. The premature neonate has impaired tubular reabsorption of sodium and limited sodium retention, so frequently requires sodium supplements to avoid hyponatremia.

Babies obtain their calories from a liquid diet, and have an immature urinary concentrating ability so they produce relatively large volumes of dilute urine that is isotonic with plasma (300 mOsmol kg^{-1}). They are therefore prone to dehydration if they are starved for excessive periods of time, and renal failure is common in sick infants. The renal tubular system and concentrating abilities mature over the first few months of life, and infants are able to produce concentrated urine (1200–1400 mOsmol kg^{-1}) and withstand fluid deprivation by 1 year of age.

Hepatic function and drug handling

Children have been described as 'therapeutic orphans' in that many drugs, especially new drugs, have not been studied in this age group; we can hope that this will be rectified in future. The liver in the newborn infant contains 20% of the hepatocytes found in adults and continues to grow until early adulthood. The liver is the principal site of drug metabolism, some evidence of which can be found in fetal life, albeit at low levels.

Phase I processes (metabolic, e.g. the cytochrome P-450 system) are significantly reduced at birth whilst phase II processes (conjugation) may be well developed (sulfation) or limited (glucuronidation). Paracetamol is excreted by sulfation in the neonate and glucuronidation in adults. In general, drug effects are prolonged in neonates, and drugs should be titrated to effect, given by bolus rather than infusion, or plasma levels monitored as appropriate. Maturation of enzymatic processes increases over the first few weeks of life, and the half-life of drugs such as morphine reaches adult levels at 2 months of life. Neonates require significantly less morphine than older children, especially in the first week of life. Plasma protein binding is reduced in neonates and infants (low levels of α1-acid glycoprotein), and drugs that are plasma protein bound (such as local anaesthetics) may demonstrate increased toxicity.

Infants have reduced hepatic stores of glycogen and immature gluconeogenic enzyme systems. They have a high metabolic rate so they are susceptible to hypoglycaemia following starvation. Blood sugar should be measured routinely during surgery. An isotonic solution containing glucose should be used if the child has been hypoglycaemic or receiving parenteral nutrition pre-operatively

Coagulation

Development of the coagulation system starts *in utero* and continues until about 6 months of age. Vitamin K dependent factors are 70% of adult values at birth, and all newborn infants require vitamin

K prophylaxis to prevent haemorrhagic disease of the newborn. Platelets are present in normal numbers at birth, and reach adult reactivity at 2 weeks of age. Coagulation screening tests are prolonged in normal infants up to the age of 6 months, which is reflected in values for the normal ranges.

Temperature control

Thermoregulation in the neonate is limited and easily overwhelmed by environmental conditions. Heat production is limited and there is a greater potential for heat loss (high body surface area to body weight ratio, increased thermal conductance, increased evaporative heat loss through the skin). The newborn infant reduces heat loss by vasoconstriction and increases heat production through brown fat metabolism (non-shivering thermogenesis), although this is at the expense of increased oxygen consumption. Brown fat metabolism is inhibited by volatile agents. The preterm baby is particularly vulnerable to cooling as the immature skin is thin and allows major heat and evaporative fluid losses. Premature infants should have minimal handling and exposure to avoid excessive heat loss. Surgery is frequently performed in the neonatal unit for this reason.

Central nervous system, nociception and the stress response

The brain forms 10–15% of body weight at birth, but only 2% of body weight by the age of 8 years. The brain is reliant on glucose for metabolism but the child is also able to utilise ketones under normal conditions. The cerebral metabolic requirement for oxygen ($CMRO_2$) is higher in young children owing to the demands of growth.

Autoregulation of cerebral blood flow is present in the newborn period. The lower limit for cerebral autoregulation in neonates is not known, but is thought to be around a cerebral perfusion pressure of 30 mmHg. The appropriate mean arterial blood pressure for premature neonates is controversial but it is generally accepted that the mean arterial pressure equates to the gestational age of the child during the first day of life, rising to a minimum of 30 mmHg by 3 days.

Developmental aspects of pain

Neonates, including premature neonates, show well-developed responses to painful stimuli. Indeed, the fetus shows a stress response (and behavioural changes) to nociceptive stimulation from 18–20 weeks gestation, which can be attenuated by the administration of fentanyl. It has long been known that attenuation of the stress response to surgery improves post-operative morbidity and mortality.

The neonatal period is characterised by marked sensitivity to sensory stimuli of all types, with low thresholds of response to mechanical and noxious stimulation. The nociceptive responses of neonates are significantly different from those of adults; at birth, a noxious stimulus (e.g. heel prick) will elicit an exaggerated movement of the whole body and movement of all four limbs.

The process of maturation of the nociceptive system is complex and involves interactions between the peripheral and central nervous systems, changes in receptor, ion channel and neurotransmitter expression and the effects of neurotrophins. Experimental evidence has shown widespread, functional opioid receptors in the spinal cord of newborn animals (rather than located to lamina I and II of the spinal cord as in adult life). It appears that there is a great deal of neuronal fine-tuning during early neonatal life, which may be influenced by the activity of endogenous opioids. There is a question about the long-term effects of exposure to exogenous morphine in neonates at this time of neuronal plasticity. Conversely, early pain experiences may result in sensitisation and may also have long-term effects, possibly through developmental changes in sensitivity to nociceptive stimuli.

Long-term effects of early exposure to anaesthetic agents

Recent work has investigated the effects of exposure of the developing brain to drugs that block NMDA receptors or potentiate GABA receptors in animal models. All anaesthetic drugs commonly used in paediatric practice (midazolam, propofol, barbiturates, all volatile agents, ketamine and etomidate) are found to cause dose dependent neuronal apoptosis with deficits in hippocampal synaptic function and persistent memory/learning impairments in these animal models. The relevance to clinical practice is unclear at present. Surgery without effective anaesthesia and pain relief would be inhumane and would also have significant adverse effects. It would seem sensible to avoid surgery during infancy unless it is necessary, to avoid multiple agents and, if possible, to limit duration of anaesthesia to less than 2 hours.

Key points

- Early neonatal life is a time of rapid development and adaptation that makes the neonate particularly vulnerable during surgery.
- Neonates and infants are prone to airway obstruction and respiratory failure; respiration

should be supported with CPAP as a minimum during anaesthesia, with positive pressure ventilation for all except minor procedures.
- Neonates and infants have limited cardiac reserve, and deep anaesthesia should be avoided.
- Surgery should only be undertaken if necessary during infancy. Babies should be kept warm, should not be volume loaded or starved for excessive periods of time, and balanced anaesthesia should be used, with judicious use of opioids.

Further reading

Booker PD. Extrauterine development of the cardiovascular system. In: Lake CL and Booker PD, eds. *Pediatric Cardiac Anesthesia*, 4th edition. Lippincott Williams and Wilkins. 2005.

Haycock G. Disorders of the kidney and urinary tract. In: Rennie JM, ed.

Roberton's Textbook of Neonatology, 4th edition. Elsevier Ltd. 2005.

Motoyama ET. Respiratory physiology. In: Bissonnette B and Dalens BJ, eds. *Principles and Practice of Pediatric Anaesthesia* McGraw-Hill. 2003.

Motoyama EM, Finer JD. Respiratory physiology in infants and children.

In: Smith PJ, ed. *Smith's Anaesthesia for Infants and Children*, 8th edition. Elsevier Health Sciences. 2011, p. 62.

Stratman G. Neurotoxicity of anaesthetic agents in the developing brain. *Anes Anal* 2011;**113**:1170–9.

Chapter 2

Pharmacological issues affecting anaesthesia in neonates and young children

George H. Meakin

Introduction

Paediatric patients, especially neonates and infants, differ from adults in the way they respond to drugs. These differences became apparent in the 1950s following a number of major adverse drug events including an increase in kernicterus in newborns treated with sulfonamides, and fatal cardiovascular collapse among infants treated with chloramphenicol. Research into these conditions showed that paediatric responses to drugs are determined by a large number of factors that change independently during growth and development.

The factors that determine paediatric responses to drugs can be divided into those affecting pharmacokinetics and those affecting pharmacodynamics. This chapter reviews these factors and describes how they affect the pharmacology of selected anaesthetic drugs in neonates and young children.

Factors affecting pharmacokinetics

- Absorption
- Distribution
- Elimination

The processes of absorption, distribution and elimination of drugs are influenced by a number of age-related factors. In general, absorption and distribution of drugs tend to be increased in neonates and infants compared with older subjects, while the capacity for elimination is often reduced. Thus, there is an increased risk of drug overdose and toxicity in the very young.

Absorption

Absorption refers to the translocation of a drug from its site of administration into the systemic circulation. Many anaesthetic drugs and adjuvants are administered by intravenous injection. Absorption by this route is rapid and complete. Absorption by other routes (e.g. intramuscular, inhalation) is usually faster in neonates and infants, and this contributes to a more rapid onset of therapeutic as well as adverse effects.

Distribution

Distribution refers to the transfer of a drug from the systemic circulation into the various body compartments, and is affected by:

- Cardiac output
- Protein binding
- Body water
- Blood–brain barrier

Cardiac output: At birth, weight-normalised resting cardiac output is around $200 \, ml \, kg^{-1} \, min^{-1}$; thereafter it declines gradually to about $100 \, ml \, kg^{-1} \, min^{-1}$ by adolescence (Figure 2.1). The relatively high cardiac output in infants and young children translates into faster circulation times, so that drugs are distributed to and from their sites of action more rapidly.

Cardiac output varies with (body weight)$^{3/4}$ because it depends on metabolic rate (see section on dosing below). However, when normalised for body weight, as in Figure 2.1, it declines exponentially in relation to (body weight)$^{-1/4}$ (i.e. weight$^{(3/4-1)}$ = weight$^{-1/4}$). The same exponential decline is evident for weight-normalised extracellular fluid (ECF) volume (Figure 2.3) and the per kilogram doses of many drugs in older infants and children (Figure 2.7).

Protein binding: Plasma protein binding limits the amount of drug that is available to diffuse into the extracellular space and interact with tissue receptors. In general, acidic drugs such as barbiturates bind to

Core Topics in Paediatric Anaesthesia, ed. Ian James and Isabeau Walker. Published by Cambridge University Press. © 2013 Cambridge University Press.

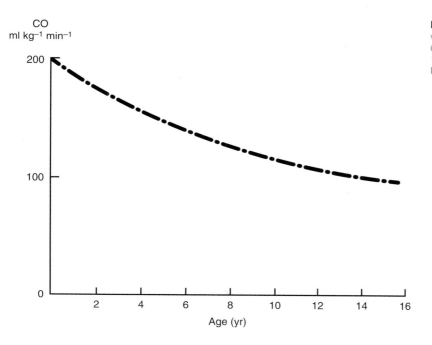

Figure 2.1 Variation in cardiac output with age. (Adapted from Rudolph AM. Congenital Diseases of the Heart. 1974, Chicago: Year Book Medical Publishers, p. 28.)

albumin, while basic drugs such as tubocurarine, morphine and local anaesthetics bind to globulins, lipoproteins and glycoproteins.

A number of factors lead to decreased protein binding of drugs in newborns and infants:

(1) Reduced concentrations of plasma proteins (Figure 2.2);

(2) The persistence of fetal albumin, which has a reduced affinity for drugs;

(3) Increased concentrations of free fatty acids and unconjugated bilirubin, which compete with acidic drugs for binding sites;

(4) A tendency to acidosis, which may alter the ionisation and binding properties of plasma proteins and of drugs.

Total plasma protein concentration and binding capacity approach adult values at about 1 year of age.

Body water: Total body water constitutes 80% of the body weight at birth, but this declines steeply in the first year to around 60% (Figure 2.3). The reduction in body water is accounted for mainly by a decrease in ECF, which declines from 45% of body weight at birth to 26% by the age of 1 year, after which there is a more gradual decline to around 19% by adulthood.

The greater volume of ECF in infants and children is important because it constitutes part of the volume of distribution of all drugs. It is also a major thoroughfare for all nutrients and metabolites in the body, so it is perhaps not surprising to find that, when expressed as a percentage of body weight, ECF volume varies in relation to (body weight)$^{-1/4}$, suggesting a relationship with metabolic rate.

The blood–brain barrier: This term is used to describe the relative impermeability of brain capillaries to most ionised substances and macromolecules. This impermeability appears to be due to tight junctions between the endothelial cells of brain capillaries, and the absence of pinocytotic vesicles in brain capillary cytoplasm. The barrier is less well developed in newborns, resulting in a greater brain uptake of partially ionised drugs such as morphine.

Elimination

Elimination refers to the removal of a drug from the body. It consists of metabolism (or biotransformation) and excretion.

Metabolism: Metabolic processes mainly transform lipid-soluble drugs into water-soluble metabolites which can be excreted more readily by the kidney. The reactions involved may be categorised as phase I (non-synthetic) or phase II (synthetic) reactions.

- Phase I reactions encompass oxidation, reduction and hydrolysis;

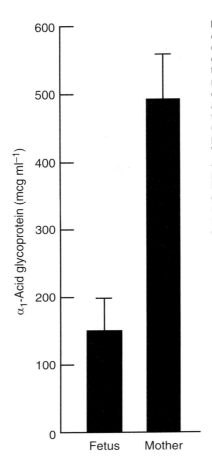

Figure 2.2 Plasma concentrations of α1-acid glycoprotein in the fetus and the mother. Fetal concentration is about one-third that of the mother. (Reproduced with permission from Wood M and Wood AJJ. Changes in plasma drug binding and glycoprotein in mother and newborn infant. *Clin Pharmacol Ther* 1981;**29**:522–6.)

- Phase II processes involve conjugation with other molecules, notably sulfate, glucuronide and glycine.

Most of the enzymes responsible for these reactions are found in the smooth endoplasmic reticulum of hepatocytes and are recovered from the microsomal fraction of cell homogenates.

The concentrations and activities of microsomal enzymes are reduced or absent in the newborn. In particular, parts of the mixed oxidase or cytochrome P-450 system are less than half as active as in adults and may take from a few weeks to several years to develop. This results in reduced metabolism of many drugs including barbiturates, diazepam and amide local anaesthetics. Similarly, the ability to form glucuronide conjugates is impaired owing to reduction in the activity of glucuronyl transferase and uridine diphosphate glucose (UDPG) dehydrogenase. This is of major importance in the metabolism of

morphine, which is greatly reduced in the neonate and takes over 6 months to approach adult levels.

Many drugs are metabolised at extrahepatic sites, frequently by esterases. Studies with neonatal plasma have shown that the rate of hydrolysis of procaine by butyrylcholinesterase (plasma cholinesterase) is half of that in adults. However, the reduction in butyryl-cholinesterase activity has no effect on the duration of action of suxamethonium in the newborn, which seems to be influenced more by the rapid redistribution of the drug from its site of action.

Atracurium is metabolised by non-enzymatic cleavage at body temperature and pH (Hofmann elimination) as well as by hydrolysis. Plasma clearance of atracurium is therefore independent of organ function and, when normalised for body weight, is somewhat greater in infants than in older children.

Excretion: Drugs and their metabolites are excreted principally by the kidney; the processes involved are glomerular filtration and tubular secretion.

Some drugs are simply filtered, in which case their rate of elimination will depend upon the glomerular filtration rate (GFR). GFR is lower in newborns and infants than in adults and, when related to body surface area, it achieves adult values at 3–5 months of age. However, when related to body weight, GFR reaches adult values at 1–2 weeks, which reflects more accurately the age at which the half-times of unmetabolised drugs approach adult values.

Proximal tubular secretion is important for the elimination of some conjugated drugs; it reaches adult levels by about 7 months of age.

Factors affecting pharmacodynamics

Drug–receptor interaction may be influenced by developmental changes in receptor number, type, affinity and the availability of natural ligands. Such changes are common in the newborn period and have been implicated in the altered responses to some anaesthetic drugs.

Nicotinic acetylcholine receptor: The nicotinic acetylcholine receptor (AChR) is a ligand-gated ion channel with a molecular weight of 260 kilodaltons, which in mammals exists in fetal and adult forms. The fetal receptor is similar to the AChR of the electric eel and consists of five protein subunits designated α, β, α, γ and δ grouped around a central pore

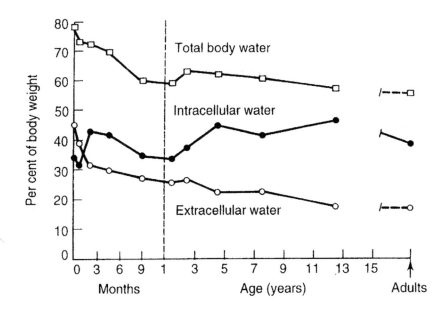

Figure 2.3 Variation in body water compartments with age. (Adapted from Friis-Hansen B. Body water compartments in children: Changes during growth related changes in body composition. *Pediatrics* 1961;**28**:169–81.)

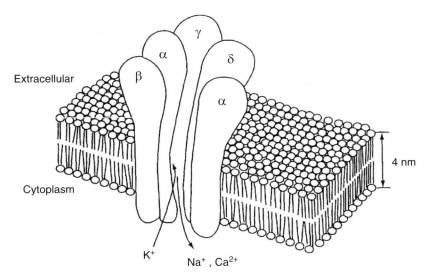

Figure 2.4 Diagram of fetal acetylcholine receptor showing five glycoprotein subunits α, β, α, γ, δ, grouped around a central pore. In the adult acetylcholine receptor subunit γ is replaced by a subunit designated ε. (Adapted from Goudsouzian NG, Standaert FG. The infant and the myoneural junction. *Anesth Analg* 1986:**65**;1208–17.)

(Figure 2.4). In the adult receptor, the γ subunit is replaced by a subunit designated ε which decreases the time it remains open after two molecules of acetylcholine (ACh) bind to its α subunits. The relatively long 'open time' of the fetal receptor increases the safety factor in neuromuscular transmission and may explain the observation that newborn rats are relatively resistant to tubocurarine. The fact that resistance to tubocurarine is not normally seen in human newborns accords with the histological finding that fetal AChRs are not present on human muscle fibres after 31 weeks of gestational age.

Combined pharmacodynamic and kinetic studies in humans suggest that the neuromuscular junction of the neonate is three times more sensitive to the effects of non-depolarising muscle relaxants than that of the adult. Evidence from young rats suggests that this sensitivity is the result of a 3-fold reduction in the release of ACh from motor nerves (Figure 2.5).

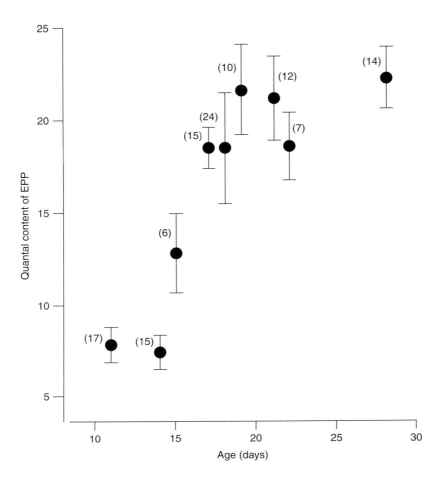

Figure 2.5 Variation in the quantal content of the endplate potential (EPP) in phrenic nerve-hemidiaphragm preparations from rats aged 11–28 days. The 3-fold *reduction* in ACh release at 11 days compared with 21 days corresponds with a 3-fold *increase* in the sensitivity of the neuromuscular junction to tubocurarine. A similar reduction in ACh release in human neonates could account for the increased sensitivity of their neuromuscular junctions to non-depolarising relaxants. (Reproduced with permission from Wareham AC, Morton RH, Meakin GH. Low quantal content of the endplate potential reduces safety factor for neuromuscular transmission in the diaphragm of the newborn rat. *Br J Anaesth* 1994;**72**:205–9.)

Opioid receptors: Radioreceptor binding studies in the rat have demonstrated age-dependence of the relative proportion of μ, κ and δ opioid receptors. Furthermore, work in mice indicates that the selectivity of the μ receptor for μ-specific ligands changes with age. As the μ and κ receptors mediate the respiratory effects of opioids, changes in the number and affinity of these receptors could be a factor in the increased susceptibility of newborns to opioid-induced respiratory depression.

GABA$_A$ and NMDA receptors: The GABA$_A$ and NMDA receptors are ligand-gated ion channels with features resembling those of the AChR. The GABA$_A$ receptor is the site of action of barbiturates and benzodiazepines, and a likely target for most general anaesthetics. The NMDA receptor regulates L-glutamate signalling and is blocked by the action of ketamine. Both receptors undergo significant developmental changes in their subunits and roles which may have

important implications for anaesthesia and neuronal development.

Paediatric dosing

Calculating the correct dose of a drug for a neonate or young child invariably involves scaling the dose according to the patient's size. However, it is important to appreciate that scaling for *size* does not take account of *age*-related differences in pharmacokinetics and pharmacodynamics, examples of which have been cited above. Furthermore, different doses will be obtained depending on which of several available size models is used.

Scaling for size: Scaling for size is often called allometrics (Greek: alo – other, metron – measure). One of the first attempts at scaling for size, other than with simple body weight, was the surface area law postulated by Sarrus and Rameaux in 1839. This law

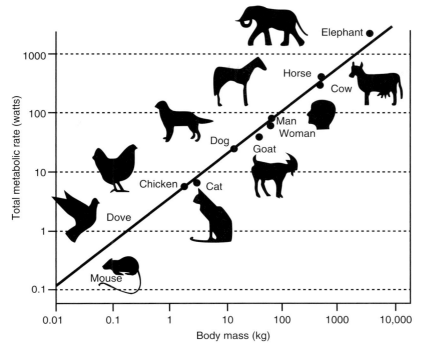

Figure 2.6 Log–log plot of metabolic rate against body mass in a wide range of animals. An empirically derived line with a slope of ¾ gives an excellent fit to the data. (Reproduced with permission from Schmidt-Nielson K. *Scaling: Why is Animal Size So Important?* Cambridge: Cambridge University Press. 1984.)

asserts that physiological functions are comparable whatever the size of the organism when related to body surface area. The rationale for this was that as most heat loss occurs through the skin, so metabolic rate, and the many physiological functions that depend on it, will vary in proportion to body surface area.

Classical scaling principles hold that the surface area of geometrically similar bodies increases in proportion to their length squared, and that their volume or mass (if they are of similar density) increases in proportion to their length cubed. Thus, in bodies of the same shape and density, surface area is proportional to mass to the power of 2/3.

If surface area = SA, length = l and mass = M then:

$$SA \propto l^2 \qquad (2.1)$$

$$M \propto l^3 \qquad (2.2)$$

$$\therefore l \propto M^{1/3}$$

Substituting $M^{1/3}$ for l in equation (2.1) gives:

$$SA \propto (M^{1/3})^2 = M^{2/3} \qquad (2.3)$$

However, it is an oversimplification to apply the surface area law to animals since young and old, small

and large, thin and fat animals differ in both bodily proportions and density. Furthermore, animal data suggest that a better estimation of metabolic rate is obtained from body mass to the power of 3/4 as shown in Figure 2.6.

Three size models

As an extension of the ideas outlined above, the size models most commonly used to scale paediatric doses are the weight model, the 2/3 power (surface area) model, and the 3/4 power model. The following equations demonstrate how these size models may be used to obtain paediatric doses from adult ones.

Weight model:

$$Dose_{paediatr} = (W_{paediatr}/W_{adult}) \times Dose_{adult} \qquad (2.4)$$

2/3 power (surface area) model:

$$Dose_{paediatr} = (W_{paediatr}/W_{adult})^{2/3} \times Dose_{adult} \qquad (2.5)$$

3/4 power model:

$$Dose_{paediatr} = (W_{paediatr}/W_{adult})^{3/4} \times Dose_{adult} \qquad (2.6)$$

Thus, using the weight model (Equation 2.4), the paediatric dose of any drug may be obtained by

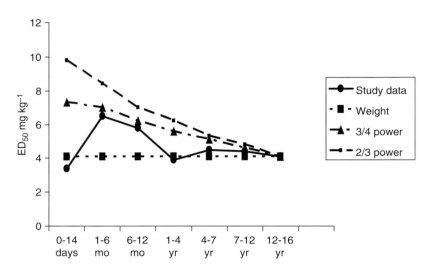

Figure 2.7 Biphasic variation in the ED_{50} sleep dose of thiopental with age (solid line). The broken lines represent paediatric doses of thiopental predicted from the adult dose of 4 mg kg^{-1} using one of three size models (weight, 3/4 power and 2/3 power). The weight model predicts the lowest doses, the 2/3 power model the highest; the 3/4 power model predicts doses intermediate between the other two and provides the best fit to the data in children aged 1–6 months and older. (Data taken from Jonmarker C, Westrin P, Larsson S *et al*. Thiopental requirements for induction of anesthesia in children. *Anesthesiology* 1987;**67**: 104–7; and Westrin P, Jonmarker C, Werner O. Thiopental requirements for induction of anesthesia in neonates and in infants 1 to 6 months of age. *Anesthesiology* 1989;**71**:344–6.)

multiplying the adult dose by the weight of the patient divided by the adult weight. When using the 2/3 and 3/4 power models (Equations 2.5 and 2.6), the calculation is similar except that the fraction $W_{paediatr}/W_{adult}$ is raised to the power of 2/3 and 3/4 respectively.

Figure 2.7 illustrates some difficulties of using size models to predict paediatric doses of anaesthetic drugs. It will be seen that the variation in the dose of thiopental required to produce sleep in 50% of subjects (ED_{50}) with age is biphasic, with an ascending limb from birth to 1–6 months followed by a gradual decline throughout infancy and childhood. Since a biphasic curve cannot be modelled by a single mathematical function, it is impossible to predict the full range of paediatric doses from the adult value using any of the available size models.

To illustrate this point, the paediatric doses of thiopental predicted by the weight model, the 2/3 power model and the 3/4 power model are represented by the three broken lines superimposed on the data in Figure 2.7.

It is evident that the weight model underdoses most of the infants and children but is the least likely to overdose the neonates. The 3/4 power model provides the best fit to the data in older infants and children, but both it and the 2/3 power model significantly overdose the neonates.

The biphasic distribution of drug dosage shown in Figure 2.7 is shared by many drugs including most volatile anaesthetic agents, non-depolarising muscle relaxants and morphine. The ascending

limb reflects age-dependent maturation of organ or enzyme systems which cannot be predicted by size models. The descending limb appears to reflect the gradual decline in weight-normalised basal metabolic rate throughout childhood, since doses in this range can best be predicted by the 3/4 power size model.

Suxamethonium is a noteworthy exception to the biphasic dosing pattern as it displays a monophasic decline in weight normalised dose requirements from birth, which is predictable by the 3/4 power model (Figure 2.8).

In summary, it appears that the best estimate of the dose of a drug in a child from that of an adult will be obtained using the 3/4 power model, which relates drug doses to basal metabolic rate. However, none of the size models is completely reliable and their use must be supported by pharmacodynamic and pharmacokinetic data. Drug doses are much less predictable in infants aged less than 1 year owing to immaturity of organs and enzyme systems. Reduced doses are frequently required in this age group.

Intravenous anaesthetic agents
Thiopental

In the newborn, plasma protein binding of thiopental is reduced, so that the fraction of unbound drug is almost twice that found in older children and adults. In addition, the elimination half-time is more than three times as long in neonates as in older children; however, as recovery depends primarily on

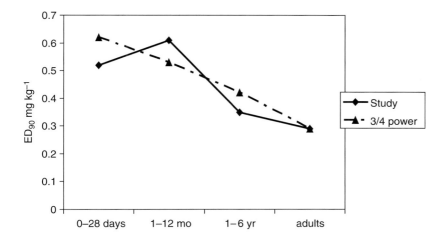

Figure 2.8 Monophasic variation in the ED_{90} dose of suxamethonium with age (solid line). The broken line represents paediatric doses of suxamethonium predicted from the adult dose of $0.3\,mg\,kg^{-1}$ using the 3/4 power size model. (Data taken from Meakin GH, McKiernan EP, Morris P et al. Dose-response curves for suxamethonium in neonates, infants and children. *Br J Anaesth* 1989;**62**:655–8; and Smith CE, Donati F, Bevan DR. Dose–response curves for succinylcholine: single versus cumulative techniques. *Anesthesiology* 1988;**69**:338–42.)

redistribution, the effect of an induction dose is not significantly prolonged.

The ED_{50} doses of thiopental are shown in Figure 2.7. As doses of about $1.3 \times ED_{50}$ are required to produce rapid, reliable induction of anaesthesia in all age groups, it is apparent that for induction with thiopental:

- Healthy neonates require 4–$5\,mg\,kg^{-1}$
- Infants require 7–$8\,mg\,kg^{-1}$
- Children require 5–$6\,mg\,kg^{-1}$

The reduced requirement for thiopental in neonates compared with infants aged 1–6 months may be explained by decreased plasma protein binding, greater penetration of the neonatal brain or increased responsiveness of neonatal receptors.

The increased induction requirements for thiopental in infants and children compared with adults (average dose $4\,mg\,kg^{-1}$) may be due to the increased cardiac output in younger patients (a function of basal metabolic rate) which should reduce the initial concentration of thiopental arriving at the brain.

The main complications of thiopental are apnoea and hypotension. These will be minimised by using the smallest practical dose, especially in small infants.

Propofol

Propofol has largely replaced thiopental as the intravenous induction agent of choice in paediatric centres because of its rapid, clear-headed recovery characteristics and an association with antiemesis. In addition, propofol suppresses laryngeal and pharyngeal reflexes, thereby facilitating tracheal intubation and the insertion of a laryngeal mask airway.

The faster and more clear-headed recovery following a single dose of propofol compared with thiopental is due to propofol's shorter distribution half-time and more rapid plasma clearance. The rapid elimination of propofol (plasma clearance approximately six times as fast as thiopental in paediatric studies) reduces the potential for accumulation, making the drug suitable for maintenance of anaesthesia. Induction and maintenance doses of propofol are greater in children than in adults because the volume of the central compartment is 50% larger and the plasma clearance 25% faster in children. Average induction doses ($1.3 \times ED_{50}$) in unpremedicated patients are:

- Infants $4\,mg\,kg^{-1}$
- Children $3\,mg\,kg^{-1}$
- Adults $2\,mg\,kg^{-1}$

When given together with an opioid, the average infusion dose of propofol for maintenance of anaesthesia in children is 0.1–$0.2\,mg\,kg^{-1}\,min^{-1}$, approximately twice the dose required in adults.

Paediatric studies have consistently demonstrated a greater reduction in systolic and diastolic blood pressure following injection of propofol compared with thiopental, which may make the latter preferable in small infants. Also, the use of propofol for prolonged sedation in paediatric intensive care units is associated with a rare syndrome comprising lipaemia, metabolic acidosis, heart failure, rhabdomyolysis and death. The cause of this syndrome is unknown, but attention has focused mainly on impairment of fatty acid oxidation by propofol as a possible cause. In view of these reports, the drug regulatory authorities of the United Kingdom, Canada and the United States have recommended that propofol should not be used for intensive care sedation of children.

Opioids

Until the late 1980s, the use of opioid drugs was avoided in newborns and young infants because of their increased susceptibility to respiratory depression. However, attitudes changed following the demonstration that neonates mount a significant stress response to surgery which can be modified by opioids.

The susceptibility of newborns to opioid-induced respiratory depression may be due to:

- Increased central nervous system (CNS) penetration by opioids;
- Reduced capacity for opioid elimination; and
- Developmental changes in the relative proportions and affinities of opioid receptors.

The recent availability of the ultra-short acting opioid remifentanil has further stimulated interest in the use of this class of drugs in infants.

Morphine

Following an intravenous injection of morphine, brain uptake is slow owing to poor lipid solubility. Similarly, the decay of CNS concentration is slow as it depends on elimination of the drug by the liver. Conjugation with glucuronide produces both active and inactive metabolites which are excreted by the kidneys. Morphine clearance in neonates is one-quarter of that in adults and takes 6 months to approach adult values. Accordingly, the elimination half-time of morphine is significantly prolonged in young infants. The fraction of protein-bound morphine is similar in all age groups (18–22%).

Morphine remains the drug of choice for the management of severe post-operative pain in infants and children. It is usually administered by continuous infusion or by patient controlled analgesia (PCA). In view of the long elimination half-time of morphine, a loading dose is required to achieve an effective plasma concentration within a reasonable time.

For children and infants aged over 6 months, a loading dose of 100 mcg kg^{-1} followed by a maintenance infusion dose 10–30 mcg kg^{-1} min^{-1} should achieve and maintain an adequate target concentration of 10–25 ng ml^{-1}.

In newborns, a plasma concentration of morphine of 10–25 ng ml^{-1} should be achieved with a loading dose of 25 mcg kg^{-1} followed by an infusion rate of 5–10 mcg kg^{-1} min^{-1}. All infants and children receiving morphine infusions should be monitored with continuous pulse oximetry, and infants aged less than 1 month should be nursed in a high dependency unit.

Fentanyl

Fentanyl is a synthetic opioid with a high lipid solubility that confers increased potency, rapid onset and short duration of action. After a dose of 1–3 mcg kg^{-1}, the clinical effects of fentanyl are terminated by redistribution and its duration of action is limited to 20–30 minutes. However, after repeated doses or a continuous infusion, progressive saturation of peripheral compartments occurs and its effects may last for several hours.

The mean plasma clearance of fentanyl in infants is greater than that in adults, although there is great interpatient variability due to age and the type of surgery. Fentanyl clearance increases during the first 2 weeks of life, reflecting rapid maturation of the cytochrome P-450 3A4 enzyme. During the same period, the volume of distribution of fentanyl is 2–3 times that in adults and there is a corresponding increase in the half-time of elimination. Accordingly, single doses of fentanyl in neonates should be reduced (e.g. 0.5–1 mcg kg^{-1}).

Remifentanil

Remifentanil is a new ultra-short acting, ester-linked synthetic opioid. Following intravenous infusion it is rapidly hydrolysed by non-specific blood and tissue esterases to produce a virtually inactive carboxylic acid compound. As remifentanil is not a substrate for butyrylcholinesterase (plasma cholinesterase), its elimination is not affected by a deficiency in this enzyme.

In a study of infants and children aged from 0 to 18 years, the elimination half-time of remifentanil was found to be short and similar in all age groups (about 9.5 min). The short elimination half-time frequently makes a loading dose unnecessary and facilitates control of the infusion. Unlike other opioids, its duration of action does not increase with increasing dose or duration of infusion, because its volume of distribution is small and its clearance is fast. The usual infusion dose of remifentanil is $0.1–0.5 \, \text{mcg kg}^{-1}$ min^{-1}. Its use in neonatal and infant anaesthesia is associated with a reduction in the requirements for volatile anaesthetic agents, stable cardiovascular conditions and a low incidence of post-operative apnoea.

Muscle relaxants

Suxamethonium

Suxamethonium is the only depolarising muscle relaxant in clinical use. A singular combination of rapid onset and short duration of action make it especially useful for emergency tracheal intubation. Elimination depends on hydrolysis by butyrylcholinesterase, hence a deficiency in this enzyme may result in prolonged block.

Studies during thiopental–fentanyl–nitrous oxide anaesthesia showed that the doses of suxamethonium for 90% depression of the twitch response (ED_{90}) in neonates, infants and children were 0.52, 0.61 and $0.35 \, \text{mg kg}^{-1}$ respectively. These values were all greater than that obtained in a comparable adult study ($0.29 \, \text{mg kg}^{-1}$) (Figure 2.8). In view of these results it was recommended that neonates and infants should be given $3 \, \text{mg kg}^{-1}$ and children $2 \, \text{mg kg}^{-1}$ of suxamethonium for tracheal intubation. The duration of action of these doses was about the same as or less than that produced by $1 \, \text{mg kg}^{-1}$ in adults (6–8 min) reflecting the shorter half-times of suxamethonium in infants and children.

When an intravenous line is not accessible, suxamethonium may be given by intramuscular injection. In this case, doses of $5 \, \text{mg kg}^{-1}$ for infants and $4 \, \text{mg kg}^{-1}$ for children will be required to produce 85–100% twitch depression. Maximum block will be achieved at 3–4 min and full recovery will occur after 15–20 min (Figure 2.8).

The increased dose requirement of suxamethonium in younger patients probably results from its distribution into a larger volume of ECF rather than an altered response to the action of the drug at post-junctional acetylcholine receptors. This suggestion is supported by the observation that the paediatric ED_{90} doses can be predicted fairly accurately from the adult dose using the 3/4 power size model, since the ECF volume bears a constant relationship to (body weight)$^{3/4}$ throughout life (Figure 2.8).

The unique mode of action of suxamethonium (sustained depolarisation) and its activity at muscarinic acetylcholine receptors are responsible for a large number of adverse effects. Of greatest concern have been reports of rare, but often fatal, hyperkalaemic cardiac arrests in boys with undiagnosed muscular dystrophy. As a result of these reports, the US Food and Drug Administration (FDA) recommends that the use of suxamethonium in children should be reserved for emergency intubation and instances where immediate securing of the airway is necessary, e.g. laryngospasm, difficult airway, full stomach, or for intramuscular use when a suitable vein is not available.

Non-depolarising muscle relaxants

Clinical studies in the 1960s and 1970s produced conflicting results about the sensitivity of paediatric patients to non-depolarising relaxants. The question was largely resolved in 1982 by a study which demonstrated that the steady state concentration of tubocurarine corresponding to 50% depression of EMG twitch (C_{pss50}) in neonates was only one-third of that in adults, while that of infants was about one-half. However, when the dose corresponding to 50% depression of EMG twitch (D_{50}) was determined for each patient by multiplying the C_{pss50} by the volume of distribution (V_{dss}) there were no significant differences between the groups (Table 2.1). It was concluded that while neonates and infants were sensitive to tubocurarine in terms of the lower plasma concentration required to produce a given effect, this was countered by an increased volume of distribution (ECF volume), such that dose did not vary significantly with age. The same appears to be true of other non-depolarising muscle relaxants.

Experimental data from young rats suggest that the increased sensitivity of the neuromuscular junction of the human neonate and infant to non-depolarising muscle relaxants is a reduction in the release of ACh from developing motor nerves (Figure 2.5). A pre-junctional locus for the weakness in neuromuscular transmission in human infants is also consistent with the mature appearance of the motor endplate from 31 weeks gestational age, the absence of fetal AChRs after this time and the apparently normal response of the motor endplate to suxamethonium in newborns (see above).

Table 2.1 Steady state concentration of tubocurarine for 50% depression of EMG twitch (C_{pss50}), steady state volume of distribution (V_{dss}) and dose for 50% depression of twitch (D_{50}) calculated from the other two parameters.

	C_{pss50} (mcg ml^{-1})	V_{dss} (l kg^{-1})	D_{50} (mcg kg^{-1})
Neonates	0.18	0.74	155
Infants	0.27	0.52	158
Children	0.42	0.41	163
Adults	0.53	0.30	152

Adapted from Fisher DM, O'Keefe C, Stanski DR *et al*. Pharmacokinetics and pharmacodynamics of D-tubocurarine in infants, children and adults. *Anesthesiology* 1982;**57**:203–8.

Atracurium

Atracurium is a bis-quaternary benzylquinolinium diester with an intermediate duration of action. The molecule is eliminated primarily by Hofmann elimination, a process dependent on pH and temperature.

When compared during thiopental–nitrous oxide–narcotic anaesthesia, the ED_{95} of atracurium has been shown to be significantly lower in neonates and infants than in children (119 and 163 vs 195 mcg kg^{-1}). Following a standard intubating dose of atracurium 0.5 mg kg^{-1} (~2 × ED_{95}), 95% depression of twitch occurred more rapidly in neonates than in children (0.9 vs. 1.4 min), while recovery to 10% of control twitch height occurred more rapidly in neonates compared with the other two groups (22.7, 29.7 vs 28.6 min; for neonates, infants and children respectively). Prompt, predictable recovery in all age groups is a major advantage of atracurium when used for paediatric anaesthesia.

The adverse effects seen with atracurium relate mainly to histamine release. Commonly, this results in a macular rash or erythema along the course of the vein of injection, which may subsequently spread peripherally. Occasionally the rash may be accompanied by more serious histamine effects such as hypotension, tachycardia or bronchospasm. The cardiovascular changes are dose-related and usually occur at doses greater than twice the ED_{95}.

Cisatracurium

Cisatracurium is one of 10 stereoisomers that make up the commercially available atracurium mixture. The ED_{95} of cisatracurium is 45 mcg kg^{-1}, therefore it is approximately three times as potent as atracurium. The increased potency of cisatracurium compared with atracurium confers greater specificity of action and fewer histamine-related side effects. The main disadvantage of increased potency is a slower onset of action. Consequently, a dose of ~3 × ED_{95} of cisatracurium (0.15 mg kg^{-1}) is required to produce intubating conditions at 2 min comparable to those obtained with 2 × ED_{95} of atracurium. Following a dose of cisatracurium 3 × ED_{95}, 25% recovery time was shown to be longer in infants than in children (43 vs. 36 min), which could have clinical importance in infants undergoing short surgical procedures.

Mivacurium

Mivacurium has a structure similar to that of atracurium but a shorter duration of action due to its metabolism by butyrylcholinesterase. When measured during halothane anaesthesia, the mean ED_{95} of mivacurium in children ranged between 89 and 95 mcg kg^{-1} while that for infants tended to be less at 65 to 85 mcg kg^{-1}. In children anaesthetised with thiopental–nitrous oxide–oxygen, mivacurium 0.2 mg kg^{-1} (~2 × ED_{95}) provided satisfactory intubating conditions in 98% of patients at 90 s. Onset of complete block occurred at 1.9 min and 25% recovery of twitch occurred at 8.5 min. Consequently, mivacurium may be an alternative to suxamethonium when neuromuscular block of short duration is required but rapid onset of action is unnecessary. Mivacurium has significant histamine releasing properties which may be evident at therapeutic doses and its duration of action can be greatly prolonged in patients with butyrylcholinesterase deficiency.

Vecuronium

Vecuronium is a monoquaternary aminosteroid relaxant of intermediate duration of action, which is largely eliminated unchanged by the liver. As with other non-depolarising relaxants, the variation in effective dose of vecuronium is biphasic with the ED_{95} in infants being similar to that in adolescents while the maximum effective dose occurs in children aged 5–7 years (Figure 2.9). Significantly, a standard intubating dose of 100 mcg kg^{-1} of vecuronium (~2 × ED_{95}) maintains over 90% neuromuscular blockade for almost an hour in newborns and infants compared with only 18 min in children. Vecuronium is therefore a *long-acting* muscle relaxant in neonates

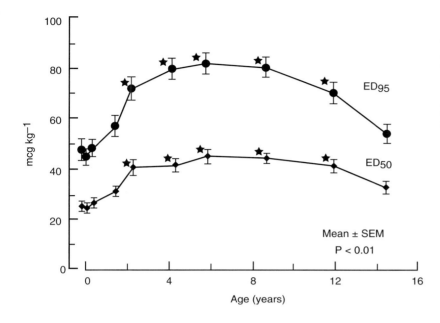

Figure 2.9 Variation in the ED_{50} and ED_{95} doses of vecuronium with age. The values are significantly greater in children aged 2 to 13 years compared with younger and older patients. (Reproduced with permission from Meretoja OA, Wirtavuori K, Neuvonen PJ. Age-dependence of the dose–response curve of vecuronium in pediatric patients during balanced anesthesia. *Anes Analg* 1988;**67**:21–6.)

and infants reflecting its dependence on hepatic function for elimination.

Rocuronium

Rocuronium is an analogue of vecuronium with a more rapid onset of action making it a suitable for rapid sequence induction in patients with normal airways. Rapid onset is the result of reduced potency, which necessitates an increase in dose, and hence the injection of a larger number of drug molecules. When compared during nitrous oxide–opioid anaesthesia, the ED_{95} of rocuronium was significantly lower in infants than in children (248 vs. 396 mcg kg^{-1}) while the duration of clinical effect following a standard intubating dose of 0.6 mg kg^{-1} (~2 × ED_{95}) was much longer (42 vs 27 min). These results confirm that rocuronium, like vecuronium, is longer-acting in infants than in children. However, unlike vecuronium, rocuronium retains the characteristics of an intermediate-acting muscle relaxant in infants.

Antagonism of non-depolarising relaxants

Any residual non-depolarising neuromuscular blockade at the end of anaesthesia should be antagonised with an anticholinesterase. This is especially important in infants in because of their reduced respiratory reserve. The anticholinesterases used commonly are neostigmine and edrophonium.

In the presence of 10% recovery of twitch height, 35 mcg kg^{-1} of neostigmine or 0.7 mg kg^{-1} edrophonium have been shown to provide maximal antagonism in both paediatric and adult patients (Figure 2.10). Recovery after edrophonium was faster than that after neostigmine for the first 2 min, but doubling the doses of the antagonists had no significant effect on recovery. Recovery after either antagonist was faster in paediatric patients compared with adults. For convenience, somewhat larger doses of 50 mcg kg^{-1} of neostigmine or 1 mg kg^{-1} of edrophonium are usually given. Atropine 20 mcg kg^{-1} or glycopyrrolate 10 mcg kg^{-1} should be administered before, or with, the anticholinesterase drug to prevent muscarinic effects.

Inhaled anaesthetics

The commonly used inhalation agents in paediatric anaesthesia are halothane, sevoflurane, isoflurane, desflurane and nitrous oxide. Because of its non-pungent odour, rapid induction characteristics and relative cardiostability, sevoflurane has mostly replaced halothane as the induction agent of choice in children. Sevoflurane and isoflurane are currently the principal agents for maintenance of anaesthesia.

Uptake and elimination of inhaled anaesthetics occur more rapidly in paediatric patients than in adults, primarily because of an increased level of

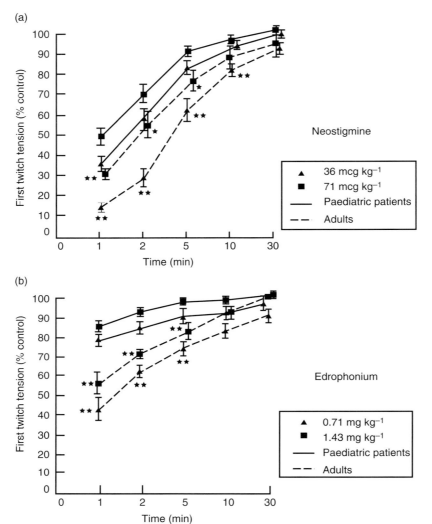

(a)

Neostigmine

▲ 36 mcg kg⁻¹
■ 71 mcg kg⁻¹
— Paediatric patients
- - Adults

(b)

Edrophonium

▲ 0.71 mg kg⁻¹
■ 1.43 mg kg⁻¹
— Paediatric patients
- - Adults

Figure 2.10 Recovery of the first twitch tension as a percentage of control twitch height in paediatric patients and adults after one of two doses of neostigmine (a) or edrophonium (b). Significant differences between paediatric and adult patients after the same dose of antagonist: * $P < 0.05$; ** $P < 0.01$. (Reproduced with permission from Meakin G, Sweet PT, Bevan JC et al. Neostigmine and edrophonium as antagonists of pancuronium in infants and children. *Anesthesiology* 1983;**59**:316–21.)

ventilation in relation to functional residual capacity (FRC) and a corresponding increase in weight-normalised cardiac output (Figure 2.2). Thus, the ratio of the alveolar-to-inspired halothane concentration measured at 20 min in infants aged 1–3 months is 0.83 compared with 0.59 in adults. The increased rate of uptake of inhaled anaesthetics in infants correlates with more rapid induction of anaesthesia and earlier development of adverse cardiovascular events.

Halothane

Halothane is a halogenated alkane with a non-pungent petrolic odour making it suitable for inhalation induction in infants and children. Induction of

anaesthesia is rapid owing to its relatively low blood–gas partition coefficient and high potency (Table 2.2).

In newborns, the minimum alveolar concentration (MAC) of halothane is 0.9%, but it increases rapidly to a maximum of 1.2% at age 1–6 months and thereafter declines gradually to 0.8% in the adult (Figure 2.11). The reduced MAC of halothane in neonates compared with infants may relate to immaturity of the central nervous system, or attenuation of the pain response due to increased plasma concentrations of endorphins. The higher MAC in infants compared with older children and adults may be due to reduced solubility of inhaled anaesthetics in brain tissue owing to an increased content of water.

Table 2.2 Properties of volatile anaesthetics.

	Halothane	Isoflurane	Sevoflurane	Desflurane
Odour	Non-pungent petrolic	Pungent ethereal	Non-pungent ethereal	Pungent ethereal
Blood–gas coefficient				
Neonates	2.1	1.2	0.7	–
Adults	2.3	1.4	0.7	0.4
MAC (%)				
Neonates	0.9	1.6	3.3	9.2
Adults	0.8	1.2	2.0	6.0
Rate of metabolism (%)	20	0.2	2.0	0.02
Myocardial depression	++	+	+	+
Peripheral vasodilation	+	++	++	++
Respiratory depression	+	++	++	++

Adapted from Meakin G. Neonatal anaesthetic pharmacology. In: Hughes DG, Mather SJ, Wolf AR, eds. *Handbook of Neonatal Anaesthesia.* Saunders. 1996;18–54.

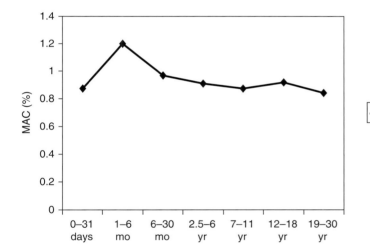

Figure 2.11 Variation in the MAC of halothane with age. (Data taken from Lerman J, Robinson S, Willis MM *et al.* Anesthetic requirements for halothane in young children 0–1 month and 1–6 months of age. *Anesthesiology* 1983;59:421–4; and Gregory GA, Eger EI, Munson ES. The relationship between age and halothane requirements in man. *Anesthesiology* 1969;**30**:488–91.)

Neonates and young infants are more sensitive to the myocardial depressant and vagotonic effects of inhaled anaesthetics than older children. Reduction in arterial pressure with halothane is due primarily to myocardial depression. Both bradycardia and hypotension due to halothane in infants can be prevented or treated by injection of atropine 20 mcg kg^{-1} IV or IM.

Sevoflurane

Sevoflurane is trifluoromethyl isopropyl ether, one of two newer ether anaesthetics halogenated solely with fluorine (the other being desflurane). Fluorination decreases solubility in fat and blood, thereby reducing anaesthetic potency while increasing the rate of uptake and elimination. Sevoflurane is minimally pungent and appears to be better tolerated than halothane for induction of anaesthesia. Because of its lower blood solubility (Table 2.2), induction and recovery are more rapid with sevoflurane than with halothane.

The MAC of sevoflurane varies with age, being higher in neonates and young children than in adults (Table 2.2). Sevoflurane produces less myocardial depression and bradycardia than halothane; however, significant hypotension may still occur in neonates.

Although an estimated 5% of the inhaled dose of sevoflurane is metabolised producing inorganic fluorides, peak concentrations of fluoride in paediatric studies have not exceeded two-thirds of the suggested nephrotoxic level of 50 mmol l^{-1} and there have been no reported cases of sevoflurane nephrotoxicity.

Emergence agitation is a significant problem with sevoflurane. The reported incidence varies from 30 to 80% and it affects mainly pre-school children. Episodes typically last for 10–12 min during which the child appears to be agitated, restless, combative, frightened and inconsolable. It cannot be attributed solely to pain or rapid emergence from anaesthesia and has been described as a short-lived acute organic mental state (paranoid delusion) of uncertain aetiology. It may be the result of different washout times between excitatory and inhibitory centres in the central nervous system. The incidence of emergence agitation following sevoflurane can be reduced by the use of sedatives and short-acting opioids: e.g. intravenous induction with propofol, administration of 1 mcg kg^{-1} of fentanyl 10 min before the end of anaesthesia.

Isoflurane

Isoflurane is halogenated methyl-ethyl ether with an irritant odour which results in a high incidence of respiratory complications during induction and recovery from anaesthesia. The MAC of isoflurane varies with age in a similar manner to that of halothane. Thus, it is approximately 1.6% in neonates, 1.9% at age 1–6 months and thereafter declines gradually to about 1.2% in adults. The MAC of isoflurane is further reduced in premature infants: at 32 weeks gestational age it is approximately 1.3% while at 32–37 weeks it is 1.4%. Equipotent concentrations of isoflurane and halothane produce similar reductions in blood pressure in infants and children, although heart rate and myocardial function are better preserved with isoflurane.

Desflurane

Desflurane is created by the replacement of the single chorine atom of isoflurane with fluorine. Like isoflurane, desflurane has a pungent ethereal odour making it unsuitable for inhalation induction of anaesthesia. However, because of its lower blood solubility (Table 2.2) recovery after desflurane anaesthesia is faster than that after halothane or sevoflurane. The MAC of desflurane varies with age in a way similar to that of most other volatile anaesthetics, being 9.2% in newborns, 9.9% in infants aged 6–12 months and thereafter declining gradually to 6.0% in adults. The cardiovascular profile of desflurane is similar to that of halothane, metabolism is negligible and the drug resists degradation by soda lime. The rapid recovery seen after desflurane may be of special benefit in neonates and ex-premature infants in view of their increased susceptibility to post-operative apnoea and ventilatory depression.

Nitrous oxide

Nitrous oxide is a sweet smelling, non-irritant, anaesthetic gas with a low blood–gas partition coefficient (0.47) resulting in rapid uptake and elimination. When used as a carrier gas with oxygen it speeds the uptake and elimination of potent volatile anaesthetics by the second gas effect and reduces their MAC requirement for anaesthesia. The low potency of nitrous oxide may be an added safety factor when the agent is used in neonates, who generally tolerate anaesthetics poorly.

In recent years there have been calls for the abandonment of nitrous oxide in routine anaesthesia owing to a greater appreciation of its disadvantages (e.g. potential for delivering a hypoxic mixture, distension of air pockets in the body, increase in intracranial pressure, contribution to greenhouse gas effect). Although paediatric anaesthetists at the author's institution still find nitrous oxide useful for inhalation induction of anaesthesia, its use for maintenance of anaesthesia is declining in line with recent trends in adult anaesthetic practice.

Local anaesthetics

Local anaesthetics are commonly used for wound infiltration and peri-operative nerve blocks as part of a multimodal approach to analgesia. Drugs of the amino-amide type are used most frequently. Lower concentrations of α-1-acid glycoprotein in young infants increase the amount of unbound local anaesthetic and the potential for central nervous system (CNS) and cardiovascular toxicity. Total body clearance is also reduced in young infants as a result of the limited oxidising capacity of the liver which, together with an increase in the volume of distribution, leads to a prolonged elimination half-time. Accordingly,

Table 2.3 Doses of local anaesthetics in infants and children

Drug	Age (months)	Initial dose (mg kg^{-1})	Maintenance dose (mg kg^{-1} h^{-1})	Duration (h)
Bupivacaine and Levobupivacaine	0–6	0.5–1.25	0.2–0.25	36
	> 6	1–2.5	0.25–0.5	
Ropivacaine	0–6	0.5–1.5	0.2	36
	> 6	1–3	0.4	

Reproduced with permission from Morton NS. Local and regional anaesthesia in infants. *Cont Educ Anaes Crit Care Pain* 2004;**4**:148–51.

the maximum permitted single and infusion doses of local anaesthetics should be reduced in young infants.

Bupivacaine is a racemic mixture of R (+) and S (−) enantiomers. Its chief advantage is its long duration of action (e.g. 4–6 hours after a single epidural injection). For patients aged over 6 months, the maximum single injection dose (plain or with adrenaline) is 2.5 mg kg^{-1} and the maximum epidural infusion rate is 0.5 mg kg^{-1} h^{-1} for a maximum of 36 hours (Table 2.3). In infants aged less than 6 months these doses should be halved and consideration should be given to reducing the rate of infusions by a further one-third after 24 hours as there is evidence of drug accumulation even with the reduced doses.

Bupivacaine toxicity is a particular concern in children since most blocks are carried out under anaesthesia when early signs of impending catastrophe are absent. Demonstration in the 1970s that the S (−) enantiomer of bupivacaine was significantly less cardio-depressant than the R (+) enantiomer led to the development of ropivacaine and levobupivacaine. In view of their wider safety margins, these S (−) enantiomer drugs should be the local anaesthetics of choice for paediatric anaesthetic practice. In comparative trials, ropivacaine, levobupivacaine and bupivacaine were found to be equally effective when given in equal doses and concentrations to children for caudal and epidural analgesia, but ropivacaine and levobupivacaine were associated with less motor block. The maximum recommended doses for ropivacaine and levobupivacaine are shown in Table 2.3.

Key points

- The relatively high cardiac output in infants and young children translates into faster circulation times, so that drugs are distributed to and from their sites of action more rapidly.
- The blood–brain barrier is less well developed in newborns resulting in a greater brain uptake of partially ionised drugs such as morphine.
- Estimating the dose of a drug for a neonate or small child usually involves scaling from the adult dose according to weight and allowing for any age-related sensitivity.
- The best estimate of the dose of a drug in an older child will be obtained by scaling the adult dose using the 3/4 power model.
- The ED$_{50}$ of many drugs and the MAC of most volatile agents rises to a peak at about 6 months then declines gradually to adult levels.

Further reading

Blumer JL, Reed MD. Principles of neonatal pharmacology. In: Yaffe SJ, Aranda JV, eds. *Neonatal and Pediatric Pharmacology.* Lippincott Williams & Wilkins. 2005;146–58.

Kearns GL, Reed MD. Clinical pharmacokinetics in infants and children: A reappraisal. *Clin Pharmacokin* 1989;**17** (suppl.1):29–67.

Meakin GH. Developmental pharmacology. In: Holzman RS, Mancuso TJ, Polander DM, eds. *A Practical Approach to Pediatric Anesthesia.* Lippincott Williams & Wilkins. 2008;17–47.

Meakin GH. Muscle relaxants. In: Bingham R, Lloyd-Thomas A, Sury M, eds. *Hatch and Sumner's Textbook of Paediatric Anaesthesia.* Hodder Arnold. 2007;227–42.

Meakin G. Neonatal anaesthetic pharmacology. In: Hughes DG, Mather SJ, Wolf AR, eds. *Handbook of Neonatal Anaesthesia.* Saunders. 1996;18–54.

Morselli PL. Clinical pharmacology of the perinatal period and early infancy. *Clin Pharmacokin* 1989;**17** (suppl 1.):13–28.

Developmental psychology and communicating with children and families

Judith A. Short

Introduction

Children make fascinating patients but they can also present huge challenges, particularly in the area of communication. A child's ability to understand and respond to changes in their health and the need for medical treatment evolves as they become older and gather life experience. A flexible approach to communication and explanation is therefore necessary, which can be adapted to the age and development of each child. For some doctors, developing a rapport with children seems a natural skill, but for others age-appropriate communication with young patients proves much less easy.

The aims of good communication are to gain the trust and cooperation of children, and to help them understand the reasons for some of the procedures they have to face, so that they might tolerate them more easily. It is also important that children are provided with the means to be able to contribute where possible to the decisions that affect their health and wellbeing, even if they are not considered competent to give formal consent for their treatment.

This chapter provides some background on the developmental psychology of health and illness understanding, and discusses some basic techniques and strategies for communication with children and families, including those with special needs.

Developmental psychology

It is impossible to do justice to the complex study of developmental psychology in a few short paragraphs, but a brief summary of some key concepts may help to illustrate the ways in which children begin to understand their world as they grow and develop.

Developmental theory

The field of developmental psychology was revolutionised by the theories of Jean Piaget in the 1960s. Prior to Piaget, it was felt that children's development was a passive result of their upbringing, but Piaget asserted that children are active agents in shaping their own development. As a result of continual interaction and cognitive adaptation, they become better able to understand their world. Piaget described four stages of development through which children progress, characterised by qualitatively different ways of thinking, as they develop an increasing ability to engage logical (operational) thought and to separate internal realities such as wishes, needs and thoughts from the outside world.

- The first stage is the sensorimotor stage of infancy (from birth to 2 years) during which the child is particularly concerned with coordinating movement and action. As language begins to appear, words come to represent objects and things, and the child learns that objects continue to exist even when they cannot be seen or heard.
- The second stage is the pre-operational stage (from 2–7 years) during which children are able to solve problems by the use of tools, communication and ideas, although they may not be able to generalise from one experience or observation to another similar one. They remain egocentric, with difficulty in seeing another's point of view, and display animism, attributing life and lifelike qualities to inanimate objects. They may also demonstrate illogical, often magical thinking: for instance they usually believe in the tooth fairy and Father Christmas.
- The third stage is the concrete operations stage (7–11 years) when children are able to use

Core Topics in Paediatric Anaesthesia, ed. Ian James and Isabeau Walker. Published by Cambridge University Press. © 2013 Cambridge University Press.

elementary logic to solve problems and understand much more about the physical world, but are limited by their inexperience in the realm of possibilities. They are, however, able to combine performance with a verbal explanation or an attempt to reason out the problem.

- The fourth stage is the formal operations stage (from 11 years) in which children are able to reason scientifically, think hypothetically and consider abstract concepts.

Further information processing theories suggest that these aspects of development do not occur in discrete stages, but occur as a continuous process. Information is received, registered, processed and manipulated, allowing the child to develop increasingly complex ways of interacting with the world. As a child develops, both their capacity for information storage and their processing power increase, allowing them to consider a greater range of strategies, manage increasingly complex thought and hold more than one concept in mind simultaneously.

A child's cognitive, motor, emotional, personality and social development all occur simultaneously, each influencing the progress of the others. The Russian psychologist Vygotsky described the importance of knowledgeable adults in helping children to explore ideas which are just beyond their current stage of development, bridging the gap between what they know and what they can be taught. Erik Erikson's theory of psychosocial development suggests that children develop in response to experiences they have in interaction with their world. Of major importance in early life is the interaction between children and the adults who care for them. Play is also important to human development as children work toward organising their inner perceptions to fit the external world in which they must function. According to Erikson, every individual moves through an orderly sequence of stages, each of which is more complex. Maturation occurs as the individual ascends from one stage to another. At each stage the individual is faced with a psychosocial conflict, which must be resolved before moving on to the next stage of development. In early childhood (age 18 months to 3 years) children work on achieving autonomy and become more aware of adults other than their parents. In middle childhood (age 3 to 6 years) children develop initiative and are increasingly expected to be responsible for themselves and their toys and other possessions. They may develop an understanding of cultural norms and the beginnings of a conscience, and ask many questions in an attempt to understand things that had previously been a mystery to them. In later childhood and adolescence, children may adhere to a wide range of beliefs and ideologies until they achieve a stable identity and self-concept as young adults.

Emotional development theory is complex but suggests that infants may be able to distinguish between different facial expressions at an early stage, and toddlers with developing language skills may rapidly begin to use words associated with emotion. Children's understanding of the rich complexity of human emotion continues to develop through childhood, and the ability to sympathise and empathise probably continues to evolve throughout the human lifespan. Children imitate behaviours observed in adults, and this may include actions that are aggressive or comforting. It is unclear what triggers cause different emotional reactions to the same stimulus in different children of the same age, so it may be difficult to predict how individual children may respond to a stressful or challenging situation.

Children's understanding of health and disease

Children differ greatly from adults in their understanding about the cause of illness and its treatment and prevention, as well as their perceptions of hospitals. It is useful to appreciate some of the apparent misconceptions children may hold when trying to find ways to inform and educate them about their condition and its management. As children's understanding becomes more complete and scientific, they develop increasing competence and capability to share in medical decision-making and informed consent.

- Children under 3 have very limited understanding of health and disease and an incomplete sense of time. They respond well to distraction, play and the calm presence of a carer, more than to comprehensive explanations.
- Between 3 and 6 years, when a child's understanding of the world is dominated by fantasy and magic, they have a poor sense of cause and effect and may be unable to distinguish between inner and outer reality. They have very limited understanding of the makeup of the body, but fear injury and may imagine that an isolated

condition or injury will affect their whole body. They often perceive illness to be a consequence of their own actions – the outcome of wrongdoing – and may also believe aspects of medical treatment to be a form of punishment. It is important to emphasise to children of this age that the illness or situation is not their fault, and also to explain which part of the body is affected and that other parts are not involved. They respond well to rehearsal of unfamiliar procedures in the form of role play, especially if they are to encounter people wearing masks, or play therapy, where the feelings of a doll or toy can be expressed and medical equipment can be introduced and handled.

- Between 6 and 12 years, fantasy and reality become distinguished and children develop a better understanding of structure and function. Illness is understood as an internal dysfunction rather than just as external bodily trauma, and children begin to understand about infection and contagion, although they may misinterpret every illness as being caused by germs. They begin to correctly perceive medical treatment as the means to become well, but they may fear surgery as a form of mutilation and worry about anaesthesia because of confusion between sleep and death. They may also find it difficult to express their concerns, and worry that nobody else will understand how they are feeling, particularly when they are in pain. Children of this age group require comprehensive explanations and reassurance, but respond less well to play therapy.

- Teenagers have a much more physiological understanding of illness and health prevention and will be able to rationalise enough to contribute to discussions about consent. They fear loss of autonomy and control, and worry about awareness and risk. They need much more adult-orientated explanations, with allowance for their limited experience.

It may be tempting to imagine that a child with a complicated medical history and many previous admissions to hospital will have an increased level of understanding and a large range of coping strategies, but in fact neither may be any further developed than those of a child experiencing their first anaesthetic. In addition, children may regress behaviourally and emotionally to an earlier stage of development when anxious or unwell.

The child in the context of the family

In general, children are not treated in isolation, but access healthcare with the assistance of their family. Parents usually consider themselves to be their child's advocate, and may have a clear view regarding the level of information they wish their child to receive. In elective circumstances, it would be unusual for an anaesthetist to talk to or examine a child without a parent or family member present, although it may sometimes be appropriate to afford adolescent patients privacy and confidentiality. Some parents may encourage their child to answer and ask questions themselves, whereas others may dominate the clinical encounter.

Many parents will have talked reassuringly with their child about having an operation and an anaesthetic and are pleased to meet the anaesthetist at the pre-operative visit and to have the opportunity, along with their child, to ask questions and clarify any issues. However, there are a number of situations in which the pre-operative assessment may not be so straightforward. It is not uncommon for parents to have avoided any discussion of the reason for the child's admission, because they wished to spare the child any worry. Occasionally parents may even have misled their child entirely about their expectations of the hospital visit. Unfortunately, there will usually be a moment when the child realises that all is not as it seemed and an acute loss of trust ensues. If it becomes clear at the pre-operative visit that a school-age child is unaware that they are due to have an anaesthetic, it may be appropriate to seek the parent's permission to explain gently to the child the purpose of their visit to the hospital, the procedures involved in having an anaesthetic and the measures taken to avoid anxiety and discomfort. It is not usually advisable, except perhaps with some children with special needs, to perpetuate a situation where the child is given no information or is deliberately misinformed.

There may also be occasions when a parent's anxiety or previous personal experience has led them to develop prejudices against certain treatment options and to transfer these to the child. An example of this would be a parent declaring a child to be needle phobic, when it is actually the parent who has the fear of needles. It is sometimes difficult to unpick such situations, but it may be necessary to explore a parent's reasoning, especially if there are reasons why an undesired option may be clinically appropriate. It may be that parents are unaware of the methods available to ameliorate discomfort, such as the use of local anaesthetic cream prior to cannulation.

It is common to use parents as proxies when gathering and providing information regarding paediatric patients. However, parents' perceptions of their child's responses may not accurately reflect the child's feelings, anxieties and needs, especially as the child becomes more independent. A partnership approach may often have to be adopted, which gives the child a voice, while allowing decision-making to be shared by parent, child and anaesthetist together.

Communicating with parents

When a child is injured, unwell or facing surgery, parents often experience a high level of anxiety, vulnerability and responsibility. They may look for reassurance and guidance, and may actively seek a number of different opinions on their child's treatment and prognosis. Parental anxiety is easily transmitted to the child, so it is important to allay as many of a parent's fears as possible and to keep them well informed at every stage. Such information should give a comprehensive and accurate account of the anaesthetic process and the measures taken to ensure safety and comfort. It has a number of aims: to educate and empower, to assist parents in their supportive role, to provide a starting point for discussion and to facilitate consent or authorisation for treatment. Specific explanations may be required if complex monitoring techniques, local anaesthetic blocks or rectal drug administration are to be used. In general, parents wish to be reassured that there will be someone looking after their child at all times, that they will be allowed to be with their child as soon as possible in recovery, and that steps will be taken to keep their child pain-free. It is very important that parents who are to accompany their child to the anaesthetic room understand their role and are ready to leave at the appropriate moment.

Written information leaflets can be very useful, especially if offered in advance of admission. Examples of such resources are available from the Royal College of Anaesthetists patient information website (http://www.youranaesthetic.info).

Communicating with children

There are many potential barriers to effective communication with children. There are inevitable time constraints; five or more patients may all need to be assessed in the short time between admission and the start of the list. In the limited time available, the anaesthetist must locate the patient, provide introductions, gather all the medical details required, formulate an anaesthetic plan and discuss any options which may require a decision from the patient and family. Having these discussions exclusively with the parent or carer may save time, but will fail to allow the anaesthetist to build a rapport with the child. Parental advocacy, as discussed above, may also prevent the anaesthetist from communicating directly with the child, and children may already have misconceptions or fears about their impending treatment that interfere with their ability to interact positively with the stranger before them. It is therefore important to create an atmosphere of trust that is non-threatening and friendly from the outset.

Environment

The setting in which we meet children and their families is important. If children can be made to feel at ease, they are more open to accepting and interacting with someone new. It is useful to make the waiting and consulting areas for children inviting and not too clinical, with child-sized furniture, appropriate decoration and activities to reduce boredom. Young children may have brought a favourite toy with them, and drawing attention to this can be a useful way of breaking the ice. It is worth bearing in mind that the clothing worn by the anaesthetist has the potential to cause confusion. If the anaesthetist conducts the anaesthetic assessment wearing street clothes, the child may not recognize them later when they are wearing scrubs and a hat in the anaesthetic room, and some warning of the change is useful.

Separate facilities should be available for older children and adolescents who have different needs compared with younger children. Although it would be usual to talk to older children in the presence of their parents, it may be appropriate to offer them the option of privacy before introducing sensitive issues, such as smoking, alcohol or recreational drug use and sexual activity.

Non-verbal communication

Children have the ability to pick up a large amount of non-verbal communication. Their first impression is made as the anaesthetist approaches them. It is therefore important to smile, to have open facial expressions, to use friendly open gestures, to appear confident and to make eye contact with the child. It is also very effective to adopt a sitting position at the level of the child, so they do not feel threatened by someone towering above them. It is helpful to direct most of the conversation to the child and to maintain intermittent eye contact with them, even when the discussion is mainly being held with the parent.

It is possible to begin to assess how easily the child might cooperate with further procedures by observing their non-verbal communication. A child who will not make eye contact, or who spends the entire assessment clinging to his mother, is unlikely to tolerate cannulation or an inhalational induction as easily as one who has been interactive, lively and open to suggestion.

Verbal communication

Even very small children can pick up on the tone, character and speed of speech, so it is important that these do not sound impatient or unfriendly. It is also important to use simple age-appropriate language, avoiding medical jargon, abbreviations or complicated technical explanations. It may be necessary to explain some simple words, where misinterpretation could occur. For instance, the word 'mask' is unlikely to conjure up the image of an anaesthetic mask in a child's mind, but is more likely to make them think of a snorkelling mask, the mask used as a disguise by a superhero or the gas mask they have seen in a museum, none of which would seem a sensible way to start an anaesthetic.

The use of positive language is also very helpful, avoiding words which trigger fear or anxiety. Instead of the word 'needle', a cannula can be described as a 'tiny plastic tube' and anaesthetic gas can be described as 'sleepy air'. Using the phrase 'I'll give you medicines to keep you comfortable' may sound more reassuring than 'to stop you feeling pain'. It is important not to mislead children or to make promises that cannot be kept. For example, it is unwise to tell a child that cannulation will not hurt, but acceptable to say that most people do not feel much when they have had local anaesthetic cream on their hand first.

Explanations and information

It is sometimes difficult to gauge how much information and explanation to offer a child about anaesthesia and the various procedures and potential risks involved. It may be tempting to try to keep explanations brief and superficial, but consultation with children has revealed that they actually have sophisticated information needs, with concerns and fears which mirror those of adults. Children as young as 7 years may have concerns that they might die or wake up during the operation. As well as an expression of general nervousness, children's common concerns include the fear of pain (cannulation as well as post-operative pain), awareness, separation from family, the duration of surgery and anaesthesia, and a need to know how the anaesthetic works. They therefore need reassuring explanations that are comprehensive, honest and accurate, while appropriate to their age and level of understanding. It may be worth noting that children may better understand the concept of risk, and the probability of an event occurring, if the information is presented diagrammatically, such as in the form of a pie chart, rather than by the use of verbal labels (rarely, sometimes) or proportions (1 in 10, 1:10).

Behavioural and psychological techniques

For many children, simple explanations may not be sufficient to encourage them to cooperate with or tolerate the processes involved in anaesthetic induction. The reassuring presence of a calm parent is helpful and will avoid separation anxiety. In addition, play specialists may be able to help prepare children for anaesthesia by demystifying some of the equipment and procedures. A child who has been allowed to handle a mask and anaesthetic tubing and pretend to give their teddy bear an anaesthetic may be more willing to accept a mask themselves in the anaesthetic room. Similarly, showing a child a cannula with the needle removed may make the prospect of cannulation less frightening.

Distraction techniques are also very effective, whether provided by simple measures such as a book, blowing bubbles or a noisy toy, or more sophisticated equipment such as DVDs or handheld games consoles. Children may respond very positively to guided imagery, which is the conscious use of the imagination to create positive images and a calm relaxed state. It can be particularly useful during inhalational induction if children can be persuaded to engage with a story in which the introduction of the odour of sevoflurane seems a natural element. One example might be drawing an imaginary picture of a princess or racing car with different coloured felt-tip pens (see boxed text on page 34). Alternatively children might be persuaded to play a game which involves blowing up the reservoir bag of the breathing system to try to burst the balloon, or to take deep breaths as if they were about to blow out their birthday candles. Cannulation can also be subject to imagery, with the cannula variously described as a butterfly, an aeroplane or even a 'Spiderman web-shooter'. Utilisation of these techniques depends on open lines of communication with the child and builds on the rapport developed during the pre-operative visit.

Written information for children

Children may be more accepting of anaesthesia if preparation has begun at home. Children have a right to receive information that is meaningful to them and there is therefore a need for age-appropriate, accurate, written information, presented in an appealing and accessible form. There are several published children's books which can be recommended for general preparation for the hospital visit (see Further reading), and the Royal College of Anaesthetists information leaflets for children and young people provide more specific detail about anaesthesia. The best timing for discussions at home varies with the age of the child. Children between 2 and 3 years old should be told about the hospital visit 2–3 days before and then again on the day, whereas for children between 4 and 7 years old, up to a week in advance is appropriate. Older children and young people have usually been more involved in making decisions about the operation or investigation and so are likely to have been talking about it for weeks before the day of admission.

The difficult child

In spite of the utilisation of some or all of the techniques already described, a small proportion of children will refuse to cooperate with anaesthetic induction. For some children this is a manifestation of extreme anxiety; for others it is a form of power play. In either situation, non-cooperation may be predictable in advance and sedative premedication will reduce anxiety and promote a smooth and calm induction.

Recognising anxiety

Some children may demonstrate anxiety overtly by their behaviour. They may be withdrawn, non-communicative, tearful or unwilling to make eye contact, or may verbally express their nervousness and its causes. Others may actively resist any interventions from the start, refusing to cooperate with being weighed, having local anaesthetic cream applied or changing into a hospital gown. Occasionally parents may indicate that apparently calm children have been expressing concern at home and showing symptoms of anxiety, such as sleep disturbance. It is well recognised that in addition to a more difficult anaesthetic induction, high levels of pre-operative anxiety can lead to adverse emotional and behavioural sequelae at home post-operatively, such as separation anxiety, sleep disturbance, emotional regression, bed-wetting and even an increase in post-operative pain. It is therefore important to recognise susceptible children and intervene, by appropriate psychological interventions, sedative premedication, or both. The repetition of information about anaesthetic processes, no matter how carefully delivered, is insufficient preparation for these children. A variety of coping strategies and relaxation techniques, such as distraction, breathing exercises and imagery, can be used successfully, even when time is limited.

Non-cooperation in the anaesthetic room

Occasionally children, in spite of preparation and/or premedication, refuse to allow anaesthetic induction. The options available to manage this situation then depend on the age and developmental level of the child, the level of urgency of the planned surgery and, to an extent, the views of the parents.

- Very young children, who are clearly unable to rationalise or contribute to the consent process, and who can be held safely by their parents, can often be rapidly induced by an inhalational technique.
- A forced induction of this nature is inappropriate for older children who are able to express their refusal clearly and who would require restraint to allow induction to proceed. In elective circumstances, a 'time-out' is required, to allow a distressed child to become calm, or to allow a rational child to express the reasons for their change of mind. Options then include negotiation about the mode of induction, offering sedative premedication if it has not already been given, and postponing the surgery for another day to allow further discussion and pre-operative preparation.

- It would be unacceptable to use physical restraint or a forced induction using sevoflurane or intramuscular ketamine, unless the child was refusing life-saving emergency surgery, or the child had a learning disability which would prevent them from responding to the options outlined above.

Children with special needs

There are about 75 000 children in the UK with moderate to severe learning difficulties who will have an increased need for healthcare interventions compared with the rest of the population. It is common for such children to find the process of anaesthesia particularly difficult.

There are some relatively simple strategies that can be used to improve the experience of children with special needs, such as placing them first on the operating list to minimise waiting and fasting times, the judicious use of sedative premedication, providing a quiet waiting area or a single room, and using an anaesthetic technique that promotes rapid recovery with little postoperative discomfort, low rates of nausea and vomiting, and early discharge to the home environment.

Pre-operative preparation may prove difficult, as the conventional information resources available may not be appropriate or accessible for these children. Anaesthetists may have to become familiar with alternative forms of communication, or be prepared to be flexible in their approach to ensure that they have given children with special needs the best opportunity to share their views and receive information. Such children will often receive the best service if there has been contact between the hospital ward and the family prior to admission, in order to establish the child's particular needs and requirements, both for physical issues such as mobility and nutrition, and also for likes, dislikes and phobias.

- Many children have a health passport, which gives a brief but useful summary of their usual level of function including communication.
- If children have had a previous anaesthetic experience, their parents may have particular requests for a subsequent anaesthetic plan.
- Occasionally a child may even require premedication at home to make the journey to hospital possible.

Individualised approaches such as these may require extensive discussion between the family and the child's regular carers, the child's usual medical team, the admitting team and ward and the anaesthetist, and will usually need considerable advance planning.

Language and communication disorders

Children with learning disability and/or language and communication disorders may use forms of augmentative and alternative communication (AAC). AAC is the term used to describe methods of communication which can be used to add to the more usual methods of speech and writing when these are impaired. AAC is particularly useful when there are physical difficulties with speech production rather than with cognition. AAC methods may be unaided or aided:

- Unaided AAC
  o Body language, facial expressions, gestures, signing
- Aided AAC
  o Low tech – writing, drawing, picture boards, symbols, objects
  o High tech (requiring a power source) computers, switches, voice output communication aids (VOCA)

Using a form of AAC, a child may be able to indicate 'yes' and 'no' and thus may be able to contribute to discussions in which there is a choice, for instance the options for anaesthetic induction. Parents and carers are usually keen to assist healthcare providers in communicating effectively with their child and will be able to explain the form of AAC used at home and at school. They may also be able to offer a degree of interpretation if, for example, the child uses a sign language such as Makaton. AAC methods can be used to help children to understand the unfamiliar procedures associated with hospital treatment, if verbal explanations are insufficient. One example is the use of a symbol system to create a time-line of a hospital visit, where each step in the process is represented by a symbol which is used as a prompt and a form of explanation (see Figure 3.1).

Autistic spectrum disorder (ASD)

Patients with ASD may present a particular challenge in terms of communication. They often struggle with the loss of their usual, often very rigid routine on the day of admission, and may become very agitated in large, noisy, open waiting areas.

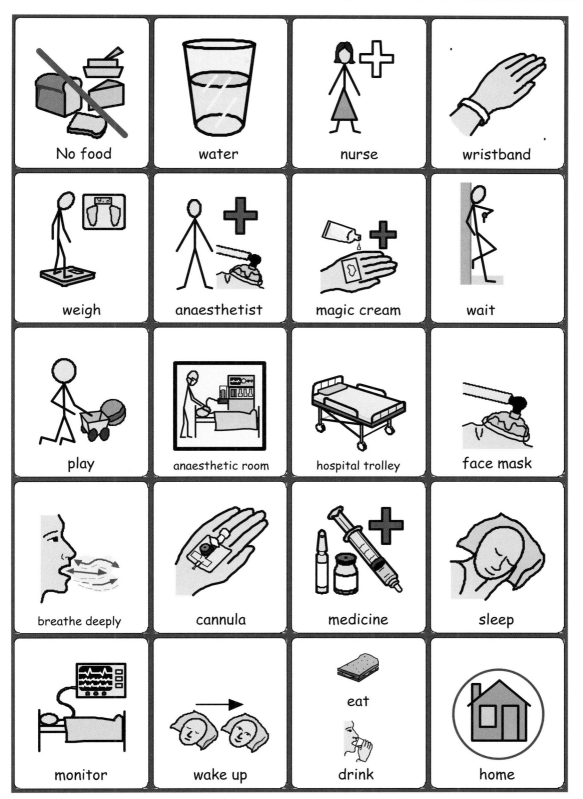

Figure 3.1 An example of a symbol system, used to create a time-line of a hospital visit. See plate section for colour version. Used with permission from Widgit Symbols © Widgit Software. 2002–2011 www.widgit.com

They may struggle to interact with strangers, and may resist being touched or examined in any way. In terms of offering explanations for some of the procedures with which they are expected to comply, a different approach may be necessary. In general, children with ASD respond best to communication techniques which help them to learn *how* to manage a hospital visit, rather than methods which enhance our ability to explain *why*. Such techniques might include behavioural modification strategies, structured symbol time-line approaches or social stories which supply details of the social situation, social cues and expected behaviour. A suggested symbol time-line for a day case admission is available from the Royal College of Anaesthetists patient information website, in the approved leaflets section (see also Figure 3.1).

Key points

- Efficient communication with young patients and their families plays a large part in the quality of anaesthetic care.
- Children require age- and developmentally appropriate information and explanations.
- Good pre-operative preparation may reduce adverse post-operative emotional and behavioural sequelae.
- Advanced communication strategies may be helpful in reducing anxiety and promoting cooperation.
- Children with special needs may need a flexible approach, including the use of augmentative and alternative communication methods to ensure their ability to interact is maximised.

Further reading

Cyna AM, Andrew MI, Tan SG. Communication skills for the anaesthetist. *Anaesthesia* 2009;**64**:658–65.

Rawlinson SC, Short JA. The representation of anaesthesia in children's literature. *Anaesthesia* 2007;**62**:1033–8.

Slater A, Bremner G, eds. *An Introduction to Developmental Psychology*. Blackwell Publishing. 2003.

Smith L, Callery P. Children's accounts of their pre-operative information needs. *J Clin Nurs* 2005;**14**:230–8.

The Royal College of Anaesthetists patient information series: http://www.youranaesthetic.info

Information about Makaton: http://www.makaton.org

Information about symbol resources: http://www.widgit.com

General information on AAC: http://www.communicationmatters.org.uk

Guided imagery story for inhalational induction – led by the anaesthetist with the focus provided by the child.

The breathing system is flushed with oxygen or pre-loaded with nitrous oxide in oxygen, to create odourless gas flow. Then the mask is introduced:

'I've got a mask here that's like a plastic bubble. It has a soft bit that fits on your nose and your chin. Do you think it's the right size for you? Shall we check? That looks just right to me. I'm just going to hold it near your nose like this and I'd like you to tell me your favourite colour. [PINK] In a minute, there's going to be a smell as if you just took the lid off a pink felt-tip pen. We're going to draw a picture in our minds. What would you like to draw? [PRINCESS] Here's your pink felt-tip pen… (*introduce 2% sevoflurane*) Let's draw a beautiful pink princess with a lovely dress and pretty shoes. Now she's going to need a friend. What's your second favourite colour? [PURPLE] Well, here's a purple felt-tip pen to draw another princess in a lovely purple dress (*increase sevoflurane to 4%*). Now we'll need some blue for the sky (*increase sevoflurane to 6%*) and some green for the grass (*increase to 8%*) and some yellow for the sunshine, and soon we'll have a whole rainbow of colours for your picture. Perhaps you can finish it when you wake up later.'

Chapter 4

Consent and the law, including research and restraint, in paediatric anaesthesia

Lisa Flewin

Introduction

A 9-year-old boy is listed for circumcision. You pre-assess him on the paediatric day ward. He appears nervous but cooperative. He is tearful as you collect him from reception but he walks to the anaesthetic room with his mother. He refuses to accept either inhalational induction or insertion of a cannula or indeed to get on the trolley. His mother is insistent that you proceed. Would you continue, and if so how?

This chapter aims to give you a legal and ethical framework on which to base your decision and your approach to such clinical problems. It relates to practice in the United Kingdom. There are differences between English and Scottish law.

Consent
Self-determination

Self-determination with respect to one's body is a fundamental human right. From the 1960s the rights of those under 18 to self-determination have been progressively recognised and protected in law. Medical examinations, treatments and investigations all represent intrusion of bodily integrity, and as such require consent from the child or their guardian. Only in limited circumstances can a doctor proceed without it. Consent may be expressed or implied, and it can be written, verbal or even non-verbal. Consent can make the physical intrusion of treatment or investigation lawful, but not always. It will not necessarily make an act lawful where it results in serious injury. For consent to be valid, the person giving consent must be capable of taking that particular decision, be acting voluntarily and be provided with enough information to make an informed decision.

Consent serves several purposes. It recognises the individual's rights of autonomy and self-determination. It demonstrates cooperation and belief in a treatment modality, which in itself is integral to the success of many treatments. It also offers some protection to the medical practitioner where disputes arise.

Battery

Failure to obtain consent can result in an action for battery or a claim on the tort of negligence. It can also result in disciplinary action for the professional concerned from their regulatory body. An action for battery arises where the defendant has been touched and for which there has been no consent, either expressed or implied. No actual physical harm need arise, and the intentions of the aggressor are irrelevant. For the plaintiff, an action for battery is often likely to be successful. They need only to show that they were wrongfully touched by the defendant. An action of battery will be pursued where a doctor has proceeded in the face of a refusal to a procedure, or has undertaken an additional procedure unconnected to the one for which consent was obtained.

Negligence

In an action based on negligence, on the other hand, the plaintiff must prove causation. The plaintiff must show that the defendant proceeded without consent, and that this resulted in the injury for which they are seeking damages. The Court must be satisfied that the patient would not have given his or her consent had they been properly informed of what was to be done. Where a patient has consented to a procedure but the doctor failed to mention a complication that the patient subsequently suffered there is a basis for a

Core Topics in Paediatric Anaesthesia, ed. Ian James and Isabeau Walker. Published by Cambridge University Press. © 2013 Cambridge University Press.

claim in negligence. The negligence refers to the failure to inform rather than the way in which the procedure was performed.

Minors 16–18 years

A child becomes competent to accept medical treatment independently of their parents' rights of determination when they achieve sufficient understanding and intelligence to enable them to understand fully what is proposed. Under the age of 18 years, a child is referred to as a minor. A minor is presumed competent when they attain 16 years of age. This is referred to as the presumptive test of competence and is defined by the Family Law Reform Act 1969 in England and Wales, or the Age of Legal Capacity (Scotland) Act 1991.

Minors under 16 years: Gillick competence

Below the age of 16 years a minor can give valid consent if they demonstrate Gillick competence. This is an evidential test of competence derived from the case of Gillick v W. Norfolk & Wisbech AHA (1985). This case set a precedent that permitted children of sufficient maturity to seek contraceptive advice without the knowledge of their parents, but was subsequently applied more generally to allow children who fulfilled the criteria to consent to other forms of medical treatment. The age at which Gillick competence can be demonstrated will depend on the child and the complexity of the treatment or procedure. Where a Gillick-competent child requests non-disclosure to their parents their confidentiality must be respected. Where possible it is good practice to encourage children to involve parents.

In order to demonstrate Gillick competence the child should understand that there is a choice to be made and demonstrate a willingness to make it. The child should be able to understand the nature of the proposed treatment and the risks involved. They should appreciate what the effects of non-treatment might be. It is important that the child can retain the information long enough to come to a decision.

'Assent' to treatment

The term 'assent' is sometimes used to describe an agreement by the child to participate with a degree of explanation and understanding appropriate to their age and development, but falling short of fully valid consent. It serves as evidence of a child's willingness to participate but does not replace the need for full consent.

Parental responsibility

Where the child does not have the capacity to give consent it must be sought from someone with parental responsibility. Legally, consent need only be obtained from one person with parental responsibility; however, it is good practice to involve all relevant parties.

The Children Act 1989 defines who has parental responsibility:

- The child's mother;
- The child's father if married to the mother at the time of conception or birth;
- If unmarried, then the father can obtain parental responsibility:
  - by jointly registering the birth with the mother,
  - by making a parental responsibility agreement with the mother,
  - by court order,
  - if the couple subsequently marry;
- A legally appointed guardian;
- A person awarded a residence order concerning that child;
- A local authority designated in a care order, except where the child is being 'accommodated' or in 'voluntary care' (see Section 20 of the Children Act);
- A person or authority holding an emergency protection order in respect of the child.

In 2009 the law was amended such that it became a legal right for both parents, regardless of gender, to have their names on the birth certificate, giving them both parental rights.

Delegation of parental responsibility

Parents have parental responsibility toward their children to safeguard and promote the child's health, welfare and development. Parental rights only exist to enable them to fulfil their responsibilities. Parental rights therefore terminate 'if and when the child achieves a sufficient understanding and intelligence to enable him or her to understand fully what is proposed'. Persons with parental responsibility can arrange for some or all of that responsibility to be met by others, a grandparent who is regularly involved in the child's care, for example. Although it is helpful for this to be in writing, the Children Act does not specify that it must be so. Where such responsibility has been explicitly delegated, then that person's consent is valid. It may be that those with parental responsibility do not themselves have the capacity to consent on behalf of the child owing to mental illness or special needs, in which case legal advice should be sought.

Emergency treatment

In the situation where no one is able to give valid consent it is lawful to provide emergency treatment in the absence of consent on the basis that it is in the child's best interests. Assessment of best interests should be based on the physical, emotional, social, cultural and psychological needs of the individual. The views of, and the effect on, other family members may need to be considered. Evidence of the effectiveness of the proposed treatment, risks of treatment, and of delaying or withholding treatment, must be taken into account. Where possible, treatments that maximise the patient's future choices should be offered so that the child can exercise his or her autonomy when they do attain competency. It is not necessarily the case that any treatment that prolongs life is in a child's best interests.

Refusal of treatment

It seems logical that competence to consent to treatment would extend to assuming competence to refuse treatment. Indeed in the House of Lords decision in Gillick, both Lord Fraser and Lord Scarman agreed that once a child had developed 'sufficient understanding and intelligence to enable him or her to understand fully what is proposed' then he/she could give consent without the consent of his/her parents. Lord Scarman took this point further to conclude that when a minor became Gillick-competent the parent and indeed the court would no longer be able to determine whether or not the child could undergo medical investigation and treatment. However, this principle has not been upheld in case law and it is Lord Fraser's view that prevails, that there would remain circumstances in which the parents or the courts could override a decision by a minor if it is in their best interests. Consent to treatment is in agreement with medical opinion whereas refusal of treatment goes against a body of medical opinion and therefore arguably requires a greater level of understanding.

Determining Gillick competence

After Gillick the British Medical Association (BMA) and the Law Society attempted to define more precisely what level of understanding the individual should have in order to be deemed Gillick-competent. It can be argued that a greater level of understanding is asked of children compared with adults. The case of ReE in 1990 demonstrates this point. The patient was 15 years old and like his parents a Jehovah's Witness. He was suffering from leukaemia. The case arose when he and his parents refused a treatment regimen that offered a high chance of cure, but involved blood transfusions, in favour of a less successful treatment avoiding the use of blood products. Although impressed with his level of understanding and conviction to his faith, the judge declared that he did not adequately appreciate the pain and distress that would arise nor the effect on his family. Moreover he felt the details were too distressing to even contemplate telling the boy. So the Court was unwilling to arm him with the information to allow him to make an informed choice. The ruling resulted in the boy receiving blood transfusions as part of his treatment. He continued to voice his objection until ultimately he reached adulthood when he refused further blood transfusions and died.

An adult who is not suffering from a mentally incapacitating illness has a right to choose to consent to or refuse treatment, however irrational their choices, and even if it is clearly not in their best interests. By contrast a child who is considered mature enough that their capacity to consent should be considered 'as effective as it would be if [the child] were of full age' appears to forgo their right to refuse treatment where the consequences are serious and restrict future choices. The legal position in Scotland differs and a refusal of treatment by a competent minor is more likely to be upheld.

ReW, in 1992, concerned refusal of treatment by a minor suffering from anorexia nervosa. It was recognised that the condition itself fundamentally interferes with a person's ability to consent to aspects of treatment, for example around the issue of force-feeding. This perhaps justifies subjecting some sufferers of anorexia nervosa to general anaesthesia in order to overcome a refusal of nasogastric tube placement to facilitate feeding.

Advance directives, living wills

It follows from the above that in the United Kingdom where a young person's refusal may not be legally upheld, advance directives and living wills are not legally binding. They are, however, useful as evidence to that individual's wishes.

In 2008 the story of Hannah Jones hit the headlines. Hannah had developed a cardiomyopathy as a result of chemotherapy she had received, aged 4 years, for the treatment of acute myeloid leukaemia. At the age of 12 years with worsening heart failure Hannah was told that she needed a heart transplant to survive. Hannah firmly refused a transplant and her parents supported her decision, as did her doctors initially. In 2007 she was again offered a transplant, which she continued to refuse but this time the hospital authorities initiated High Court Proceedings to override her decision. The case never reached the High Court as the hospital abandoned legal action. Hannah later came to the decision herself to accept a heart transplant. It is not certain whether or not the hospital would have been successful in overriding Hannah's refusal. It is true that the Courts have overridden many teenagers refusing treatment for life-threatening conditions. They would have had to weigh up the effect of breaching Hannah's autonomy with what was considered her best interests. If Hannah was deemed Gillick-competent and her parents also withheld consent then this presents a strong legal position. However, only once has expert medical opinion been rejected in favour of the parents' refusal of life-saving treatment. A role for paternalism still exists. Reasons given for treatment being enforced in the past have included concerns that convictions strongly held as a teenager may be regretted later and that coming to terms with a serious health condition involves a process, part of which is denial, which may in itself result in a fluctuating capacity. It can only be speculated as to whether Hannah's change of mind is evidence of these.

Obtaining consent

The responsibility for seeking a patient's consent lies with the doctor undertaking the procedure. This task can be delegated to someone else provided that individual is suitably trained and qualified and has sufficient knowledge of the proposed procedure. Currently in the United Kingdom a separate consent is not required for general anaesthesia, and the information imparted and the recording of such is subject to guidance from the professional bodies. The question of who takes consent for radiological investigations under general anaesthesia has been the subject of debate and is still not resolved. It has been argued that the risk associated with anaesthesia is greater than the risk of the investigation. However, this can also be said of some minor surgical procedures, yet there is no suggestion that the anaesthetist should take consent in those situations. Also the risk of anaesthesia can only be taken into context when one understands the implications of the investigation, and that can only be imparted by the clinician requesting the test.

'Bolam test' vs 'reasonable or prudent patient' test

In the United States informed consent prevails and all information is disclosed to the patient. In the United Kingdom failure to disclose information has been judged on a professional standard which has its origins in the Bolam case in 1985, that is that 'a doctor is not negligent if he has acted in accordance with practice accepted as proper by a responsible body of men skilled in that particular art'. Increasingly the courts have modified this standard patient to encompass a 'reasonable or prudent patient test' in which 'material risks' must be disclosed and this has been endorsed by the General Medical Council (GMC). The 'reasonable patient' test still allows the doctor some discretion in terms of a therapeutic privilege that allows him or her to withhold information. The doctor may exercise this therapeutic privilege if 'risk disclosure poses such a threat of detriment to the patient as to become unfeasible or contraindicated from a medical point of view'. Few cases have supported the therapeutic privilege as a defence for failure to disclose risk. An example might be where disclosing the risks of an antipsychotic treatment was likely to deter a patient from treatment when the underlying condition itself threatened the patient's life and altered their judgement. It is not sufficient just to give information. There is an obligation on the physician to ensure the patient or parent understands what has been said to them.

Non-disclosure of medical conditions

If a patient wants to leave the decision about his or her care to someone else or states that s/he does not want to be given details of his/her condition or treatment then as far as possible this should be respected. However, it is advisable to try and understand why and offer as much basic information as possible together with insight as to the consequences of not having it. The validity of consent must be questioned if no information has been imparted. It is key to the development of a therapeutic relationship that the child trusts the physician treating him or her. It is important that age-appropriate information is given. The welfare of the child is the priority even if the parents express a wish for them not to know anything.

Proof of consent

There is no legal requirement for a signed consent form except for living organ donation and fertility treatment. A signed consent form serves as a record that a discussion took place but it is not proof of valid consent. It is always wise to document, however, especially where it is hospital policy to do so. Where a competent child has given consent their signature alone is sufficient.

Court Orders

The Courts have the power to consent to treatment on behalf of a minor. If agreement among child, parents and medical team cannot be reached within a reasonable time period then it may be necessary to seek a Court Order in relation to parental rights and responsibilities (Children Act 1989). If the parents disagree about certain procedures such as organ donation, sterilisation or circumcision, these specific cases should also be referred to court. In addition, the High Court has an inherent *parens patriae* jurisdiction over children. Its powers include being able to give consent or forbid a doctor from carrying out a procedure, or authorise withdrawal of treatment. No child, parent or court has the power to enforce a doctor to perform a procedure that the doctor does not feel is clinically justified. A child can be made a Ward of the High Court, which ensures that no important decisions in the child's life can be made without referral to the Court. Wardship is granted for 21 days in the first instance. Court decisions can be sought in emergency situations in and out of office hours by a lawyer, the judge sometimes advising over the phone.

Any Court decision must be made with the child's welfare of paramount importance. Section 1 (3) of the 1989 Children Act defines the factors to be considered. These include:

- The ascertainable wishes of the child
- Physical, emotional and educational needs
- Likely effect of any change in circumstances
- Age, sex and background
- Any harm suffered or at risk of being suffered
- How capable his or her parents or other relevant persons are of meeting his/her needs

Due consideration must also be given to complying with the European Convention of Human Rights.

Research

Society as a whole benefits from good quality research. However, the extent to which individuals should be subjected to risks for the good of others, especially where those individuals lack the ability to consent, is a difficult ethical dilemma. The Nuremberg Code of 1947 suggests that those who cannot express their views should be excluded from research. It can be argued, however, that excluding children from research is unjust because it breaches their right to the best attainable healthcare. There is a paucity of law protecting individuals involved in human research.

Research in children

As previously stated, the degree of understanding sought from a child is higher than from an adult. The law and those bodies involved with advising on consent adopt a paternalistic approach. Treatment can be administered to a child in the absence of consent if it is in their best interests. Using the same argument, therapeutic research can be in a child's best interests but non-therapeutic research is difficult to justify. However, if the purpose of research is ultimately to improve diagnosis and treatment of patients, then to refuse child subjects participation in research is to deny the paediatric population advances in clinical management.

Guidance from professional bodies

The Royal College of Paediatrics and Child Heath (RCPCH) Ethics Advisory Committee bases its guidelines on six principles.

- Research involving children is important for the benefit of all children and should be supported, encouraged and conducted in an ethical manner.
- Children are not small adults; they have an additional, unique set of interests.
- Research should only be done on children if comparable research on adults could not answer the same question.
- A research procedure that is not intended directly to benefit the child subject is not necessarily either unethical or illegal.
- All proposals involving medical research on children should be submitted to a research ethics committee.
- Legally valid consent should be obtained from the child, parent or guardian as appropriate.

When parental consent is obtained, the agreement of school-age children who take part in research should also be requested by researchers.

In order to be ethical, research must be based on sound scientific principles. The aim should be clearly defined, and the methodology should be expected to answer the question asked. The project should be completed and submitted for publication. Authors should declare any conflicts of interest and identify sources of funding for projects. Anonymity of the research participants should be protected.

The Medical Defence Union and British Medical Association offer practical advice to those involved in research on children. This involves getting expert advice in drawing up the consent form. The procedure should be explained very carefully and fully, preferably in the presence of an independent witness. A patient's participation in a research project should be documented in the medical notes. In addition to meeting the requirements and obtaining the approval of the local research ethics committee (LREC), the research should also comply with relevant advice from the Royal Colleges, research bodies and professional associations. For therapeutic research, it is important to emphasise to the patient and family that they are free to withdraw at any time without care being affected. There is no specific legal ruling in respect of healthy non-competent children being volunteered for non-therapeutic research. The law has been interpreted to imply that parents cannot authorise such involvement. However, the MDU and RCPCH have suggested that this should be slightly modified to allow parents to give authority where the procedure entails only negligible risk and discomfort. A parent cannot override a Gillick-competent child's refusal to consent for non-therapeutic research.

'Acceptable risk'

It is generally accepted that a lower degree of risk is acceptable for children subjected to research compared with adults. There is little consensus, however, as to how to define acceptable risk. Everyday life has risk associated with it. Minimal risk describes procedures such as non-invasive urine sampling or using blood or tissue taken as part of management of a clinical condition. Low risk describes procedures that cause brief pain, emotional distress or small bruises such as blood sampling. Low-risk procedures are unlikely to be considered acceptable if there is no benefit to the child. However, if the child shows altruism and on careful explanation is willing to accept this discomfort, then it may be reasonable to proceed. High-risk invasive procedures may only be justifiable for research when the procedure is part of diagnosis or treatment intended to benefit the child subject.

Restraint

The Department of Health defines restraint as 'the positive application of force with the intention of overpowering the child.' Restraint implies a restriction of liberty or freedom of movement. It therefore constitutes a breach of an individual's autonomy. Restraint also breaches the Human Rights Act Articles 3, 5 and 9. Justification for using restraint in limited circumstances in healthcare can be argued ethically on the principles of beneficence, acting in the patient's best interests, and non-maleficence, preventing harm.

Restraint in anaesthesia practice

It is common for a child to demonstrate varying degrees of resistance to aspects of medical management. The causes may be many and include a wariness of strangers, unfamiliar settings, anxiety, frustration, phobia or a genuine refusal. Management in the setting of surgery and anaesthesia is made more difficult because the anaesthetist will often not have a pre-existing relationship with the child, starvation results in distress to the child, and it can involve separation from the carer. Decisions as to whether to proceed often have to be made in a very narrow time frame. It is important to try to interpret the child's behaviour in light of his or her developmental age. In addition to the views of the child, consideration must also be given to the urgency of the procedure, the presence of valid consent from someone with parental responsibility and the consequences of not proceeding or delaying treatment. Proceeding with treatment against the child's wish may be legal, but may require either physical and/or pharmacological restraint and may have unwanted psychological sequelae.

If a decision has been made to override a young person's refusal that is both ethical and legal then it may seem logical that any amount of force can be used to achieve this. However, merely because treatment is in a competent patient's best interests does not mean that force is.

Using restraint or force to impose a treatment on an unwilling patient is in practice very difficult and fortunately rarely necessary. With sufficient time and explanation most will accept and cooperate with treatment. Most of the medical literature regarding restraint appears in relation to psychiatry and some articles relating to dentistry for those with special needs.

The Department of Health and Royal College of Nursing gives guidance on the appropriate use of restraint. If it proves impossible to gain a child's cooperation and the clinician decides that restraint is appropriate:

- The degree of restraint should be the minimum necessary to achieve the aim;
- Restraint, without court order, should only be employed for essential treatment or to prevent significant harm;
- For less urgent treatment of a competent minor, court approval should be sought even if the parents give permission to proceed;
- Where possible the staff involved should have an established relationship with the child;
- A full explanation as to the nature and need for restraint should be given to child and parents;
- Staff involved should be prepared and appropriately trained;
- All parties involved may benefit from an opportunity to discuss the incident soon after;
- Use of restraint should be recorded in the medical notes, including witness reports from other staff involved;
- It is important to remember that restraint is being utilised to facilitate care of the child, not as a means of punishment.

The inappropriate use of restraint may result in criminal charges, action in civil law or prosecution under health and safety legislation. As well as understanding when it is appropriate to use restraint, it is also important to have some measure of what constitutes reasonable force. Case law has yet to provide us with a test for assessing this. It is helpful to look to other areas of medical law. The Bolam test if applied would suggest that if restraint was accepted medical practice in that situation, then it would be legal. The case of Bolam v Friern Hospital Management Committee, from which this test is derived, involved a psychiatric patient sustaining injuries as a result of not being restrained during ECT treatment; this lack of restraint was accepted practice in 1957. We have seen since Bolam, however, that the courts are not bound by professional standards, in Bolitho v City and Hackney Health authority (1998), and that the test of reasonableness should also be satisfied. If there is a necessity to act, then the force may be justifiable in order to ensure patient and staff safety and facilitate effective treatment. It has been suggested that the same standards as apply in Criminal Law, for instance in police arrests, may need to be satisfied. In such circumstances, the force employed should not be excessive and it should be in proportion to the perceived benefit.

Returning to the opening clinical example of the 9-year-old boy listed for circumcision: one approach would be to remove the child from the stressful environment or alternatively remove all the unnecessary staff from the room so it appears less threatening. Ascertain whether the child is anxious about a particular aspect of the procedure, such as insertion of the cannula, or fundamentally does not want the operation. It can be very helpful to involve the surgeon who may already have a rapport with the child from a previous clinic appointment. It is also an opportunity to establish with the child how strong the indication for surgery is. It may be that his symptoms have subsided and that he is rightfully questioning the need for surgery. If he is fearful of a particular element of the procedure but in agreement with the need for surgery, returning to the ward for an anxiolytic premedication might be an acceptable way to proceed. Alternatively postpone surgery to allow a play therapist or clinical psychologist to work with the child. This would have the advantage of hopefully arming the child with coping strategies to deal with similar stressful situations in the future. If the child demonstrates a determined refusal to acknowledge the need for surgery then restraint, whether it be chemical or physical, is inappropriate and the child should be reviewed in clinic.

Key points

- A child is presumed competent to accept medical treatment independently of their parents when they attain an age of 16 years.
- Below the age of 16 a child can give consent if they demonstrate Gillick-competence. They should understand the nature and risks of the proposed treatment and non-treatment, and that there is a choice to be made.
- If a child's parents are unmarried the father has consent if he is named on the birth certificate or a parental responsibility agreement is in effect.

Further reading

Association of Anaesthetists of Great Britain and Ireland. Consent for anaesthesia. *Anaesthesia*. AAGBI. 2006.

BMA. *Assessment of Mental Capacity: Guidance for Doctors and Lawyers. A Report by the British Medical Association and The Law Society.* BMA. 1996.

BMA. *Consent, Rights and Choices in Health Care for Children and Young People.* BMJ Books. 2001.

General Medical Council. *Consent: Patients And Doctors Making Decisions Together*. General Medical Council. 2008.

McIntosh N. Guidelines for the ethical conduct of medical research involving children. *Arch Dis Child* 2000;**82**:177–182.

The Medical Defence Union. *Consent to Treatment*. Medical Defence Union. 1996.

The Parental Responsibility Agreement (Amendment) Regulations 2009, no. 2026 and The Parental Responsibilities and Parental Rights Agreement (Scotland). Amendment Regulations 2009, SSI/2009/191.

The Royal College of Nursing. *Restraining, Holding Still and Containing Children: Guidance for Good Practice.* RCN. 1999.

Safeguarding Children and the anaesthetist

Kathy A. Wilkinson

Introduction

'Safeguarding Children', by which is meant their protection from maltreatment or neglect, is essential core knowledge for all healthcare workers. The Children Act 2004 was introduced in England and Wales following the Laming report of 2003 into the death through maltreatment of a young girl. Safeguarding policy and practice is central to the National Service Frameworks for Children and equivalent initiatives in all parts of the UK. The National Institute for Health and Clinical Excellence (NICE) has published guidance that is referenced within this chapter to assist in the recognition of maltreatment.

Anaesthetists need to be fully aware of local safeguarding processes as they may be involved in the following circumstances:

(1) When a baby or child is admitted as an emergency for resuscitation or surgery and the cause of the presenting illness is unclear, e.g. severe head injury;

(2) When a baby or child is admitted for investigation of Safeguarding concerns, e.g. a child protection plan is in place and forensic investigations are needed;

(3) When a baby or child is admitted for urgent or elective surgery and coincidental suspicious signs are noted that may be the result of abuse or neglect;

(4) When a child or parent discloses concerns that prompt one to believe there may be maltreatment within a family.

Box 5.1   Definitions and terminology

Age
- Infant: <1 year
- Child: <13 years
- Young person: 13–17 years

Box 5.2   In relation to maltreatment (Working Together to Safeguard Children, 2010)

- *Suspect* means a serious level of concern about the possibility of maltreatment but is not proof of it.
- *Consider* means that maltreatment is one possible explanation for the alerting feature or is included in the differential diagnosis.
- *Physical abuse* may involve hitting, shaking, throwing, poisoning, burning or scalding, drowning, suffocating or otherwise causing physical harm to a child.
- *Physical harm* may also be caused when a parent or carer fabricates the symptoms of, or deliberately induces, illness in a child they are looking after.
- *Emotional abuse* is the persistent emotional ill treatment of a child such as to cause severe or persistent adverse effects on the child's emotional development. It may involve conveying to children that they are worthless or unloved, inadequate, or valued only insofar as they meet the needs of another person.
- *Sexual abuse* involves forcing or enticing a child or young person to take part in sexual activities, including prostitution, whether or not the child is aware of what is happening. The activities may involve physical contact, including penetrative (e.g. rape, anal or oral sex) or non-penetrative acts. This may include non-contact activities, such as children looking at, or involved in the production of pornographic material, or watching sexual activities, or children being encouraged to behave in sexually inappropriate ways.
- *Neglect* is the persistent failure to meet a child's basic physical and/or psychological needs, likely to result in the most serious impairment of the

Core Topics in Paediatric Anaesthesia, ed. Ian James and Isabeau Walker. Published by Cambridge University Press. © 2013 Cambridge University Press.

Box 5.2 *(cont.)*

child's health and development. Neglect may occur during pregnancy as a result of maternal substance abuse. It may involve a parent or carer failing to provide adequate food, shelter and clothing, failure to ensure adequate supervision, or failure to provide access to appropriate medical care or treatment.

Box 5.3 **Under Section 31(9) of the Children Act 1989 as amended by the Adoption and Children Act 2002**

Harm means ill-treatment or the impairment of health or development, including, for example, impairment suffered from seeing or hearing the ill-treatment of another;
Development means physical, intellectual, emotional, social or behavioural development;
Health means physical or mental health; and
Ill-treatment includes sexual abuse and forms of ill-treatment which are not physical.

Under Section 31(10) of the Act:

Where the question of whether harm suffered by a child is significant turns on the child's health and development, his or her health or development shall be compared with that which could reasonably be expected of a similar child.

Signs of child maltreatment
Physical abuse

A full account of abusive injuries is beyond this review, and general features are presented.

Infants under 1 year have the highest rate of notification on Child Protection Registers in the UK and are four times as likely as older children to suffer severe injuries that lead to their death. Physical abuse may present in many forms.

Bruises, bites, lacerations and burns

Children, particularly those under 5 years, often present to hospital with injuries – most are relatively minor, and most are accidental. A basic knowledge of normal child behaviour and development is useful in making an assessment, and the context of the

injury is important. Clinicians should consider for each infant or child:

- What is the level of independent activity?
- Are there predisposing medical conditions or disabilities?
- Is the mechanism of injury consistent with the explanation of how it occurred?
- Has there been a delay in presentation?

For the anaesthetist who sees just a 'snapshot' of the child and family dynamics this may be particularly difficult, and usually other members of the team have already interviewed the family, asked these questions and documented their analysis. If you are unsure you should also ask and you should document your concerns in the child's medical record.

With regard to bruises, it is extremely difficult to date their occurrence from appearance alone. However, multiple regular bruises of the same shape and size may be of concern, particularly if the shape is one made by an object that the child may have been hit with or gripped forcefully with, e.g. finger tip marks. Bruises in soft tissue areas away from bony prominences are unusual. Bruises on a baby or child who is not independently mobile always require explanation.

Human bites are of concern (other than those obviously caused by a young child). Lacerations which have been inflicted may have a characteristic shape, can be symmetrical and may be hidden under clothing or include the face and/or neck. With burns, consider how usual it is for the particular part of the body to be in contact with hot structures or materials, and again whether the explanation offered and the developmental level of the child is consistent with this. Symmetrical burns and scalds with sharply delineated edges are less likely to be accidental and imply that the child has been placed in a hot bath, for example (rather than falling or stepping in accidentally). Cigarette burns may appear as small circular blisters, or deep craters (dependent on the age and severity of the burn) which if multiple may be difficult to distinguish from excoriated insect bites.

Fractures

The context is vital, and discussion should include an explanation of mechanism of injury, current motor development, the timing of the injury in relation to presentation and whether there may be associated bone fragility. Fractures of different ages are unusual, as are fractures in a non-ambulant infant and those picked up by coincidental investigation, for example rib fractures noted on a chest X-ray. These should raise suspicions of non-accidental aetiology.

Torn frenum

For some time it has been believed that injury to the upper labial frenum in children is pathognomonic of physical abuse. This has recently been questioned and the evidence base challenged. Facial injuries are common in children of all ages. A torn frenum is relatively common in toddlers or young children who fall on their face, onto low-lying furniture, or have a blow to the face, for example from a swing. There are also many cases in the literature of children who present with a torn frenum in association with other physical and skeletal injuries, some of whom have been very seriously abused. History is therefore all-important, and it is particularly important that if seen in isolation this injury is assessed in context. However, if the explanation of injury is inadequate or implausible it may be necessary to perform additional investigations, particularly in very young children. (See also Further reading.)

Head injuries

Head injuries are the leading cause of death from child maltreatment. If there is no history of major accidental trauma and no underlying predisposing condition, it is extremely unusual for a child to present with an intracranial haematoma (subdural or subarachnoid), and the presence of such an injury should raise suspicions. Similarly, hypoxic/ischaemic brain damage may present as the first sign of abuse, for example on a diagnostic CT scan in a baby who presents with new seizures. In infants under the age of 1 year, up to 95% of severe head injuries may be non-accidental. Mortality in babies under 6 months is particularly high (approximately 30%) and many survivors have residual disability.

The role of the radiologist is often important in the context of physical abuse in childhood and there are useful UK joint guidelines in this area.

Fabricated or induced illness

This may be especially difficult to diagnose, but should be suspected if the presenting symptoms and/or signs seem to be at odds with a recognised clinical picture. Further suspicion should be aroused if symptoms and signs only appear or reappear when the carer is present, and are only observed by that person. Other features of fabricated illness include a tendency to consult many different doctors, and new symptoms appearing as soon as old ones disappear.

Near death events

Child maltreatment should be suspected when repeated life-threatening events occur which have no obvious medical explanation, and are witnessed by only one parent or caregiver. In infants these events may be accompanied by bleeding from the nose or mouth, which may be a result of attempted asphyxiation.

Submersions

As in all cases of abuse, if the history of submersion is inconsistent, delayed and/or unrealistic in the detail given, suspect maltreatment. The history may also reveal a degree of lack of supervision which in itself constitutes neglect.

Sexual abuse

This may present as an injury (genital or anal), sexually transmitted infection (including anogenital warts), pregnancy and/or inappropriate 'sexualised' behaviour. The significance of many symptoms and signs depends on the age of the child or young person and that of any sexual partner; for example pregnancy in a girl of 15 would not generally constitute abuse if the partner is of a similar age, whereas it may well if the partner is considerably older.

The recognition, investigation and management of sexual abuse in childhood are highly specialised areas in which only a small number of the safeguarding team participate. Careful and meticulous history taking is essential. Examination and investigation can be particularly difficult in children, and on occasion may require general anaesthesia.

Anal dilation

Great care is required in the interpretation of anal signs, such as anal fissures, and in particular an isolated finding of anal dilation. There are very few absolutely diagnostic signs of abuse, and in interpreting this sign it is important to know what constitutes normal anal appearance. It is also important to bear in mind that anal tone may be markedly altered by the effects of general and regional anaesthesia, as well as relatively common childhood problems such as chronic constipation.

> **Box 5.4** Clinical features which may cause concern or suspicion
>
> Suspicious signs which may be indicative of abuse (see also www.core-info.cf.ac.uk)
> - Unusual or excessive bruising, particularly in the non-ambulant baby/child
> - Cigarette burns
> - Bite marks
> - Unusual injuries in inaccessible places e.g. neck, ear, hands, feet and buttocks
> - Intra-oral trauma
> - Damage to intra-oral frena, or unexplained frenum injury in a non-ambulant child
> - Genital/anal trauma (where no clear history of direct trauma is offered or part of the clinical presentation)
> - Trauma without adequate history e.g. intra-abdominal trauma
>
> If anaesthetists have real concerns they are advised to discuss these at an early stage with key child-protection workers. A suggested form of words might be:
>
> 'Whilst James was asleep some unusual marks were noticed. We aren't sure what caused this and need to ask for a second opinion. Another doctor/ nurse should take a look.'

> **Box 5.5** Duties of the anaesthetist
> 1. To act in the best interests of the child which are always paramount
> 2. To be aware of the child's rights to be protected
> 3. To respect the rights of the child to confidentiality
> 4. To contact a paediatrician with experience of child protection for advice (on-call paediatrician for child protection, named or designated doctor/nurse)
> 5. To be aware of the local CP mechanisms
> 6. To be aware of the rights of those with parental responsibility

Neglect

Neglect may or may not be deliberate. It constitutes a situation in which the child or young person is put at risk as a result of the persistent failure to meet his or her basic physical or psychological needs. This may in turn result in impairment of health and development, which leads to harm. It may on occasion be very difficult to decide whether one is looking at neglect or the results of poverty (clearly both can coexist). For the anaesthetist, particularly if seeing the child and family in a day-case setting, it may be particularly difficult to make this distinction. Suspicions might be raised if the young child is inappropriately dressed or smelly, or if there is no emotional rapport between the carer and the child.

Suspected child maltreatment: the referral process

If there is a suspicion of child maltreatment, there are formal processes of assessment, planning, intervention and review, the speed of which depends on the urgency of the situation. These are outlined in the HM Government document 'Working Together to Safeguard Children' (see Further reading), and in the accompanying flow charts 'What to do if you are concerned a child is being abused'. The initial processes are summarised for anaesthetists in the 2007 Intercollegiate document 'Child Protection and the Anaesthetist: Safeguarding children in the operating theatre' (see also Figure 5.1). *At all times the child's best interests are paramount.*

Assessment

NICE guidance stresses the importance of carefully listening to and observing children and their families in the context of assessing possible maltreatment. This is to gain a fuller picture of the situation and information may come from several sources. The next step would normally be to seek an explanation from the parent or carer, and then to record exactly what has been observed or heard (from whom and when) and why you have concerns. In the case of the anaesthetist some information may have come to light at pre-assessment, for example. Seeking an explanation should be conducted jointly with a consultant paediatrician who agrees there is a need for consideration of possible maltreatment. It may be the preliminary step prior to referral to a child protection professional (in England the named or designated doctor or nurse for child protection). Any discussion with the parent and/or child or young person requires careful planning as to when and where this should be conducted, and who needs to be present. A very clear form of words is also necessary. Remember at this stage you and colleagues may well be unsure about aetiology, so it may be helpful to think and speak about referrals to

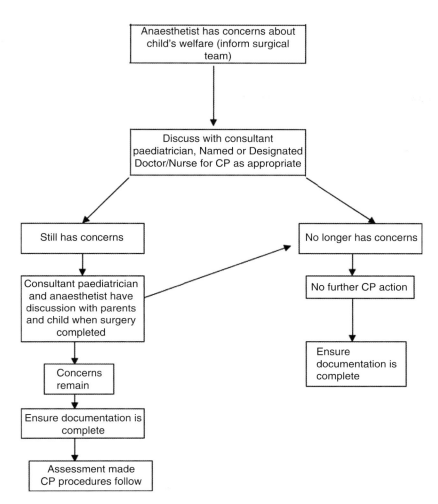

Figure 5.1 Flow chart showing the steps an anaesthetist should take if they have concerns about the welfare of a child.

the child protection team in terms of wanting a second opinion.

The next steps depend on the urgency and the level of understanding of the situation at that point, and will not generally involve the anaesthetist directly. However, this may involve discussion with child protection professionals and others who are involved with the child and family. The suspicion of child maltreatment may be high or low in the differential diagnosis. If suspicion is low, maltreatment should be excluded from the list of possible diagnoses (as much as is feasible). If this cannot be done, if further information is required, or if suspicion is high, a formal review should be arranged involving colleagues from social services. The recommendation in England and Wales is that this should always be within 7 days of referral.

The initial process includes an assessment of risk and possible protective factors within the context of the child's family and environment (including the quality of parenting), being aware of the developmental level and needs of the child.

Planning and action phases

Following this there are three possible outcomes in England (these do not differ in principle in other parts of the UK):

- No further action;
- A voluntary programme of support for the child and family (in England and Wales as described in Section 17 of the 1989 Children Act. This may be described as a 'Child in Need Plan');

- If there is 'actual or likely significant harm', a compulsory child protection investigation, strategy discussion and action is conducted in England and Wales by the Local Safeguarding Children's Board (LSCB), as described in Section 47 of the 1989 Act (a 'Child Protection Plan'). In Scotland a Serious case review is conducted by the Child Protection Committee, and in Northern Ireland the Area Child Protection Committee.

If there is a need for *urgent* action, an immediate strategy discussion is required involving other agencies such as social services and police. This aims to decide rapidly on how best to provide immediate protection for the child (and any other children in the same family). Rarely this may require direct police intervention, such as the detention of a parent.

Review

In England and Wales if a child is subject to a Child Protection Plan, a core group including a key worker is appointed. This group will be responsible for commissioning further specialist assessments and intervention, and further reviews occur at a minimum of 3 and 6 months, and thereafter until there is no longer a safeguarding issue.

Keeping records

If child abuse or neglect is suspected, it is essential that clear records are kept of all information relating to the child, including location, times, dates and those involved. If an anaesthetist is involved in a resuscitation episode and abuse is a possible causative factor, it is particularly important to make sure that the records are complete and accurate with times, names and designations of all staff noted. It is useful to check these records personally for clarity and accuracy, and it may be helpful to keep a personal record for future use. These records may form the basis of a medical report or police statement at a later date. Always stick to your own area of expertise and restrict suggestions about management to your area of responsibility.

Sharing information, consent and confidentiality

The child's safety and wellbeing is paramount. Information may need to be shared with healthcare professionals within the hospital setting, being aware of best practice with regard to maintaining confidentiality. If possible you should seek consent to do so, explaining why information sharing is necessary. If there is a need to disclose information to outside agencies such as police and social services this should generally be specifically explained to the parent and child or young person and documented. In general the responsibility for both this discussion and disclosing medical records, including sensitive information, will be with the safeguarding team. If written consent is taken it should include specific permission to share medical records including photography.

When a child dies

In England, Wales and Northern Ireland when a child dies this may result in one of two responses from the relevant Safeguarding Board or committee. If the death is clearly the result of abuse it will also automatically trigger a serious case review. However, if it is 'unexpected' (defined as all deaths in children and young people 0–18 years which were not anticipated 24 hours beforehand) it will also be reviewed by a child death review panel, which may also discover safeguarding issues. The procedure for these investigations in England is outlined in the 'Working Together' document of 2010, and there are similar although not identical systems in place in Scotland, Wales and Northern Ireland (see Further reading).

Child protection legislation

The law relating to child protection varies across the UK. In England and Wales the most important legislation around child protection is contained in the 1989 Children Act.

Section 17 of the 1989 Children Act sets out the statutory responsibilities of the local authority to maintain a child's health and development. It may be used to justify the need for additional resources when a child is deemed 'in need' and is not invoked exclusively in the context of maltreatment.

Section 47 of the 1989 Children Act is invoked when there is sufficient concern about a child or young person to require Children's Social Care to undertake a formal investigation, which may also involve the police. This will mean talking to people known to the family, interviewing the child or young person alone, and performing a medical examination. A formal assessment of risk forms part of this process.

In Scotland the relevant legislation is the Children (Scotland) Act and the cases are referred via the Scottish Children's Reporter system (see www.scra. gov.uk).

Possible outcomes from a Section 47 enquiry are as below:

- *Child assessment order* – allows social services to investigate to see whether any further action is needed.
- *Child protection order* – emergency protection order that allows social services to remove the child from the family home for a limited time or while investigation continues.
- *Child protection case conference* – follows investigation under Section 47. Attended by professionals who know the family, or who have specialist information or knowledge. Parents and carers are encouraged to attend.
- *Child protection plan* – assesses risk, ways of protection, short and long term aims, roles and responsibilities, monitoring and evaluation.
- *Care order* – commits the child to the care of the local authority.
- *Supervision order* – places the child under the supervision of a social worker or probation officer.
- *Emergency protection order* – allows social services to remove child from home if believed to be at significant risk, granting parental responsibility to social services. Lasts up to 8 days, can be extended once.
- *Child protection register* – confidential list of all children who have been identified at a child protection conference to be at significant risk of harm. Reviewed at least every 6 months.

Who has parental responsibility?

Within a care order the parents may still share parental responsibility but the local authority will decide to what extent they may exercise this. Within a supervision order the parental responsibility remains with the parents. If the child is under a care order and is being cared for foster parents, the local authority usually consents to medical treatment. Note that a care order may occasionally be in force from birth, based on previous parental behaviour.

Documentation of the child protection plan

Local Safeguarding Children's Boards/Child Protection committees may suggest a proforma to facilitate clear documentation in cases of child maltreatment. If there is a formal 'child protection plan' this should also be available. These documents should be accessible as they provide important background information for the anaesthetist, for instance before interviewing a child and parent on the ward prior to elective surgery. They are likely to be more detailed and accurate than word of mouth and they should be filed at the front of the patient's notes. Be aware that material within these notes is of a confidential nature and is available on a 'need to know' basis.

Key points

Safeguarding children and vulnerable adults is currently a high profile issue within health, social care and education in the UK.

The responsibilities of anaesthetists are not dissimilar from those of many other groups of medical and nursing staff who work with children, be it occasionally or regularly.

A team approach involving child protection professionals is essential.

Key responsibilities are:
- Always putting the child first
- Awareness and identification of risk
- Awareness of the process of referral
- Appropriate referral
- Clear and complete documentation
- Maintaining confidentiality

Box 5.6 Safeguarding vignettes

- An 11-month-old infant presents to the accident and emergency department at 06:00. Mother reports that she has been found in her cot at 04:00 having a seizure. On arrival she is unresponsive to stimulation, pale and hypotensive. After intubation and fluid resuscitation a CT scan of the head reveals bilateral subdural haemorrhages and raised intracranial pressure, and a chest X-ray shows bilateral callus formation in old rib fractures. She is transferred immediately to the regional PICU where care is managed jointly with neurosurgery.

Box 5.6 *(cont.)*

A serious case review is held 2 weeks later and there are subsequent court proceedings. You are asked to provide a statement by the police. The consultant paediatric neurologist relies on the very clear notes made immediately after initial resuscitation and prior to transfer.

- A 7-year-old child requires colposcopy and vaginal swabs within 24 hours for forensic investigation of possible sexual abuse by mother's partner. The child is fitted in at the end of a routine list, and you are informed that examination will be performed jointly by a consultant paediatrician and gynaecologist. The regular theatre team is surprised to find that the case takes almost 1 hour, as clinical photographs are also required. You are asked to take blood for HIV and Hepatitis C serology for which consent has also been obtained.

- A 4-year-old presents for dental extraction of several carious teeth. The child is unkempt and has dirty clothes, and both he and his mother are distraught in the anaesthetic room. When his heavy pullover is removed after induction he is noted to have three regular burns <1 cm in diameter on his right arm. The anaesthetist and dentist ask a consultant paediatrician to attend theatre, and a decision is made to discuss the marks with the mother back on the day ward. No satisfactory explanation is forthcoming and therefore the designated/nominated doctor is asked to advise, and attends the unit later that day. The child goes home with mother and subsequent discussions reveal that the child's 11-year-old sibling has burnt him with a cigarette. Additional support and follow up is provided for the child and family in the community.

Further reading

A Guide to Getting it Right for Every Child. 2008. http://scotland.gov.uk/resource/Doc/238985/0065813.pdf

All Wales Child Protection Procedures: Children in Wales. http://www.childreninwales.org.uk/areasofwork/safeguardingchildren/index.html

Association of Paediatric Anaesthetists of Great Britain and Ireland. *Safeguarding Resources.* http://www.apagbi.org.uk/professionals/professional-standards/safeguarding

Department for Education. *The Protection of Children in England: A Progress Report. Lord Laming.* The Stationery Office Limited. 2009. www.dcsf.gov.uk

DH England. *Working Together to Safeguard Children.* 2010. https://www.education.gov.uk/publications/eOrderingDownload/00305-2010DOM-EN.pdf

DH England e-learning Health. Safeguarding Children and Young People, Level 2 and 3.

https://e-learningforhealthcare.org.uk (updated 2012).

DHSSPSNI. *Understanding the Needs of Children in Northern Ireland (UNOCINI) guidance,* 2011. www.dhsspsni.gov.uk

General Medical Council. *0–18 years: Guidance for Doctors.* 2007. www.gmc-uk.org

General Medical Council. *Protecting Children and Young People. The Responsibilities of All Doctors.* 2012. www.gmc-uk.org.uk

National Institute for Health and Clinical Excellence. *When to Suspect Child Maltreatment.* (Guideline 89). 2009. Available at www.nice.org.uk

Royal College of Anaesthetists. *Safeguarding Children and Young People: Roles and Competencies for Healthcare Staff.* (Intercollegiate document) September 2010. http://www.rcoa.ac.uk/document-store/safeguarding-children-and-young-people-roles-and-competences-health-care-staff

Royal College of Paediatrics and Child Health. *Child Protection Companion.* London. 2006. www.rcpch.ac.uk (currently being updated)

Royal College of Paediatrics and Child Health. *Child Protection Reader.* 2007. www.rcpch.ac.uk

Royal College of Radiologists and Royal College of Paediatrics and Child Health, 2008. *Standards for Radiological Investigations of Suspected Non-accidental Injury.* www.rcr.ac.uk/docs/radiology/pdf/RCPCH_RCR_final.pdf.

The National Guidance for Child Protection in Scotland. 2010. http://www.scotland.gov.uk/Publications/2010/12/09134441/0

The Victoria Climbié Inquiry Report. The Stationery Office Limited. 2003.

Welsh Child Protection Systematic Review Group. www.core-info.cardiff.ac.uk

Also see publications at www.nspcc.org.uk

Chapter

6

Pre-operative assessment for paediatric anaesthesia

Reema Nandi

Introduction

Anaesthetists are responsible for the pre-operative assessment of their patients, all of whom should be seen before receiving a general anaesthetic, ideally by the anaesthetist administering it. The aim in assessing patients before anaesthesia and surgery is to improve outcome by:

- identifying pre-existing medical conditions;
- identifying potential anaesthetic difficulties;
- assessing and quantifying risk;
- planning peri-operative care.

The pre-operative assessment visit is also a useful time to discuss peri-operative management with the child and parent and can be an opportunity to allay fears and anxiety.

Good pre-operative assessment should improve efficient use of operating theatre time by reducing the cancellation of surgery on the day for clinical reasons, and it may reduce the number of patients who fail to attend on the day of surgery. Excellent team working among health professionals is essential to achieve this.

The ideal of the anaesthetist who will anaesthetise the child conducting a pre-operative assessment well in advance of the proposed procedure is not always possible. Pre-operative assessment clinics, possibly nurse-led, using carefully constructed questionnaires have been used effectively for healthy children undergoing minor and intermediate procedures. Questionnaires are an effective way of gaining background information and should reduce the time spent asking basic questions, allowing more time to discuss actual problems and the operation. Although pre-operative assessment is believed to be a basic element of anaesthetic care there are no controlled trials on the clinical effect of provision

of a pre-anaesthetic review of medical records, or an adequate physical examination. Nevertheless, even if seen in an assessment clinic, all children should be reviewed by the anaesthetist on the day of surgery.

The assessment of children for general anaesthesia differs in several ways from the assessment of an adult.

- Young children are not able to give a history and must be assessed in conjunction with their parents or caregivers.
- Even when assessing older children a discussion with parents is important.
- Discussion with both the child and caregiver is an essential aspect of informed consent.
- Co-morbidity in childhood is predominantly the consequence of congenital disorders or acute illnesses, particularly infectious diseases, compared with adults where the anaesthetist is primarily concerned with the consequences of chronic disorders usually involving the cardio-respiratory system.
- Chronic disorders in children are less common, although the incidence of problems such as morbid obesity is increasing.
- Thorough assessment in small children is particularly important as they often have less physiological reserve than adults.

Clinical evaluation

This is based on a careful medical history, including current medication and any drug allergies, physical examination and review of relevant clinical investigations. The clinical notes and previous anaesthetic records will usually provide information on known medical problems and treatment. The indication for surgical procedures and surgical history should be noted.

Core Topics in Paediatric Anaesthesia, ed. Ian James and Isabeau Walker. Published by Cambridge University Press. © 2013 Cambridge University Press.

Interview

The pre-operative interview is the anaesthetist's first introduction to a patient and is an opportunity to develop a rapport with the child and parents. This is usually the most efficient and productive component of pre-operative assessment. In children who are basically healthy this is often short and its objective is to clarify details obtained from the notes and detect unrecognised disease that could increase the risk of surgery above the baseline. In infants, an antenatal and neonatal history, including gestational age and any need for respiratory support, should be taken. The ex-preterm infant requires careful pre-operative preparation by experienced medical staff (see Chapter 9). There should be a review of issues pertinent to the planned anaesthetic procedure including functional status, cardiopulmonary function and homeostatic status. A personal or family history of anaesthetic problems can be helpful in identifying children with a susceptibility to malignant hyperthermia, at risk of an atypical pseudocholinesterase, an unknown bleeding disorder or muscular dystrophy, for example. A medication history should include those that have been stopped recently, particularly steroids as it may be necessary to provide peri-operative supplementation. Undesirable side effects, including allergy, to medication or other agents should be noted. Discussion about current medications should include over-the-counter medications. Recent vaccinations and laboratory tests should be recorded. In older children and adolescents, smoking and drinking habits and the possibility of pregnancy may be relevant. It may be helpful or necessary to interview older children away from their carers.

The anaesthetist should ask about previous anaesthetic inductions and their acceptability to the child. This will lead naturally to discussion about the induction technique to be used for the current event. Most anaesthetists will endeavour to accommodate preferences of the child and parent, within reason. The pre-operative visit provides an opportunity to discuss the potential risks encountered in children during anaesthesia.

Jehovah's Witnesses

For families who are Jehovah's Witnesses, discussions about possible blood transfusion should take place well in advance of elective surgery and involve the surgeon and a representative of the Local Hospital Liaison committee for Jehovah's Witnesses. In the UK, if the parents refuse to give permission for a blood transfusion a 'Specific Issue Order' under Section 8 of The Children's Act 1989 can be obtained from the High Court. In an emergency, where a child may die without immediate transfusion, the clinician must obtain a second opinion from a colleague and document the details in the medical notes before proceeding with the transfusion. The courts are highly likely to uphold the decision of the clinician to transfuse under these circumstances.

Herbal medicine

A significant and increasing proportion of the paediatric population receives or has received herbal preparations, approximately 16% in children presenting for ambulatory surgery. There should be direct questioning about use of these agents as 70% of patients taking herbal medications do not report their use and such medications have the potential to produce undesirable peri-operative consequences. For example Ma huang (*Ephedra sinica*) used for the treatment of a variety of symptoms, and as an agent to promote weight loss because it increases the metabolic rate, is an ephedrine-containing drug. It is a cardiovascular stimulant, acting as an alpha- and beta-adrenergic agonist, and is a potent bronchodilator. Ephedra can potentially interact with volatile anaesthetic agents and promote arrhythmias and has been associated with numerous fatalities. Furthermore, there can be profound intra-operative hypotension in patients who have used ephedra on a long-term basis. Other common herbal remedies that may impair coagulation, particularly when taken with medications such as NSAIDs, are listed in Table 6.1.

Even though adverse events related to the consumption of herbal medication are likely to be under-reported, a report of the World Health Organization Monitoring Centre into nearly 5000 cases of adverse events associated with herbal medications before 1996 included approximately 100 events in children below 10 years. The American Society of Anesthesiologists has recommended that the use of herbal medication should be discontinued 2–3 weeks before surgery, although the impact on morbidity and mortality of this is not known.

Vaccinations

Anaesthesia and surgery exert immunomodulatory effects and it has been suggested that they may exert additive or synergistic influences on vaccine efficacy

Table 6.1 Herbal medicines that may affect coagulation

Bilberry
Ginkgo biloba
Bromelain
Dong quai
Ginseng
Ginger
Feverfew
Garlic
Chamomile
Fish oil
Grape seed extract
Horse chestnut

and safety. Alternatively, inflammatory responses and fever elicited by vaccines may interfere with the post-operative course. Few studies have assessed the influence of anaesthesia and surgery on paediatric vaccine responses. It appears that the immuno-modulatory influence of anaesthesia during elective surgery is both minor and transient (around 48 hours), and the current evidence does not provide any contraindication to the immunisation of healthy children scheduled for elective surgery. However, respecting a minimal delay of 2 days for inactivated vaccines or 14–21 days for live attenuated viral vaccines between immunisation and anaesthesia may be useful to avoid the risk of misinterpretation of vaccine-driven adverse events as post-operative complications.

Allergies

Along with a history of current medication a history of known allergies must be sought. Latex allergy accounts for 19% of allergic reactions in children and is the most common cause of intra-operative anaphylaxis, as opposed to muscle relaxants in adults. Particular care should be taken questioning children at high risk for latex allergy such as those with:

- spina bifida
- urinary tract malformations
- history of atopy
- previous repeated exposures to latex

- allergy to foods that have cross reactivity with latex proteins, e.g. kiwi, banana, avocado, chestnuts

Physical examination

All children should be examined before a general anaesthetic. This examination should include:

- main vital observations, including blood pressure, pulse (rate and regularity) and respiratory rate;
- cardiac and respiratory examination;
- weight and height.

There may be emergency situations when it is not possible to weigh a child, and an estimate is necessary. The formula taught by the Resuscitation Council (UK) is, for weight in kg:

$$Wt = 2(age + 4).$$

This may underestimate weight and the newer Luscombe formula may be more accurate (again, weight is in kg):

$$Wt = (3 \times age) + 7$$

Whichever formula is used it is important to remember that this is only an estimate, and an accurate weight should be obtained as soon as is practical.

In addition, there should be assessments for specific anaesthetic procedures, such as intubation (airway examination including dentition), regional anaesthesia and venous access. If loose teeth are identified the parents and child should be warned that it may be necessary to remove them during anaesthesia.

Examination of the child reassures anxious parents that the anaesthetist has made a thorough assessment of the child prior to surgery, and it allows the anaesthetist to familiarise themselves with the child. During the physical examination, the anaesthetist should respect the modesty of older children.

Investigations

There is no good evidence to show that routine pre-operative testing, e.g. urinalysis, haemoglobin and serum electrolytes, in healthy children (or adults for that matter) undergoing minor to intermediate surgery is beneficial. The literature does not address the issue of whether practice changes as a result of the tests; as a result of this there have been consensus developments around pre-operative testing. Routine testing is unnecessary for the healthy child undergoing minor or intermediate surgery. The current practice is to target investigations at specific patient groups who have pre-existing medical problems that may influence peri-operative management. This will include those with an underlying disease such as renal or hepatic impairment or who take medications that might influence water and electrolyte balance.

Mild anaemia, found in up to 10% of healthy children, is not associated with increased peri-operative morbidity, nor does it change the anaesthetic management; checking haemoglobin is therefore not warranted in most cases. An exception is the neonate less than 60 weeks post-conceptual age; those with a haematocrit less than 30% may be at greater risk of post-operative apnoea, and pre-operative haemoglobin testing in this group is considered to be essential by most anaesthetists.

There is clear evidence that pre-operative coagulation profiles have a very low positive predictive value in detecting occult bleeding disorders or an increased risk for peri-operative haemorrhage. However, where even minimal bleeding could be critical, for example neurosurgery, coagulation screening is justified.

Sickle status should be established in children from racial groups susceptible to sickle cell disease, such as those from west and central Africa and northeast Saudi Arabia. If this is unknown a sickledex test should be performed. If the sickledex test is positive, haemoglobin electrophoresis should be performed to determine the precise genotype. This should be done well in advance of surgery as electrophoresis takes some time to perform.

The sickledex test is not effective in neonates owing to the presence of high levels of fetal haemoglobin. In the UK sickle cell disease screening is included in the blood spot test undertaken shortly after birth.

Chest X-ray is generally unnecessary unless there are specific respiratory issues or respiratory symptoms.

Heart murmur

Heart murmurs are common in pre-school children, with a reported incidence of up to 80%. Their detection is common during routine pre-operative assessments and although most are not clinically significant, a small proportion may be due to a lesion that may result in cardiovascular compromise under anaesthesia.

The majority of children with congenital heart disease are diagnosed in the first few months of life. Any child under 1 year of age with a previously unheard murmur should be referred for assessment by a cardiologist as signs and symptoms may be unreliable in this age group, particularly those with syndromes that are associated with cardiac disease e.g. Down syndrome, CHARGE association, VACTERL (Vertebral, Anal, Cardiac, Tracheo-oEsophageal fistula, Renal, Limb) association, Turner syndrome and DiGeorge syndrome.

It can be difficult to discriminate between an innocent and a pathological murmur on purely clinical grounds. Innocent murmurs are usually:

- Soft, early systolic, or
- Continuous (venous hum)
- Without any precordial thrill

The murmur is also unlikely to be important or to complicate anaesthesia if there are no symptoms such as:

- Failure to thrive
- Feeding difficulties
- Dyspnoea or tachypnoea
- Sweating episodes
- Poor exercise tolerance
- Recurrent respiratory infection
- Cyanotic episodes
- Syncope or chest pain

An ECG should be obtained in patients with a murmur. Children over 1 year with features of an innocent murmur, without signs or symptoms of clinical disease and who have no ECG abnormalities, can be anaesthetised safely and should be referred for cardiology review at a later date. In the asymptomatic child with a murmur two conditions that need to be excluded are hypertrophic obstructive cardiomyopathy and critical aortic stenosis. The ECG shows left axis deviation and left ventricular hypertrophy in both of these conditions and cardiological review is essential.

A commonly used algorithm for pre-operative management of cardiac murmurs is shown in Figure 6.1.

Antibiotic prophylaxis for infective endocarditis

Guidance has changed recently, and the routine administration of antibiotics is no longer recommended for patients at risk of infective endocarditis,

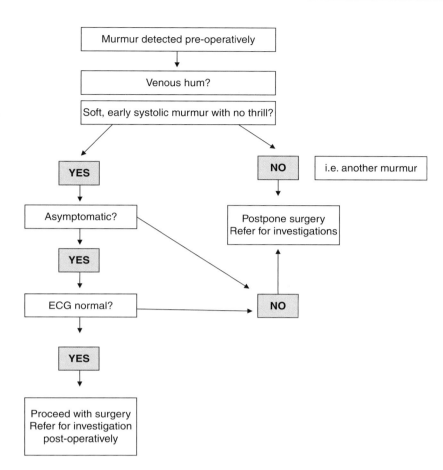

Figure 6.1 Management of a child with a cardiac murmur.

even for those children undergoing dental procedures. Antibiotic prophylaxis is now only recommended for susceptible patients undergoing gastrointestinal or genito-urinary procedures at a site with suspected infection. The organisms most likely to cause endocarditis are *Staphylococcus aureus*, streptococci and enterococci. Local protocols will dictate the choice of antibiotics to cover these organisms.

Patients at risk are those with:

- Acquired valve disease with stenosis or regurgitation
- Valve replacement
- Structural congenital heart disease, including surgically corrected or palliated structural conditions (excluding isolated atrial septal defect, fully repaired ventricular septal defect or patent ductus arteriosus, and endothelialised closure devices)
- Previous infective endocarditis
- Hypertrophic cardiomyopathy

Known cardiac disease

Management of the child with known cardiac disease is covered in Chapter 33. It is important to be aware of the cardiac lesions that are most likely to give rise to problems during anaesthesia and that need detailed investigation and expert management:

- Left ventricular outflow tract obstruction
- Cardiomyopathy
- Pulmonary hypertension
- Single ventricle circulations

Upper respiratory tract infection (URTI)

The incidence of URTI in children presenting for anaesthesia is very high since a normal child will experience two to nine episodes of URTI per year. Despite the importance of this clinical problem, there is still no consensus or any evidence-based practice guidelines regarding optimal anaesthetic management of children with URTIs who require elective surgery. Children with active and recent URTIs are at increased risk of peri-operative airway complications, such as:

- Laryngospasm
- Bronchospasm
- Atelectasis
- Arterial oxygen desaturation

Evidence also suggests these events are mostly manageable and without long-term, adverse sequelae in otherwise well children, and that children with an acute, uncomplicated URTI have no increased morbidity.

In a longitudinal study of over 1000 children who had had an URTI in the 4 weeks preceding surgery, risk factors for adverse respiratory events were identified as:

- Use of tracheal tube
- History of prematurity
- History of asthma
- Airway surgery
- Parental smoking
- Copious secretions

Importantly, there were no significant problems for these children following discharge. This evidence suggests that a blanket policy of cancellation of all procedures in children with URTIs is inappropriate. As well as lack of evidence of any clinical benefit from such a policy, repeated cancellation of surgery carries significant adverse economic and emotional consequences. From a practical point of view, in a child that suffers an average six to eight URTIs per year, if all recent URTIs are a reason for postponing surgery there will be only a few weeks in which the child is asymptomatic and considered fit for surgery. Also, children with an URTI may have altered airway reactivity for up to 6 weeks following infection, and there is clinical uncertainty as to how long the procedure should be postponed following an URTI.

A child with an URTI should be carefully assessed by the anaesthetist to establish suitability for surgery. Decisions should be made on a case-by-case basis, and when considering the risk/benefit ratio for each individual child, the child's presenting symptoms and age, the urgency of the surgery, co-morbid conditions (e.g. asthma or cardiac disease), and the type of surgery should be taken into consideration. As well as

thorough examination of the child, it is vital that the anaesthetist questions the parents about the child's respiratory symptoms and the child's general level of 'wellness'. Surgery should be postponed in a child with signs and symptoms of a severe URTI:

- Unwell, or 'not quite themselves'
- Lethargic
- Pyrexia of greater than $37.5\,^{\circ}C$
- Purulent nasal secretions
- Productive cough

In a child who is essentially well, with minimal respiratory symptoms, minor surgery should proceed. If the child's condition is between these two levels, which is more often the case, the decision is more difficult. Children with a history of asthma or prematurity or requiring airway surgery or tracheal intubation should be treated with greater caution as all of these factors are associated with greater peri-operative complications. Investigations are not always helpful as a normal white blood cell count or normal chest X-ray does not exclude a significant URTI. The decision to proceed or not depends on the clinical judgement of the anaesthetist.

If the procedure is postponed there is no consensus as to when the operation should be rescheduled. The risk of respiratory complications remains increased for at least 4 weeks after an URTI and therefore this is the time frame suggested for deferring surgery.

Premedication

As well as gaining information about the physical condition of the child the pre-operative visit is an opportunity to assess the child's psychological status and level of anxiety. The pre-operative visit itself is well known to reduce anxiety, by providing information and reassurance, and may help to determine the factors associated with anxiety. Further preparation such as visits to the operating theatre, written information and videos can all be offered pre-operatively and, although valuable, are time-consuming. Early assessment of children may be able to direct anxious children and parents to behavioural therapy or anxiolytic premedication or both.

Midazolam is the drug of choice for reducing anxiety in children less than 20 kg. It has a short onset of action and should be administered in a dose of $0.5\,\mathrm{mg\,kg^{-1}}$ (max dose 20 mg) around 30 minutes before anaesthesia. The onset of marked anxiolysis has been reported to occur within 15 minutes of administration. Its bitter taste can be masked by sweetening agents and its popularity can be attributed to a low frequency of serious side effects. It has been associated, however, with paradoxical excitement, the cause and incidence of which are not known.

Temazepam, 0.5–1.0 mg kg^{-1} (max 30 mg), given orally 1 hour before anaesthesia is a useful short-acting benzodiazepine in older children. It has a variable calming effect but has few side effects and little effect on recovery time.

Chloral hydrate (30–60 mg kg^{-1}) or *triclofos* (25–50 mg kg^{-1}) can be effective but is impractical in children over 12 kg owing to the large volume required.

Clonidine 4 mcg kg^{-1} given orally is as effective as midazolam and has analgesic, antiemetic and calming properties. However, it takes 60–90 minutes to work and prolongs recovery.

Melatonin 0.2 mg kg^{-1} given 50 minutes before induction reduces anxiety with few if any side effects, and produces fewer post-operative behavioural problems than midazolam as well as reducing the dose of propofol required for induction.

Other pre-operative medication
Topical local anaesthetic agents

These are used to reduce the pain of intravenous cannulation.

EMLA® cream (eutectic mixture of local anaesthetics) contains 2.5% prilocaine and 2.5% lidocaine and needs to be applied for at least 1 hour. It is effective for over 120 minutes after removal but can cause blanching of the skin and vasoconstriction.

Ametop® gel is 4% amethocaine and works after 30–45 minutes. It is more effective than EMLA and results in less vasoconstriction.

LMX 4®, lidocaine 4% cream, is a newer agent that works after 30 minutes.

Ethyl chloride (Cryogesic®) is a vapo-coolant spray that has no pure analgesic properties, but causes a diminution of skin sensation within a few seconds lasting for a minute or so. It is flammable so needs to be used with care.

Simple analgesics

Paracetamol, 20 mg kg^{-1}, given orally 30 minutes pre-operatively can aid post-operative analgesia. Non-steroidal anti-inflammatory agents ibuprofen (5 mg kg^{-1}) and diclofenac (1 mg kg^{-1}) can also be helpful.

Antimuscarinics

Atropine and glycopyrrolate are used when an anti-sialagogue is required, e.g. prior to airway surgery.

H2-receptor antagonists

These are rarely used in paediatric anaesthetic practice as acid aspiration pneumonitis is very unusual in children. Ranitidine may have a place in reducing the effects of anaphylaxis in children with a history of latex allergy.

Non-pharmacological methods of reducing anxiety

These include the presence of parents at induction, play therapy, hypnotherapy, music therapy, visits to the operating theatre before surgery, written information, videos and interactive websites.

Pre-operative fasting

Pre-operative fasting is required to minimise the volume of gastric contents, thus reducing the risk of regurgitation and pulmonary aspiration under anaesthesia. However, prolonged pre-operative fasting results in thirst, hunger and irritability, and puts neonates and small infants at risk of hypoglycaemia. A Cochrane Database review of pre-operative fasting for preventing peri-operative complications in children was conducted in 2005 and updated in 2009.

- Only one incidence of regurgitation and aspiration was reported in 2543 children considered to be at normal risk for such events during anaesthesia.
- Children permitted fluids up to 120 minutes pre-operatively were not found to experience higher gastric volumes or lower gastric pH values than those who fasted.
- The children permitted fluids were less thirsty and hungry, better behaved and more comfortable than those who fasted.
- Evidence relating to the pre-operative intake of milk was sparse.
- The volume of fluid permitted during the pre-operative period did not appear to impact on children's intra-operative gastric volume or pH contents.

The authors concluded that there is no evidence that children who are denied oral fluids for more than 6 hours pre-operatively benefit in terms of intra-operative gastric volume and pH compared with children permitted unlimited fluids up to 2 hours pre-operatively. Children permitted fluids have a more comfortable pre-operative experience in terms of thirst and hunger. This evidence applies only to children who are considered to be at normal risk of regurgitation and aspiration during anaesthesia. Our standard starvation policy is:

- Clear fluids can be given up to 2 hours
- Breast milk can be given up to 3–4 hours and
- Formula milk and food can be given up to 6 hours before surgery.

Delayed gastric emptying

Children who sustain a traumatic injury have delayed gastric emptying, and gastric residual volume depends largely on time taken from food intake to time of injury. Therefore a child that requires urgent surgery after a major injury should be managed as if they have a full stomach. Anxiety and pain can also affect gastric emptying although this has not been extensively studied in children.

Prevention of peri-operative venous thromboembolism

Although the incidence of peri-operative deep vein thrombosis and pulmonary embolus is low in children, if they do occur they are associated with significant morbidity and mortality. The incidence is probably one-tenth of that seen in the adult population but is increasing. This may be due to increased awareness and the improved survival of children with complex congenital conditions which are associated with thromboembolism. Factor V mutation, anti-thrombin deficiency and protein C deficiency are all independent risk factors for childhood venous thrombosis.

Central venous catheters, which are used increasingly, are probably the single most important risk factor for thrombosis of the larger central veins. They can damage vessel walls and affect blood flow as well as being used to infuse thrombogenic fluids. Sub-clavian vein catheters are at greater risk of thrombosis than internal jugular lines as are those placed percutaneously rather by a venous cut-down technique.

Prophylaxis

Early mobilisation should be encouraged in the post-operative period, dehydration should be avoided and central venous catheters removed as soon as possible. Most children undergoing surgery do not require any other preventative measures. Older children at risk, including those undergoing long procedures, should wear elastic compression stockings, and pneumatic compression boots should be used intra-operatively.

Children with a known risk of thromboembolism should receive subcutaneous low-molecular-weight heparin such as:

- Enoxaparin, 0.5 mg kg^{-1} every 12 hours for children over 5 kg or 0.75 mg kg^{-1} every 12 hours for infants below 5 kg;

or

- Reviparan, 30 U kg^{-1} every 12 hours for children over 3 months or 50 U kg^{-1} every 12 hours for infants less than 3 months.

As the anticoagulant action of low-molecular-weight heparin is largely mediated by anti-factor-Xa activity this effect should be monitored by assaying anti-factor-Xa. Bleeding complications tend to be minor with the recommended prophylaxis doses.

Key points

- Children with a previously unheard murmur or ECG signs of left ventricular strain should be referred for cardiological review before anaesthesia.
- There is no evidence to suggest that recent vaccination interferes with anaesthesia.
- It is rarely necessary to postpone children with signs of minor upper respiratory tract infection, unless there is a history of asthma or congenital heart disease.

Further reading

Brady MC, Kinn S, Ness V *et al.* Pre-operative fasting for preventing perioperative complications in children (Review). *Cochrane Database Syst Rev* 2009;Oct 7;(4):CD005285.

Luscombe M, Owens B. Weight estimation in resuscitation: is the current formula still valid? *Arch Dis Child* 2007;**92**:412–15.

Murat I, Constant I, Maud'huy H. Perioperative anaesthetic morbidity in children: a database of 24,165 anaesthetics over a 30-month period. *Paed Anaes* 2004;**14**(2): 158–66.

Siebert JN, Posfay-Barbe KM, Habre W, Siegrist CA. Influence of anesthesia on immune responses and its effect on vaccination in children: review of evidence. *Paed Anaes* 2007;**17**(5):410–20.

Tait AR, Malviya S, Voepel-Lewis T *et al.* Risk factors for peri-operative adverse respiratory events in children with upper respiratory tract infections. *Anesthesiology* 2001;**95**(2):299–306.

Anaesthesia for children with common medical conditions of childhood

Nargis Ahmad and Ian James

Introduction

An understanding of the common acute and chronic conditions of childhood, and associated anaesthetic considerations, is essential knowledge for the paediatric anaesthetist.

When children with medical co-morbidity present for operative care outside of specialist centres, liaison between local and specialist paediatric teams can be beneficial. Clinical networks can extend the reach of specialist advice and provide a vehicle for supporting local clinical services. Parents and other carers can be an invaluable source of information and often have copies of clinical correspondence that contain detailed summaries of their child's current and past treatment. Management of the child with cardiac disease is covered in Chapter 33. This chapter will cover some of the other common conditions of childhood.

Obstructive sleep apnoea syndrome (OSAS)

Up to 12% of pre-school children snore. Adenotonsillar hypertrophy is the most common cause, although obesity is increasingly common. Less common causes of snoring include anatomical abnormalities which crowd the upper airway, such as midfacial hypoplasia, macroglossia, micro- or retrognathia, and pharyngeal hypotonia. When not accompanied by OSAS it is generally referred to as 'primary snoring'.

Increased upper airway (UAW) resistance can lead to obstructive hypoventilation and OSAS. In adults OSAS is defined as cessation of airflow for 10 seconds or more during sleep, but this is not applicable to infants in whom apnoeas of only a few seconds can cause desaturation. A more useful definition in children might be:

A disorder of breathing during sleep characterised by prolonged partial upper airway obstruction and/or intermittent complete obstruction (obstructive apnoea) that disrupts normal ventilation during sleep and normal sleep patterns.

About 15% of children who snore have OSAS, which can lead to failure to thrive, poor learning and behavioural problems. In prolonged, severe OSAS chronic hypoventilation can lead to pulmonary hypertension, right ventricular hypertrophy and cor pulmonale, although this is rare. Mild pulmonary hypertension is likely to be asymptomatic.

Parents who report that their child snores habitually should be asked whether they have noticed:

- Laboured breathing during sleep
- Apnoea
- Cyanosis
- Restless sleep
- Diaphoresis
- Excessive daytime sleepiness
- Behavioural difficulties
- Enuresis

A clinical history of sleep-disordered breathing does not reliably distinguish children with primary snoring from those with OSAS. Overnight oximetry has been used to assist identification of children with obstructive hypoventilation but whilst it has a high positive predictive value its utility is limited by the low negative predictive value. The history does have some value where polysomnography (sleep study) is not available. If parents describe a cycle of apnoea, cyanosis and parental intervention (such as shaking the child to start breathing) then this is highly suggestive of OSAS.

Criteria for the diagnosis of OSAS vary internationally and the role of polysomnography is controversial.

Core Topics in Paediatric Anaesthesia, ed. Ian James and Isabeau Walker. Published by Cambridge University Press. © 2013 Cambridge University Press.

In the United Kingdom it is regarded as the gold standard. During polysomnography a coordinated study of the stage of sleep, episodes of arousal and ECG is performed with concurrent respiratory monitoring of abdominal and chest wall movements, respiratory effort, airflow, ventilation and oxygenation.

OSAS occurs when elevated UAW resistance leads to intermittent complete UAW obstruction. The prevalence of OSAS is between 1 and 3% with a peak at around 3–6 years of age.

OSAS should always be considered in the following conditions:

- Craniofacial abnormalities
- Down syndrome
- Cerebral palsy
- Neuromuscular disorders
- Sickle cell disease
- Genetic/metabolic/storage diseases

Anaesthesia for children with OSAS

In children with OSAS, sedative premedication is usually avoided as it can provoke airway obstruction. During induction of anaesthesia, airway obstruction is likely and the anaesthetist should be prepared to manage this with conventional airway manoeuvres and adjuncts prior to placement of a tracheal tube or supraglottic device. The laryngeal mask (LMA) is often useful in relieving obstruction and may also be suitable for use during maintenance of anaesthesia.

If pulmonary hypertension has been identified pre-operatively this needs to be fully evaluated and managed appropriately (see Chapter 33).

Post-operative management will to some extent be determined by the on-going therapy for OSAS and the nature of the surgery. The tendency to obstructive hypoventilation can worsen in the post-operative period and hence these patients need close monitoring, for example in a high dependency unit. A nasal prong and/or CPAP may help maintain airway patency. If CPAP is usually needed at night then it will be necessary in the post-operative phase. These patients are generally not suitable for day case surgery. Post-operative opiates are best avoided if non-opiate analgesics will suffice.

Asthma

The incidence of asthma in children is increasing but the risk of peri-operative bronchospasm is low in stable asthmatics. Classical asthma has genetic and

Table 7.1 Severity of asthma in children 5–12 years

Grade	Steroids	Add-on therapy
1	None	Inhaled β2 agonist e.g. salbutamol as required
2	BDP up to 400 mcg d^{-1}	
3	BDP up to 400 mcg d^{-1}	LABA or LTRA
4	BDP up to 800 mcg d^{-1}	LABA or LTRA or aminophylline
5	BDP >800 mcg d^{-1} plus oral steroids	Oral steroids

Adapted from British Thoracic Society Guidelines.
BDP, beclamethasone; LABA long-acting β2 agonist, e.g. salmeterol; LTRA, leukotriene receptor agonist, e.g. montelukast

environmental influences and is associated with IgE mediated hypersensitivity. Such children usually have a wheeze and a dry non-productive cough; they are sometimes described as atopic wheezers. It is important to recognise that not all children who wheeze have atopic asthma. Wheeze is a common presentation in infants and pre-school children who have a respiratory viral infection, and wheeze may also be associated with tracheo- or bronchomalacia. However, all children who wheeze are best considered as being at risk of peri-operative bronchial hyperreactivity.

Well-controlled asthmatics tolerate anaesthesia well but poorly controlled asthmatics or those with severe disease are at risk of complications, so it is important to establish disease severity and efficacy of management. Peak flow and lung function tests are not usually possible in small children and hence their role is limited. Guidelines, such as those from the British Thoracic Society (BTS), are widely available and should be consulted if necessary. They define the severity of asthma according to the treatment required for symptom control (see Table 7.1). Questions to be asked of parents in the pre-operative assessment should include:

- How frequently is the wheeze present?
- Is the child using an inhaler regularly (usually beclomethasone) or only intermittently when wheezy (usually salbutamol)?
- How often is the salbutamol required?
- Has the child had to be admitted to hospital for their asthma? If so was an intensive care admission with ventilation required?

- Are they taking medications other than beclomethasone and salbutamol?
- Are they taking or have they ever needed oral steroids?

In an atopic child a careful allergy history is also essential.

In the majority of patients, the wheeze will be managed well with regular beclomethasone and intermittent salbutamol, and anaesthesia will generally be uneventful, provided measures are taken to minimise airway irritation.

A history of frequent admissions to hospital or life-threatening episodes of bronchospasm generally reflects severe underlying disease or poor disease management and suggests high peri-operative risk. These children may well be taking oral steroids. It is important to ensure that in these children symptoms are optimal at the time of elective surgery. Elective surgery should be postponed if symptoms are poorly controlled or if there has been a recent worsening of symptoms. Bronchial hyperreactivity is present for several weeks after an acute exacerbation of asthma or respiratory tract infection; this should be borne in mind when assessing readiness for anaesthesia. If symptoms are poorly controlled or major surgery is planned there may be merit in starting steroids a few days before surgery, but this decision should be undertaken in conjunction with the respiratory team. Chest X-rays are rarely useful in determining fitness for anaesthesia in such cases.

Anaesthesia for children with asthma

For those children who are using bronchodilator and steroid inhalers, these should be continued. Consider changing from inhaled to nebulised bronchodilators in the peri-operative period. It is useful to administer an additional puff of bronchodilator inhaler and nebulised salbutamol just prior to transfer to theatre.

Sevoflurane, propofol or ketamine are all suitable for induction. Ketamine, with its recognised bronchodilation, may have some advantages in the child with severe asthma; an antisialagogue may also be required to minimise secretions.

Airway instrumentation should be limited where feasible and use of a LMA may be appropriate (or facemask if the procedure is very short). If intubation is necessary it should be timely, i.e. when there is an adequate depth of anaesthesia. Use of topical local anaesthesia or opioids should be considered. The tracheal tube position should be carefully checked and carinal irritation avoided.

Drugs that lead to mast cell degranulation and histamine release are best avoided, particularly in those children with more severe asthma. These include atracurium, mivacurium and morphine.

For children on oral or high-dose inhaled steroids it may be necessary to provide peri-operative supplementation, although this is rarely necessary for short procedures.

Regional techniques should be considered where appropriate for provision of analgesia. Deep extubation may be appropriate but the timing of extubation will be influenced by the age of the patient and the nature of surgery.

There is uncertainty about the use of NSAIDs in children with asthma, as they may exacerbate symptoms in some children. Parents can usually advise whether ibuprofen has been taken previously without ill effect. It is our practice to avoid them only in patients with severe asthma (grade 3–5).

Peri-operative bronchospasm

The anaesthetist should always be on the alert for and ready to treat peri-operative bronchospasm. This may manifest itself initially by subtle adverse changes in ventilatory parameters such as a fall in tidal volume and/or a rise in airway pressure, and a rise in end-tidal CO_2. If severe it may progress to hypoxaemia. Treatment should be prompt. Increasing the inspired oxygen will not solve the problem but will buy some time. It is essential to ensure that the tracheal tube is not at the carina or beyond, and that it is not blocked. If other causes of bronchospasm, such as acute anaphylaxis, and other causes of hypoventilation, including equipment issues, have been excluded, treatment may include the following:

- Increase the concentration of the volatile agent, which may help alleviate the bronchospasm.
- It may be possible to administer an inhaled β2 agonist or ipratropium via the tracheal tube.
- If unresolved, administer intravenous salbutamol (5 mcg kg^{-1}) or aminophylline (5 mg kg^{-1}), both given over 10 minutes. It may be necessary to start infusions of these drugs.
- The ECG should be monitored closely as aminophylline may cause dysrhythmias, particularly in the presence of high concentrations of volatile agents.

- Resistant bronchospasm should be treated with intravenous hydrocortisone (4 mg kg^{-1}) and adrenaline (1 mcg kg^{-1}).
- When ventilation has to be increased substantially to overcome the bronchospasm it is important to maintain a slow ventilator rate and to adjust the I:E ratio to allow adequate time for expiration.
- Increasing airway pressure to overcome the bronchospasm may reduce cardiac output and blood pressure owing to a rise in intrathoracic pressure so fluid administration may be necessary.

Patients should be managed in a high dependency or intensive care setting post-operatively if there has been a period of significant peri-operative bronchospasm.

Cystic fibrosis (CF)

Cystic fibrosis is an autosomal recessive disorder in which a defective transmembrane receptor leads to defective exocrine gland ion transport, affecting the components of mucus, digestive juices and sweat. Over 8000 people in the UK currently have CF.

About 1 in 2500 babies born in the UK will have CF. Screening is offered to all neonates born in England.

The presentation of CF is highly variable. It can present with:

- Neonatal bowel obstruction
- Recurrent respiratory symptoms
- Malabsorption
- Failure to thrive
- Abnormal stools

The diagnosis is not always made in early childhood; 10% of CF patients present after their tenth birthday.

The multidisciplinary care that these patients receive has made a considerable impact on the prognosis for this patient group, and survival without lung transplantation has improved in the past 20 years. CF patients have annual multisystem reviews. Timely liaison with the patient's CF team is always advised if these patients present for surgery.

CF is a complex multisystem disease but concerns during anaesthesia are primarily respiratory. Lung function is thought to be essentially normal at birth but deteriorates with age. Patients are likely to have V/Q (ventilation/perfusion) mismatch. Patients have viscid mucus and mucociliary clearance is impaired; airway obstruction and cycles of infection and inflammation lead to bronchiectasis. Patients are initially susceptible to infection with *Staphylococcus aureus* and *Haemophilus influenzae* but eventually become colonised with *Pseudomonas aeruginosa*. Patients are increasingly colonised with rarer microorganisms, and infection control measures should be considered when planning the operating list.

Pre-operative treatment goals are to target infection with antibiotics and improve mucus clearance with strategies such as physiotherapy and mucolytic therapy. Where possible physiotherapy should be scheduled for just before surgery; on occasion it can be helpful to undertake endobronchial toilet during anaesthesia. Bronchial hyperreactivity can be a feature of CF and bronchodilators may be useful. Coughing frequently occurs at induction and emergence from anaesthesia.

Diabetes mellitus is a common accompaniment to CF in older children and patients may be on insulin. This often can be difficult to manage because of recurrent infection and the not infrequent use of steroids in the management of CF.

Chronic lung disease of prematurity/ bronchopulmonary dysplasia (BPD)

BPD is but one of many co-morbidities associated with prematurity; others include necrotising enterocolitis, intraventricular haemorrhage, periventricular leukomalacia and retinopathy of prematurity.

BPD is a chronic lung disease which should be suspected in ex-premature infants who received mechanical ventilation in the neonatal period. Injury to the immature lung is believed to be a consequence of the combination of impaired lung development and ventilator associated injury.

Later in infancy, symptoms may be minimal and parents may not always alert the anaesthetist to the presence of BPD. When assessing ex-premature patients, information should be specifically sought about the length of time spent being ventilated, and how long supplemental oxygen therapy was necessary. Some patients continue on home oxygen for many months.

Patients with BPD are at risk of desaturation and bronchospasm and may need higher peak pressures and higher PEEP to achieve adequate minute ventilation. Permissive hypercapnia is usually appropriate and patients are likely to need higher inspired oxygen. Respiratory function may be improved by the use of bronchodilators and steroids. Diuretics may also be used to treat BPD. In severe cases right ventricular function may be affected by the development of pulmonary vascular disease.

These patients are rarely suitable for day-case procedures. Many will need supplemental oxygen for the first post-operative night, particularly those currently receiving or who have only recently stopped home oxygen.

Diabetes mellitus (DM)

About 1 in 1000 children in the UK have diabetes, in 95% of whom it is insulin-dependent type 1 (IDDM). With rising levels of childhood obesity the prevalence of type 2 diabetes is increasing.

There are a variety of insulin regimens (Table 7.2), and most children will be on one of the following:

- Multiple dose insulin regimens (MDI)
  - o Usually short-acting insulin with meals, with a long-acting insulin, typically glargine, at night
- Twice daily insulin
- Continuous subcutaneous insulin infusion (CSII)
  - o CSII is increasingly common in children over 12 years, providing basal insulin with boluses at meal times

The wide variety of insulin regimens makes it increasingly difficult to set out a prescriptive protocol for the management of insulin-dependent children undergoing anaesthesia and surgery.

Peri-operative management is aimed at avoiding hypoglycaemia and ketoacidosis and will be influenced by:

- Whether surgery is elective or emergency;
- The nature of surgery, i.e. a minor or major procedure;
- Whether surgery will delay normal oral intake post-operatively, e.g. gastrointestinal surgery;
- Whether nausea and vomiting is anticipated, which may also delay post-operative oral intake;
- The usual insulin regimen;
- Whether the DM is well controlled. Management of diabetes in adolescent patients can be challenging, and this group may have poor control.

In general, minor surgery in well-controlled diabetic patients, over 5 years of age, who will rapidly return

Table 7.2 Examples of types of insulin in use

Insulin type		Onset (h)	Peak (h)	Duration (h)
Ultra-short	Novorapid®, Humalog®	<0.5	1	3–4
Short	Humulin S®, Actrapid®	0.5–1	2–6	3–8
Long-acting	Insulatard®, Humulin I®	3–4	4–12	10–20
	Glargine	1	none	24
	Detemir	1	none	12

to a normal eating pattern can be undertaken on a day-case basis.

Key principles are:

- Children with IDDM cannot be fasted without running the risk of hypoglycaemia;
- They will still need insulin even though they are being fasted for surgery;
- They should be scheduled first on the operating list (preferably in the morning) to avoid unnecessarily long starvation periods;
- The aim is to maintain blood sugar at 5–10 mmol l^{-1} throughout the peri-operative period, avoiding both hypoglycaemia and hyperglycaemia;
- Those on a MDI regimen should receive half their long-acting insulin the night before surgery;
- As a general rule, patients having surgery in the morning should omit their morning dose of insulin;
- Patients having surgery in the afternoon should omit their midday insulin.

Children undergoing major surgery or who have poorly controlled IDDM should be managed in conjunction with the endocrinology service. For these patients it is usually safest and easiest to run an insulin infusion titrated to regular blood sugar levels (see Table 7.3) together with a 5% glucose/0.45% saline infusion.

Emergency surgery in children with diabetes

Acute illness may precipitate diabetic ketoacidosis (DKA) and this may present as an acute abdomen. General anaesthesia in the presence of DKA is extremely hazardous.

Always check weight, electrolytes, glucose, venous pH/bicarbonate and urine for ketones pre-operatively.

Table 7.3 Insulin infusion regime. Adjust insulin infusion according to blood glucose concentrations

Blood glucose	Suggested insulin infusion rates
> 12 mmol l^{-1}	0.05 Units kg^{-1} h^{-1}
9 to 12 mmol l^{-1}	0.04 Units kg^{-1} h^{-1}
7 to 8.9 mmol l^{-1}	0.03 Units kg^{-1} h^{-1}
4 to 6.9 mmol l^{-1}	0.02 Units kg^{-1} h^{-1}
<4 mmol l^{-1}	0.01 Units kg^{-1} h^{-1} with 2 ml kg^{-1} of 10% glucose

These doses may need to be revised in severely ill patients and children who were on high doses of insulin or receiving steroids. **Do not** stop the insulin infusion if the blood glucose is lower than 4 mmol l^{-1} as this will cause hyperglycaemia. Reduce the rate of the insulin infusion further. Continue with glucose infusion and increase the rate if required.

If ketoacidosis is present, treatment should proceed in accordance with an established protocol for diabetic ketoacidosis. Surgery should be deferred until circulating volume and electrolyte deficit are corrected and the patient is rehydrated and haemodynamically stable. Rehydration of a patient with DKA must be done very slowly using isotonic fluids (see Chapter 14).

For a detailed guide to the management of IDDM see Further reading.

Adrenal insufficiency

Children receiving glucocorticoids as part of their treatment are at risk of adrenal insufficiency due to chronic suppression of the pituitary–hypothalamic–adrenal axis. This includes children using inhaled steroids for asthma and allergic rhinitis. Peri-operative steroid supplementation should be considered:

- For those who are on long-term treatment;
- For those who have been receiving systemic steroids for more than 3 weeks;
- For those who have recently finished such a course, and where adrenal insufficiency has a pituitary origin, e.g. anterior pituitary disease.

In adults, those receiving more than 20 mg per day of prednisolone, or equivalent, are generally thought to need supplementation. In children this would equate to about 0.3–0.5 mg kg^{-1} prednisolone per day. Table 7.4 shows the equivalent doses of corticosteroids.

Table 7.4 Equivalent anti-inflammatory doses of some corticosteroids

Prednisolone 1 mg is equivalent to		
	Betamethasone	150 mcg
	Dexamethasone	150 mcg
	Hydrocortisone	4 mg
	Methylprednisolone	800 mcg

It is usual to administer hydrocortisone 2 mg kg^{-1} at induction for those deemed at risk of adrenal suppression.

Congenital adrenal hyperplasia

Defective cortisol biosynthesis leads to increased levels of adrenocorticotrophic hormone (ACTH) and disordered mineralocorticoid and androgen production. Most cases are due to 21-hydroxlase deficiency with a small proportion arising as a result of defective 11β-hydroxylase production. Those with 21-hydroxylase deficiency may have disordered glucose and electrolyte homeostasis often with severe salt wasting. Early virilisation and precocious puberty may be present.

Peri-operatively, careful monitoring of electrolytes, glucose and fluids is essential. These patients cannot respond to stressors such as surgery, and normal steroid intake must be maintained in the peri-operative period; this may need to be administered parenterally. Additional cover for surgery must also be given to prevent a crisis, usually hydrocortisone 2 mg kg^{-1} at induction. Further doses should be given at 4-hourly intervals during prolonged, major surgery.

Obesity

The prevalence of obesity in children is increasing. It is usually idiopathic but rarely may be associated with endocrine or genetic syndromes such as Prader–Willi. Obese children have a significantly higher prevalence of co-morbidities compared with non-obese children, including:

- Asthma
- Hypertension
- OSAS
- Gastro-oesophageal reflux
- Type 2 diabetes

There is therefore an increased risk of adverse events with anaesthesia and surgery. These are primarily respiratory events as it can be more difficult to maintain an airway and to ventilate by facemask. Forced vital capacity (FVC) and functional residual capacity (FRC) are lower, hence there is an increased likelihood and rapidity of oxygen desaturation. Also, bronchospasm and laryngospasm occur more readily. Lung compliance can be poor and a tracheal tube is safer than a LMA. However, there is often a poorer view at laryngoscopy. Patients should be pre-oxygenated at the start of anaesthesia. Venous access can be difficult.

It is difficult to define obesity in children, as body mass index (BMI) varies with age and sex. It is usually defined therefore in terms of deviation from established reference data for mean BMI. Lean body weight (LBW) should be used for most drug dose calculations, especially paracetamol, although determining this requires access to gender-specific reference charts (see Further reading).

A quick estimate for ideal body weight (IBW) can be obtained by using standard growth charts to determine the predicted weight that corresponds to the child's height. In an obese child, lean body tissues such as muscle contribute approximately a third of the excess weight.

LBW can therefore be assumed to be:

$$IBW + 0.3 \times (TBW - IBW)$$

Total body weight (TBW) should be used to calculate the dose of suxamethonium and opioids.

Haemoglobinopathies

There are a large number of variants of haemoglobin, the majority of which are exceedingly rare. Only a very few have any real significance for anaesthesia, namely sickle cell disease (and its variants) and thalassaemia. These will be discussed below.

Some of the rare, abnormal haemoglobins have increased affinity for oxygen which may result in impaired oxygen release, tissue hypoxia and polycythaemia. Other haemoglobin variants have reduced oxygen affinity causing asymptomatic, mild benign cyanosis. There may also be an altered absorption spectrum leading to inaccurate readings when using pulse oximetry. A rare haemoglobinopathy such as Hb Koln or the presence of excess methaemoglobin should be suspected in the unusual situation when pulse oximetry readings are inexplicably low in an otherwise stable child and readings do not improve with increased inspired oxygen.

Sickle cell disease

About 1 in 2500 babies born in the UK has a sickle cell disorder in which an abnormal β-globin chain results in the production of haemoglobin HbS. This is a consequence of an abnormal gene which has an autosomal co-dominant pattern of inheritance. Sickle cell disease (SCD) refers to those who are homozygous for the gene, HbSS. Those with heterozygous expression, HbAS, are said to have sickle cell trait.

In the presence of hypoxia HbS changes into a brittle sickle shape and can cause painful, vaso-occlusive ischaemic multisystem injury, most notably in bones, hands and feet, spleen and the bowel. Cerebrovascular events and acute chest syndrome are severe complications. In some patients there may be renal dysfunction from recurrent vascular injury. There is some evidence that an increased thrombotic tendency of sickle erythrocytes and an associated endothelial component may account for the vascular occlusive complications. Haemolysis and splenic sequestration leads to chronic anaemia. Sickling and its effects are compounded by acidosis and dehydration.

Who is at risk?

The erythrocytes of heterozygous sickle cell individuals confer some protection from *Plasmodium falciparum* malaria, and the offending gene is frequently found in areas where malaria is endemic. Those at highest risk of having sickle cell disease are thus of African, Afro-Caribbean, Asian and Mediterranean origin, and the sickle status of these patients should always be determined prior to anaesthesia. In many countries, including the United Kingdom, sickle status is routinely tested at birth as part of the neonatal dried blood spot test. If the status is unknown, a rapid sickle solubility test can be undertaken (sickledex). This cannot distinguish between HbAS and HbSS, so if it is positive haemoglobin electrophoresis should be performed.

- The sickledex test is unreliable in the presence of significant levels of fetal haemoglobin (HbF) although as HbF does not sickle infants under the age of about 4 months are not at risk.

- In sickle cell trait, the low level of HbS is insufficient to produce sickling unless there is profound hypoxia so no particular risks are associated with anaesthesia.
- In SCD, and variants such as HbSC and HbS-beta thalassaemia, anaesthesia does carry risks. Patients may be anaemic pre-operatively and are at risk of peri-operative sickling. HbSS cells begin to sickle at oxygen saturations below 85%, but hypothermia, acidosis and dehydration also contribute to the development of complications.
- The risk of peri-operative complications is increased in patients undergoing major surgery or those who have a history of chest crises, OSAS, CNS disease or frequent painful bone crises. Children who have had a previous stroke as a result of SCD are at a particularly high risk of peri-operative morbidity.

Anaesthesia for children with sickle cell disease

Pre-operative management of patients with SCD should include consultation with a haematologist and exchange or top-up transfusion as appropriate. Transfusion policies to reduce the level of HbS or raise the haematocrit are associated with a high incidence of transfusion-related complications, so a modified approach should be taken (see Table 7.5). Where pre-operative transfusion is indicated this may take several weeks. For emergency surgery, children should be given a top-up transfusion as in Group 2.

- Evidence of OSAS should always be sought because patients with sickle disease have impaired splenic function and may have hypertrophy of other lymphoid tissue, e.g. tonsils and adenoids.
- Patients should be scheduled first on the operating list and good hydration maintained until normal oral intake is re-established.
- Anaesthetic technique should minimise exposure to hypoxaemia, hypercapnia, acidosis, hypothermia and hypovolaemia, during and following surgery. Overtransfusion and hyperviscosity must be avoided. The majority of crises occur post-operatively. Supplemental oxygen should be administered to keep oxygen saturations above 95% until the child is mobilising freely.
- Care with positioning is important to minimise venous stasis, and tourniquets should be avoided if possible.

Table 7.5 Transfusion recommendations for SCD and elective surgery

Group 1	Well child, no special risk factors, short procedure – e.g. grommets *Top-up transfusion only if Hb <6 g dl^{-1}*
Group 2	Well child, no special risk factors, intermediate surgery – e.g. hernia repair, adenotonsillectomy for mild OSAS *Top-up transfusion to Hb 9–11 g dl^{-1}*
Group 3	Child with previous acute chest syndrome, frequent painful crises, or undergoing major surgery – e.g. abdominal surgery, thoracic surgery *Exchange transfusion to achieve HbS < 30%; Hb < 12 g dl^{-1}*

- Effective post-operative analgesia is essential, which may be challenging in patients already on opioids for painful sickle crises.

Thalassaemia

The thalassaemias are a heterogeneous group of anaemias caused by defective globin chain production, and are one of the commonest genetic defects worldwide.

Who is at risk?

As the phenotype confers some resistance to malaria, affected individuals are usually of Mediterranean, Middle Eastern or African descent.

There are four genes for α-globin and two genes for β-globin. Alpha-thalassaemias involve deletion of one or more of the four α-globin genes. Deletion of one or two of these causes mild anaemia, deletion of three causes HbH disease (variable chronic anaemia) and deletion of all four leads to fetal hydrops.

Beta-thalassaemia may be minor or major depending on whether one or two abnormal globin genes are inherited. Beta-thalassaemia major presents after 6 months with anaemia, as HbF production declines. Management of the anaemia includes regular blood transfusions. Bone marrow transplantation is potentially curative.

Anaesthesia for children with thalassaemia

Repeated transfusion and consequent chronic iron loading causes end organ damage, so there may be hepatic or cardiac dysfunction, including conduction disturbances. Extramedullary haemopoiesis may lead to maxillary hyperplasia with the potential for difficulty with airway management.

Glucose-6-phosphate dehydrogenase (G6PD) deficiency

This hereditary red cell disease is the most common enzyme defect in humans.

Who is at risk?

It is particularly common in Mediterranean countries, Africa, the Middle East, southeast Asia and some of the Pacific Islands. Most patients are asymptomatic but haemolytic anaemia and jaundice may be present. Acute haemolysis is promoted by infection or exposure to certain drugs including:

- Dapsone, and other sulfones
- Quinolones, such as ciprofloxacin
- Sulfonamides, such as co-trimoxazole
- Nitrofurantoin
- Methylene blue

There is considerable heterogeneity in G6PD deficiency, so not all patients will be equally affected. It is prudent nevertheless to avoid all these drugs. High dose aspirin and some of the quinines may also cause haemolysis in some patients.

Coagulation disorders

Von Willebrand's disease (VWD), a defect or deficiency of Von Willebrand factor, is the most common coagulation disorder, and is of varying severity. It is frequently mild and may not be recognised.

Haemophilia A is a sex-linked recessive disorder in which there is defective production of factor VIII. Patients bruise easily with risk of spontaneous bleeding into joints, muscles, the renal tracts and the brain.

Haemophilia B is less common and due to deficiency of factor IX.

Coagulation screening will reveal a prolonged activated partial thromboplastin time (APTT) with normal thrombin time and prothrombin time, though this may be normal in VWD.

Patients undergoing surgery should be managed in conjunction with the haematology department. For haemophilia, appropriate factor concentrate should be given to raise levels to 30–50% prior to surgery. Desmopressin (DDAVP), a synthetic analogue of vasopressin, increases plasma levels of Von Willebrand factor and Factor VIII and is the mainstay of treatment for VWD. It can be used in mild cases of haemophilia A where resistance has developed to factor concentrates, but is ineffective in haemophilia B.

Epilepsy

Epilepsy occurs in about 2% of children and may be idiopathic, with a small genetic predisposition, or secondary to events in the pre-, peri- or post-natal period. Many congenital syndromes and inherited metabolic disorders are associated with seizures. Seizures in children may be generalised or focal (partial). Partial seizures can be associated with impaired consciousness (complex partial seizures) and can progress to generalised convulsions. Petit mal epilepsy, infantile spasms and myoclonic epilepsy are forms of epilepsy which occur in the paediatric population.

Numerous antiepileptic drugs are in use, many of which may interact with anaesthetic agents. The more common anticonvulsants e.g. phenobarbitone, phenytoin, carbamazepine and sodium valproate induce liver enzymes and the metabolism of aminosteroid type muscle relaxants may be accelerated. Larger or more frequent doses may be required. Sodium valproate, carbamazepine, primidone and ethosuximide can cause thrombocytopenia.

Parents will usually be able to advise about the form of convulsions and how well they are controlled by anticonvulsant medication. Carers also may have 'rescue' benzodiazepine medication and can advise whether this has been needed for prolonged convulsions and how frequently it has been used.

Ideally elective surgery should occur when seizure control is optimal. For patients who have epilepsy refractory to medical therapy this may not be realistic. There does not appear to be a problem using sevoflurane for induction in children with epilepsy, but it is probably sensible to avoid ketamine.

In order to maintain anticonvulsant levels, antiepileptic medication should be continued pre-operatively and consideration given as to how anticonvulsant levels will be maintained in the post-operative period if it is likely there will be a prolonged period before oral intake can be restarted. It may be necessary to liaise with the neurology service. Rescue medication should be available post-operatively for patients in whom seizure control is poor. Sedative premedication may be helpful if behavioural difficulties are encountered.

Ketogenic diets

Intractable epilepsy may be managed with a high fat, low carbohydrate ketogenic diet. The carbohydrate intake should not be increased in the peri-operative period as this could provoke a relapse. Glucose-free intravenous fluids should be used initially, and blood sugar should be monitored hourly aiming to maintain blood glucose in the range 3–4 mmol l^{-1}. Excessive ketosis should also be avoided as this may lead to nausea and vomiting and acidosis. Measurement of plasma pH and biochemistry is advisable as in long surgical procedures metabolic acidosis may develop which may require bicarbonate administration. Monitoring urinary ketones will help confirm that the ketones are in the correct range, 8–16 mmol l^{-1}.

Cerebral palsy (CP)

CP is a chronic disorder of movement and posture caused by an injury to the developing brain.

Spasticity, ataxia and choreoathetosis may be present in varying degrees. Intellectual impairment may be present but some patients will have normal intelligence which may be masked by expressive language disorders.

Patients with CP often have sensory impairment, epilepsy and need nutritional support. Muscle spasms and contractures are common. Patients are likely to be taking anticonvulsants and antispasticity medication and these should not be abruptly discontinued.

If assessment is challenging, the patient's carers are usually best placed to advise about intellectual function, communication and positioning. Careful consideration must be given to positioning to support deformed limbs and fragile skin.

Patients may have chronic respiratory impairment secondary to weak respiratory muscles, gastro-oesophageal reflux and chronic aspiration. Secretions and drooling are often an issue, and drying agents e.g. hyoscine patches may be prescribed. Respiratory function may be further compromised by scoliosis.

Nutrition may be poor with supplemental nutrition given via a gastrostomy. Often little subcutaneous fat is present, and temperature should be monitored under anaesthesia.

It is difficult to evaluate whether this patient group is sensitive to the respiratory depressant effects of opioids. Assessment of pain can be challenging and appropriate scoring systems should be used with analgesia carefully titrated to ensure optimal pain relief. Opioid analgesia should be carefully titrated but it should not be withheld where indicated.

Chronic renal failure (CRF)

The care of patients with CRF should always be coordinated with the renal team. Most children are asymptomatic until glomerular filtration rate (GFR) is severely reduced. Patients may have anaemia, hypertension, electrolyte disturbance, renal osteodystrophy and failure to thrive. The anaesthetist should consider the cause of CRF, how the CRF is managed e.g. how the dialysis is performed – peritoneal or haemodialysis- and whether transplantation has been attempted or is planned. The patient may be oliguric or anuric.

Cardiorespiratory function should be fully evaluated. Peritoneal dialysis can be associated with basal atelectasis, pleural effusions and pneumonias. Hypertension may be present, and the normal blood pressure for the patient and use of antihypertensives should be noted. Left ventricular hypertrophy (LVH) and diastolic dysfunction has been noted in older children. Chronic anaemia may be well tolerated and transfusion may not be indicated.

Volume status, fluid overload or volume depletion, may be evident from examination findings. Timing of dialysis in relation to induction of anaesthesia is critical owing to the considerable fluid shifts. Allow approximately 6 h after dialysis for equilibration between fluid compartments. Electrolyte levels must be checked with particular attention to potassium levels.

Heparin may be present after dialysis. Uraemia can prolong bleeding time, and correction is by infusion of cryoprecipitate or DDAVP and not platelet infusion.

Avoid the non-dominant arm for venepuncture and IV access, as arteriovenous fistula at wrist or elbow may be needed for haemodialysis. Vascular access may be extremely challenging if multiple sites have been used for haemodialysis catheters, as thrombosis of vessels is not uncommon.

Key points

- Children with poorly controlled asthma or with recent upper respiratory tract infection are at high risk of peri-operative bronchospasm. Surgery may need to be delayed until symptoms are controlled.
- The prevalence of diabetes in children is increasing, some of whom will be on a continuous subcutaneous insulin infusion regimen. It is important to maintain blood sugar at 5–10 mmol l^{-1} throughout the peri-operative period, and this may necessitate liaison with the endocrinology team.
- For children with epilepsy on a ketogenic diet, blood sugar should be monitored hourly aiming to maintain peri-operative blood glucose in the range 3–4 mmol l^{-1}. Glucose-containing intravenous fluids should be used sparingly.
- Lean body weight should be determined for obese children and used to calculate most drug doses, especially paracetamol.

Further reading

British Thoracic Society Guidelines on Asthma, 2011. http://www.brit-thoracic.org.uk/Portals/0/Guidelines/AsthmaGuidelines/sign101%20Jan%202012.pdf

Mortensen A, Lenz K, Abildstrom H, Lauritsen TLB. Anesthetizing the obese child. *Ped Anes* 2011;**21**:623–9.

Peri-operative management of IDDM: http://www.gosh.nhs.uk/health-professionals/clinical-guidelines/management-of-children-and-young-people-with-diabetes-during-surgery/

Chapter

8

Congenital and inherited disorders affecting anaesthesia in children

Nargis Ahmad and Ian James

Introduction

Children with congenital anomalies or inherited metabolic disorders can be a challenge to the paediatric anaesthetist. An encyclopaedic knowledge of these conditions, however desirable, is unrealistic for most practising paediatric anaesthetists. For some of the rarer disorders the evidence base on which to plan an optimal anaesthetic technique is usually limited to single case reports or small series. This synopsis does not intend to provide comprehensive details of all these conditions, but will cover some of the more common conditions. For the rarer anomalies the reader should consider a more comprehensive text or one of the web-based resources, such as the Online Mendelian Inheritance in Man® database accessible via the National Center for Biotechnology Information (NCBI) website.

Congenital anomalies

When faced with a patient with an unusual congenital syndrome a systematic approach to pre-operative assessment will usually identify issues that are likely to be of direct relevance to the anaesthetic technique. These most commonly involve the airway and the cardiovascular system. In some conditions there may be endocrine or metabolic issues that need to be considered, glucose and steroid management in particular. Limb abnormalities or fragile skin require careful assessment of potential sites for intravenous access, and protection of skin and joints during positioning. Evaluation will be assisted by accessing information about the usual features of the condition that should help identify areas that should be considered in more detail in any individual patient. It is worth bearing in mind that most conditions were

originally classified from phenotypes with inheritance patterns observed and described. Whilst great progress has been made in understanding the genetic basis of many of these conditions both phenotypic and genetic heterogeneity are not uncommon.

Many conditions are associated with dysmorphic features, abnormal growth parameters, developmental delay and learning disability. These should be evident during the pre-operative assessment, and it is assumed that the behavioural aspects of care will be considered pre-operatively in all cases. Some conditions are associated with seizures and it is important to determine how well these are controlled. Intractable seizures may be treated with a ketogenic diet. For these patients strict glucose control is essential in the peri-operative period. For the sake of brevity such considerations are not highlighted individually for each condition in the table.

Inborn errors of metabolism

An overview of the more common inborn errors of metabolism is shown in Table 8.1. The signs and symptoms of inherited metabolic disease (IMD) arise as a consequence of a failure of one or more steps within a metabolic process. In essence they result in one or more of the following:

- Accumulation of substrate
- Accumulation of metabolite
- Deficiency of normal product of metabolic pathway
- General metabolic derangement e.g. acidosis

The inherited disorders of metabolism constitute a diverse group and as a consequence the general information provided is limited to broad principles. They

Core Topics in Paediatric Anaesthesia, ed. Ian James and Isabeau Walker. Published by Cambridge University Press. © 2013 Cambridge University Press.

Table 8.1 Overview of inherited metabolic disorders

Classification	Example	Anaesthetic considerations
Disorders of amino acid metabolism	Phenylketonuria (PKU) Homocystinuria Maple-syrup urine disease (MSUD)	Seizure medication, maintain special diet. Marfanoid, thrombosis risk high so maintain hydration, thrombosis prophylaxis. Hypotonic, hypoglycaemia, seizures.
Urea cycle disorders	Carbamyl phosphate synthase deficiency	Prone to hyperammonaemia and encephalopathy. Avoid catabolism and dehydration during fasting. Maintain high carbohydrate, low protein diet. Avoid blood in the stomach as this is a protein load. Infusion of substrate to optimise non-urea cycles for nitrogen removal is often necessary; specialist advice should be taken.
Disorders of organic acid metabolism	Methylmalonic acidaemia, Propionic acidaemia	Prone to hypoglycaemia, ketoacidosis, hyperammonaemia. Maintain normoglycaemia, hydration and acid-base status. Restrict protein.
Disorders of carbohydrate metabolism	Glycogen storage diseases e.g. von Gierke, Pompe, Cori, Andersen, McArdle Galactosaemia	Minimise fasting, maintain normoglycaemia and acid base homeostasis. Avoid lactate-containing fluid. Pompe may have hypertrophic cardiomyopathy. Hepatic dysfunction.
Lysosomal storage disorders	Mucopolysaccharidoses (MPS) Lipidoses e.g. Tay–Sachs, Fabry, Niemann–Pick	High risk airway, cervical spine, cardiac complications. Seizures. Lysosomal accumulation of sphingolipid substrates, hepatomegaly, developmental delay.
Disorders of fatty acid oxidation	Medium chain acyl–CoA dehydrogenase deficiency	Avoid metabolic consequences of fasting with infusion of dextrose, maintain acid–base homeostasis.
Mitochondrial disorders	Genetic and phenotypic heterogeneous group with reduced capacity for oxidative phosphorylation	Myopathic, often with cardiomyopathy and neurodevelopmental delay. Avoid prolonged propofol infusion, avoid lactate-containing fluids, maintain normoglycaemia. May have disordered control of respiration.
Peroxisomal disorders	Zellweger syndrome	Hypotonia, hepatic and renal impairment, chronic respiratory dysfunction. Zellweger associated with congenital heart disease.

may present with acute encephalopathy or seizures, or other neurological symptoms such as stroke, hypotonia or movement disorders. Hypoglycaemia or a metabolic acidosis may also be the first presentation. Myopathy is not uncommon.

The IMDs that are likely to cause most problems for anaesthetists are the mucopolysaccharidoses (MPS), in which there is abnormal sequestration into connective tissue of partially degraded glycosaminoglycans. These are discussed in more detail below.

The broad principles of anaesthetic management of IMDs include:

- Assessment of the patient's condition and any organ dysfunction;

- Avoiding prolonged fasting times, and maintaining hydration;
- Maintaining metabolic homeostasis peri-operatively by limitation of metabolism via the abnormal metabolic pathway; this may involve prevention of the catabolic state and provision of glucose during 'starvation';
- Consideration of strategies to correct severe acidosis pre-operatively, e.g. haemodialysis;
- Limiting acidosis and avoiding lactate-containing fluids;
- Monitoring glucose and acid–base state peri-operatively;
- Avoiding the accumulation of blood in the stomach; the protein content of blood can trigger

acute decompensation in many IMDs, especially those involving amino acid metabolism;

- Avoiding hypothermia.

Close collaboration with relevant IMD specialists will assist in this management.

Pre-operative assessment

As is commonly the case in paediatric anaesthesia, the family can often provide a wealth of information about their child. For many of the rarer conditions families may have accessed web-based resources extensively and have joined condition-specific support groups. It is not uncommon for them to be more knowledgeable about the syndrome and its ramifications than non-specialist clinical staff. Many of these children may need repeated surgical procedures; previous anaesthetic records may be a further source of valuable information and should always be examined.

Airway

Airway assessment is critical. Some disorders distort the normal anatomy of the bones and soft tissues associated with the airway. Those seen most commonly are due to:

- Maxillary hypoplasia, as in some of the craniosynostoses, e.g. Apert syndrome;
- Mandibular hypoplasia, as in the Pierre Robin anomalad;
- Mandibular and maxillary hypoplasia, such as Treacher–Collins syndrome;
- Hemifacial microsomia, as in Goldenhar syndrome;
- MPS, with thickened, stiff, abnormal tissues;
- Macroglossia, as in Beckwith–Wiedemann and Down syndromes.

As a consequence:

- Facemasks may be difficult to fit;
- The upper airway may be crowded and prone to obstruction on induction of anaesthesia;
- Mouth opening may be limited;
- Oral airways may be difficult to insert;
- Nasal passages may be too small for a nasopharyngeal airway;
- Laryngoscopy and intubation may be very difficult.

Cleft palate may also be present, compounding any difficulty with laryngoscopy.

Growth and development and medical and surgical treatment will be pertinent to any assessment. Some airway abnormalities improve with age, e.g. Pierre Robin sequence, but may worsen in others such as MPS. A full evaluation is necessary prior to any anaesthetic.

A history of disordered breathing may be suggestive of obstructive apnoea. This is usually during sleep (OSAS) but in rare cases may occur when awake. Assessment of the nasal passages, mouth opening, oropharynx including palate, tongue, maxilla, mandible and mandibular space, temporomandibular joint and cervical spine is essential and may predict whether difficulty in airway management or direct laryngoscopy intubation is likely.

A range of tracheal tube sizes should always be available because the size required may differ from that predicted by conventional formulae. The laryngeal mask airway (LMA) has been found to be a useful device for airway maintenance in patients with MPS, and also as a conduit for fibre optic intubation (FOI). Management of the difficult airway is covered in Chapter 22.

Cervical spine

The craniocervical junction (CCJ) is the site of a wide range of developmental and acquired anomalies in the paediatric population. The CCJ may be compromised by:

- Deformity
- Instability
- Compression

Deformity may arise as a result of distortion of normal anatomy or anomalous vertebral segmentation. Anomalous segmentation often coexists with craniovertebral anomalies such as craniosynostosis and disorders of branchial arch development. For example, cervical hemivertebrae are a feature of Goldenhar syndrome. In Klippel–Feil syndrome, fusion of cervical vertebrae results in a short neck with very limited mobility, which can result in intubation difficulties.

Instability of the CCJ may occur at the occipitoatlanto and atlanto-axial joints. Anomalies of the odontoid process leading to atlanto-axial instability are well recognised in Down syndrome, Morquio syndrome, Hurler syndrome and Klippel–Feil syndrome. Excessive movement of the neck may lead to cervical spine injury, and airway manoeuvres and patient positioning are times of great vulnerability during general anaesthesia.

Compression of the cervicomedullary junction is a feature of some of the MPS syndromes, when tissue infiltration leads to stenosis of the cervical canal. Cervical cord compression is also a common feature of achondroplasia.

Breathing

Respiratory muscle and bulbar weakness are features of myopathic conditions, and chronic aspiration and recurrent infections are common.

Generalised hypotonia may be present, and some conditions are associated with kyphoscoliosis which may progressively limit respiration. Limited respiratory reserve may be masked by a low level of activity in patients who are not ambulant.

Cardiovascular

Many congenital syndromes have an associated cardiac lesion, such as a ventricular septal defect (VSD) or valve stenosis. In older patients it is most likely that this will have been repaired or palliated. It is unusual for syndromic patients to present for non-cardiac surgery with an undiagnosed or unstable cardiac defect. The implications for anaesthesia in the presence of a cardiac lesion are dealt with in Chapter 33.

Particular care should be taken in patients with Williams syndrome, who have supra-aortic valvar stenosis and in whom a fall in systemic vascular resistance and blood pressure can lead to profound myocardial ischaemia. In those patients in whom cardiomyopathy is an associated factor, such as those with Duchenne's muscular dystrophy, Pompe's disease or disorders of fatty acid metabolism, a full cardiovascular work-up is essential prior to anaesthesia. This should include quantitative echocardiographic assessment of cardiac function.

Endocrine, metabolic and renal systems

These systems should be considered and evaluated as indicated. In a number of syndromes patients are on steroids and may need additional cover peri-operatively. This is particularly important in adrenogenital syndrome.

Careful management of glucose is essential in the glycogen storage disorders (e.g. von Gierke, Pompe,

Cori, Andersen, McArdle) and in the Beckwith–Wiedemann syndrome. It is important that fasting time is kept to a minimum, and it may be necessary to start an infusion of glucose before anaesthesia.

Where renal dysfunction is an associated factor careful attention should be made to fluid management, and to the use of drugs that rely on the kidney for excretion.

Skin, bone and joint disorders

Great care must be taken with patient positioning in patients with fixed deformities of their joints, or where there is abnormal joint laxity as in Marfan's syndrome. As noted earlier some patients have a fixed or potentially unstable neck which must be positioned carefully. The same applies to patients with fragile bones, such as in osteogenesis imperfecta.

In Ehlers–Danlos syndrome abnormal collagen leads not only to joint laxity but also to extremely fragile skin and other tissues. It can be very difficult to site and maintain intravenous access.

Epidermolysis bullosa is also a syndrome in which management of skin and mucosal surfaces is particularly challenging, and is discussed below.

Some specific syndromes

Down syndrome

This is one of the commonest congenital syndromes, occurring in approximately 1 in 600–700 live births; 95% are trisomy 21 and 2% are mosaic. The incidence increases with advancing maternal age. The characteristic phenotype includes features of low-set ears, up-slanting eyes, a small nose, large tongue, brachycephaly, short neck, clinodactyly, a single palmar crease and a varying degree of intellectual impairment. Forty to fifty per cent have congenital heart disease, most commonly an atrial or ventricular septal defect, frequently as part of an endocardial cushion defect. Duodenal atresia may occur. Children with Down syndrome may be moderately hypotonic and are often hypothyroid. They have an increased risk of leukaemia.

Associated features of relevance to anaesthesia include a significant incidence of occipito-atlantoaxial instability, and great care is needed with manipulation of the head and neck during intubation and subsequent positioning. A history of recurrent chest infections should raise concern about pulmonary aspiration secondary to cervical cord compression and should prompt radiological investigation of the cervical spine. The large tongue and a narrow nasopharynx result in easy upper airway obstruction. The larynx is often slightly small and it is common to need a tracheal tube 0.5 mm narrower than usual for the age.

Epidermolysis bullosa (EB)

This is a group of disorders in which the epidermis and mucous membranes separate readily from the underlying tissues. The patient is at risk of formation of bullae with trivial trauma, particularly on exposure to shearing forces. Three major types of EB are recognised: simplex, junctional and dystrophic. In the severe forms, such as recessive dystrophic EB, recurrent skin damage and scarring of the fingers and toes leads to pseudosyndactyly and severe contractures, so called 'mitten hands'. Scarring of the corners of the mouth leads to progressive microstomia, and oropharyngeal mucosal scarring leads to fixation of the tongue within the mouth. There is frequently very poor dentition, and oesophageal strictures are common. Cardiomyopathy has been reported but this is rare.

These patients usually present for repair of their fused digits, oesophageal dilation or dental restoration. They are a particularly challenging group and must be treated with great care. Surgical procedures should only be undertaken in specialist units where there is ward-based nursing expertise. Patients are often colonised with methicillin resistant *Staphylococcus aureus* (MRSA).

Anaesthesia for children with EB

Careful handling is essential for these patients. Friction and sliding during transfer must be avoided, and adhesive tapes should not be used. Intravenous lines should be secured with a non-adhesive dressing. There are now self-adhesive silicon based products suitable for this, e.g. Mepiform®. Arterial and central lines, if required, should be sutured in. Gel should be used to cover the eyes. These patients can lose heat readily so a warm theatre environment is advisable.

Airway management

Careful airway assessment is imperative to assess limitation of mouth opening and degree of neck movement. All airway equipment, including the facemask, airway and laryngoscope, should be generously lubricated with paraffin jelly or Vaseline gauze. Vaseline gauze should be placed under the chin where the anaesthetist places their fingers. An oral airway may not be needed as the immobility of the tongue usually allows an unobstructed airway. Laryngoscopy and intubation can be difficult because of limited mouth opening, which tends to get worse with increasing age. Tracheal intubation does not appear to cause laryngeal or tracheal bullae and is generally considered safe. Nasal intubation may be preferable for extensive dental work or oesophageal dilation, but whichever route is used it is essential that great care is taken to avoid sliding or shearing forces. The tube can be secured with ribbon gauze or clingfilm. A well-lubricated LMA may be used with caution.

Monitoring

Small ECG electrodes can be secured with non-adhesive silicon dressings as with intravenous lines, or with clingfilm. Clip-on oximeter probes should be used. Blood pressure cuffs can be used safely as they do not produce a shearing force, but should be well padded.

Post-operative care

Effective post-operative analgesia is essential as it will reduce the likelihood of restlessness and agitation during emergence from anaesthesia, although this is not always possible to achieve. Intravenous analgesia may be the most effective route. Regional analgesia, single dose or by continuous infusion, has been utilised successfully and will be useful in some patients. The increasing use of ultrasound to improve the success rate of regional nerve blockade may be beneficial. Many patients have difficulty with oral medications, and rectal analgesia may be necessary.

Mucopolysaccharidoses

Patients with MPS present a very high risk for anaesthesia. Abnormal sequestration of partially degraded glycosaminoglycans results in a progressive, multisystem disease with organomegaly, visual, auditory and intellectual deficits, airway abnormalities, cardiovascular impairment, joint and bony deformities, and characteristic coarse facial features.

Treatment options now include haematopoietic stem cell transplantation and recombinant enzyme replacement therapy. Stem cell transplantation halts progression of these diseases, and reduces hepatosplenomegaly, joint stiffness, obstructive sleep apnoea, facial dysmorphism, heart disease, hydrocephalus and hearing loss. Skeletal and ocular abnormalities are not corrected and neurological outcomes remain poor. Enzyme replacement therapy may be of benefit in MPS I, II and VI.

Anaesthesia for children with MPS

Behavioural problems are common but sedative premedication should be used with extreme caution. Pre-operative assessment should include thorough clinical evaluation of the cardiac and respiratory systems. Cardiomyopathy, valvular heart disease and coronary artery disease may be present. A recent echocardiogram should be reviewed. Active respiratory tract infection is a contraindication to elective surgery. Close post-operative monitoring is essential.

Airway management

The overall incidence of airway difficulties is 25%, with failure to intubate in 8% of MPS cases (rising to 54% and 23% respectively in Hurler's syndrome). Contributory factors include:

- Airway tissue deposition of glycosaminoglycans;
- A short and often unstable neck;
- Poor joint mobility including the cervical spine and temporo-mandibular joints;
- Macroglossia;
- Micrognathia.

Previous anaesthetic records should be evaluated but as all of these factors get worse with age a difficult airway must always be expected. Careful preparation and planning, including the full range of difficult airway adjuncts, is essential. Pre-operative sleep studies may be required as OSAS is often present.

Cervical spine instability most often occurs in MPS I (Hurler) and IV (Morquio). Flexion–extension cervical spine images taken under specialist supervision should be considered. In Morquio syndrome potential cervical myelopathy secondary to canal stenosis should be evaluated with magnetic resonance (MR) imaging. Neck manipulation should be avoided. Manual inline stabilisation is recommended.

The use of an antisialagogue may be helpful. As a result of tissue distortion facemasks may not fit well, oral airways may worsen airway obstruction and nasopharyngeal airways may be difficult to place. The LMA has been found to be particularly useful and its use as a conduit for intubation is well

described. FOI may be necessary in which case it is important to anticipate that the correct size tracheal tube may be smaller than that expected.

Airway obstruction following tracheal extubation can result in pulmonary oedema. Awake extubation is advised and dexamethasone may be helpful.

Malignant hyperthermia susceptibility (MHS)

MHS is a genetic disorder of skeletal muscle calcium regulation in which uncontrolled skeletal muscle hypermetabolism, triggered by volatile agents alone or in conjunction with suxamethonium, leads to a life-threatening state known as malignant hyperthermia (MH). The triggering substances release calcium stores from the sarcoplasmic reticulum causing muscle contracture, glycogenolysis, ATP consumption and heat production. Oxygen demand soon outstrips supply and ATP stores are depleted leading to lactic acidosis and rhabdomyolysis. If treated promptly most patients recover although there remains a mortality rate of around 5%.

Who is at risk?

This condition is usually inherited in an autosomal dominant pattern, so all closely related members of a family in which MH has occurred must be considered susceptible. The defective gene affects the ryanodine receptor (RyR1) allowing abnormal calcium flux across the sarcoplasmic reticulum, and it is possible to identify some people with MHS on genetic testing. Unfortunately MHS cannot reliably be excluded on the basis of a genetic test as MH has a high level of locus heterogeneity and not all MH genes have been completely described. For new cases or for those with a family history the gold standard for diagnosis is a muscle biopsy and in vitro contracture test (IVCT). The sample size required is such that muscle biopsies are not performed on children less than 10–12 years old (30 kg). Anaesthesia for muscle biopsy is covered in detail in Chapter 37.

Anaesthesia for children with MHS

It is important to be aware that a previous history of uneventful anaesthesia does not exclude risk. If MHS is suspected, all volatile agents and suxamethonium should be avoided. The anaesthetic machine should have vaporizers removed, and it is usual to flush the machine and circuits with oxygen for about 30 minutes prior to use to remove residual traces of volatile agent. Propofol, opioids, benzodiazepines, nitrous oxide, local anaesthetics and barbiturates can all be used as part of a trigger-free technique. In addition to usual minimal monitoring it is essential to include central temperature. Dantrolene should be available and its location confirmed.

Recognition and management of MH

Protocols for the treatment of MH in all patient groups are widely circulated and should be readily available in all anaesthetic areas.

At the start of an episode of MH the patients may exhibit generalised muscle spasm, often first noticed as masseter spasm. Subsequently they develop:

- Unexplained hypercapnia, including tachypnoea in the spontaneously breathing patient;
- Unexplained tachycardia, possibly with arrhythmias;
- Hyperthermia, classically rising $>1\,^\circ$C every 5 minutes;
- Hypoxaemia;
- Acidosis and hyperkalaemia.

It is important to note that there is a variable onset of these symptoms, which may only manifest themselves in the recovery period.

Myoglobinuria and raised plasma creatine kinase may develop later.

Treatment must be prompt and includes:

- Discontinuation of volatile agents;
- Administration of 100% oxygen via a clean breathing circuit;
- Active cooling with ice packs; cold gastric and bladder lavage may be helpful;
- Dantrolene, 2–3 mg kg^{-1}; this may need to be repeated in doses of 1 mg kg^{-1} to a maximum of 10 mg kg^{-1}. Dantrolene requires mixing and can take some time to dissolve so assistance may be required;
- If surgery cannot be stopped, maintenance of anaesthesia should continue with intravenous agents;
- Sodium bicarbonate, calcium chloride, insulin and glucose as necessary to treat acidosis and hyperkalaemia;
- Antiarrhythmics may be necessary, but calcium channel blockers must be avoided;
- Encourage a diuresis if there is any myoglobinuria;
- Treat disseminated intravascular coagulation as necessary.

In due course the patient should be referred for further investigation.

Associated conditions

There are a small number of very rare muscle disorders that are closely linked and exhibit MHS. These conditions are:

- Central core disease
- Multi-minicore disease
- King–Denborough syndrome

MHS is not a feature of other neuromuscular diseases such as the muscular dystrophies or myotonias. Patients with Duchenne or Becker's muscular dystrophies are, however, at risk for hyperkalaemia and rhabdomyolysis on exposure to volatile anaesthetic agents and suxamethonium, but this complication is a different entity which has been termed anaesthesia-induced rhabdomyolysis (AIR).

Muscular dystrophy

The muscular dystrophies (MD) are a group of X-linked genetic disorders in which there is absent or abnormal dystrophin, leading to muscle weakness and atrophy. Duchenne muscular dystrophy (DMD) is the most common form, with an incidence of 1 in 3500 males. Becker MD is a milder form which does not usually present until the teenage years.

Patients with DMD experience progressive degeneration and fibrosis of all muscle types with onset from the age of about 3 years. It is rapidly progressive, and patients are frequently wheelchair-bound by adolescence. Life expectancy has increased with advances in supportive therapies and use of steroids.

Anaesthesia for children with muscular dystrophy

MD patients are especially at risk during and after general anaesthesia because of:

- Restrictive lung disease, from respiratory muscle weakness and scoliosis;
- Dilated cardiomyopathy (DCM), which is common, although the history may not always reveal symptoms if the patient is inactive;
- Risk of rhabdomyolysis and hyperkalaemia;
- Fibrosis of the conduction system, which may lead to rhythm disturbances.

Multidisciplinary assessment is essential prior to elective surgery. Lung function tests, sleep studies, and echocardiograms should be regularly undertaken as part of the management of these patients. Cardio-respiratory review should be organised prior to surgery with a repeat of any investigations that are not recent. Full assessment may necessitate admission a day or two prior to surgery to optimise respiratory function. Non-invasive ventilation (NPPV) may need to be started prior to surgery and continued afterwards.

Peri-operative steroid replacement should be used in all patients who have been on steroids in the previous 6 months.

Gastrointestinal smooth muscle is affected in DMD, so gastric stasis may occur. H2 antagonists should be administered the night before surgery and the morning of surgery, e.g. ranitidine 3 mg kg^{-1}, max 150 mg.

Post-operative respiratory support for patients with DMD

The post-operative period is a particularly challenging time in the care of these patients. PICU will be required for all but the most minor surgery. Forced vital capacity (FVC) is useful for predicting respiratory insufficiency post-operatively:

- <50% indicates an increased risk of respiratory complications;
- <30% is considered high risk, probably requiring ventilatory support.

Anaesthesia-induced rhabdomyolysis

Although patients with muscular dystrophy are not MH susceptible, life-threatening rhabdomyolysis and hyperkalaemia can occur following the administration of suxamethonium or exposure to volatile inhalational anaesthetic agents, probably owing to an abnormal resting permeability in the unstable sarcolemma.

Suxamethonium is totally contraindicated, and there should be minimal exposure to volatile anaesthetic agents. Total intravenous anaesthesia (TIVA) is desirable.

Riley–Day syndrome (familial dysautonomia)

This is a rare, inherited, autonomic and sensory neuropathy seen most commonly in people with an Eastern European Jewish ancestry. Clinical features include reduced pain perception, gastro-oesophageal reflux with recurrent aspiration, seizures, hypotonia and scoliosis. An inability to form tears leads to dry eyes. They also have impaired haemodynamic reflexes which seem to be pronounced under anaesthesia, resulting in a very labile blood pressure, with exaggerated vaso-vagal responses. Hypovolaemia is poorly tolerated. Epidural anaesthesia has been shown to provide cardiovascular and autonomic stability and should be used where appropriate. Temperature control may also be poor and should be monitored.

Key points

- Many congenital disorders have an associated cardiac defect or a difficult airway problem.
- Children with mucopolysaccharidoses are high risk cases for anaesthesia. They can present major airway difficulties and may have an unstable cervical spine.
- Children with muscular dystrophies and myotonias are not generally at risk of malignant hyperthermia, but are at risk of hyperkalaemia and rhabdomyolysis if exposed to suxamethonium or volatile agents.

Further reading

Goldschneider K, Lucky AW, Mellerio JE et al. Perioperative care of patients with epidermolysis bullosa. Proceedings of the 5th International Symposium in Epidermolysis Bullosa, Santiago, Chile, December 4–6, 2008; Ped Anes 2010;**20**:797–804.

Online Mendelian Inheritance in Man (OMIM); http://www.ncbi.nlm.nih.gov/omim

Rosenberg H, Sambuughin N, Dirksen R. Malignant Hyperthermia Susceptibility. www.ncbi.nih.gov/books/NBK1146

Stuart G, Ahmad N. Perioperative care of children with inherited metabolic disorders. Cont Edu Anaes Crit Care Pain 2011;**11**:62–8.

Walker R, Belani KG, Braunlin EA et al. Anaesthesia and airway management in mucopolysaccharidosis. J Inherit Metab Dis (Epub ahead of print 30 November 2012).

Walker RWM, Darowski M, Morris P, Wrailt JE. Anaesthesia and mucopolysaccharidoses. A review of airway problems in children. Anaesthesia 1994;**49**: 1078–84.

Chapter

9

The premature and ex-premature infant

Isabeau Walker

Introduction

The impact of premature birth is life-long, and although the risk of acute complications recedes throughout infancy and early childhood, long-term morbidity remains high. Low gestational age at birth is an independent risk factor for increased mortality from respiratory, cardiovascular, endocrine and congenital disorders in childhood and early adulthood. This chapter will describe the clinical conditions unique to the premature and ex-premature infant, and special considerations for the conduct of anaesthesia in this vulnerable population.

Definitions

Definitions in common use are as follows:

Gestational age: time from the first day of the last normal menstrual period to the day of delivery. Gestational age is described in completed weeks.

Conceptional age: time between conception and day of delivery. Gestational age is equal to conceptional age +2 weeks. Gestational age is the preferred term.

Chronological age: time elapsed since birth.

Post-menstrual age: gestational age + chronological age. Used to describe age during the perinatal hospital stay. A baby born at 28 weeks who is now 4 weeks of age has a post-menstrual age of 32 weeks.

Corrected age: chronological age reduced by the number of weeks born before 40 weeks of gestation. Used to describe the age of children who were born preterm up to the age of 3 years. A baby born at 28 weeks who has a chronological age of 6 months has a corrected age of (26 weeks − (40−28 weeks) = 14 weeks.

Full term neonate: 37–42 weeks gestation and aged <1 month

Premature neonate: <37 weeks gestation
Extreme preterm neonate: <28 weeks gestation
Low birthweight (LBW): <2500 g
Very low birthweight (VLBW): <1500 g
Extremely low birth weight (ELBW): <1000 g

Risk factors for premature delivery

The risk factors for premature delivery include maternal factors, complications of pregnancy and fetal factors:

- Maternal age <20 years or >40 years
- Low socioeconomic status
- Maternal diabetes
- Smoking
- History of previous premature labour
- Premature rupture of membranes
- Chorioamnionitis
- Placental abruption
- Pre-eclampsia
- Multiple gestation pregnancies
- Congenital abnormalities
- Intrauterine growth retardation

Clinical consequences of premature delivery

Delivery before 37 weeks gestation affects multiple systems as important aspects of organ development are not complete until this time. The clinical consequences of prematurity depend on the gestational age at birth and any underlying abnormalities that may have resulted in premature delivery. The premature infant is particularly vulnerable to:

- Thermoregulatory instability
- Disorders of glucose, fluid and electrolyte balance and renal function

---

Core Topics in Paediatric Anaesthesia, ed. Ian James and Isabeau Walker. Published by Cambridge University Press. © 2013 Cambridge University Press.

- Respiratory distress syndrome
- Bronchopulmonary dysplasia
- Sepsis
- Pulmonary haemorrhage
- Apnoea
- Chronic lung disease
- Patent ductus arteriosus (PDA)
- Necrotising enterocolitis (NEC)
- Retinopathy of prematurity (ROP)
- Intraventricular haemorrhage (IVH)
- Failure to thrive
- Neurodevelopmental complications

Mortality due to premature delivery decreased markedly in the 1990s after the introduction of exogenous surfactant therapy for respiratory distress syndrome. Advances in neonatal intensive care have extended the survival of premature infants such that around 50% of babies born at 24 weeks and around 90% of those born at 27 weeks survive, but the levels of morbidity are high. Outcomes are better in female babies, singleton pregnancies and when antenatal steroids have been used. Babies with ELBW are more susceptible to complications. First-year survival for babies with a birth weight of <500 g is approximately 15%, 500–749 g 50% and >750 g 85%.

Thermoregulatory instability

Thermoregulation in the premature neonate is limited and easily overwhelmed by environmental conditions. There is a great potential for heat loss (high body surface area to body weight ratio, increased thermal conductance, increased evaporative heat loss through non-keratinised skin) and limited heat production through brown fat metabolism. The principle of anaesthesia in these infants is for minimal handling in a warm environment, preferably with surgery performed in the neonatal unit.

Renal function, fluid and electrolyte balance and glucose

Nephrogenesis is completed at 35 weeks and premature babies have impaired renal function with reduced glomerular filtration rate, and limited ability to concentrate urine, excrete potassium and reabsorb bicarbonate. Plasma creatinine initially reflects that of the mother. Renal function is usually normal in childhood, but ex-premature neonates have an increased incidence of hypertension in later life.

The extracellular fluid compartment is relatively expanded at birth, and the post-natal diuresis may be associated with 10–20% weight loss. Fluid requirements are increased by the use of radiant heaters (increased evaporative heat loss) and reduced by the use of heated incubators. Antidiuretic hormone is elevated in the first few days of life and as a result of the stress response.

Premature babies may develop hyponatraemia due to water overload or excess sodium loss, or hypernatraemia due to excess water loss. Premature infants are also susceptible to hypoglycaemia, defined as blood glucose <2.5 mmol l^{-1}. Maintenance fluids containing 10% dextrose are usually required, with added sodium after 24 hours. Rapid infusion of concentrated glucose solutions should be avoided as these are hyperosmolar and cause damage to peripheral veins, and are a risk factor for hyperglycaemia and cerebral haemorrhage.

Excessive fluid administration is a risk factor for patent ductus arteriosus, bronchopulmonary dysplasia and intraventricular haemorrhage. Fluids are restricted in the first few days of life and liberalised thereafter. Fluid and electrolyte balance is complex and should be closely monitored using daily weights and frequent monitoring of electrolytes.

Nutrition

The high nutritional requirements in the developing fetus are met via the placenta, and it is difficult to match these in the premature neonate owing to gut immaturity. Early enteral feeding may be a risk factor for NEC and parenteral nutrition is often required. Anaesthetists should take care to preserve peripheral veins in these vulnerable infants as these will be required to insert intravenous long lines for feeding. Trophic feeds (very small volumes of enterally administered nutrients to stimulate the development of the immature gastrointestinal tract) are started when the baby is medically stable and then increased as tolerated. Feed is ideally breast milk fortified with calories, protein and minerals, particularly calcium, phosphate and sodium, to promote growth and avoid protein malnutrition, osteopenia of prematurity, rickets and hyponatraemia.

Respiratory distress syndrome and bronchopulmonary dysplasia

The incidence of respiratory distress syndrome (RDS) is inversely proportional to gestational age, and occurs in 60% of infants born at <30 weeks gestation. It is due to the immaturity of the lungs combined with absence of pulmonary surfactant, normally produced in the type II pulmonary pneumocytes from 24 weeks gestation.

RDS presents with increased work of breathing with tachypnoea, dyspnoea, chest retractions, and cyanosis and 'grunting'. The lungs are non-compliant, and there is widespread atelectasis on chest X-ray (CXR) with a granular appearance and widespread air bronchograms. Histologically, the lungs contain hyaline membranes in terminal airways, hence the previous terminology hyaline membrane disease.

RDS may be complicated by air leak (pneumothorax, pneumomediastinum, pulmonary interstitial emphysema) and is the precursor to bronchopulmonary dysplasia (BPD) and chronic lung disease (CLD).

BPD is defined by the requirement for supplemental oxygen or ventilatory support at 36 weeks postmenstrual age. Typical CXR changes include a ground glass appearance in early stages, later progressing to patchy atelectasis, cystic changes, hyperexpansion and areas of emphysema. Modern obstetric and neonatal intensive care practice has improved the course of RDS but unfortunately the incidence of BPD has not been reduced, possibly owing to the improved survival of extreme premature infants.

Antenatal corticosteroids are administered to mothers in preterm labour to induce surfactant production. This is associated with better outcomes from RDS and does not produce adverse neurodevelopmental effects. Exogenous surfactant is administered prophylactically to infants <28 weeks gestation within hours of birth, or as rescue in RDS, and this has an additive effect to antenatal steroids. Long-term intubation and positive pressure ventilation are avoided if possible as they are more likely to be associated with barotrauma, oxygen toxicity and the development of BPD. The baby may be briefly intubated for the administration of surfactant, but is rapidly weaned to nasal continuous positive airway pressure (nCPAP) if possible. Longer-term intubation is more likely to be required in VLBW infants <28 weeks, and if oxygenation with nCPAP is inadequate with inspired oxygen >50–60%. Of note, post-natal steroids have been found to have an adverse effect on development of the brain in premature infants and are no longer recommended to facilitate weaning from long-term ventilation.

Ventilation strategy in premature infants is chosen to minimise ventilator induced lung injury and includes:

- Permissive hypercapnia
- Minimal FiO_2, oxygen saturation 88–95%
- Minimal peak inspiratory pressures
- PEEP 3–5 cmH_2O
- I:E ratio 1:1
- Respiratory rate 60 breaths/minute

High frequency oscillatory ventilation (HFOV) is used to reduce barotrauma and oxygen requirements. Inhaled nitric oxide may be used as rescue therapy, but may increase intraventricular haemorrhage and does not appear to improve long-term outcomes.

The mortality from RDS is 5–10% and is rare in babies >1.5 kg at birth. BPD occurs in 15–50% of VLBW infants and is associated with long-term morbidity that continues into later life. Infants may remain oxygen-dependent for many months, although it is unusual to require oxygen after 2 years of age. The ex-premature infant is susceptible to respiratory infection in childhood; hospital admission due to infection with respiratory syncytial virus is common in the first 2 years of life. Some may remain symptomatic into adult life. Asthma is common, and ex-premature infants may have acquired subglottic stenosis as a consequence of prolonged intubation.

Apnoea of prematurity

Apnoea of prematurity is defined as a pause in breathing of more than 20 seconds or a pause associated with bradycardia and/or desaturation. Apnoeas may be:

- Central (brainstem or peripheral chemoreceptor immaturity);
- Obstructive (reduced airway tone, asynchrony of diaphragmatic or upper airway activity, excessive neck flexion or structural abnormalities);
- Mixed central and obstructive (most common).

Central control of ventilation matures with age, and apnoea of prematurity is seen in 90% of premature infants <1000 g at birth. In utero, the fetus responds to hypoxia by suppressing ventilation, whereas the mature response to hypoxia and hypercapnia is to increase ventilation. Premature and newborn term babies respond to hypoxia by a brief increase in ventilation followed by apnoea and have a blunted response to hypercapnia. In the term infant, normal responses to hypercapnia and hypoxia are seen by 3 weeks of age, but this is delayed in premature infants.

Apnoea may be triggered by hypoxia, sepsis, intracranial haemorrhage, metabolic abnormalities, hypo/hyperthermia, upper airway obstruction, heart failure, anaemia, vaso-vagal reflexes and drugs, including prostaglandins and anaesthetic agents.

Apnoeas are treated by stimulation, bag-mask ventilation, nCPAP or intubation and ventilation. The underlying cause should be treated. Caffeine may be used as a respiratory stimulant. It has a wide therapeutic range and may reduce BPD and neurodevelopmental disability.

Apnoea of prematurity usually resolves by 43 weeks post-menstrual age. Term neonates are at low risk of post-operative apnoea after routine minor surgery at 44 weeks post-menstrual age, but the probability of post-operative apnoeas decreases to less than 1% only at 60 weeks post-menstrual age in premature neonates (i.e. for a baby born at 28 weeks, at 8 months chronological age).

Sepsis

Infection is a major cause of morbidity and mortality in premature infants and may present with non-specific signs including hypothermia, hyperthermia, tachycardia, apnoea, bradycardia, feeding problems, increased oxygen requirements or metabolic acidosis. A fall in platelet count of >30% is frequently seen, for which the differential diagnosis is intraventricular haemorrhage or NEC.

Early onset infection is usually acquired from the mother (group B streptococci, *Escherichia coli*), after the first week of life due to nosocomial infection (*Staphylococcus aureus*, Klebsiella, Pseudomonas). Late onset sepsis may be due to *Candida albicans* or Gram-negative organisms, particularly in association with in-dwelling catheters. Ideally cultures should dictate antibiotic treatment.

Patent ductus arteriosus

The arterial duct is one of the fetal shunts and closes in response to increased oxygen levels and a fall in circulating prostaglandins by 48 hours in 90% of term and 'well' premature babies. Patent ductus arteriosus (PDA) is seen in 50% of VLBW infants owing to low oxygen tension, continuing high prostaglandin levels, acidosis or expansion of the circulating volume.

Blood is shunted left-to-right across the PDA and causes high pulmonary blood flow, worsening RDS, cardiac failure and a low diastolic pressure. PDA is a risk factor for intraventricular haemorrhage, necrotising enterocolitis (NEC) and chronic lung disease (CLD).

PDA typically becomes symptomatic at 5–10 days as pulmonary vascular resistance falls. Clinical signs include increased work of breathing and increased ventilatory requirements, bounding pulses, and a continuous murmur with CXR cardiomegaly and increased vascular markings on CXR. Diagnosis is confirmed by echocardiography.

Treatment for symptomatic PDA includes fluid restriction, diuretics, and 'medical' closure with indomethacin or ibuprofen. NSAIDs may cause renal impairment, gastrointestinal haemorrhage and perforation and are contraindicated in the presence of thrombocytopenia. Surgical closure is indicated if symptoms persist, medical treatment fails or NSAIDs are contraindicated.

Necrotising enterocolitis

NEC is a disease of prematurity, and the incidence is inversely proportional to gestational age. It is seen in up to 8% of neonates admitted to NICU and is associated with a high mortality, up to 50%, depending on severity.

NEC is associated with hypoxic or ischaemic injury to the gut mucosa, causing inflammation and transmural necrosis affecting any part of the intestine, typically the terminal ileum, caecum or ascending colon. NEC is associated with early feeding with formula milk and colonisation with pathogenic bacteria; breast milk may be protective, but does not prevent NEC.

NEC classically presents with abdominal distension, bloody stool and bile-stained aspirates during the second to third week of life as full feeds are started. Signs of sepsis may predominate and progress to apnoea with shock and disseminated intravascular coagulation. The abdominal wall may be reddened and intestinal perforation may cause a localised mass. Abdominal X-ray shows characteristic thickened dilated loops of bowel, with intramural gas or portal venous gas. Free gas indicates gut perforation and a poor outcome. There may be a low platelet count, raised C-reactive protein and metabolic acidosis.

Medical treatment includes fluid resuscitation, +/− inotropes and correction of coagulopathy, with withdrawal of feeds and 7–10 days of broad-spectrum antibiotics and total parenteral nutrition. Fifty per cent of infants with NEC require surgery for intestinal perforation or failure of medical treatment. Surgical options include resection of necrotic bowel and formation of a proximal stoma and distal mucous fistula, or gut resection and primary anastomoses. Critically ill babies may be treated with a peritoneal drain, or proximal defunctioning jejunostomy and 'second look' laparotomy at 24 hours if the baby survives.

Intraventricular haemorrhage

Severe disability may be seen in premature infants, usually due to germinal matrix intraventricular haemorrhage (IVH), which may be classified into four grades:

- Grade I   Germinal matrix haemorrhage
- Grade II   IVH without ventricular enlargement
- Grade II   IVH with ventricular enlargement
- Grade III   IVH with extension into the parenchyma

The prognosis in grade I and II IVH is good; grade III IVH is associated with severe impairment in 40% and grade IV IVH is associated with severe impairment in 90% of infants.

Major IVH usually occurs within the first few days of life; the risk is inversely proportional to gestational age as cerebral autoregulation has not yet developed. Risk factors for IVH therefore include hypotension, fluctuating blood pressure, morphine infusion (causing hypotension), hypertonic infusions, hypoxia and hypocapnia.

Mean arterial pressure (MAP) should be maintained within normal range as much as possible by judicious use of volume expansion, early use of inotropic agents such as adrenaline or dopamine, and avoidance of aggressive volume expansion, especially in the first few days of life. The normal lower limit of MAP is roughly equivalent to the gestational age on the first day of life, and is at least 30 mmHg by day 3 of life.

Periventricular leukomalacia (PVL) describes histological changes in periventricular white matter seen in premature infants. PVL is associated with hypoxic–ischaemic or toxic injury, infection, impaired cerebral autoregulation, cerebral 'steal' due to a large PDA and severe hypocapnia. Bilateral occipital cystic PVL is a very strong predictor of cerebral palsy, particularly spastic diplegia.

Retinopathy of prematurity and oxygen toxicity

Retinopathy of prematurity (ROP) is seen in LBW infants less than 32 weeks gestation, and is due to hyperoxia in the first weeks of life, which causes vasoconstriction of retinal vessels leading to retinal ischaemia and subsequent vasoproliferation. Good neonatal care and ophthalmic screening and treatment can largely prevent ROP.

There is concern that even brief exposure to high oxygen levels is associated with increased morbidity and mortality in VLBW infants; fluctuations in oxygen levels should be avoided and oxygen saturation maintained between 88 and 95%, not exceeding 95%. Newborn resuscitation should be carried out with room air rather than 100% oxygen.

Pain perception and early brain development

Neonates, including premature neonates, show well-developed responses to painful stimuli. Attenuation of the stress response to surgery and other painful interventions has been shown to improve morbidity and mortality.

Recent work has investigated the effects of anaesthetic drugs such as midazolam, nitrous oxide, isoflurane and ketamine on the developing brain. In animal experiments these agents were found to cause widespread apoptosis with persistent memory and learning impairment. The relevance to clinical practice is unclear, but only essential surgery should be performed in early life.

Conduct of anaesthesia in the premature infant
General considerations

Anaesthesia and surgery in the premature neonate are high risk. They require close collaboration with the neonatologists and careful attention to detail for successful outcomes. Consent should be discussed with the parents and questions answered fully.

In some situations it is possible for surgery to take place in the NICU. This has the advantage of providing a thermoneutral environment, minimal handling and access to a neonatal ventilator, but potentially limited access for the surgeon. PDA ligation is frequently performed in the NICU but laparotomy for NEC is more challenging and usually reserved for babies *in extremis*. If babies are transported to theatre, they must be kept warm, with minimal handling and extreme care not to displace intravenous lines or the tracheal tube during transport.

Particular factors that should be taken into account when anaesthetising premature infants:

- The temperature of the operating room should be raised to 25 °C and there should be a means of heating the baby (overhead heater or hot air) and heating all fluids.
- The surgical drapes should be lightweight, ideally plastic, so that the baby (and the tracheal tube) can be seen at all times. Drapes should not be stuck to the fragile skin, and the surgeons must not rest their hands on the infant.
- Invasive monitoring is useful in the septic patient receiving inotropes, or when cardiovascular stability is anticipated, and is ideally inserted prior to surgery.
- End-tidal CO_2 may significantly under-read.
- An air/oxygen mix should be used and hyperoxia avoided (oxygen saturation <95%).

Anaesthesia should only be induced when all are fully prepared. An oral uncuffed tracheal tube (2.5–3 mm internal diameter) is usual, or a shouldered tracheal tube (Cole tube). The advantage of the latter is that there is less resistance to ventilation, the disadvantage that the wide portion of the tube may be displaced between the cords to cause subglottic stenosis. The tracheal tube is often tied to a bonnet, and the position should be rechecked every time the infant is moved.

Avoid hyperventilation, oxygen saturation >95%, high peak inspiratory pressures and barotrauma. Permissive hypercapnia is acceptable. Isotonic fluids should be used during surgery (0.9% saline, Hartmann's or Ringers lactate), given as boluses of 10 ml kg^{-1} and titrated to blood pressure, heart rate, capillary refill time and base excess if available. Avoid swings in blood pressure and excessive volume

loading. Blood should be transfused to maintain a haematocrit of 36% in the newborn infant (high levels of HbF); 30% in the chronically transfused infant.

Blood glucose should be monitored and glucose-containing maintenance fluids continued during surgery. This fluid should not be used for bolus administration.

Multimodal analgesia should be used for pain relief.

Special situations
Anaesthesia for NEC

- Babies require careful pre-operative resuscitation and correction of acid–base balance and coagulopathy, and may require blood, platelets and fresh frozen plasma during surgery.
- Fluid shifts during surgery may be significant, up to 60–80 ml kg^{-1}, but avoid excessive fluid volumes.

Anaesthesia for PDA ligation

- The position of the aortic arch should be checked before the child is positioned for thoracotomy to clip the PDA.
- It is occasionally difficult to identify anatomical structures during surgery, and it is possible to place the clip incorrectly. Correct placement of clip is indicated by rise in blood pressure, particularly diastolic blood pressure. A pulse oximeter should be placed on the lower half of the body to detect accidental ligation of the descending aorta. Persistent desaturation after reinflation of the lung indicates accidental ligation of the pulmonary artery.
- Intercostal nerve blocks placed by the surgeon under direct vision are useful (limit dose of L-bupivacaine to 1.5 mg kg^{-1}).

Conduct of anaesthesia in the ex-premature infant
General considerations

The child may have chronic lung disease, reduced lung compliance, asthma, gastro-oesophageal reflux, impaired renal concentrating ability, chronic anaemia, failure to thrive, neurodevelopmental delay and/or seizures, subglottic stenosis and difficult venous access.

The child will be susceptible to post-operative apnoeas up to 60 weeks post-menstrual age and may require post-operative nCPAP or ventilation; oral caffeine may be considered, particularly if previously used.

Anaesthesia for hernia repair

- Inhalational anaesthesia using sevoflurane or desflurane for maintenance, with caudal anaesthesia or ilioinguinal nerve block and paracetamol for post-operative analgesia.
- Spinal anaesthesia may be suitable in experienced hands and may reduce post-operative apnoeas, provided supplemental sedation is avoided.

Anaesthesia for ventriculo-peritoneal (VP) shunt

- The theatre should be warmed and prolonged exposure avoided as the baby is at risk of hypothermia.

- The surgery is painful, and judicious use of opioids is required for post-operative analgesia in combination with paracetamol and ibuprofen; the baby is at risk for post-operative apnoeas and should be monitored carefully post-operatively.

Key points

- The impact of premature birth is life-long, affects multiple organ systems and is associated with reduced life expectancy.
- Modern neonatal intensive care has improved survival of extreme premature and low birthweight babies, although problems associated with chronic lung disease, poor growth and developmental delay are common.
- Premature babies commonly present for surgery in association with patent ductus, necrotising entercolitis or retinopathy of prematurity; surgery is high risk, and close collaboration with the neonatal team is required to ensure the baby is in optimal condition for surgery.
- Ex-premature infants may have a wide range of disabilities, and poor venous access is to be expected.

Further reading

Bingham R, Lloyd Thomas A, Sury M, eds. *Hatch and Sumner's Textbook of Paediatric Anaesthesia*. Churchill Livingstone. 2007.

Rennie J, ed. *Roberton's Textbook of Neonatology*, 4th edition. Elsevier Ltd. 2005.

Subramanian S. Extremely low birth weight infant. Medscape reference:

Drugs, diseases and procedures. http://emedicine.medscape.com/article/979717

Chapter

10

Day-case anaesthesia in children

Peter A. Stoddart

Introduction

Most children undergoing elective surgery or diagnostic procedures are discharged home on the same day. The development of day surgery was primarily driven by the need to reduce cost and improve utilisation of resources, but there are significant benefits for children, particularly as day-case surgery limits the separation of an otherwise healthy child from their home and family environment. Children with chronic or complex healthcare needs also benefit as day-case surgery reduces the time spent in hospital and risk of hospital acquired infections. Successful day-case surgery requires the anaesthetist to work as part of a multidisciplinary team and to use techniques to minimise peri-operative morbidity, particularly post-operative nausea and vomiting (PONV) and pain. It works well both in a specialist paediatric setting and at the local district hospital where most children continue to be managed.

Standards for day-case surgery and anaesthesia

A paediatric day-case service needs clear leadership, organisation and infrastructure based on the guidance and standards set by the Department of Health and professional bodies. A multidisciplinary report published by Action for Sick Children in 1991, 'Just for the Day', set 12 quality standards describing the ethos, staffing, facilities and information required for children and families needing day-case procedures, and these standards are still relevant today. Key recommendations include:

- Admission should be planned in an integrated way to include pre-admission, day of admission and post-admission periods.
- The child must not be admitted or treated alongside adults.
- Medical, nursing and all other staff must have received specific training and be skilled in working with children and their families.
- Specific written information must be provided to ensure parents understand their role and responsibilities throughout the episode.

Many day units are freestanding or organised as separate units within a larger hospital. In a non-specialist hospital it is important to foster child-centred care, and in the day unit this may be achieved by reserving dedicated sessions for children. Staff should have the appropriate skills and experience in paediatric day-case surgery, and should not be required to look after children of higher acuity (or adult patients) at the same time.

Clinical standards have been further defined by the Department of Health (DH) 'Getting the right start: National Service Framework for Children' and incorporated into guidance documents from the professional colleges, the Royal College of Nursing, Royal College of Surgeons Children's Surgical Forum, and the Royal College of Anaesthetists. The delivery of these standards is challenging, particularly with respect to pain management and training in child protection and paediatric resuscitation. The Royal College of Anaesthetists has recognised this; it supports local competency based resuscitation training programmes and has developed a specific e-learning module for child protection (http://www.e-lfh.org.uk/projects/safeguarding/index.html).

Core Topics in Paediatric Anaesthesia, ed. Ian James and Isabeau Walker. Published by Cambridge University Press. © 2013 Cambridge University Press.

Organisation – patient selection and preparation

Patient selection

The Department of Health has set a target to achieve more than 75% of surgery as day-case care. The DH publication 'Day surgery: operational guide' suggests that the default question should be 'Is there any justification for admitting this case as an inpatient?' rather than 'Is this patient suitable for day surgery?' Clearly this change in emphasis will increase the proportion of children undergoing day-case procedures. Careful patient selection is fundamental to safe, efficient day-case services. Procedures regularly undertaken as day cases are listed in Table 10.1.

Clear exclusions for day-surgery in children include:

- Major invasive operations;
- Surgery associated with significant physiological derangement or prolonged post-operative pain;
- Children needing specialist nursing or nutritional care.

Many patients are excluded because of their age, prematurity, co-existing medical conditions, previous anaesthetic problems or social circumstances. Children should be discharged home to an environment where they will receive at least the same level of care they would have by remaining in hospital. Typical exclusions are listed in Table 10.2. Some exclusions are relative, and decisions may have to be made on a case-by-case basis after discussion with an anaesthetist.

The lower age limit for day surgery depends on the individual unit. A specialist paediatric centre may accept term babies and healthy ex-premature infants > 60 weeks post-conceptional age for day surgery but many district hospitals have a 6- or 12-month minimum age limit because of their infrequent experience with younger infants.

The inclusion of tonsillectomy as a day-case procedure has been controversial in the United Kingdom owing to concerns about post-operative haemorrhage, pain control and PONV. However, many centres now undertake this procedure as a routine using clearly defined day-case tonsillectomy guidelines for anaesthesia, surgery and post-operative care delivered by an experienced consultant-led team. Exclusions include children under 3 years old, or with obstructive sleep apnoea or syndromes that affect the airway, e.g. Down

Table 10.1 Procedures and surgery commonly undertaken as day cases

General
- Excision of minor lumps and bumps including lymph nodes
- Herniotomy
- Excision of hyrocoele
- Umbilical hernia repair

Urology
- Circumcision
- Orchidopexy
- Cystoscopy including removal of ureteric stents
- Minor hypospadias

ENT
- Adenotonsillectomy
- Myringotomy
- Diagnostic microlaryngoscopy
- Removal of foreign body
- Nose manipulation under anaesthetic (MUA)

Dental
- Extraction
- Conservation

Ophthalmic
- Strabismus/ptosis correction
- Examination under anaesthetic
- Tear duct probing

Orthopaedic
- Botox injections
- Change of plaster
- Arthroscopy
- Removal of metalwork

Plastic
- Dressing changes, removal sutures
- Excision of skin lesion including laser therapy
- Pinnaplasty

Medical
- Diagnostic cardiac catheterisation
- Bone marrow sampling
- Lumbar puncture and intrathecal cytotoxics
- Radiotherapy
- MRI, CT scan

syndrome or mucopolysaccharidosis. Surgery is performed in the morning so that children can remain in hospital for at least 6 hours to ensure that they are pain-free, drinking and not bleeding before discharge home. Community follow-up and communication with the general practitioner is essential for all day cases, particularly for children undergoing day-case tonsillectomy.

Table 10.2 Common exclusions for day-case anaesthesia

Surgical
- Open cavity surgery involving cranium, thorax or abdomen
- Associated with significant or prolonged pain requiring more than simple analgesia
- Requirement for specialist nursing e.g. risk of compartment syndrome
- Prolonged procedure > 90 mins
- Airway surgery e.g. laryngeal papillomas
- Risk of significant post-operative haemorrhage

Patient
- Prematurity with post-conceptional age <60 weeks
- Poorly controlled systemic disease e.g. epilepsy, asthma, metabolic disease and diabetes
- Acute viral or bacterial respiratory infection
- Obstructive sleep apnoea especially in association with obesity or Down syndrome
- Complex congenital cardiac disease or cardiac failure
- Sickle cell disease
- Neuromuscular disease e.g. Duchenne muscular dystrophy or history of malignant hyperthermia

Social
- Parents unable to cope with an additional sick child
- Single parent with poor local support
- Lack of telephone
- Inadequate transport home. Public transport may be acceptable e.g. for a child in a pushchair
- Prolonged journey home e.g. greater than 1 hour

Pre-admission preparation

Good organisation and planning by the admission clerks, ward nurses, play therapists, theatre staff, surgeons and anaesthetists is essential to ensure the smooth running of a unit that is welcoming and friendly and minimises potential upset to the child and their family. Adequate preparation for the family is required, with clear written information about what to expect, what to bring and what to do on the day, especially in terms of fasting guidelines and routine medication. For the child, information may be presented in the form of a story or interactive book, DVD or Internet material. The Royal College of Anaesthetists and Association of Paediatric Anaesthetists of Great Britain and Ireland have published an excellent series of patient information leaflets for children and young people of different ages (http://www.youranaesthetic.info).

Nurse-led assessment using a pre-admission screening questionnaire should be used to identify any potential problems that need to be discussed or assessed by a senior anaesthetist pre-operatively, and will prevent unexpected cancellations on the day. Pre-admission assessment may be carried out at initial booking, on the phone using standardised questionnaires, or during a visit to the day unit to meet the nurses and play specialists, and to see the ward and possibly the recovery unit. Many families find this particularly beneficial, and such pre-operative visits have been shown to reduce anxiety on admission. Some units offer families visits on a weekend in the form of a Saturday Club. Fit healthy ASA 1 or 2 children do not need any pre-anaesthetic screening investigations except for a sickle cell test in those at risk.

All children must be seen on the day of admission by the surgeon (or paediatrician for medical procedures) and anaesthetist, to confirm that the procedure is still required and that the child remains fit for anaesthesia, and to finalise consent.

Day surgery and the child with a cold

The child with a 'runny nose' or low-grade fever can cause concern. These symptoms are common and are reported in 20–30% of children presenting for day surgery, especially ENT surgery. The child who is fractious, clearly unwell or pyrexial (temperature >37.5 °C), or has clinical signs on chest auscultation, should be cancelled, as the additional anaesthetic risk is unwarranted for an elective procedure. However, most children are well and otherwise asymptomatic with a simple rhinitis, so delay is not required. The decision to postpone must rest with the anaesthetist and will be guided by their experience and expertise and by any co-morbidity of the child, particularly a history of asthma, atopy or prematurity, or the presence of other risk factors for peri-operative adverse respiratory events (parents who smoke, or the need for intubation, or surgery on the airway). Children who are cancelled because of an upper respiratory tract infection (URTI) in our unit have their surgery postponed for at least 2 weeks so that any airway irritability is likely to have recovered.

After admission to the day unit, children are encouraged to play, read, draw, watch TV/DVDs or play video games to pass the time prior to anaesthesia. In our unit most children come to the induction room in their own clothes or nightwear. It is standard UK practice for one or two parents to accompany the

Pre-admission clinic
Check for contraindications/allergies
Anaesthetist/ENT SHO to prescribe the following, unless contraindicated:

Premedication
Paracetamol 20 mg kg^{-1} (max 1 g)
Ametop to both hands

Take home medication
Paracetamol 20 mg kg^{-1} (max 1 g) 6 hourly for 10 days
Ibuprofen 10 mg kg^{-1} (max 200 mg) 8 hourly for 7 days
Codeine 1 mg kg^{-1} (max dose 60 mg) 6 hourly for 7 days (10 days if no NSAIDs)

Day of admission
Give premed as prescribed

Peri-operative analgesia
Fentanyl 1–2 mcg kg^{-1}
Diclofenac 1 mg kg^{-1} (max dose 100 mg)

Post-operative analgesia
Regular:
Paracetamol 20 mg kg^{-1} (max 1 g) 6 hourly
Ibuprofen 10 mg kg^{-1} (max 200 mg) 8 hourly
Codeine 1 mg kg^{-1} (max dose 60 mg) 6 hourly

Discharge medication
Take home medication as prescribed at pre-admission with **ibuprofen unless contraindicated**

Pain information leaflet and diary – **record medication given in diary up to time of discharge**

Ward contact details

Figure 10.1 Pain management guideline for day-case tonsillectomy patients at the Bristol Royal Hospital for Children NHS Trust.

child to the anaesthetic room, and to remain with them until after induction of anaesthesia. This usually avoids the need for pre-operative sedation. However, this may be stressful for the parents, and they must understand their role and what to expect, and a member of staff must accompany them. Parents are also encouraged to collect the child from the recovery room as soon as the child is awake.

Anaesthesia techniques

Planning and attention to detail improve outcomes after anaesthesia. The development of guidelines helps to standardise performance. An example of a guideline for the management of analgesia in hospital and at home after tonsillectomy is shown in Figure 10.1.

Premedication

Sedative premedication is occasionally needed because of high anxiety levels, even if the child and family are well prepared, and particularly for children with behavioural problems or poor previous experiences.

Oral midazolam 0.5 mg kg^{-1} is commonly used. The bitter taste may be disguised by mixing in flavoured syrup, and the child will usually be sedated or at least more cooperative after about 20–30 minutes. Midazolam may sometimes cause paradoxical excitation and poor emergence, particularly in pre-school children. This may be because midazolam blocks explicit memory but not implicit memory (the memory of being anxious). Midazolam premedication may also be responsible for anxiety and prolonged behavioural changes after discharge. Oral clonidine 4 mcg kg^{-1} at least 45 minutes before induction is a useful alternative; it does not taste unpleasant, and although it causes more sedation, it is associated with less behavioural disruption both in recovery and at home, and in a recent study was preferred by most parents.

The pain of cannulation for induction of anaesthesia is greatly reduced with topical anaesthesia with local anaesthetic creams or ethyl chloride spray. There are a number of local anaesthetic creams available for use pre-operatively, but until there are direct comparison decisions about which should be used, decisions are often based on cost.

- EMLA®. This was the first widely used local anaesthetic cream. It is a 5% eutectic mixture of lidocaine and prilocaine. It needs to be applied for an hour prior to cannulation and often causes vasoconstriction of the vein and surrounding skin.
- Ametop®. This is a 4% gel of tetracaine that produces topical anaesthesia for venepuncture in about 45 minutes that lasts up to 4–6 h after removal. Some children develop erythema and skin oedema that may obscure the vein.
- LMX 4®. This is a new liposomal preparation of 4% lidocaine that is effective 30 minutes after application but may also cause erythema and skin oedema.

Induction of anaesthesia

Many older children prefer intravenous induction. Venepuncture is better tolerated in a young child if they are sitting on their parent's knee whilst distracted with a familiar comfort toy, blanket, video games or DVD. Alternatively, inhalational induction with sevoflurane in oxygen or nitrous oxide may be preferred, particularly in small infants with difficult venous access or at the request of an older child. Inhalation induction is frequently combined with directed imagery and hypnotic relaxation techniques. Experienced anaesthetic teams are adaptable and use any or a combination of these induction techniques depending on the child and their own preferences.

Children undergoing day-case anaesthesia require straightforward general anaesthesia combined with a local anaesthetic block and/or non-opioid analgesia using paracetamol and a NSAID. Propofol 3–5 mg kg^{-1} is the intravenous induction agent of choice, as it suppresses upper airway reflexes thereby aiding insertion of a LMA or a tracheal tube if required. Pain on injection can be reduced with the newer preparations and a small dose of lidocaine 0.2 mg kg^{-1}. The antiemetic and recovery properties of propofol are particularly useful in a day-case setting.

Maintenance of anaesthesia

Maintenance is usually with an inhalational agent, the choice of which is governed by cost and airway irritability. Compared with isoflurane, the expensive newer agents sevoflurane and desflurane allow rapid awakening but not necessarily earlier discharge from recovery. Both are associated with episodes of agitated emergence, although these are less common in children who have good analgesia. Emergence delirium in recovery can be treated with a judicious dose of fentanyl 0.5 mcg kg^{-1}. Desflurane is an airway irritant, particularly in children with asthma, and is best avoided if the child has had a recent URTI. Total intravenous anaesthesia (TIVA), using a target-controlled infusion of propofol, sometimes with remifentanil, is particularly useful where there is a high risk of emesis as in pinnaplasty or strabismus surgery.

Airway management

Very short procedures, e.g. bone marrow sampling or lumbar puncture for chemotherapy, may be managed with simple mask anaesthesia. Anaesthesia for most body surface surgery may be administered with the child breathing spontaneously through a LMA or other supraglottic airway device. There are many different types of supraglottic airways in use, with a clear move to single-use disposable products because of the expense of sterilisation and risk of transmissible agents, although few have been trialled specifically in children. The flexible reinforced LMA is useful for head and neck surgery including tonsillectomy or strabismus surgery.

Tracheal intubation is not usually required for day surgery, but is not contraindicated, provided the correct size tube is selected and inserted and removed atraumatically. The intubation technique depends on the personal preference of the anaesthetist, commonly using deep sevoflurane or propofol anaesthesia followed by either controlled or spontaneous ventilation. Non-depolarising neuromuscular blocking agents may be also be used; 0.5 mg kg^{-1} atracurium can be easily reversed after 20 minutes with 0.05 mg kg^{-1} neostigmine and 0.01 mg kg^{-1} glycopyrrolate. The use of aminosteroid-based agents such as vecuronium and rocuronium may increase with the recent introduction of sugammadex, as this offers reversal of any depth of neuromuscular block with minimal side effects. Unfortunately the current high cost of sugammadex precludes the routine use of this drug. Suxamethonium has many minor and some rare life-threatening side effects, so routine use is avoided in current day case anaesthesia practice.

Analgesia

Good pain control with a low risk of PONV is fundamental to good day-case anaesthesia. Nursing staff must be trained and empowered to routinely monitor, record and treat pain. Long-acting opioids should be avoided, and even fentanyl can increase the risk of emesis, although low doses may avoid poor emergence in recovery.

Paracetamol is usually used in combination with a NSAID and provides good pain relief with minimal side effects. Pre-operative administration by mouth is convenient as most children have good experience of these analgesics and antipyretics at home. The recent introduction of an intravenous preparation of paracetamol increases the options for anaesthetists concerned about a large volume of oral paracetamol syrup before induction of anaesthesia (oral dose paracetamol 20–30 mg kg^{-1}). The NSAIDs, ibuprofen 5–10 mg kg^{-1} PO, or diclofenac 1–1.5 mg kg^{-1} PO, PR or IV are well tolerated and frequently used. Nevertheless the recognised contraindications and side effects must be remembered when prescribing, for example in leukaemia patients with thrombocytopenia, or children with a family history of aspirin induced asthma. NSAIDs can be used safely for most non-aspirin sensitive asthmatic children. If NSAIDs are precluded or rescue analgesia needed, codeine 1 mg kg^{-1} PO can be used. Tramadol 1–2 mg kg^{-1} is an alternative and has the added advantage of oral and intravenous formulations. Codeine or tramadol may be prescribed for oral use to take home if necessary.

Local anaesthetic blocks are the mainstay of post-operative analgesic management especially for infra-umbilical surgery. All children's anaesthetists should be practised at both caudal and simple nerve blocks e.g. penile and ilioinguinal/iliohypogastric blocks. The addition of clonidine 2 mcg kg^{-1} will increase the duration of caudal bupivacaine with minimal additional side effects. Caudal blocks alter both motor and proprioceptive function in the legs and are probably best reserved for non-ambulatory infants, as older children may find these side effects troublesome. Peripheral nerve and fascial blocks, e.g. rectus sheath or transversus abdominis plane (TAP) blocks, are associated with lower risk of major complications compared with neuroaxial blocks, and act for much longer than simple wound infiltration.

A number of studies have demonstrated high success rates of ultrasound-guided blocks using low volumes of local anaesthetic compared with the traditional surface landmark techniques, and ultrasound is routinely used in many centres (see Chapter 16). Low volume blocks minimise dose requirements of local anaesthetic and improve safety. Specific nerve blocks for limb surgery, e.g. femoral or sciatic/popliteal blocks, may also be performed using ultrasound guidance or peripheral nerve stimulators. These blocks produce excellent analgesia but also an associated motor block, so if used for day-case procedures, parents must be given explicit nursing advice with regard to mobilisation and to avoid the risk of the child developing pressure sores. Parents should be given clear advice about starting supplemental oral analgesia post-operatively to cope with the loss of pain relief at home when a local anaesthetic block wears off.

Post-operative nausea and vomiting

In adult practice, PONV after day surgery may result in unplanned admissions, but this is less of a problem in paediatric practice (see Chapter 19). Routine antiemetic administration is not indicated for young children, but should be targeted to high-risk patients, namely those with one or more risk factors for PONV:

- History of PONV or motion sickness;
- Older children, particularly adolescent girls;

- Children undergoing strabismus surgery, pinnaplasty or adenotonsillectomy;
- Children who have received peri-operative opioids.

Ondansetron 0.15 mg kg^{-1} IV or PO appears to be the most efficacious drug for the prevention of PONV, either alone, or in high-risk children combined with dexamethasone up to 0.15 mg kg^{-1} IV (maximum 4 mg). Dexamethasone should be avoided in those at risk of tumour lysis or diabetes in which case the recent reintroduction of droperidol 20 mcg kg^{-1} is a useful third line drug in the absence of contraindications (such as prolonged QT syndrome).

Dehydration and early fluid intake may provoke PONV. Children should be encouraged to drink clear fluids until 2 h pre-operatively and given intra-operative intravenous fluids, at least 10 ml kg^{-1} Hartmann's solution if they have not had a drink or are undergoing anaesthesia >30 min. After surgery, making children drink before discharge will increase the risk of vomiting, but they should be encouraged to drink if they are thirsty. Avoiding inhalational agents by using TIVA should be considered for high-risk patients, and newer techniques, including acupressure, are future possibilities.

Discharge after surgery

Before discharge the child must have returned to their pre-anaesthetic state and be pain-free, and there should be a clear plan for post-operative pain relief. They should be encouraged to drink and have a light snack before leaving. The time for discharge varies with the child and the procedure undertaken. Most children are ready to leave between 1.5 and 3 h after returning to the ward.

A benchmark of less than 3% of patients should need overnight admission because of an unforeseen surgical complication (typically bleeding) or anaesthetic complication (typically prolonged PONV or poor pain control). The management of unexpected admission needs a clear plan to be in place, particularly if the day unit is separate from an inpatient paediatric unit.

Care at home

Parents should be given clear advice about pain relief at home. This is simplified if analgesic combinations are dispensed pre-packed from the day-case unit (see Figure 10.1). The parents should be given both verbal and written post-operative advice concerning analgesic management and wound care, e.g. bathing, return to school, sporting activities, and also the possibility of time-limited behavioural and sleep changes (see Figure 10.2). The surgeon and anaesthetist should review the family post-operatively, or if nurse-led discharge, agreed protocols should be used. A discharge letter for the GP and community nurse should be given to the parents to ensure good communication with the primary healthcare team. A contact telephone number for parents to seek further advice is essential, and many units routinely contact families within 24/48 h for further support and feedback.

A successful day-case anaesthetic service is dependent on a multitude of often simple but inter-related issues e.g. good local anaesthetic blocks, avoiding tight bandaging for pinnaplasty to reduce PONV, or ensuring the child brings in (and takes home!) their favourite toy to reduce stress and anxiety in the anaesthetic room. Regular multidisciplinary audit and review of outcomes including patient and staff satisfaction is therefore a prerequisite for continued development.

Key points

- Paediatric day-case care is beneficial from both a cost and efficiency point of view and reduces disruption for the child and family.
- Child-centred care pathways are needed, with good organisation and clear information and instructions for families.
- Simple uncomplicated general anaesthesia with supplemental local analgesia is required to provide good pain control and low risk of emesis.
- Plans for unexpected admission, a written discharge summary and guidance for post-procedural symptom control with a telephone contact number are needed.
- Guidelines and standards have been written and set by the RCoA, RCN, RCS and Department of Health. Regular patient satisfaction surveys and audit of quality and safety of care should be conducted using these standards.

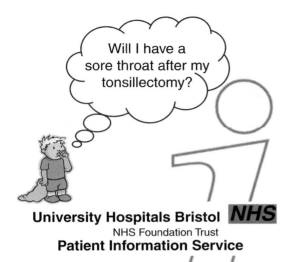

Will I have a sore throat after my tonsillectomy?

University Hospitals Bristol **NHS**
NHS Foundation Trust
Patient Information Service

Contact details for advice
Ward 36
On 0117 342 8336

Paediatric Pain Service
Bristol Royal Hospital for Children
Upper Maudlin Street
Bristol BS2 8BJ

Patient Information is
Supported by
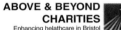
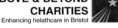
**ABOVE & BEYOND
CHARITIES**
Enhancing helathcare in Bristol

August 2008

**Hospital Switchboard: 0117 923 0000
Minicom: 0117 934 9869
www.uhbristol.nhs.uk**

For an Interpreter or Signer contact the telephone number
on your appointment letter.
For this leaflet in Large Print, in Braille,
Audio Format, Email, please call:
0117 342 3728

© UH Bristol NHS Foundation Trust   August 2008   CHILDREN/SORETONSIL/Aug08

What pain will my child experience?

Your child's throat will be sore for approximately seven to
ten days after the operation. Ear pain and 'smelly breath' are
also common during the first week. The ear pain can be more
of a nuisance especially at night. Chewing gum or sucking on a
sweet / ice pop may help reduce the discomfort in the throat
and ears as well as improve the taste. You should encourage
your child to continue to eat and drink as this helps them
recover and their throat to heal.

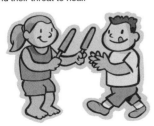

What medication will my child have?

During your child's stay in hospital a combination of
Paracetamol, Ibuprofen and Codeine will be used as pain
relief. It is normal practice for these to be given either
orally or rectally until your child is settled. Staff will ensure
that the medication is given regularly as this is the best way
to maintain comfort.

Will my child have pain relief to take home?

Yes, we will give you enough analgesia for ten days. This will
be a combination of Paracetamol, Ibuprofen and Codeine
or Paracetamol and Codeine. We advise both Paracetamol
and Ibuprofen are given daily for the first week as the
combination gives better pain relief. Codeine can be used if
your child is still experiencing pain.

If Ibuprofen is not suitable for your child we advise that the
codeine is given regularly with the Paracetamol for the first
week and then reduced as your child recovers.

Pain relief for home

There is guidance below on how often each of the medications
should be given; a pain assessment tool and a diary to help
you keep a record of the time and number of doses you give
your child.

Paracetamol

You will be given ten days supply of Paracetamol, four doses
a day are allowed. We advise that a dose is given before bed
and on waking. The other two doses should be given an hour
before lunch and tea so that your child is comfortable and
able to eat.

2

3

Figure 10.2 Patient information booklet for tonsillectomy at Bristol Royal Hospital for Children.

Ibuprofen

You will be given 7 days supply of Ibuprofen and your child will be **allowed only 3 doses a day.** This is a slightly higher dose than normal and that's why we have restricted it to 3 doses a day. We advise that the dose is given at meal times to maintain maximum comfort for eating and drinking.

The Ibuprofen should be stopped and the GP seen if your child develops 'tummy' pain, vomits blood or has blood in their motion.

Codeine

You will be given 7 days supply of Codeine. This medicine is to be used if regular Paracetamol and Ibuprofen are not keeping your child comfortable. Your child will be allowed up to 4 doses of Codeine a day. If Ibuprofen is not suitable for your child Codeine will be prescribed regularly.

They may not need 4 doses. We usually find a dose morning and evening most effective. The further two doses may be used if necessary, e.g. if they waken with pain in the night or during the afternoon. Although you have been given 7 days supply of codeine if **given only when needed** this supply may last for 10 days.

Codeine can cause constipation so it is very important to encourage your child to drink well and eat regularly.

4

What if the medication does not keep my child comfortable?

It is very rare for children not to be comfortable and able to eat and drink if the medication is given regularly as prescribed. However if your child is still uncomfortable please contact your GP who will assess your child for any complications and review their pain medications.

Taking the pain medicine regularly will make swallowing easier and speed recovery.

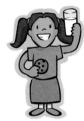

5

Pain Assessment Tool

Hurts Worst	10
Hurts WholeLot	8
Hurts EvenMore	6
Hurts LittleMore	4
Hurts Little Bit	2
No Hurt	0

6

Pain medicine diary

This diary will help you keep a record of when your child's medication is next due and see when they are improving.
(* as you give each dose)

Medication	Day 1	Day 2	Day 3	Day 4	Day 5	Day 6	Day 7	Day 8	Day 9	Day 10
Paracetamol										
Ibuprofen										
Codeine										
Average daily pain score 0 = no pain 10 = worst pain										
Sleeping through the night										
Drinking regularly										
Eating regularly										

7

Figure 10.2 (cont.)

Further reading

Association of Paediatric Anaesthetists of Great Britain and Ireland. *Good Practice in Postop and Procedural Pain*. APAGBI. 2008; http://www.apagbi.org.uk/docs/APA_Guidelines_on_Pain_Management.pdf

Association of Paediatric Anaesthetists of Great Britain and Ireland. *APA Guidelines on the Prevention of Postoperative Vomiting in Children*. APAGBI. 2009; http://www.apagbi.org.uk/docs/Final%20APA%20POV%20Guidelines%20ASC%2002%2009%20compressed.pdf

Brennan LJ. Modern day-case anaesthesia for children. *Br J Anaes* 1999;**83**:91–103.

Department of Health. *Day surgery: Operational guide*. DH. 2002; http://www.dh.gov.uk/en/Publicationsandstatistics/Publications/PublicationsPolicyAndGuidance/DH_4005487

Department of Health. *Getting the Right Start*. National Service Framework for Children: Standard for hospital services. DH. 2003; http://www.dh.gov.uk/prod_consum_dh/groups/dh_digitalassets/@dh/@en/documents/digitalasset/dh_4067251.pdf

Ewah BN, Robb PJ, Raw M. Postoperative pain, nausea and vomiting following paediatric day-case tonsillectomy. *Anaesthesia* 2006;**61**:116–22.

Lonnqvist P-A, Morton NS. Paediatric day-case anaesthesia and pain control. *Curr Opin Anaesthesiol* 2006;**19**:617–21.

Royal College of Anaesthetists. *Guidance on the Provision of Paediatric Anaesthetic Services*. RCoA. 2004; http://www.rcoa.ac.uk/docs/GPAS-Paeds.pdf

Royal College of Surgeons of England. *Surgery for Children: Delivering a First Class Service*. The Royal College of Surgeons of England. 2007; http://www.rcseng.ac.uk/rcseng/content/publications/docs/CSF.html

Thornes R. (Caring for Children in the Health Services) *Just for the Day – A Study of Services for Children Admitted to Hospital for Day Treatment*. Action for Sick Children. 1991.

White MC, Cook TM, Stoddart PA. A critique of elective pediatric supraglottic airway devices. *Ped Anes* 2009;**19**:55–65.

General principles and safe paediatric anaesthesia

Ian James

Introduction

Safety is paramount in the provision of anaesthesia for all patients. Children comprise a quarter of the population, and many will need anaesthesia at some time during childhood. Most children undergoing surgery are fit and healthy, and in England and Wales most elective procedures and anaesthesia for minor trauma are undertaken outside a specialist paediatric centre. However, there are many situations where children require 'specialised paediatric anaesthesia', for instance neonates and infants, those undergoing complex surgery, or those with significant co-morbidity. It is essential that wherever children are cared for, staff are appropriately trained, there is suitable equipment and the child is in an environment that is child- and family-friendly. Ideally, specialist and non-specialist centres should work closely together in clinical networks to provide comprehensive services for children. Regular clinical attachments help to foster links and enable non-specialist anaesthetists to maintain their skills.

Guidance on the provision of appropriate anaesthetic services for children has been published (see Further reading). The main principles include:

- Children should be separated from and not treated alongside adults. The specific needs of adolescents and young people should be recognised.
- Anaesthesia should be undertaken or overseen by staff who have undergone appropriate training and maintain regular paediatric practice.
- The anaesthetic assistant, recovery and ward staff must possess specific paediatric skills.
- Staff should undergo regular paediatric resuscitation training.

- There should be acute pain services for children.
- There should be neonatal, high dependency and intensive care services as determined by the nature of the surgery undertaken in that hospital.
- Where a child presents to a non-specialist centre with a life-threatening condition, and it is not feasible to transfer the child, the most senior appropriately experienced anaesthetist available should care for that child.
- Guidelines for the management of common emergencies in children, including resuscitation, anaphylaxis and management of the head injured child should be readily available.
- Wherever possible, parents (or carers) should be involved in care and decisions about the child.

Risks of anaesthesia

Mortality

General anaesthesia in healthy children without co-morbidity undergoing elective surgery is very safe, with a risk of death related to anaesthesia generally quoted as about 1 in 200 000 anaesthetics. Some specialist centres have reported zero mortality in large series of children in this category. In one large North American survey, the most common cause of peri-operative cardiac arrest was cardiovascular, most commonly due to hypovolaemia from blood loss or hyperkalaemia from transfusion of stored blood. Respiratory causes were the next most frequent, most commonly due to airway obstruction in recovery due to laryngospasm. Equipment-related cardiac arrest occurred mainly owing to vascular injury from central venous lines. Medication-associated cardiac arrest is less frequent since the decline in the use of halothane. Children at greatest risk of peri-operative

Core Topics in Paediatric Anaesthesia, ed. Ian James and Isabeau Walker. Published by Cambridge University Press. © 2013 Cambridge University Press.

cardiac arrest and mortality due to anaesthesia are those with heart disease, or pulmonary hypertension, and those under 1 year of age, with the highest risk group being neonates undergoing cardiac surgery.

Where there is increased risk due to co-morbidity or anticipated anaesthetic or surgical difficulty, it is essential that this is discussed with the parents or carers and that this is documented in the medical records.

Morbidity

Parents frequently ask about the side effects of anaesthetics. There are common and very common side effects (1:10–1:100 children); these include nausea and vomiting (particularly in older children), sore throat and dizziness. Uncommon side effects (1:1000–1:10 000) include post-operative respiratory depression (higher risk in neonates, especially ex-premature neonates), awareness or damage to teeth. Awareness may occur more commonly in children than adults, although fortunately children rarely develop symptoms of post-traumatic stress disorder. Risk factors for awareness appear to be intubation (greater stimulation) and the use of nitrous oxide (possibly associated with use of a lower concentration of inhaled volatile agent). Rare complications (1:10 000–1:100 000) include peri-operative cardiac arrest, as described above.

Occasionally parents may ask whether anaesthetics, especially repeated anaesthetics, can have a detrimental effect on their child's development. In the past few years, concerns have been raised from animal experiments suggesting that anaesthesia agents that function as NMDA antagonists or GABA agonists cause neuro-apoptosis in the immature mammalian brain. This has led to concerns about general anaesthesia in preterm and newborn infants. There is inadequate information at present to suggest that this is a problem in humans. Recent studies suggest that there are no adverse long-term effects on the brain of a single short anaesthetic in young children, but some have suggested that multiple anaesthetics before the age of 4 years may be associated with learning difficulties, although this is not proven. The general consensus of experts is that it is unethical and harmful to deny anaesthesia to neonates and small infants if they need it, and there is no reason to change practice at present. This is now an active field of research.

Preparation for theatre

It is essential that all children undergo anaesthesia assessment prior to coming to theatre (see Chapter 6). As well as establishing fitness for anaesthesia and determining co-morbidity, this will allow an opportunity to discuss the plan for and the risks of anaesthesia. The need for premedication will depend on the preference of the anaesthetist and the type of surgery being undertaken and of course on the perceived state of anxiety of the child. Parents may be able to offer advice on their child's likely behaviour, but it is not uncommon for a child to appear calm and unperturbed during the pre-operative visit yet to become extremely distressed and uncooperative on arriving in the anaesthetic room. If premedication and/or topical analgesia is prescribed, it is important to try to get the timing right for its administration. The most common premedication is oral midazolam $0.5 \, \text{mg kg}^{-1}$ given approximately 30 minutes before induction, although occasionally the children who would most benefit from some form of anxiolysis will refuse it or spit it out. Midazolam can also be given intranasally ($0.2 \, \text{mg kg}^{-1}$) but it can cause an unpleasant burning sensation in the nose. Intranasal dexmedetomidine $1 \, \text{mcg kg}^{-1}$ has been suggested as an alternative but may take over 60 minutes to take effect.

For topical analgesia tetracaine 4% gel (Ametop®) and lidocaine 4% cream (LMX 4®) work within 45 minutes, while EMLA® may take an hour to be effective. Ethyl chloride spray can make the skin less sensitive for a few minutes and is favoured by some older children but is flammable and should be used with caution in environments with a lot of electrical equipment.

If the procedure is being undertaken in a theatre that is not regularly used for children, the anaesthetist must take particular care to ensure that the appropriate equipment for a child is available and is in working order. This includes appropriate ventilator settings; for most children pressure-controlled ventilation is used, and the default settings for volume-controlled ventilation suitable for an adult will cause harm. Theatre temperature may need to be increased if a small child is to be operated on. Children can lose heat rapidly, and warming equipment should be employed for all children, other than perhaps for very short cases. Modern warming equipment can be very effective and should never be used without monitoring core temperature.

All children must be weighed accurately before theatre as all drug and fluid prescriptions are weight-based. In very obese children, lean body weight (LBW) should be calculated as most drug doses should be based on lean rather than actual body weight. Drugs and fluids should be drawn up and prepared carefully, using appropriately sized syringes and giving sets. An obsessive-compulsive personality trait is beneficial.

Surgical Safety Checklist

The WHO Surgical Safety Checklist should be used for all cases. There should also be a team brief prior to the case or the list starting to ensure that team members are acquainted, that all are clear what operation is to be done before surgery starts, and any equipment that may be needed is available. Figure 11.1 shows our standard routine.

Parental presence during induction

This can be extremely helpful, and we generally allow both parents to remain until the child is asleep unless there is expected airway difficulty or a rapid sequence induction is planned, when it may be preferable to ask parents to leave prior to induction. Many studies have shown that parental presence leads to reduction in both the child's and parent's anxiety. For small children, induction is usually undertaken in the parent's arms or sitting on their lap. Both parents and children overwhelmingly support parental presence at induction, although some parents may find the experience upsetting. It is important to let them know what to expect, and also that they do not have to be present if they do not wish to be.

For children who are particularly anxious it may be less distressing if they are allowed to come to theatre in normal clothes. For adolescent children anxieties about modesty should be anticipated; they too may feel more comfortable if not compelled to wear a revealing theatre gown. Hair clips and other accessories, if still in place, can be removed once the child is asleep.

Induction

The choice of intravenous or gas induction is generally determined by the preference of the child, parent and anaesthetist, although a lack of suitable veins in small infants often dictates an inhalational induction. Where appropriate, the child should be given the choice. Many children are frightened of needles while others may have previous experience of a gas induction and do not want to repeat it. Many children of course want neither, and it can sometimes be challenging to proceed without some form of restraint. Having the parent present to assist can be helpful. For very anxious children it can sometimes help to insert a cannula on the ward prior to transfer to theatre.

Sevoflurane is the most common means of gas induction. There is no 'correct' or 'best' means of using it. For some children a gradual increase of the vapour works well, for others moving rapidly to or starting at 8% is better. Nitrous oxide speeds up induction, and initial sedation with nitrous oxide and oxygen may make acceptance of a facemask easier.

Some children will tolerate a mask relatively happily, others less so. Applying a mask forcibly to a small child is oppressive and can lead to a more challenging induction at the time and at future surgery. It is often easier to use the cupped hand as a 'mask', holding it close to the nose and mouth.

There are some masks with fruit aromas that may help tolerance of a gas induction. There are also liquid essences of fruit or other pleasant aromas such as mint or chocolate available which can be added to the HME filter.

The most commonly used IV induction agent is propofol, although this can be very painful, especially in small veins. Higher doses, $3-5\,\mathrm{mg\,kg^{-1}}$, are needed in small children than adults. Thiopentone ($5-7\,\mathrm{mg\,kg^{-1}}$) is not commonly used but remains a useful alternative, as it is not associated with pain on injection.

Airway management

Many small infants partially obstruct readily during induction, and inserting a Guedel airway will generally be beneficial.

Airway management will depend on the type of surgery. Many tubes are secured with adhesive tape; it is important to ensure this does not stick to the mucosa of the lips. In small infants the skin can be fragile and tape should be removed with care at the end of surgery. It is very easy to inflate the stomach

Surgical Safety Checklist: aide memoire GOSH *NHS*

Figure 11.1 Surgical Safety Checklist. See plate section for colour version.

Theatre team brief at start of the session:

- Who is on the team today?
- What are we doing?
- Do we have the equipment?
- Are there any staffing issues?
- Any outside issues?
- Any time issues?
- Is the list order correct?

Sign-in: immediately prior to induction, led by the anaesthetist

- Consent form checked
- Surgical site marking checked
- Ward checks completed
- Allergies checked
- Metal check (MRI)
- Anaesthesia drugs and equipment checks completed
- Check blood available in fridge (if applicable)
- Airway/aspiration risk assessed – assistance and equipment available (if necessary)

- Remember stop before you block

Time-out: immediately prior to incision, led by the circulating nurse

- **Surgeon, anaesthetist and scrub nurse/ODP: confirm consent and site. Refer to the relevant imaging (if applicable)**
- Discuss the procedure briefly:
  - Anaesthetist: introduce case, confirm allergies, ASA score; any concerns?
  - Surgeon: review case; any critical or unusual steps?
  - Scrub nurse/ODP: confirm sterile equipment available, any other concerns?
- If relevant – perfusionist: bypass plans, any other concerns?
- Confirm antibiotic prophylaxis has been given (if necessary)
- Confirm appropriate warming measures in place
- Confirm thromboembolic prophylaxis undertaken (if necessary)
- Are there any new team members?

Sign-out: at completion of surgery, led by the circulating nurse

- Confirm swab, needle and instrument counts are correct
- Confirm procedure to be written in Theatre book
- Confirm specimen has been labelled (if appropriate)
- Any equipment issues to address/incident form to complete?
- Surgeon/Anaesthetist/Nurse: review the post-operative plans

Checklist Group 2011

with air when ventilating a small child by facemask. This can impede ventilation and a nasogastric tube should be inserted to deflate the stomach.

It is common practice to extubate neonates and infants fully 'awake', when their airway reflexes have returned and they are breathing regularly. For some older infants who are breathing spontaneously it may be appropriate to extubate 'deep', but this will usually require the MAC of the volatile agent to be around 1.5. Extubating an infant between these two extremes can lead to breath-holding or laryngospasm.

Laryngospasm

This occurs much more commonly in children than in adults, particularly in small infants. It most frequently occurs during induction or immediately after extubation, sometimes with no apparent precipitating cause. Often it is because the airway is stimulated too early during induction, or the tracheal tube is removed too early at the end of surgery. Blood or secretions at the larynx can precipitate laryngospasm.

Partial laryngospasm is characterised by a high-pitched inspiratory noise with increased respiratory effort but minimal visible sign of airflow. If laryngo-spasm is complete there will be no noise. It is important to recognise both quickly as hypoxia can rapidly ensue.

Management of laryngospasm involves prompt action:

- Ensure there is a tight-fitting facemask. Give high-flow 100% oxygen and apply CPAP to the circuit; the reservoir bag should be 'tight'.
- Apply jaw thrust and small rapid breaths, avoiding gastric inflation if possible.
- Alert the anaesthetic assistant, who should prepare the appropriate intubation equipment and tracheal tube as quickly as possible.
- Make sure the oximeter and ECG remain attached.
- If the laryngospasm does not resolve quickly, consider deepening anaesthesia with a volatile agent or give propofol $1 \, \text{mg} \, \text{kg}^{-1}$.
- If no improvement, give suxamethonium $1 \, \text{mg} \, \text{kg}^{-1}$ IV and atropine 20 mcg kg^{-1} and ventilate by hand; it may not be necessary to intubate. Suxamethonium $4 \, \text{mg} \, \text{kg}^{-1}$ IM may be used if the IV cannula has been displaced at the end of surgery.
- Consider passing a nasogastric tube after laryngospasm has resolved

Laryngospasm will usually settle without the need for intervention other than maintaining high-flow oxygen with positive pressure in the breathing circuit. Occasionally, at the end of surgery, it may be difficult to break the laryngospasm, and it may be necessary to re-institute anaesthesia, re-intubate and leave the tracheal tube in place until the patient is fully awake. Negative pressure pulmonary oedema may occur in young people after severe laryngospasm.

Rapid sequence induction

In theory, classic rapid sequence induction (RSI) should be used in all children at risk of regurgitation and aspiration. This includes those requiring emergency surgery that are not appropriately fasted, particularly those with proximal bowel obstruction, and in the child with post-tonsillectomy haemorrhage who may have a stomach full of blood. However, there are practical limitations that make classic

RSI difficult in infants, and in some instances inappropriate:

- Attempts to pre-oxygenate a frightened and uncooperative small child may be counter-productive.
- It is not always possible to obtain venous access in small infants to administer an intravenous induction agent and a rapidly acting muscle relaxant. Inhalational induction may be necessary.
- The high oxygen consumption seen in infants leads rapidly to hypoxia if ventilation is avoided before intubation.
- The cricoid ring is higher. Cricoid pressure can make intubation more difficult, and may not actually 'obstruct' the oesophagus effectively.

For these reasons many experienced paediatric anaesthetists will adopt a pragmatic approach in small infants with a potentially full stomach, and will gently ventilate while waiting for the muscle relaxant to work, with gently applied cricoid pressure. Suxamethonium $2 \, \text{mg} \, \text{kg}^{-1}$ remains the standard muscle relaxant, but as apnoea is not a fundamental component of this 'controlled RSI', many will use a slower, non-depolarising agent such as atracurium or rocuronium. For the older child classic RSI should be utilised.

Teeth

For children in the middle of orthodontic treatment it is important to establish whether their braces are fixed or can be removed. It is also very important to establish whether a child has any loose deciduous teeth. If very loose, it may be necessary to remove a tooth after induction to prevent it being dislodged during airway insertion and lost or inhaled. This possibility should be explained to the parents during the pre-operative visit. The tooth must be kept safe and handed to the parents after the procedure.

Occasionally a permanent tooth may be unintentionally avulsed during airway manipulation. It is important to be aware that this can be successfully salvaged if acted upon immediately. There is a 30-minute golden window for this, and a guideline such as that in Figure 11.2 should be followed.

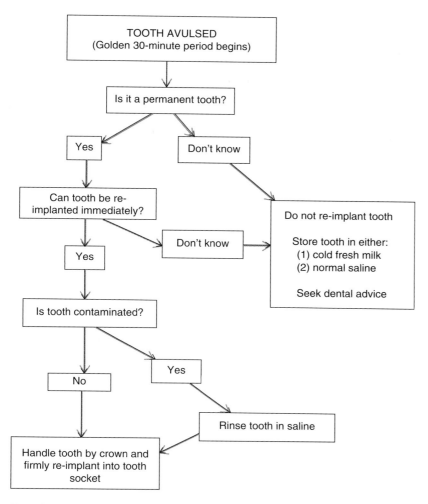

Figure 11.2 Management of avulsed tooth during general anaesthesia.

From Soneji B, Forde K, Mason C, Dental Department, Great Ormond Street Hospital NHS Foundation Trust.

Intravenous lines

These should be well-secured and preferably visible throughout the procedure. It is surprisingly easy for extravasation to occur in small infants, especially if fluid boluses are given rapidly under high pressure. Where a child arrives in theatre with an IV line already in place, it must be inspected carefully before being used for induction. The skin over the cannula tip should be visible and this will necessitate removing any dressings that may have been applied to prevent the child displacing the cannula. Pain on injection of saline should give rise to suspicion that the line has 'tissued', although it may also be due to phlebitis in a long-standing line.

It is not always possible of course for IV lines to be visible throughout the procedure. Before the child is covered with drapes it is important to ensure the line is working well. Many cannulae in children are placed over or near wrist and ankle joints, and ease of injection can be very positional. This must be resolved before the child is covered. If a line becomes more difficult to inject into or if fluids slow down during the procedure the possibility of extravasation should be considered.

At the end of the operation, all IV lines must be flushed with saline to avoid the possibility of later flushing of residual drugs into the circulation. There have been a number of reports to National Reporting and Learning Service in England of harm due to flushing of residual anaesthetic drugs in IV cannulae in children.

Extravasation

There are some drugs that will cause severe tissue injury if extravasation occurs which in some cases can lead to skin necrosis and nerve or tendon injury. Severe injury may necessitate later surgical release of contractures and skin grafting. Tissue damage occurs from cytotoxic drugs, hyperosmolar substances, highly acid or alkaline solutions, drugs formulated in alcohol or polyethylene glycol, or vasoconstrictor drugs causing local ischaemia. Occasionally damage occurs as a result of high volume extravasation causing mechanical tissue ischaemia.

Drugs most likely to cause problems during anaesthesia include:

- X-ray contrast media
- Thiopentone
- Atracurium
- Sodium bicarbonate
- Calcium chloride or gluconate
- Vasoactive drugs

There are established treatment protocols for extravasation injury that must be readily available. Immediate management involves minimising the concentration of drug at the site of extravasation by stopping the injection, and aspirating as much drug as possible from the cannula.

Where there has been significant leakage of a tissue-damaging drug, saline washout should be performed. This involves making multiple skin incisions around the site of extravasation. Saline is then injected through one or more of the incisions with a blunt needle to flush extravasated drug out through the other puncture sites. It may be necessary to obtain input from the plastic surgery service.

Positioning

This will be dictated largely by the surgical procedure and the majority of cases will be supine. The head should not be rotated beyond 65°, particularly in paralysed children, as this can lead to C1–2 facet dislocation. This atlanto-axial rotary subluxation can occur in children because of ligamentous laxity, poorly developed cervical musculature, horizontally orientated facet joints and wedge-shaped cervical

vertebrae. The head should be supported in a gel ring to prevent abnormal rotation.

Care should be taken to ensure that all pressure points are well padded, particularly when the patient is prone or on their side. Particular care must be taken to protect the eyes when the patient is prone.

If the arms are extended above the head, which may be necessary in some radiological investigations, they should be supported in such a way that there is no tension at the shoulder to avoid the possibility of a brachial plexus injury.

Latex allergy

There appears to be a substantial increase in the number of patients and medical staff who have developed sensitivity, and in some cases an allergy, to latex. All departments should have a protocol for managing such patients, the most important measure being establishing a latex-free environment. Ideally this should become standard in all operating theatres. Patients should be scheduled first on the list so that the presence of aerosolised latex particles is minimised. If this is not possible the theatre should be unused for at least 30 minutes prior to starting.

Those at high risk for serious reactions fall into three groups:

(1) Those with a history of latex anaphylaxis, confirmed by positive antibody testing;
(2) Those with a history of allergy to latex, with urticaria, eye swelling, central dermatitis or bronchospasm;
(3) Those with no previous reaction, but who have:
  - Spina bifida
  - Genito-urinary anomalies
  - Multiple surgical procedures
  - Documented reactions to IV drugs.

There appears to be cross-sensitivity to peanuts and to some fruits such as kiwi, banana or avocado, so allergy to these should raise an index of suspicion. Previous recommendations for premedication of latex-sensitive patients with steroids, antihistamine and H2 receptor blockers are no longer advised as this does not prevent a reaction nor does it affect the severity of reaction.

Departments should have well-documented protocols in the operating theatres and recovery areas detailing what equipment is latex-safe and what should be avoided. Latex-free anaesthetic equipment is now widely available. Items such as the operating table or transport trolley mattress should be fully covered, breathing circuit reservoir bags can be enclosed in a polythene bag, and blood pressure cuff hoses can be covered in tape. Elastoplast should be avoided. Drugs must not be drawn up by injecting through a rubber bung. Should a severe reaction occur, management is as below.

Acute major anaphylaxis during anaesthesia

Anaphylaxis is a severe life-threatening generalised or systemic hypersensitivity reaction, usually characterised by:

- Pharyngeal or laryngeal oedema
- Acute severe bronchospasm
- Hypotension
- Tachycardia
- Skin/mucosal changes

Hypotension may occur rapidly, although frequently the first indication to the alert anaesthetist is a change in the ventilatory parameters. This may be a rise in airway pressure or more commonly a fall in delivered tidal volume. Severe bronchospasm, with difficulty ventilating the lungs, will lead rapidly to a fall in oxygen saturation. In severe cases it can be exceedingly difficult to ventilate the lungs, and end-tidal CO_2 may rise owing to hypoventilation. A fall in end-tidal CO_2 may be seen if the bronchospasm is so severe that there is little alveolar ventilation.

The most likely causes of a drug-induced anaphylactic reaction in a child are antibiotics (penicillins or cephalosporins), lidocaine, radiological contrast media and latex. Reaction to muscle relaxants does not appear to be as common in children as in adults.

The treatment of a severe anaphylactic reaction is summarised in Figure 11.3. Adrenaline should be administered early. Where the treatment has been

- Discontinue suspected agent
- Summon help
- 100% oxygen, intubate if necessary
- Give adrenaline, 1 mcg kg^{-1} IV (0.1 ml kg^{-1} of 1:100 000)
- Give rapid volume bolus, 10–20 ml kg^{-1}, Hartmann's solution or similar
- Repeat adrenaline as necessary for resistant hypotension or bronchospasm; start continuous infusion if multiple boluses required
- CPR if necessary

For adrenaline-resistant bronchospasm:

- Salbutamol, 5–15 mcg kg^{-1} IV

or

- Aminophylline, 5 mg kg^{-1} IV over 20 minutes

Consider:

Hydrocortisone	4 mg kg^{-1} IV	
Chlorpheniramine	<6 months:	250 mcg kg^{-1} IV
	6 m–6 y:	2.5 mg
	6–12 y:	5 mg
	>12 y:	10 mg

For resistant hypotension, start noradrenaline infusion, 0.05–0.5 mcg kg^{-1} min^{-1}

Check blood gas and treat acidosis if present.

Check coagulation, treat as appropriate.

Figure 11.3 Emergency management of severe anaphylaxis.

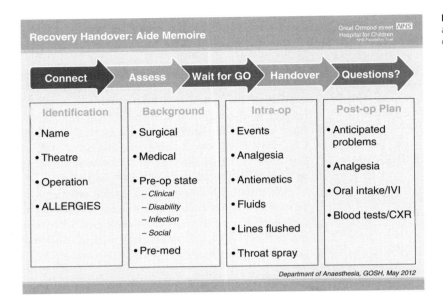

Figure 11.4 Recovery handover aide-memoire. See plate section for colour version.

prolonged, or infusions of adrenaline or noradrenaline have been necessary, the patient should be admitted to a high dependency or intensive care unit for post-operative monitoring.

Even in cases where the situation is resolved promptly the patient should remain in hospital overnight, as in up to 20% of cases there can be a biphasic reaction with recurrence of symptoms up to 12 hours later.

Full documentation of the episode is essential. If possible, as soon as the patient has stabilised, blood samples for mast-cell tryptase (5 ml into plain tube) should be taken as these will help to determine whether there was mast-cell degranulation. Peak levels occur at 1–2 hours, and repeat samples should be taken at 1, 2, 4 and 12 hours to document the reaction. The Immunology service should be contacted to investigate the patient further.

Recovery

It is important to provide a thorough handover to the recovery room or intensive care staff at the end of the procedure. This should include details of intra-operative analgesia, antiemetics and antibiotics that have been given or charted for post-operative administration, any airway or venous access difficulties that have been encountered, and any other adverse events. If topical anaesthesia has been applied to the larynx it is important to advise when the patient can drink.

We usually advise that this should be at least 2 hours after the larynx was sprayed. A simple aide-memoire such as that shown in Figure 11.4 works well in ensuring that no vital information is missed out. It is also essential to ensure all intravenous lines have been adequately flushed with saline to avoid later inadvertent administration of residual anaesthetic agents.

Emergence delirium

Behavioural disturbance during early emergence from anaesthesia, usually involving inconsolable crying, thrashing about and disorientation, has been recognised for many years, and a 'Paediatric Anaesthesia Emergence Delirium' (PAED) scale has been developed. It is particularly common in pre-school children, and appears to be more common following the use of sevoflurane and desflurane. It can be very distressing to recovery staff and to parents who witness it and who usually assume their child is in pain. However, it appears to be unrelated to post-operative pain as it can occur in non-painful procedures such as radiological investigations. There is still no clear understanding of the aetiology of emergence delirium and consequently no widely accepted prophylactic strategy. Midazolam does not appear to prevent it, whether given as premedication or during anaesthesia. Some studies have shown that propofol, fentanyl, ketamine and clonidine may be effective. Emergence delirium usually resolves over a period of 10–15 minutes, but when a child is very agitated it can be ameliorated with a bolus of propofol, $1\,mg\,kg^{-1}$.

Key points

- Safe paediatric anaesthesia requires meticulous attention to detail and constant vigilance.

- A modified rapid sequence induction technique may be necessary in infants at risk of regurgitation to avoid hypoxia.
- Laryngospasm at the end of anaesthesia is more common in infants than in adults. It is generally safer to wait until the child is fully awake before extubation.

Further reading

Bhanaker SM, Ramamoorthy C, Geiduschek JM *et al.* Anesthesia-related cardiac arrest in children: update from the pediatric perioperative cardiac arrest registry. *Anes Analg* 2007;**105**:344–50.

Dahmani S, Stany I, Brasher C *et al.* Pharmacological prevention of sevoflurane- and desflurane-related emergence agitation in children: a meta-analysis of published studies. *Br J Anaes* 2010;**104**:216–23.

Davidson AJ, Smith KR, Bkusse van Oud-Alblas HT *et al.* Awareness in children: a secondary analysis of five cohort studies. *Anaesthesia* 2011;**66**:446–54

Department of Health. *The Acutely or Critically Sick or Injured Child in the District General Hospital: A Team Response.* DH. 2006. www.dh.gov.uk/en/Consultations/Closedconsultations/DH_4124412

Lake C, Beecroft CL. Extravasation injuries and accidental intra-arterial injection. *Cont Ed Anaes Crit Care Pain* 2010;**10**:109–13.

Rappaport B, Mellon RD, Simone A, Woodcock J. Defining safe use of anesthesia in children. *New Eng J Med* 2011;**364**:1387–90.

Royal College of Anaesthetists. *Guidance on the Provision of Paediatric Anaesthesia Services 2010.* Ch 8. http://www.rcoa.ac.uk/node/714 (accessed 14 August 2012).

SmartTots (*Strategies for Mitigating Anesthesia-Related Neuro-Toxicity in Tots*). http://www.smarttots.org (accessed 16 August 2012).

van der Griend BF, Lister NA, McKenzie IM *et al.* Postoperative mortality in children after 101,885 anesthetics at a tertiary pediatric hospital. *Anes Analg* 2011;**112**:1440–7.

Chapter

12

Equipment and monitoring in paediatric anaesthesia

Philippa Evans

Introduction

It is important that correct equipment and monitoring are available to provide safe anaesthesia for children. Equipment and monitoring specifications need to take into account the anatomical and physiological differences between adults and children, particularly in relation to infants and young children.

Airway equipment

Facemasks

Inhalational induction of anaesthesia is commonly performed in paediatric practice. It is important that facemasks are acceptable to the child. Ideally they should be constructed from clear plastic and have a soft rim. Some manufacturers produce scented masks in order to make them more attractive to children.

Paediatric facemasks exist in a range of sizes. The appropriate size should be used so that the facemask sits comfortably over the mouth and nose, pressure on the eyes is avoided, there are no gas leaks and there is minimal dead space. A well-designed facemask facilitates the appropriate technique for maintaining the airway ('chin lift' or 'jaw thrust').

Oropharyngeal airways

Infants and young children have a relatively large tongue, and airway obstruction tends to occur early during induction of anaesthesia as airway tone is lost. This may be overcome with simple manoeuvres such as the application of CPAP via the breathing circuit, by a jaw thrust manoeuvre, or by the insertion of an oropharyngeal airway once anaesthesia has been deepened. Oropharyngeal airways are available in sizes 000 to 4. The correct size is selected by placing

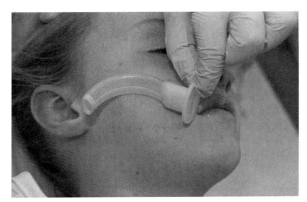

Figure 12.1 Sizing an oral airway – from the angle of the mandible to the centre of the incisors.

the airway against the side of the mouth; the airway should reach from the angle of the mandible to the centre of the incisors (see Figure 12.1). Too large an airway will protrude from the mouth and be ineffective; one that is too small may cause obstruction by pushing the tongue back.

Nasopharyngeal airways

Nasopharyngeal airways (NPA) are well tolerated in the awake child and may be useful in a variety of circumstances:

- Children with congenital abnormalities associated with midface hypoplasia (e.g. Apert's and Crouzon's syndrome), or severe micrognathia (e.g. Pierre Robin sequence);
- Airway management under anaesthesia e.g. to avoid problems with poor mouth opening or loose teeth and to aid fibre-optic intubation (FOI);
- Post-operatively to relieve obstruction at the palato-pharyngeal junction e.g. post-tonsillectomy

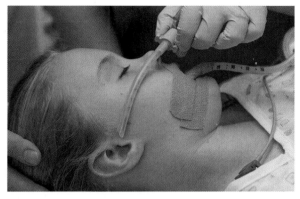

Figure 12.2 Sizing a nasopharyngeal airway – from the tip of the nose to the tragus of the ear.

in children with severe OSA, or palate repair in children with severe micrognathia.

The length of the NPA should be such that it can be fixed securely to the face whilst the tip should just protrude from behind the soft palate. Nasopharyngeal airways are commercially available for all ages, but have the disadvantage of being of fixed length. Alternatively, a NPA of specific length can be constructed from a cut tracheal tube (TT), the same size or one size smaller than the age-appropriate TT for intubation. Ideally, a flanged TT connector is used to secure the NPA to the face. It is important that the NPA is not too long or it will protrude from the nose or cause laryngeal irritation and coughing; and not too short as it will be ineffective in relieving airway obstruction at the palato-pharyngeal junction. The length should be approximately the distance from the tip of the nose to the tragus of the ear (see Figure 12.2). For some patients the NPA can be cut to length under direct vision at the end of surgery. It is important that the length of the NPA is recorded and that the NPA is suctioned to this depth regularly, particularly in post-operative patients.

Laryngeal mask airways

The paediatric LMA is sized according to patient weight (see Table 12.1). The classic paediatric LMA was not specifically designed for use in children but is merely a scaled-down version of the adult LMA. This has implications for its use in the paediatric population.

Both the classic and single-use LMAs are available in paediatric sizes 1–3. There is a learning curve when

Table 12.1 Laryngeal mask airway sizes

LMA size	Patient weight (kg)
1	>5
1.5	5–10
2	10–20
2.5	20–30
3	30–50

using the LMA in children. The complication rate is inversely proportional to patient size; displacement and airway obstruction occur most frequently with the size 1 and 1.5 LMAs. The LMA has an important role in the management of the difficult paediatric airway (see Chapter 22), and the size 1 LMA has a role in neonatal resuscitation. In infants, airway obstruction may occur if the LMA pushes the large floppy epiglottis down to obstruct the laryngeal inlet.

Difficulty can be encountered when using the traditional adult technique for LMA insertion in children. This may be due to adenotonsillar hypertrophy in older children, or due to the epiglottis impinging on the LMA grille. Different techniques for LMA insertion and removal have been described. The LMA can be inserted partially inflated against the lateral side of the tongue and gently advanced until resistance from the tonsil is met, and then moved back into the midline. Alternatively, a rotational technique may be used where the LMA is inserted 'back-to-front' with the cuff facing the palate, and turned through 180° once the hypopharynx is reached. The rotational and lateral techniques are both associated with high success rates for insertion in children less than 6 years of age.

Cuff inflation after insertion of LMAs may be according to the manufacturer's guidelines for volume and cuff pressure (<60 cmH$_2$O), or by clinical endpoints such as forward movement of the LMA and ability to ventilate with a good seal. The use of a cuff pressure monitor has been recommended to avoid hyperinflation of the cuff and improve the overall positioning of the LMA (often at lower cuff inflation volumes than suggested by manufacturers).

There is no consensus for the optimal timing for removal of LMAs in children. However, young children have reactive airways and show rapid emergence from anaesthesia. They may be more liable to develop laryngospasm if removal is delayed, and many practitioners prefer to remove the LMA while the patient is still deeply anaesthetised.

- Flexible LMAs are available in size 2 and above. They have a non-kinking flexometallic tube that is longer and has a smaller internal diameter than in the standard LMA. This increases airway resistance and may increase the work of breathing if used with spontaneous breathing in longer cases.
- The intubating LMA is available in size 3 and above. It can be a useful aid for fibre-optic intubation in children over about 25 kg.
- The Pro-Seal LMA is available from size 1.5. It has a modified cuff that has been specifically designed for children. It has an additional lumen running from the tip in parallel with the main airway that acts as an oesophageal drainage tube. This allows passive drainage of oropharyngeal contents and minimises gastric insufflation during positive pressure ventilation. The drainage tube also provides a route for nasogastric tube insertion and may prevent the epiglottis from obstructing the mask aperture. There is a high success rate for first insertion and overall high success rate for insertion in children.

Whichever of the LMA devices is used, displacement is common in children, particularly during patient transfer. The risk of displacement may be reduced by robust fixation of the device using an adhesive tape together with disconnection from the anaesthetic circuit during patient positioning.

Tracheal tubes

The narrowest part of the airway in children is at the level of the cricoid cartilage, which is the only cartilage that forms a complete ring around the airway. It has been traditional teaching to use uncuffed TTs in children under the age of 8 years. The ideal size of TT is one that will fit snugly at the level of the cricoid to allow assisted ventilation without excessive leak and prevent aspiration, whilst avoiding pressure on the tracheal mucosa, particularly in the vulnerable subglottic area. Traditionally this has been achieved by ensuring that there is a small audible leak around the TT at $20\,cmH_2O$ inflation pressure. Damage to the underlying mucosa can result in airway oedema and post-extubation stridor or, in the most serious cases, mucosal ulceration and necrosis leading to acquired

Table 12.2 Uncuffed tracheal tube sizes

Age	Internal diameter TT (mm)	Length oral TT (cm)	Length nasal TT (cm)
Neonate (3 kg)	3.0–3.5	10–10.5	12
6 months (6 kg)	4.0	11.5–12.5	13
1 year (10 kg)	4.5	13–13.5	15
> 1 year	(Age in years/4) + 4.5	(Age/2) + 12	(Age/2) + 15

subglottic stenosis. The formula for the selection of the correct size and length of TTs is based on age. These formulae are merely guides, and TTs half a size smaller and larger than the tube selected should always be available. The formulae are less reliable in children under the age of 1 year (see Table 12.2).

There have been improvements in tracheal tube technology in recent years, and there is currently much debate concerning the routine use of cuffed versus uncuffed TTs in children. Cuffed TTs are specifically indicated in intensive care for children with poor lung compliance where a large airway leak would seriously compromise ventilation. There are also a number of advantages in the use of cuffed tubes for routine anaesthesia:

- Increases likelihood of selection of the correct size tube at the first intubation; avoids potential trauma associated with multiple intubations;
- Reduces risk of aspiration;
- Allows accurate measurement of $ETCO_2$;
- Facilitates low flow anaesthesia and reduces environmental pollution and costs.

However, there is currently no international standard for tracheal tube marking or for the position or length of the cuff of a tracheal tube. There is thus great variability between manufacturers in the design of cuffed paediatric TTs, especially with regards to the position of the cuff and its relationship to the laryngeal inlet when inflated. Ideally a TT with a high volume, low pressure cuff should be used, and care should be taken that the correct size TT is chosen, that the cuff is inflated in the mid-trachea, not in the subglottic region or between the vocal cords (nor to obstruct the right upper lobe bronchus) and also that

Table 12.3 Cuffed tracheal tube sizes

Age	Internal diameter TT (mm)
Neonate (3 kg)	2.5–3.0
6 months (6 kg)	3.0–3.5
1 year (10 kg)	3.5–4.0
> 1 years	(Age in years/4) +3.5

the minimum cuff inflation pressure is used to seal the TT. The cuff pressure should be monitored and should not exceed 20 cmH$_2$O. The formula for sizing cuffed TTs is shown in Table 12.3.

Careful selection and placement of an appropriate TT, whether cuffed or not, is important in minimizing airway injury. It should be remembered that all TTs can be associated with airway trauma. It is our practice to use uncut TTs so that the tube connector can be seen, and the head can be placed to one side so that the TT will not kink. An oropharyngeal airway can be inserted along the side of the TT in order to provide some stability. Once in place it is important that the TT is fixed securely in position. There are many suitable methods. We use two pieces of adhesive tape cut into a 'trouser shape' to secure the TT. One 'trouser leg' of each piece should be attached to the TT, with the other 'leg' attached to the upper or lower lip (see Figure 12.3). It is important to make sure the tape is clear of the lip mucosa.

Polar (RAE) tracheal tube

These are useful in head and neck surgery, and are named after their inventors, Ring, Adair and Elwin. They are manufactured in a preformed shape, either 'south facing' for oral intubation for cleft surgery or tonsillectomy, or 'north facing' for nasal intubation for dental or maxillofacial surgery. The lengths of the intra-oral or intra-nasal sections are fixed. If these proportions are too long there is a risk of endobronchial intubation. There is currently no international standard for the length of preformed tracheal tubes, and different manufacturers produce tubes of different lengths. Difficulties may also be encountered in a child with failure to thrive where the larynx will be the age-appropriate size, but the child will be small for their age. The length of preformed tubes should therefore be checked after insertion by careful auscultation for bilateral breath

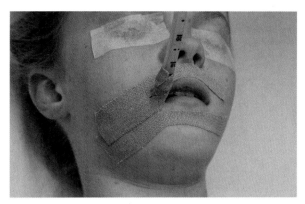

Figure 12.3 Fixation of tracheal tube. Two pieces of adhesive tape cut into a 'trouser shape'. One 'trouser leg' is attached to either the upper lip or the lower lip and the other end to the TT. An oropharyngeal airway can be inserted along the side of the TT in order to improve stability.

sounds, and if necessary the tube should be withdrawn. If using an oral preformed tube, a dental roll taped to the chin under the curve of the tube may be useful to fix the tube at the correct length. Note that extension of the head and neck reduces the length of the tube in the trachea; flexion of the neck will push the tube down towards the carina. Whatever design of tube is used, the position of the tube should be checked carefully after intubation, and again after repositioning for surgery.

Armoured tracheal tubes

These tubes are indicated in neurosurgery, for surgery in the prone position and in cases where the head position is changed during surgery. A metallic spiral in the wall of the tube provides increased flexibility and reduces the chance of kinking. This increased flexibility may necessitate the use of an introducer or stylet for intubation. They have a greater external diameter than standard TTs and a tube size half a size smaller than anticipated should be used.

Laser tracheal tubes

Flexometallic laser TTs are available in paediatric sizes for use in laser surgery in and around the airway. All polyvinyl chloride (PVC) TTs are flammable and can ignite and vaporise when in contact with the laser beam. The outer diameter of these metal laser TTs is considerably greater than their PVC counterparts, which is an important consideration when selecting an appropriately sized TT (see Table 12.4).

Table 12.4 Laser tracheal tubes, external diameter

Tube size (internal diameter) (mm)	External diameter	
	PVC tracheal tube (mm)	Metal laser tube (mm)
3.0 uncuffed	4.3	5.2
3.5 uncuffed	4.9	5.7
4.0 uncuffed	5.5	6.1
4.5 cuffed	6.2	7.0
5.0 cuffed	6.8	7.5
5.5 cuffed	7.5	7.9
6.0 cuffed	8.2	8.5

Cole tracheal tube

These tubes have a wide intra-oral section that narrows to the appropriate size distally to pass through the vocal cords. The wider portion affords them more stability than the equivalent size of TT and makes them easier to manipulate. They are popular in neonatal units. The shouldered portion sits against the vocal cords thus reducing the risk of endobronchial intubation. However, the wide portion of the Cole TT must not be allowed to move against or through the vocal cords as this may lead to vocal cord injury or subglottic stenosis.

Double-lumen tracheal tubes (DLT)

DLTs are used in adults to facilitate single lung ventilation for a variety of thoracic procedures, including video-assisted thoracoscopic surgery. The smallest commercially available DLTs are 26 Fr gauge, which is roughly equivalent in external diameter to a size 6.5 mm TT. DLTs are therefore only suitable for children from the age of 8–10 years upwards. They are available as left- or right-sided DLTs, referring to which main bronchus is intubated. When used, left-sided DLTs are preferred to avoid the bronchial cuff occluding the right upper lobe bronchus.

Laryngoscopes and blades
Straight laryngoscope blades

Straight laryngoscope blades are useful in infants up to about 6 months of age. Infants have a relatively large tongue, the larynx is relatively cephalad, and the epiglottis is long and floppy and may be angled into the lumen of the airway to cover the laryngeal inlet. This combination of factors may make it difficult to visualise the laryngeal inlet by conventional laryngoscopy (i.e. indirect elevation of the epiglottis with the tip of the laryngoscope blade placed in the vallecula above the epiglottis). The straight blade takes up less space in the mouth and allows the epiglottis to be lifted directly in order to reveal the glottic opening. Two different techniques have been described to visualise the larynx in infants: the laryngoscope blade is slid underneath the epiglottis and the tip of the blade lifted so that the glottis is exposed; or the laryngoscope blade is deliberately advanced into the oesophagus and then, with the tip lifted anteriorly, withdrawn slowly until the larynx drops into view. Both techniques bring the blade into direct contact with the under surface of the epiglottis, which may cause intense vagal stimulation.

There are a number of different straight blade laryngoscopes available (see Figure 12.4). The type selected is often based on personal preference. The Robertshaw and Seward blades have an open cross-section profile that allows for easier intra-oral manipulation of the TT. The Miller laryngoscope blade is C-shaped in cross-section, which reduces the ease of such manipulation but the extended curve at the tip of the blade facilitates anterior lifting of the epiglottis.

Curved laryngoscope blade (Macintosh blade)

These are used from the age of 6 months. The conventional technique for laryngoscopy should be employed. There are five sizes available: small infant size 0, infant size 1, child size 2, adult size 3 and large adult size 4. Polio blades and short-handled laryngoscopes may be useful.

Specialised laryngoscopes
The McCoy blade

This is a standard Macintosh blade with a hinged tip that is useful for elevating the epiglottis if it is obstructing the view of the laryngeal inlet.

The Bullard laryngoscope

This is a rigid fibre-optic laryngoscope available in three sizes: newborns/infants, paediatric and adult. It aids in glottic visualisation when the oral, pharyngeal and laryngeal axes are poorly aligned. It requires

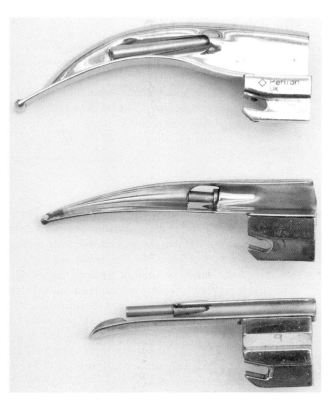

Figure 12.4 Selection of laryngoscope blades used in paediatric anaesthesia.

(a) Macintosh

(b) Robertshaw

(c) Miller

minimal neck movement for use and can be used in patients with mouth opening of just 6 mm.

Videolaryngoscopy

This describes the transmission of the view from the tip of the blade via a fibre-optic endoscope to a video display. Videolaryngoscopes are available in sizes suitable for all ages, and are useful teaching aids when learning the techniques of paediatric intubation. Some such as the Glidescope® provide an angulated view of the larynx and may be useful in difficult intubation.

Aids to intubation

Bougies and stylets are available in paediatric sizes. The smaller-sized bougies are rigid and often difficult to manipulate, and care must be taken to avoid trauma to the distal airway. A well-described technique in infants is a 'two person' technique, where the first operator obtains the best possible laryngeal view during laryngoscopy using external pressure to the larynx, and a second anaesthetist passes the bougie. Stylets are useful for the introduction of flexible tubes. Care must be taken not to allow the hard tip of the stylet to protrude beyond the end of the TT in order to avoid trauma to the airway.

Airway exchange catheters

Airway exchange catheters, for example manufactured by Cook®, are useful when employing fibre-optic techniques to manage a difficult airway. Their hollow central channel allows insufflation of oxygen and monitoring of end-tidal carbon dioxide ($ETCO_2$). The smallest size available is an 8 Fr catheter, which can be used to exchange a size 3 TT (see Table 12.5).

Suction catheters

Suction catheters are available in a range of sizes. The following formula describes the relationship between the size of suction catheter and TT:

$$\text{Suction catheter (French size)} = 2 \times \text{internal diameter (mm) of TT}$$

Breathing systems

The ideal paediatric breathing system should have minimal functional or apparatus dead space, be either valveless or fitted with very low resistance valves and

111

Table 12.5 Airway exchange catheters

Catheter gauge (French)	Catheter internal diameter (mm)	For replacement of TT with internal diameter (mm)
8	1.6	=/> 3.0
11	2.3	=/> 4.0
14	3.0	=/> 5.0

be constructed in such a way as to minimise gas turbulence and subsequent flow resistance.

Mapleson classified breathing systems into five types (A to E) according to their efficiency in eliminating carbon dioxide during spontaneous ventilation. Mapleson D, E and F systems are the most commonly used in paediatric practice as they most closely meet the criteria for an ideal paediatric system.

The Jackson Rees modification of the Ayre's T-piece

The Mapleson E system is the Ayre's T-piece. This is a valveless breathing system used for children up to 25–30 kg. It consists of a T-shaped tubing with three opening ports: one port receives fresh gas from the anaesthetic machine, the second port leads to the patient's mask, LMA or TT, the third port leads to reservoir tubing (see Figure 12.5). Mapleson F describes the Jackson Rees modification of system E by the addition of the open-ended reservoir bag to the end of the reservoir tubing.

The system requires a fresh gas flow (FGF) of 2.5 to 3 times the minute volume to prevent rebreathing with a minimum FGF flow of 4 litre min^{-1}. The open-ended bag has a number of functions: it acts as a visual monitor during spontaneous ventilation, it can be used to provide CPAP during spontaneous ventilation and it can be used to provide controlled ventilation, although experience is required to master the technique. The T-piece is not ideal for use in resuscitation for this reason.

The T-piece may also be used with a closed-ended reservoir bag and an adjustable pressure-limiting (APL) valve that allows for effective scavenging. It is too cumbersome to use during induction of anaesthesia but is useful during maintenance of anaesthesia.

The Bain system

This is the coaxial version of the Mapleson D system. It may be used during induction of anaesthesia in children over 25–30 kg. The fresh gas flow to prevent rebreathing during spontaneous ventilation is 1.5 to 2 times the minute volume. Thus a flow rate of 100 to 200 ml kg^{-1} min^{-1} is required. During controlled ventilation a fresh gas flow rate of 70–100 ml kg^{-1} min^{-1} is required.

The circle system

In this breathing system soda lime is used to absorb the patient's exhaled carbon dioxide. The paediatric circle consists of lightweight 15 mm diameter tubing and a small 500 ml reservoir bag; adult tubing and reservoir bags should be used in patients over 50 kg. The circle system/low-flow anaesthesia allows for improved preservation of heat and moisture, greater economy with less volatile agent used, and reduced environmental pollution compared with the non-absorber systems. It is important to be vigilant if an uncuffed tube with a significant leak is used and very low flow rates are employed.

Humidification

Humidification of inspired gases is important to prevent damage from dry gases and to minimise heat loss via the respiratory tract. The heat moisture exchanger (HME) is available in a range of sizes (volumes 7.8–100 ml) and is inserted at the point of connection of the airway device to the breathing circuit. The HME conserves approximately 50% of the water normally lost via the respiratory tract and prevents corresponding heat loss. This is of particular importance in neonates and small infants who lose heat more rapidly than older children and adults because their ratio of minute volume to body surface area is higher. In addition the HME protects against the inhalation of infective or hazardous particles and prevents cross-contamination between patients if reusable breathing circuits are used. The HME is most efficient with smaller tidal volumes and higher respiratory rates and so is well suited to paediatric practice.

Ventilators

The majority of children can be ventilated using modern adult circle ventilators provided:

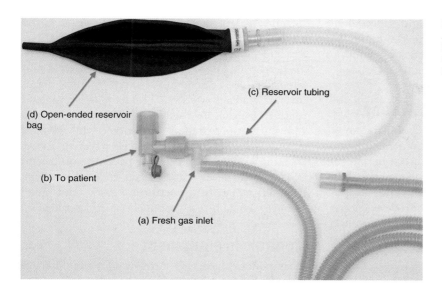

Figure 12.5 The Ayre's T-piece with Jackson Rees modification. (a) Fresh gas inlet port, (b) port to patient, (c), port to reservoir tubing, with open-ended bag (d) attached (Jackson Rees modification).

(c) Reservoir tubing

(d) Open-ended reservoir bag

(b) To patient

(a) Fresh gas inlet

- The ventilator can deliver high respiratory rates using pressure or volume controlled ventilation;
- It allows adjustment of the I:E ratio;
- Lightweight 15 mm paediatric tubing is used.

Pressure-controlled ventilation is the preferred mode of ventilation in children as it can be adjusted more easily to compensate for leaks in the breathing circuit and minimises the risk of barotrauma.

The Penlon Nuffield 200 ventilator was historically used in paediatric practice, but has largely fallen out of use as it is much less economical than a modern circle ventilator. It is a 'bag-squeezer' type of ventilator and is compatible with the T-piece, the Bain and circle systems. It is driven by compressed gas that is independent of the fresh gas flow. It is a volume preset, time-cycled flow generator in adult use. When used with a paediatric (Newton) valve, which introduces a fixed 'leak' into the system, the ventilator changes to a time-cycled pressure generator capable of delivering tidal volumes of 10–300 ml. It is recommended that the Newton valve be used for children of less than 20 kg.

Equipment for vascular access

Intravenous access

A range of sizes of cannula should be available. A 22-gauge cannula will suffice for the administration of drugs and fluid in most young children and infants. A 24-gauge cannula may be more appropriate in premature infants or those with difficult venous access. Larger-gauge cannulae are indicated for cases where significant blood loss is anticipated.

Specialised equipment is available for central venous access in children; catheters vary in length and size. A 4 Fr catheter is suitable for infants under 5 kg, 7 Fr for adolescents, and 5 Fr catheters for all other ages. Ultrasound guidance should be used with a strict aseptic technique for the placement of central venous catheters in children, commonly via the internal jugular route or via the femoral vein.

Intraosseous access

Intraosseous (IO) access provides rapid, safe and effective vascular access in situations when intravenous access is difficult, for example during resuscitation. Various purpose made needles are available in 18G (0 to 6 months), 16G and 14G sizes. They possess a trocar that prevents bone from plugging the lumen of the needle. Traditional intraosseous needles (Cook®-type) are placed manually, the site, force required and depth of insertion being determined by the operator. Since 2006, a second type of device has been used in adult and paediatric practice. The EZ-IO® (Vidacare) has a battery powered drill handle that powers needle insertion. Three different needle lengths are available, suitable for patients from 3 kg upwards.

Any drug or solution that can be given intravenously can be given by the IO route. Manual injection rather then passive infusion of fluid is required because of increased resistance. The resistance felt during injection is similar to that encountered during injection via an epidural catheter.

Equipment for fluid administration

It is important that intra-operative administration of fluids is carefully controlled and documented. Intravenous giving sets should incorporate a burette in order that accurately measured aliquots of fluid can be administered. A standard burette dispenses fluid at 20 drops per ml and a microdrop burette dispenses fluid at 60 drops per ml. Blood and blood products should be infused using a system with an integral 170–200 micrometre filter.

Fluid warmers should be used in cases where large volumes of fluid or blood transfusion is anticipated. Many of the systems used in adult practice are not appropriate for use in the paediatric setting owing to cooling along the length of the IV tubing and relatively slow infusion rates in children. This problem is overcome by the use of counter-current warming systems (e.g. Hotline®) where warm water circulates around the entire length of the delivery line up to the point of administration to the patient.

Drug administration

Drug doses in paediatric practice are based on patient weight. Often only very small volumes of standard formulations of drug are required. Smaller-sized ampoules or paediatric formulations are available for some drugs, which help to reduce waste. It is important that a range of syringes from 1 ml upwards is available in order that dosing is accurate.

Temperature maintenance

Infants and small children are at particular risk of developing hypothermia owing to their large body surface area to volume ratio. It is important to avoid hypothermia as it increases post-operative oxygen consumption, affects recovery from anaesthetic drugs, impairs coagulation, may depress ventilation and can result in arrhythmias.

The ambient temperature in the operating theatre may be raised, which will help reduce heat loss due to radiation. However, the theatre should not be heated to such an extent as to compromise staff comfort. The ideal theatre temperature is between 19 and 21 °C and it should not exceed 23 °C.

Care should be taken during induction of anaesthesia to avoid unnecessary exposure of the child. It is important to remember to keep infants' heads covered. Radiant overhead heaters with servo temperature control are useful in the anaesthetic room and during preparation for surgery in neonatal patients. Intra-operatively, forced air warming devices are most widely used. In smaller patients most benefit is derived if the device is placed under the patient. Humidification of anaesthetic gases and fluid warmers should be used routinely, as discussed above.

Monitoring equipment

Most monitors have been developed for adult practice and adapted for use in children. Essential monitoring is mandatory in all anaesthetised patients, but monitors are not a substitute for the presence of a vigilant anaesthetist who should combine the information provided by the monitors with their own observations in order to direct the management of the patient. Essential monitoring for anaesthesia includes:

- Oximetry
- ECG
- Non-invasive blood pressure
- Capnography
- Airway pressure

Pulse oximetry

This provides a non-invasive measurement of peripheral saturation of arterial blood (SpO_2). It enables the detection of incipient and unsuspected arterial hypoxaemia allowing early intervention before tissue damage occurs.

The 'peg-like' probes used in adult practice are suitable for use in older children. A more reliable device for use in younger children is a wrap-around probe in an adhesive strip. The strip can be attached to a digit, palm of hand or sole of foot, the site depending on the size of the patient. The sensors should be protected from interference from outside light sources. Motion artefact can also be a significant problem in the awake patient.

The presence of fetal haemoglobin or hyperbilirubinaemia in young infants has no clinical effect on the detection of hypoxaemia by the pulse oximeter. In patients with cyanotic congenital heart disease the oximeter tends to overestimate readings at lower saturations. It should be remembered that in neonates with duct-dependent systemic circulation, the saturation measured may be appreciably different depending on the site of the probe; shunting of deoxygenated blood through a patent ductus arteriosus will result in lower saturations in the left hand and lower body.

Electrocardiography

The electrocardiogram (ECG) provides a monitor of heart rate and rhythm, and can indicate myocardial ischaemia. Neonates and young children display right ventricular dominance on their ECG. This gradually declines with age; the QRS axis becomes similar to that of an adult by the age of 5 years. Neonatal and paediatric electrodes are available for babies and small infants.

Infants and young children are prone to bradycardia during anaesthesia and surgery. Continuous ECG monitoring allows prompt intervention. Infants and young children desaturate rapidly and develop a bradycardia in response to hypoxia. Many practitioners advocate leaving both the pulse oximeter and ECG in place during emergence from anaesthesia; if technical problems are encountered with the saturation probe and its accuracy is questioned, a slowing of heart rate will alert the practitioner to a 'patient' rather than 'equipment' problem.

Capnography

Gases with molecules that contain at least two dissimilar atoms absorb radiation in the infrared region of the spectrum. This property forms the basis of capnography and the measurement of expired carbon dioxide concentration throughout the respiratory cycle. Capnography is an invaluable aid to detect oesophageal intubation, disconnection of the breathing circuit, rebreathing and hypoventilation and is a useful monitor to indicate low cardiac output.

The capnograph sampling chamber can be either positioned within the patient's gas stream (main stream version) or connected to the distal end of the breathing system via a sampling tube (side stream version). The latter is the most common arrangement. However, both systems have their drawbacks. With side stream analysis the $ETCO_2$ may be underestimated when the tidal volumes are very small (standard rate of sampling 150–200 ml min^{-1}).

Mainstream (or in line) analysis is more accurate, but the sample cell is heavy and bulky and risks kinking the TT. The measurement of $ETCO_2$ levels in children may also be inaccurate if respiration is rapid or shallow, if there is a leak around the TT or when there is a large volume of apparatus dead space. In patients with cyanotic congenital heart disease the $ETCO_2$ readings will be lower than arterial $PaCO_2$, sometimes by 2 kPa.

Transcutaneous carbon dioxide measurement

Arterial CO_2 tension can also be estimated from the continuous measurement of transcutaneous CO_2 ($TcCO_2$). This is a useful tool in the PICU but is of limited use in anaesthesia as calibration of the apparatus takes 10 minutes for each patient, and it requires good and constant skin perfusion. It may be useful in situations where $ETCO_2$ measurement is inaccurate, for instance during laparoscopic surgery in neonates. The position of the heated sensor (43–44 °C) has to be changed every 3 to 4 hours in order to avoid thermal injury.

Non-invasive blood pressure measurement

An appropriately sized blood pressure cuff is one that occupies two-thirds of the upper arm. A width of 4 cm is recommended in full-term neonates. If the cuff is too small it overestimates blood pressure, if it too large readings are falsely low.

Invasive blood pressure measurement

An arterial line provides direct measurement of blood pressure and allows for intermittent blood sampling. The radial or the femoral arteries are the most common sites that are cannulated. The axillary artery can be used as an alternative but the brachial route should be avoided as it has poor collateral vessels. A 22-gauge cannula is suitable for most infants and small children, a 24-gauge cannula should be used in neonates and preterm babies if the radial site is accessed. A cannula in the femoral artery can compromise blood flow to the leg, especially in infants of less than 3 kg, and placement of a cannula in this site should have a strong indication in these patients. Likewise, blood flow to the leg should be monitored when combined femoral venous and arterial access is employed in older infants. Ultrasound is a useful tool for locating and confirming patency of arteries and with practice can be used to guide cannula insertion in peripheral sites even in very small babies. It is imperative that an arterial cannula does not possess an injection port and is clearly labelled. The transducer systems are the same as those used in adult practice and incorporate a column of bubble-free heparinised saline at a pressure of 300 mmHg. Care should be taken with the volume of fluid administered by the arterial flush system, and for this reason, an infusion pump delivering 1 ml hour^{-1} is commonly used in the ICU.

Monitoring cardiac output in children

Monitoring cardiac output (CO) is technically challenging in children, and most paediatric anaesthetists monitor surrogates of flow such as pressure (arterial, central venous), capillary refill, or markers of tissue oxygen delivery (base excess, lactate, central venous oxygen saturation). However, technology is improving, and a number of techniques used in adults are now directly applicable to infants and children and provide accurate measurements of cardiac output:

- Thermal dilution – catheters limited to children >5 kg
- Lithium dilution (LiDCO)
- Transoesophageal, transthoracic echocardiography
- Transoesophageal Doppler – probes limited to children >3 kg
- Pulse contour analysis (PiCCO)
- Venous oximetry
- Near-infrared spectroscopy (NIRS)

Transoesophageal Doppler

Transoesophageal Doppler is used to measure the flow velocity in the descending aorta to estimate cardiac output. Aortic diameter may be measured directly or may be derived from an inbuilt nomogram by entering age, height and weight. Placement in the oesophagus is operator-dependent, and CO values show reasonable correlation with those obtained by thermal dilution. Probes suitable for children >3 kg are now available.

Pulse contour analysis

Cardiac output may be derived from arterial waveform analysis, and there are a number of different techniques available that measure real-time CO.

However, they depend on complex mathematical and physiological calculations, and few studies have been performed in children. These techniques may be useful during stable conditions, but monitors require recalibration and may have limited accuracy when vascular tone changes or with rapidly changing haemodynamics during surgery.

Near-infrared spectroscopy

NIRS is a non-invasive optical method for continuous measurement of tissue oxygenation, and has been used as a measure of cerebral and somatic perfusion in adults and children, particularly during cardiac surgery and intensive care. It relies on the principle that haemoglobin absorbs infrared light close to the visual spectrum, and that the absorption of light depends on the oxygenation status of haemoglobin, as most other biological tissues do not absorb light of this wavelength. Whereas pulse oximetry requires a pulsatile flow and provides a measure of arterial saturation, tissue oximetry does not require a pulsatile flow and the value is mainly determined by venous oxygen saturation, haemoglobin and blood flow. Provided oxygen extraction and haemoglobin remain constant, the NIRS value becomes a surrogate measure of flow. The precise design of the equipment and the algorithms used to determine tissue oxygenation vary between manufacturers. Probes, including infant probes, are specifically designed for different tissue areas (cerebral, abdominal, renal, muscle), and will give inaccurate results if not used according to the manufacturer's instructions. The sensitivity and specificity of NIRS-derived measurements of low perfusion compared with invasive measurements of cardiac output are improved by monitoring at multiple sites. The technology is improving, but absolute values vary between manufacturers, and the upper and lower NIRS values are not clearly defined. The probes are expensive, and controversy remains about the value of NIRS in improving outcomes. However, NIRS does appear to have a role in monitoring trends in tissue perfusion, particularly as an early warning of low cardiac output or to detect catastrophic events, for instance during aortic cannulation in cardiac surgery.

Depth of anaesthesia monitors

Traditionally, clinical signs (breathing pattern, pupillary size and reactivity, eye movement) and physiological response to surgical stimulation have been used to assess depth of anaesthesia. A number of monitors have been developed by different manufacturers to assess depth of anaesthesia, based on analysis of the EEG using information derived from adult EEG data. The Bispectral Index (BIS) has been studied extensively, but other monitors include the Narcotrend™, Cerebral State Monitor™, AEP/2 and M-entropy monitor. These monitors should ideally avoid awareness in high-risk patients, and by avoiding unnecessarily deep anaesthesia, may improve recovery from anaesthesia. However, depth of anaesthesia monitors are affected by the use of neuromuscular agents, the specific anaesthetic agents used (BIS is unaffected by nitrous oxide and high-dose opioids), and there may be paradoxical changes during sevoflurane anaesthesia (increased EEG activity associated with deep sevoflurane anaesthesia results in higher BIS values). Furthermore, the EEG changes during development, and since monitors have been developed using adult data, depth of anaesthesia monitors may not be reliable in infants and younger children. No monitor has a particular advantage over another, and use in infants cannot be supported currently.

Temperature monitoring

Temperature monitoring is essential to detect both hypothermia and inadvertent hyperthermia in children undergoing general anaesthesia. The temperature is usually monitored in the nasopharynx, oesophagus, rectum or at a peripheral site. Oesophageal temperatures should be recorded in the lower third of the oesophagus to avoid falsely low readings caused by a leak around the tracheal tube. Rectal probes can cause perforation in neonates and should not be used in neutropenic patients.

Urine output

This should be monitored in all cases of major surgery or when significant blood loss is anticipated. Silastic catheters are used. The smaller catheters have a stylet, which should be removed prior to insertion to avoid creating a false passage. The smallest balloon catheter available is 6 Fr; this has a 1.5 ml balloon which is appropriate for most term neonates onwards. If a balloon catheter cannot be passed then a 6 Fr feeding tube should be used (this is stiffer and smaller than the 6 Fr Foley as it does not have the extra thickness at the balloon). The balloon should always be inflated with water, not saline (and only after urine has been identified), as saline may crystallise which can then block the channel and prevent balloon deflation. The same catheters are used for girls and boys. In male infants the preputial orifice overlies the glandular meatus and thus the prepuce does not need to be fully retracted during catheter insertion. Once inserted, the catheter should be connected to a urometer that is capable of collecting and measuring small volumes of urine.

Anaesthetic record and configuration of monitors

A clear record of all drugs and the doses administered should be part of the information recorded on the anaesthetic chart. The chart should also record the method of induction, airway management, monitoring equipment used and patient position in addition to documenting the physiological parameters measured throughout the procedure. Any problems encountered should be clearly documented as they may act as an alert for future anaesthetists.

The presence of monitoring is not a substitute for an anaesthetist. Age-appropriate alarm limits should be set for each physiological variable in order to increase vigilance. The information provided by the monitors must be integrated with the anaesthetist's own observations in order that appropriate interventions are made.

Key points

- It is imperative that the correct equipment and monitoring are available in order to provide safe anaesthesia for children.
- Laryngeal mask airway size selection is based on patient weight; tracheal tube size selection is based on patient age.
- Most children can be ventilated using modern adult circle ventilators as long as the appropriate settings are selected.
- Temperature monitoring and heat conservation techniques are important as infants and small children are at particular risk of developing hypothermia.
- Increasingly sophisticated monitors have been developed that are suitable for use in children, but no monitor is a substitute for the presence and vigilance of the anaesthetist.

Further reading

Association of Anaesthetists of Great Britain and Ireland. *Recommendations for Standards of Monitoring during Anaesthesia and Recovery.* http://www.aagbi.org/sites/default/files/standardsofmonitoring07.pdf

Bingham R, Patel P. Laryngeal mask airway and other supraglottic devices in paediatric practice. *Cont Educ Anaes Crit Care Pain* 2009;**9**(1):6–9.

Davidson A. Monitoring anaesthetic depth in children – an update. *Curr Opin Anaesthesiol* 2007;**20**:236–43.

James I. Cuffed tubes in children. *Ped Anes* 2001;**11**:259–63.

Leong L, Black A. The design of pediatric tracheal tubes. *Ped Anes* 2009;**19**:38–45.

Mariano ER, Ramamoorthy C, Chu LF, Chen M, Hammer GB. A comparison of three methods for estimating appropriate tracheal tube depth in children. *Ped Anes* 2005;**15**:846–51.

Mittnacht AC. Near infrared spectroscopy in children at high risk of low perfusion. *Curr Opin Anaesthesiol* 2010;**23**:342–7.

Skwono J, Broadhead M. Cardiac output measurement in pediatric anesthesia. *Ped Anes* 2008;**18**:1019–28.

Weiss M, Dullenkopf A, Fischer JE, Keller C, Gerber AC. European Paediatric Endotracheal Intubation Study Group. Prospective randomized controlled multi-centre trial of cuffed or uncuffed endotracheal tubes in small children. *Br J Anaes* 2009;**103**:867–73.

Whitelock D, de Beer DAH. The use of filters with small infants. *Respir Care Clin North Am* 2006;**12**(2):307–20.

Chapter

13

Venous access in children

David Chisholm

Introduction

A substantial proportion of children will require venous access at some time during their lives. This may be for resuscitation within minutes of being born, for intravenous antibiotics as an infant or perhaps to administer a course of chemotherapy for treatment of leukaemia. This chapter will outline the routes available for venous access, the factors influencing the choice of catheters and devices used, and their associated complications. Choosing the most appropriate site and type of venous access must be specific to each child and to their treatment requirements (see Table 13.1).

The correct care of venous access devices both during and following insertion is extremely important and will have a major impact on functioning of the catheter as well as reducing potentially life-threatening complications. The use of specific care bundles incorporating evidence-based measures greatly reduces both infective and non-infective complications.

Peripheral venous catheters and midline catheters

Short-term peripheral venous access is widely used in children of all ages. Short, peripherally inserted catheters can be used for drug delivery, fluid infusion and blood sampling. Total parenteral nutrition (TPN) of sufficiently low osmolarity and non-vesicant chemotherapy can also be given via this route. These catheters are usually sited into small veins on the hands, forearms, feet and scalp in infants. Catheters inserted over joints tend to cause more discomfort and are more prone to phlebitis. Larger veins at the antecubital fossa should be preserved if a subsequent midline catheter or a peripherally inserted central catheter

(PICC) is anticipated. In neonates the long saphenous veins at the ankle or knee may also be required for PICC insertion at a later date.

Peripheral catheters

Traditionally, peripheral catheters were used for only 72–96 hours but insertion duration alone is not grounds for removing functioning catheters if there is no evidence of phlebitis. Peripheral catheters are short (2.5 to 7 cm) catheter over needle devices available in a wide variety of diameters (14 to 26G) and materials (Teflon™ and polyurethane). The choice of catheter size depends on the diameter of the intended vein and also the flow requirements. In general small catheters cause less phlebitis, are more comfortable and last longer. Catheters made of Vialon™, a type of polyurethane, have been shown to cause less phlebitis than catheters made of Teflon™.

Children requiring peripheral venous access require skilled management involving both appropriate age-related behavioural techniques and suitable analgesia. Poorly managed pain during cannulation causes distress at the time, more pain during future episodes and long-term phobic behaviour. Topical anaesthesia, using a eutectic mixture of local anaesthetics (EMLA®), topical tetracaine 4% gel (Ametop®) or lidocaine 4% cream (LMX 4®), is effective if given sufficient time to work, although the removal of the occlusive plastic dressings can cause significant distress. EMLA™ should not be used in preterm neonates or any other children at risk of methaemoglobinaemia. There are also needleless injection systems of ionised lidocaine (J-tip) available that have the advantage of almost instant analgesia and compare favourably with EMLA. Ethyl chloride spray is effective, but its flammability precludes its use in environments with electrical equipment. Nitrous oxide

Core Topics in Paediatric Anaesthesia, ed. Ian James and Isabeau Walker. Published by Cambridge University Press. © 2013 Cambridge University Press.

Table 13.1 Types of venous catheters

Catheter type	Entry site	Duration of use
Peripheral venous catheters	Veins on hands, feet and forearms. Scalp veins in infants	72 to 96 hours
Midline catheters	Basilic or cephalic veins at the antecubital fossa. Tip of catheter stops short of axillary vein	Up to 28 days
Peripherally inserted central venous catheters (PICCs)	Basilic or cephalic veins at the antecubital fossa. Long saphenous vein in infants. Tip of catheter in central vein	Weeks to months
Umbilical catheters	Umbilical vein used within 1 week of birth	Up to 14 days
Non-tunnelled central venous catheters	Percutaneous insertion into internal jugular, subclavian or femoral veins	Days to weeks
Tunnelled central venous catheters	Subcutaneous tunnel with cuffed catheter into central vein	Months to years
Totally implantable devices	Port positioned on chest wall, abdomen or forearm with subcutaneous tunnelled access to central vein	Months to years
Intraosseous cannula	Proximal anterior tibia. Distal end of femur. Medial malleolus	Up to 24 hours

(Entonox) has also been used successfully for pain control during cannulation. In difficult cases, the use of real-time ultrasound has been shown to improve success rates and decrease insertion times.

Midline catheters

These are longer, soft peripheral catheters made of polyurethane or silicone, usually 3 to 4 French gauge (Fr) in diameter. They are inserted into the cephalic or basilic veins at the antecubital fossa through a specific micro-introducer kit which has a sheath that is peeled apart to leave the catheter in the vein. The midline catheter is cut to the correct length and should be positioned to stop short of the axillary vein. Midline catheters cause less phlebitis than peripheral catheters and hence may be used for up to 4 weeks. The same restriction on the osmolarity of the infusate still applies.

Complications

The commonest complication of peripheral catheters is phlebitis. This presents as redness, swelling, induration and pain around the insertion site of the catheter and necessitates removal. Phlebitis is an inflammatory reaction that is not primarily an infective process although secondary infection may occur. The incidence of catheter-related blood infection (CRBI) from peripheral catheters is about 0.2–0.5 per 1000 catheter days. Midline catheters have a lower infection rate of around 0.1–0.2 per 1000 catheter days.

Subcutaneous extravasation of infusate is another common complication with peripheral catheters. This is a particular problem in neonates where the incidence may be as high as 90%. Serious tissue damage with subsequent scarring may occur, especially with TPN and calcium-containing infusates. Rapid identification of the extravasation and treatment with injection of hyaluronidase (500 to 1000 units) and 0.9% saline irrigation can prevent tissue loss. All hospitals should have a readily accessible policy for the acute management and follow up of extravasation injuries.

Significant venous thrombosis is rare with peripheral catheters. Catheter fracture and air embolism are also rare but serious complications.

Peripherally inserted central catheters

PICCs are small diameter catheters (1.2 Fr to 5 Fr) made of silicone or polyurethane. The larger catheters may have two lumens to allow separation of incompatible infusates. PICCs allow access to the central circulation without exposing the patient to some of the serious insertion complications of direct approaches to the central veins. The dilution of the infusate by the larger volume of blood in the central veins makes them suitable for the administration of TPN and hypertonic solutions. They are also useful in the presence of coagulopathies and low platelet count as bleeding at the insertion site is rarely a serious problem and usually responds to direct pressure. Local infection and venous thrombosis proximal to the insertion site are contraindications to PICC insertion.

PICCs are most commonly inserted percutaneously into the cephalic or basilic veins in the arm. The long saphenous vein at the ankle or knee or the superficial temporal vein can be used in neonates and infants. Lower limb insertion sites in neonates have been shown to prolong catheter function and decrease overall complications when used for TPN. The use of real-time ultrasound is useful and can allow the basilic vein to be accessed above the antecubital fossa. The insertion kits are similar to the midline catheters incorporating a split sheath introducer or splittable needle for the smallest catheters. The vein can be accessed by direct cannulation or by fine needle access and the use of a Seldinger wire micro-introducer set. Most PICCs are cut to length prior to insertion using surface landmarks for the final tip position. The Groshong™ PICCs have a special valve near their tip that allows fluid to be injected or aspirated but is closed when not in use, hence must be cut to length at the hub end.

The tip of the PICC ideally is positioned in the lower third of the superior vena cava from upper limb veins or in the proximal inferior vena cava from the long saphenous vein. The use of surface landmarks with blind insertion results in a satisfactory tip position in only about 15% of cases. With fluoroscopic guidance this can be increased to 90%. If fluoroscopy is not used a post-insertion chest radiograph must be performed to verify tip position. If the tip is in the right atrium it must be withdrawn to avoid atrial perforation and cardiac tamponade, which has a mortality of over 80%. This is a particular concern in neonates having TPN or hypertonic glucose infusions and was the subject of a warning from the Department of Health in 2001. The tip of PICCs can be advanced significantly by adduction of the arm and this may precipitate serious cardiac dysrhythmias. A non-central tip position markedly increases the risk of vessel thrombosis. The reported incidence of thrombosis associated with PICCs varies widely, from around 4% if clinical signs are used, to up to 25% with surveillance venography. The cephalic venous system is reported to have a much higher thrombosis rate than the basilic system, probably owing to its tortuous course. Thrombus formation at the tip of the PICC can cause blockage requiring removal. This is a particular problem in neonates due to the small diameter of the catheters used. A continuous infusion of heparin at 0.5 IU kg^{-1} h^{-1} significantly reduces catheter occlusion.

The incidence of CRBI for outpatient PICCs is around 1.0 per 1000 catheter days. For inpatient PICCs the rate of infection is much higher at about 2.1 per 1000 catheter days. Other serious complications for PICCs include catheter fracture with associated catheter or air embolism. Catheter rupture is associated with the flushing of small catheters with syringes smaller than 10 ml as these can generate extremely high pressures.

Umbilical vein access

Central venous access in the newborn can be gained via the umbilical vein immediately after birth and for the first few days of life. The umbilical vein is a single large thin-walled vessel, compared with the smaller paired muscular umbilical arteries. It gives off several large intrahepatic branches before converging with the left portal vein and continuing as the ductus venosus. This joins the inferior vena cava with the hepatic vein. An understanding of the anatomy of the umbilical vein is crucial for avoiding some of the more serious complications associated with the use of an umbilical vein catheter (UVC).

When a UVC is used for immediate resuscitation of a neonate at birth the position of the tip cannot be verified radiologically before use, and this is the only indication for a low catheter. With the umbilicus cut to 1–2 cm the tip must not be advanced beyond 3–5 cm below the skin to avoid intrahepatic placement. UVC tips positioned within the liver have been associated with liver abscess, liver necrosis and hepatic vein thrombosis leading to portal hypertension. UVCs in the portal venous system have been implicated in causing colonic perforation and necrotising enterocolitis. UVCs should not be inserted in the presence of omphalitis, an omphalocoele or peritonitis.

For elective catheter placement the ideal tip position is just above the diaphragm in the inferior vena cava below the right atrium. There are graphs and formulae available to estimate catheter length based on umbilical to shoulder distance and weight. On a chest radiograph the catheter should be visible just to the right of the vertebral column at the level of T9–10 vertebrae above the diaphragm. Malpositioned catheters can cause cardiac perforation, cardiac arrhythmias, thrombotic endocarditis and pulmonary infarction. Great care must be taken to avoid air embolism when inserting and using UVCs because of the negative pressure in the thorax during inspiration. Haemorrhage from the umbilical stump can be a problem at insertion. This is best controlled by a circular ligature around the umbilical stump, which is subsequently released to avoid necrosis.

There are both single and double lumen UVCs available between 3 and 5 Fr in size. Double lumen catheters decrease the need for additional venous access and are not associated with a significant increase in complications. Catheters with side holes should be avoided unless being used specifically for exchange transfusion as they have a higher incidence of thrombotic complications. Correctly sited high UVCs can be used for blood sampling, drug and fluid administration, TPN and hyperosmolar infusates. They can also be used for measuring central venous pressure (CVP).

Infection of UVCs occurs in up to 15% of patients and is related to prematurity, insertion duration and catheter handling. Prophylactic antibiotics do not seem to have a role in preventing infection. As well as a cause of general sepsis, infected UVCs can also cause widespread infective emboli. Transfer of infective emboli between the venous circulation and the systemic circulation can occur through a patent foramen ovale. UVCs should be removed as soon they are no longer required and should not be left in place for more than 14 days.

Short-term central venous access

Secure access to the central venous system is often required during major surgery and during admissions to intensive care. This is usually provided by short-term non-tunnelled central venous catheters (CVC) made of a relatively stiff material such as polyurethane with a wide variety of choice in diameter (3 to 8.5 Fr), length and number of lumens (one to five). The choice of catheter type and insertion site is determined by balancing the clinical need against the risk of insertion complications. Multiple lumen catheters are useful for drug infusions especially if inotropic support is required. They also facilitate the measurement of CVP and venous blood sampling. Larger diameter catheters should be used if rapid fluid administration is required as the flow is proportional to the fourth power of the radius. The length of the catheter is dependent on the size of the child and the insertion site. The tip of these short-term catheters must be in either the inferior or the superior vena cava. Because of the risk of cardiac perforation the tip

must not lie within the heart. For short-term haemodialysis and haemodiafiltration there are special large-bore double lumen catheters that are designed for high flow rates without causing haemolysis.

Access to the central venous circulation is associated with an increased risk of bleeding both during catheter insertion and at the time of removal. The platelet count should be known prior to insertion and a clotting screen performed if there is a risk of coagulopathy. Traditionally a platelet count of greater than $50 \times 10^9 \ l^{-1}$ has been used as a safe level. However, there are studies of CVC insertions with platelet counts of above $20 \times 10^9 \ l^{-1}$ without any significant increase in haemorrhagic complications.

The most common insertion sites for short-term CVCs are the:

- Femoral vein
- Internal jugular vein
- External jugular vein
- Subclavian vein

For multi-lumen catheters the Seldinger technique is utilised. Most catheter insertion kits have a J-tip Seldinger wire. In neonates and infants the radius of the J-tip may be greater than the diameter of the vein, impeding advancement of the wire; often the other end of the wire is a soft straight tip which may be easier to insert.

It is recommended that all short-term central catheters are connected to a pressure transducer to exclude arterial placement. This should be done prior to dilation of the vein if there is any suspicion of arterial puncture. Blood gas analysis is not helpful to differentiate between arterial and venous placement especially if the child is hypoxic or supplementary oxygen is being administered. Full asepsis should be used during insertion.

Femoral vein

This is the commonest site for short-term central venous access in children. The femoral approach has the major advantage of consistent anatomy with the vein found medial to the femoral artery and accessed below the inguinal ligament. There is no risk of pneumothorax in contrast to insertion sites in the neck. The major insertion complication is arterial puncture, which occurs in up to 10% of insertions using surface landmarks and femoral arterial pulsation as guidance. The use of ultrasound significantly reduces arterial puncture rates and decreases the number of insertion attempts. Bleeding from attempts at femoral venous access is usually easily controlled by digital pressure, but there are reports of substantial retroperitoneal bleeding causing cardiovascular collapse. The femoral vein is the preferred site for short-term haemodialysis catheters owing to the straight course of the femoral vein to the inferior vena cava. It is also the best route for CVC insertion during emergency resuscitation, as cardiopulmonary massage does not have to be interrupted during placement.

Internal jugular vein

This is the next most common site to be used for short-term CVCs. It requires a higher level of technical expertise and practice compared with the femoral route. The anatomy of the internal jugular vein is much more variable than that of the femoral vein. The relationship of the vein to the common carotid artery changes with age.

- In most infants the vein either partially or completely overlies the artery at the level of the cricoid cartilage; rotating the head away from the midline increases the incidence of overlap.
- In older children and adults there is substantial variation in position of the vein.
- In up to 5% of adults the internal jugular vein actually lies medial to the common carotid artery, contrary to traditional teaching.

Hence the use of the common carotid artery as a landmark for CVC insertion is potentially flawed in many patients, and arterial puncture rates are between 5 and 15%. The dome of the lung lies posterior to the vein in the neck, and this approach is associated with pneumothorax rates of around 0.5 to 1%. The use of ultrasound significantly reduces arterial puncture, improves success rates and decreases insertion duration. Ideally ultrasound should be used for visualisation during insertion as opposed to pre-insertion orientation. In the UK, NICE has recommended that ultrasound be used for all elective CVC insertion into the internal jugular vein in both adults and children.

The size of the internal jugular vein can be increased by a head-down position, Valsalva manoeuvre or hepatic compression. The right internal jugular vein has a much straighter course to the superior vena cava (SVC) than the left side and is the preferred route. The left internal jugular vein should be avoided in children with persistent left SVC that drains to the coronary sinus.

External jugular vein

This is more superficial than the internal jugular vein although it is extremely variable in size and position. It can be used for short-term CVCs. Advancing a Seldinger wire down the vein through the clavipectoral fascia into a central vein can be problematic and hence it is not often used for this purpose. The risk of pneumothorax is small but not negligible with this approach.

Subclavian vein

This is the continuation of the axillary vein from the upper limb. It becomes the subclavian vein at the outer border of the first rib then arches up over the rib in front of the lung, anterior to and slightly below the subclavian artery. It joins the internal jugular vein to form the brachiocephalic vein and then combines with the opposite brachiocephalic vein to form the SVC. The clavicle overlies the subclavian vein for a substantial part of its extrathoracic course. From this description of the anatomy it can be seen that the vein is a deep structure in close proximity both to the lung and subclavian artery. It cannot be visualised easily with ultrasound owing to the overlying clavicle. Accessing the subclavian vein percutaneously requires a high degree of skill and expertise, and it is the approach associated with the highest failure rate.

- Damage to the vein or artery is not easily amenable to external pressure and catastrophic bleeding can occur especially if the blood collects in the pleural cavity.
- Pneumothorax rates are between 0.5 and 2% for this approach. The space between the clavicle and first rib is narrow in infants and small children and restricts the size of the catheter used.
- It can be difficult to dilate the tract to the vein, and pinching of the catheter can occur causing pain, catheter malfunction and catheter damage.
- Because of the angle of entry of the subclavian vein into the thoracic cavity the Seldinger wire is required to negotiate a 90° corner to enter the SVC. This can result in wire misplacement in around 10% of insertions with final catheter tip

Table 13.2 Complications of percutaneous central venous catheter insertion

Immediate (usually within 24 hours)	Long term
Pneumothorax	Local infection at insertion site
Haemothorax	Bloodstream infection
Haemopneumothorax	Venous thrombosis and occlusion
Hydrothorax secondary to fluid infusion	Arterio-venous fistula
Chylothorax secondary to thoracic duct damage	Arterial false aneurysm formation
Arterial puncture with local haemorrhage	
Arterial endoluminal damage with flap occlusion	
Arterial thrombosis	
Arterial embolism	
Damage to great veins with massive haemorrhage	
Local haemorrhage at insertion site	
Cardiac perforation with tamponade	
Pericardial effusion	
Cardiac arrhythmias	
Pneumomediastinum	
Air embolism	
Catheter embolism	
Wire embolism	

position in the opposite subclavian vein or either internal jugular veins. A chest radiograph should always be performed to verify catheter tip position.

Short-term non-tunnelled CVCs are extremely useful in critically ill children but are associated with a large number of complications (see Table 13.2). The commonest delayed complications are CRBI and venous thrombosis. Bloodstream infection rates are 3.4–11.3 per 1000 catheter days depending on the pre-existing patient risk factors. Children with burns and neonates less than 1000 g are at the highest risk of CRBI. In children there is not a great difference between infection rates at different insertion sites as opposed to adults where the femoral route has a much higher infection rate. Thrombosis of the vein or around the catheter can occur in 2–35% of patients. In children with diabetic ketoacidosis the use of the femoral vein for CVCs has been associated with a thrombosis incidence of around 50%, so this route should probably be avoided in these patients. The recorded incidence is much higher if active surveillance is undertaken rather than relying on clinical signs. The presence of a catheter in a small vein may cause venous congestion of the distal venous system. This is particularly noticeable in neonates and infants with femoral catheters.

Long-term central venous access

A number of children will require central venous access for a period longer than a month. Consideration should be given early in their treatment to the insertion of a long-term central venous access device to avoid the trauma, both physical and emotional, of multiple short-term catheters. Cytotoxic chemotherapy, prolonged antibiotic therapy and parenteral nutrition are the commonest indications in children. The devices used for long-term access are divided into skin tunnelled catheters and implantable injection ports.

These catheters are usually made of soft silicone but can be made of polyurethane. Polyurethane catheters are stiffer, hence can have a larger lumen with the same external diameter allowing higher flow rates. They do not soften as much as silicone catheters in the blood at body temperature and thus are associated with a higher incidence of thrombosis. The catheters may be open-ended or have a valve system such as the Groshong^{TM} two-way valve.

Long-term skin tunnelled catheters

These have a Dacron^{TM} cuff that is situated in the subcutaneous tunnel 3 to 4 cm from the exit site. Subcutaneous tissue grows in and around the cuff over a period of a few weeks. This secures the catheter in place so no other external fixation is required. It also acts as a barrier to infective agents ascending the tunnel to cause bloodstream infections. The catheters may be single lumen such as the small Broviac^{TM} catheters (2.7 or 4.2 Fr) or larger double or triple lumen Hickman^{TM} style catheters (7–12 Fr).

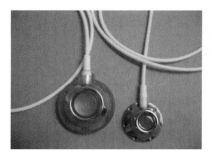

Figure 13.1
Portacath for long-term vascular access.

Implantable ports

These are made of plastic or titanium so that they are MRI compatible (see Figure 13.1). The port is usually situated in a pocket fashioned on the chest wall and secured to the fascia with non-absorbable sutures to avoid rotation in the pocket. Less commonly the port can be sited on the forearm or the upper abdomen. The port is attached to a tunnelled subcutaneous catheter (6–12 Fr) and is accessed percutaneously with a special Huber type needle. This has a non-cutting atraumatic tip with a side hole to avoid damaging the diaphragm of the port. Ports are available as either high or low profile to aid palpability with varying thickness of subcutaneous tissue. There are double lumen ports available but they are rarely used in children. The implantable port system has the advantage of essentially being a sealed system once the percutaneous needle is removed. They are associated with less local and systemic infection, and the child is not restricted on swimming and bathing when the port is not accessed.

The skin-tunnelled catheters are better for more intensive treatments such as bone marrow transplantation when multiple lumens are required. They are also preferred in needle-phobic children as accessing an implantable port is not completely painless even with local anaesthetic creams. In children less than 1 year of age and in those with very little subcutaneous fat there is a higher incidence of skin erosion over the port site, so skin-tunnelled catheters may be more suitable.

Insertion

Long-term lines can be inserted either by open surgery or by a percutaneous technique, and will require fluoroscopic support. Most children will require general anaesthesia for a port or tunnelled catheter insertion, although some older children will tolerate a percutaneous insertion with sedation and local anaesthesia. Open surgery can be used for accessing the internal and external jugular veins as well as the femoral vein. The subclavian vein is not suitable for open access. For the internal jugular and femoral veins the catheter is inserted through a venotomy under direct vision with the vessel controlled between two vascular slings. The external jugular vein can be divided and tied off with the soft catheter threaded down the proximal segment.

For percutaneous insertion the access to the vein is identical to that for the short-term catheters with the use of a Seldinger wire. Ultrasound is recommended for both internal jugular and femoral vein insertion. The subclavian vein can also be accessed with the percutaneous technique. Owing to the narrow space between the clavicle and first rib, however, the child usually needs to be above 20 kg for catheters of 7 Fr and larger. Whichever percutaneous insertion site is chosen, the position of the Seldinger wire should be confirmed with fluoroscopy prior to dilation. The catheter is then tunnelled up from the exit site for Hickman/Broviac lines or from the subcutaneous port site to a position next to the Seldinger wire. An integral vein dilator and peel-away sheath are inserted over the Seldinger wire with great care being taken not to push the stiff dilator in too far or beyond the end of the wire. Serious damage to the mediastinum or heart with fatal consequences can occur with misuse of this system. The wire and dilator are removed to leave the sheath in the vein. The soft catheter is inserted via the sheath which is then peeled away leaving the catheter in the vein. It is possible for large quantities of blood or air to flow rapidly through the peel-away sheath if the lumen is not well controlled.

The ideal position for the catheter tip of soft long-term catheters is still controversial. There have been rare reports of cardiac perforation in neonates having TPN infusions with the tip positioned within the right atrium. In larger children this seems to be much less of a concern and the catheters tend to function better if the tip is placed in the upper right atrium. The catheter can be cut to length using the intermammary line as the surface landmark for the right atrium. A better technique for use with the Seldinger wire is to position the tip of the wire in the desired position, confirmed by fluoroscopy. The amount of wire on the exterior is then measured and deducted from the known length of the wire (usually 50 cm) to give the exact length for the catheter to be cut to. This technique cannot be used for Groshong™ tip catheters, which have to be tunnelled backwards from the insertion site to the exit site or port. Fluoroscopy should always be used to confirm the final position of the catheter tip. It is not necessary to routinely perform a chest radiograph after insertion if fluoroscopy has been used, as this exposes the child to unnecessary additional radiation. A chest radiograph should be performed if there are any cardio-respiratory symptoms or signs post-operatively.

The insertion complications for long-term catheters are similar to those outlined for short-term catheters (see Table 13.2) with the addition of vascular damage and haemorrhage that can occur with any open surgery. The major long-term complications are CRBI, venous thrombosis and catheter malfunction. The incidence of CRBIs for long-term venous catheters is around 1.5–3 per 1000 catheter days for Hickman-type catheters and around 0.1–1 per 1000 catheter days for implanted ports. There is no evidence that the use of prophylactic antibiotics at the time of insertion decreases the risk of infection.

The intravascular portion of a long-term catheter is rapidly covered in a fibrin sheath that can occlude the catheter tip. This can cause infusate to track back along the catheter and cause subcutaneous extravasation despite the catheter being intact. This can be confirmed by injection of X-ray contrast solution with fluoroscopy. Fibrin sheath or thrombus formation at the catheter tip or in the catheter lumen can sometimes be dissolved by fibrinolytic therapy. This involves the instillation of urokinase 5000 IU ml^{-1} or alteplase 1 mg ml^{-1} into the dead space of the blocked lumen using a negative pressure technique. A three-way tap is connected to the catheter and an empty 10 ml syringe used to generate a negative pressure within the lumen. The tap is then opened to the syringe containing the fibrinolytic agent which is aspirated into the lumen by negative pressure and left in place for 2 to 4 hours or overnight. The catheter must then be carefully aspirated to remove any clots or remaining fibrinolytic agent prior to being flushed with heparinised saline. This procedure can be repeated if necessary, but if this is not successful the catheter should be removed. Massive thrombus formation can occur at the catheter tip, within the central veins or right atrium. This may present as pulmonary emboli, vena cava obstruction or cardiac insufficiency. The diagnosis is confirmed by ultrasound or echocardiogram. It can usually be treated effectively with systemic anticoagulation and catheter removal, but occasionally require cardiac surgery for open removal.

Care bundles for venous catheters

CRBI is a major source of morbidity and mortality in hospitalised patients, with a substantial social and economic cost. Additional hospital expenses in the United Kingdom related to a patient acquiring a CRBI have been estimated at over £15 000. Bloodstream infections account for around 6% of all hospital infections, with an estimated 42.3% of these being related to central venous catheters. Confirmation of CRBI requires the same organism to be isolated from peripheral blood culture as well as from the device in a patient with clinical signs of bacteraemia. Colonisation of venous catheters is present when an organism can be isolated from the internal lumen or the subcutaneous external surface of the catheter in the absence of clinical signs of bacteraemia. The microorganisms that colonise venous catheters are responsible for most CRBI with contamination occurring at time of insertion or by migration along the catheter track. Contamination can also occur by the transfer of microorganisms during handling of the catheter hubs. Catheter colonisation and infection by haematogenous spread from distant sites is thought to be rare. A 2006 UK prevalence study showed that coagulase-negative staphylococci were the most commonly isolated organism from all types of intravenous catheters (35%). *Staphylococcus aureus* was the second most common (25%) with methicillin-resistant organisms (MRSA) accounting for 40–45% of these infections. Candida species and enterococci are also common infective agents causing CRBI.

An evidence base compiled over the past decade resulted in the publication in 2006 of 'EPIC2: National Evidence-Based Guidelines for Preventing Healthcare-Associated Infections in NHS Hospitals in England'. These guidelines have been used to produce care bundles for both central venous catheters and peripheral intravenous cannula (Department of Health 2007 High Impact Intervention Numbers 1 and 2; see Appendices 13.1 and 13.2). The concept of a care bundle is that it brings together all the scientifically based interventions that when used together improve clinical outcome. The care bundles are divided into insertion action and ongoing care actions and are designed to be used in their entirety; assessment of compliance requires all elements to be completed for each patient. For these to be successful there must be a proactive education programme of all staff involved in the care of intravenous catheters.

In 2009 a national patient safety initiative entitled 'Matching Michigan' was launched in the NHS to reduce CRBI, involving all adult and paediatric intensive care units in England. This project aims to replicate the results of a study published in 2006 conducted in the intensive care units (ICUs) across Michigan, USA, in which evidence-based interventions resulted in a large and sustained reduction (66%) in CRBI. This reduction has been maintained during a 3 year follow-up period.

Concern has been raised that the use of care bundles has led to earlier removal of CVCs and increased use of peripheral venous cannulae on ICUs when patients still require venous access. This may be associated with an increased risk of phlebitis and subsequent CRBI. It is very important that peripheral cannulae are inspected daily and assessed for phlebitis as part of the ongoing care action. A phlebitis scoring system has been developed and is invaluable in recording the daily state of peripheral cannula insertion sites (see Appendix 13.3).

Intraosseous access

Obtaining venous access in emergency paediatric resuscitation can be extremely difficult owing to collapsed small veins, which may be impossible to visualise because of overlying fat. This is often the case in septic shock and trauma victims, particularly in infants. The tracheal route offers an alternative emergency route for drug administration but obviously requires the child to have a tracheal tube *in situ*. The absorption of drugs administered via the tracheal route is variable, and the amount of fluid permitted by this route is very limited. The highly vascularised intraosseous (IO) space functions as a non-collapsible vein into which nearly all resuscitation drugs and unrestricted volumes of fluids can be infused.

The insertion of an IO cannula is painful and if the child is not unconscious then local anaesthesia should be used. The best anatomical insertion site is the antero-medial aspect of the proximal tibia 2–3 cm below the tibial tuberosity (see Figure 13.2). The tip of the needle should be directed away from the growth plate. Other insertion sites are the distal end of the femur 3 cm above the lateral condyle and the medial

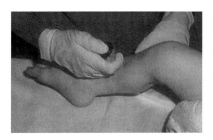

Figure 13.2
Intraosseous needle insertion on the antero-medial aspect of the proximal tibia.

malleolus at the ankle. The sternum is not recommended in children. Contraindications to IO access are a proximal fracture or severe soft tissue injury; in these cases the other side should be used. A history of osteogenesis imperfecta or osteoporosis is associated with a higher risk of bone fracture.

There are commercially available IO cannulae of variable size (14–18G) and design; some have a cutting bevel designed for a rotating insertion technique. Bone marrow aspirate needles can be used as an alternative. In neonates and small infants spinal needles have been successfully used but they tend to bend easily with the harder bones of older children. Any cannula used should have a central stylet to avoid plugging of the lumen with bone particles. Whatever the device or site chosen, a twisting technique is employed with sustained pressure until a sudden give is felt as the tip of the needle enters the medulla after passing through the harder cortex. Mechanical devices such as the EZ-IO® are available for use in children. Blood aspirated from the needle can be used for glucose and electrolyte estimation as well as cross-match and culture. Full blood count will reflect the marrow cell population rather than peripheral blood.

Infusion of fluids into the IO space requires higher pressure than normally used in intravenous infusions. Boluses of fluid can be given by syringe or the use of a pressurised system. All current resuscitation drugs and antibiotics can be given safely by the IO route. The IO route is extremely safe when used in short-term resuscitation, with complications in less than 1% of patients. Compartment syndrome requiring fasciotomy has been reported as well as injury to the growth plate, bone fracture and local haematoma formation. Osteomyelitis is a rare complication. Local extravasation is rarely serious unless vasoconstrictors or thiopentone are involved, when necrosis of the overlying skin may occur. Formal venous access should be established as soon as feasible to allow the IO access to be removed.

Key points

- Venous access is an essential element of paediatric medical practice but is associated with a high complication rate.
- The provision of venous access must be individualised to each patient to balance the risks against clinical requirements.
- The insertion complications of central venous lines are potentially life-threatening, hence

operators must be adequately trained and supervised for these procedures.
- There should be local protocols and care bundles for every type of venous access used.
- There should be an effective audit process in place to monitor complications from venous access.

Further reading

Arul GS, Lewis N, Bromley P, Bennett J. Ultrasound-guided percutaneous insertion of Hickman lines in children. Prospective study of 500 consecutive procedures. *J Ped Surg* 2009;**44**:1371–1376.

Bravery K. Paediatric intravenous therapy in practice. In: Dougherty L, Lamb J, eds. *Intravenous Therapy in Nursing Practice*, 2nd edition. Blackwell. 2008.

National Patient Safety Agency. *Minimising Central Venous Catheter Associated Bloodstream Infections: Matching Michigan*. 2009. www.npsa.nhs.uk

O'Grady NP, Alexander M, Dellinger EP *et al*. Guidelines for the prevention of intravascular catheter-related infections. *MMWR Recomm Rep* 2002;**51**(RR-10):1–29.

Pronovost P, Needham D, Berenholtz S *et al*. An intervention to decrease

catheter-related bloodstream infections in the ICU. *N Engl J Med* 2006;**355**:2725–32.

Ahluwalia JS, Brain JL, Kelsall AW. Procedures and iatrogenic disorders. In: Rennie JM, ed. *Roberton's Textbook of Neonatology*, 4th edition. Elsevier. 2005.

Appendix 13.1 Central venous catheter care bundle

Modified from: Department of Health 2007. High Impact Intervention No. 1. Central venous catheter care bundle. www.clean-safe-care.nhs.uk CR-BSI: catheter-related blood stream infection.

Insertion actions

Catheter type

- Use a single lumen catheter unless indicated otherwise.
- Consider an antimicrobial impregnated catheter if catheter to be used for 1 to 3 weeks and risk of CR-BSI is high.

Insertion site

- Subclavian or internal jugular.

Skin preparation

- Preferably use 2% chlorhexidine gluconate in 70% isopropyl alcohol. Allow to dry.
- If patient is sensitive to chlorhexidine use povidone-iodine.

Personal protective equipment

- Gloves are single-use items and should be removed and discarded immediately after the care activity.
- Eye/face protection is indicated if there is a risk of splashing with blood or body fluids.

Hand hygiene

- Decontaminate hands before and after each patient contact.
- Use correct hand hygiene procedures.

Aseptic technique

- Gown, gloves and drapes should be used for the insertion of invasive devices.

Dressing

- Use a sterile, transparent, semi-permeable dressing to allow observation of the insertion site.

Safe disposal of sharps

- A sharps container should be available at point of use and should not be overfilled; do not disassemble the needle and syringe; do not pass sharps from hand to hand.

Documentation

- Date of insertion should be recorded in the notes.

Ongoing care actions

Hand hygiene

- Decontaminate hands before and after each patient contact.
- Use correct hand hygiene procedure.

Catheter site inspection

- Observe the site for signs of infection, at least daily.

Dressing

- Ensure transparent dressing is intact, dry and adherent.

Catheter access

- Use aseptic technique and swab ports or hub with 2% chlorhexidine gluconate in 70% isopropyl alcohol prior to accessing the line for administering fluids or injections.

Administration set replacement

- Replace set immediately following administration of blood, blood products.
- Replace administration set after 24 hours following administration of TPN (up to 72 hours if no lipid).
- Replace all other sets within 72 hours.

No routine catheter replacement

Appendix 13.2 Peripheral intravenous cannula care bundle

Modified from Department of Health 2007. High Impact Intervention No. 2. Peripheral intravenous cannula care bundle. www.clean-safe-care.nhs.uk.

Insertion actions

Hand hygiene

- Decontaminate hands before and after each patient contact and before applying examination gloves.
- Use correct hand hygiene procedure.

Personal protective equipment

- Wear examination gloves if there is a risk of exposure to body fluids.
- Gloves are single-use items and should be removed and discarded immediately after the care activity.
- Gowns, aprons, eye/face protection are indicated if there is a risk of splashing with blood or body fluids.

Skin preparation

- Use 2% chlorhexidine gluconate in 70% isopropyl alcohol. Allow to dry.
- If patient is sensitive to chlorhexidine, use povidone-iodine.

Dressing

- Use a sterile, semi-permeable, transparent dressing to allow observation of insertion site.

Documentation

- Date of insertion should be recorded in notes.

Ongoing care actions

Hand hygiene

- Decontaminate hands before and after each patient contact.
- Use correct hand hygiene procedure.

Continuing clinical indication

- Check all intravenous cannulae and associated devices are still indicated.
- If there is no indication then the intravenous cannula should be removed.

Site inspection

- Observe the site for signs of infection, at least daily.

Dressing

- An intact, dry, adherent transparent dressing should be present.

Cannula access

- Use 2% chlorhexidine gluconate in 70% isopropyl alcohol, and allow to dry prior to accessing the cannula for administering fluid or injections.

Administration set replacement

- Replace set immediately after administration of blood or blood products.
- Replace all other fluid sets after 72 hours.

Routine cannula replacement

- Replace in a new site after 72–96 hours or earlier if indicated clinically.
- If venous access is limited, the cannula can remain *in situ* if there are no signs of infection.

Appendix 13.3 Visual infusion phlebitis (VIP) score

From: Jackson A. Infection control; a battle in vein infusion phlebitis. *Nursing Times* 1994;4:68–71

Appearance	Score	Comment	Action
IV site appears healthy	0	No signs of phlebitis	Observe
One of the following evident: Slight pain or redness near IV site	1	Possible first signs of phlebitis	Observe
Two of the following evident: Pain near IV site, erythema, swelling	2	Early stage of phlebitis	Resite cannula
All of the following evident: Pain along cannula, erythema, induration	3	Moderate phlebitis – consider treatment	Resite cannula
All of the following evident, and extensive: Pain along cannula, erythema, induration, palpable venous cord	4	Advanced phlebitis or start of thrombophlebitis	Resite cannula, consider treatment
All of the following are evident, and extensive: Pain along cannula, erythema, induration, palpable venous cord, pyrexia	5	Advanced stage of thrombophlebitis	Initiate treatment, resite cannula

Chapter

14

Peri-operative fluid management in children

Isabeau Walker and Dan Taylor

Introduction

Intravenous fluids are administered as a routine part of paediatric practice, but errors in fluid management may cause significant morbidity and mortality. Serious pitfalls include iatrogenic hyponatraemia (failure to prescribe appropriate fluids and monitor electrolyte balance) and inadequate fluid resuscitation (failure to assess fluid requirements). Traditional peri-operative fluid guidelines have been questioned but fortunately recent studies have started to clarify a rational approach to fluid management in children. This chapter will consider the problem of iatrogenic hyponatraemia in children, peri-operative fluid management, the management of major haemorrhage in children, and special circumstances where particular caution needs to be exercised.

Definitions

By convention, the term 'isotonic' is used for solutions containing sodium and potassium levels close to plasma (such as Hartmann's, Ringer's lactate, 0.9% saline, or 0.9% saline with added dextrose – 5% dextrose 0.9% saline or 1% dextrose 0.9% saline). Normal saline with added dextrose is hypertonic to plasma but the dextrose component is metabolised quickly so that it is effectively isotonic. Using the same rationale, the term 'hypotonic' is used for low sodium containing solutions such as 5% dextrose 0.45% saline or 4% dextrose 0.18% saline (see Table 14.1). 'Peri-operative' includes the period before, during and after surgery; intra-operative fluid requirements may differ from post-operative fluid requirements.

The problem of hyponatraemia

Hyponatraemia is defined as a plasma sodium less than 135 mmol l^{-1} and is the most common electrolyte abnormality of hospitalised children. Acute hyponatraemia that develops over a period of hours or days may have devastating consequences and unfortunately is frequently iatrogenic. Prepubertal children and women are particularly vulnerable to the effect of acute hyponatraemia as they are less able to compensate for a rapid fall in plasma sodium and develop cerebral oedema. Children have a disproportionately large brain in relation to skull size, and they are more likely to become symptomatic at a higher plasma sodium than in adults – 50% of children are likely to be symptomatic at a plasma sodium of 125 mmol l^{-1}. Symptoms of acute hyponatraemia may be subtle initially, and include increasing lethargy, headache and nausea followed by sudden onset of seizures. Once symptoms progress to respiratory arrest or coma, the prognosis is poor.

Traditional prescription of intravenous fluids is based on the formula described by Holliday and Segar in 1957. The requirement for water was linked to the calorie requirement for healthy children, and for electrolytes to the dietary intake for sodium and potassium for the 'average' child. A fluid with 4% dextrose 0.18% saline was formulated to provide the 'ideal' balance of water and electrolytes. However, a classic paper by Arieff *et al.* published in 1992 described the phenomenon of acute symptomatic hyponatraemia in previously healthy children who were treated with 'normal maintenance fluids' according to the Holliday and Segar formula during an acute illness or in the peri-operative period. Patients developed symptoms of acute hyponatraemia, in some cases over a few hours. Since then, there have been more than 60 cases reported in the literature of death or severe neurological impairment due to acute hospital-acquired hyponatraemia. The problem arises through a combination of:

- Administration of hypotonic intravenous fluids (4% dextrose 0.18% saline);

Core Topics in Paediatric Anaesthesia, ed. Ian James and Isabeau Walker. Published by Cambridge University Press. © 2013 Cambridge University Press.

Table 14.1 Composition of intravenous fluids

Fluid	Sodium (mmol l^{-1})	Potassium (mmol l^{-1})	Glucose (g dl^{-1})	Chloride (mmol l^{-1})	Osmolality (mOsmol kg^{-1})	Osmolality compared with plasma	Tonicity (after glucose metabolism)
5% dextrose	0	0	0	0	272	Isosmolar	Hypotonic
10% dextrose	0	0	0	0	555	Hyperosmolar	Hypotonic
4% dextrose 0.18% saline	30	0	40	30	282	Isosmolar	Hypotonic
2.5% dextrose 0.45% saline	77	0	25	77	293	Isosmolar	Hypotonic
5% dextrose 0.45% saline	77	0	50	77	432	Hyperosmolar	Hypotonic
Hartmann's	131	5	0	111	278	Isosmolar	Hypotonic
Polyionique B6	120	4	50	108		Hyposmolar	Hypotonic
BS-1G* (Balanced salt 1% glucose)	140	4	10	118	294	Isosmolar	Isotonic
PlasmaLyte 148	140	5	0	98	294	Isosmolar	Isotonic
0.9% saline	154	0	0	154	308	Isosmolar	Isotonic
5% dextrose 0.9% saline	154	0	50	154	560	Hyperosmolar	Isotonic
4.5% albumin	100–160	0	0	0	275	Isosmolar	Isotonic
Succinylated gelatin (Gelofusine)	154	0	0	120	274	Isosmolar	Isotonic
HES (normal saline)	154	0	0	154	308	Isosmolar	Isotonic
HES (balanced salt solution)	140	4	0	118	296	Isosmolar	Isotonic

* Elektrolyt-Infusionslösung 148 mit Glucose 1 PÄD, Serumwerk Bernburg AG, Bernburg, Germany

- Acute illness or surgery resulting in high levels of antidiuretic hormone;
- +/− increased sodium losses (e.g. intestinal/urinary losses);
- Failure to monitor plasma sodium;
- Failure to respond appropriately to low plasma sodium.

The effect of antidiuretic hormone (ADH)

Plasma sodium concentration depends on the balance between sodium and water content. In the healthy child, plasma osmolality is around 300 mOsmol kg^{-1} and water intake (determined by thirst) is matched by water loss (insensible losses and urinary losses determined by the action of antidiuretic hormone, ADH), so that the plasma sodium is maintained in the range 135–145 mmol l^{-1}. In health, if water intake is increased, ADH release is suppressed and a water diuresis occurs so that the sodium concentration is maintained in the normal range (dilute urine which may have an osmolality as low as 50 mOsmol kg^{-1} is excreted). If water intake falls, ADH is released from the posterior pituitary and activates water channels (aquaporins) in the collecting ducts of the kidney so that water is retained and small volumes of concentrated urine are produced (urine osmolality may be as high as 1400 mOsmol kg^{-1}); plasma sodium stays in the normal range.

ADH is released as part of the normal physiological response to hypovolaemia, but it is also released in response to other 'non-osmotic' stimuli commonly seen in the peri-operative period:

- Post-operative pain, stress, nausea
- Drugs (opioids, NSAID, carbamazepine, vincristine)
- Pulmonary disorders (pneumonia, bronchiolitis); IPPV
- Central nervous system (CNS) disorders (tumours, trauma, haemorrhage)

The non-osmotic release of ADH overrides osmotic control, so if the ADH levels are high because of non-osmotic causes and hypotonic fluids are administered, ADH release will not be suppressed, the 'electrolyte-free' water will be retained and the plasma sodium will fall.

Prevention of acute hyponatraemia in the peri-operative period

Acute hyponatraemia may be prevented by the use of isotonic fluids in the peri-operative period. This has been supported by a number of randomised controlled studies in recent years. Isotonic solutions also tend to correct plasma sodium concentration if the child is hyponatraemic. Conversely, administration of hypotonic fluids promotes hyponatraemia, and does not aid correction of the plasma sodium in hyponatraemic patients.

The volume of intravenous fluid is also an important consideration. The '4,2,1' formula of Holliday and Segar for maintenance fluid is a useful starting point for fluid prescription (see Box 14.1). Traditionally, many have restricted fluids to 50–70% of standard maintenance volumes in the first few days post-operatively to avoid oedema and reduce the risk of hyponatraemia. However, simple fluid restriction during this time is not sufficient to prevent hyponatraemia if patients are prescribed hypotonic fluids. Conversely, children who receive restricted isotonic fluids for a number of days post-operatively may become dehydrated so that the plasma sodium rises. This emphasises the importance of clinical monitoring to ensure that prescriptions are tailored to the individual clinical picture. It should not be assumed

Box 14.1 Prescription of intravenous fluids

- This is a suggested protocol for intravenous fluid prescription for previously well children with normal renal function. Safe fluid prescribing requires careful assessment of sodium requirements, water requirements, and close monitoring of outcomes.

Resuscitation

20 ml kg^{-1} 0.9% saline, Hartmann's, colloid or blood as indicated. Reassess and repeat as necessary.

Intra-operative fluids

10–20 ml kg^{-1} Hartmann's, colloid or blood as indicated. Reassess and repeat as necessary. Check blood glucose.

Post-operative fluids

Use oral route if possible.

Maintenance fluids
- Prescribe intravenous fluid volume according to the Holliday and Segar formula.

Weight	Daily fluid requirement	Hourly fluid requirement
<10 kg	100 ml kg^{-1}	4 ml kg^{-1}
10–20 kg	1000 ml + 50 ml kg^{-1} for each kg > 10 kg	40 ml + 2 ml kg^{-1} for each kg > 10 kg
>20 kg	1500 ml + 20 ml kg^{-1} for each kg > 20 kg (max 2500 ml day^{-1})	60 ml + 1 ml kg^{-1} for each kg > 20 kg (max 100 ml h^{-1})

Day 1 5% dextrose 0.9% saline, 100% maintenance, no added potassium chloride. Consider restriction of maintenance if child is oedematous, or requires intensive care.
Day 2 5% dextrose 0.9% saline (or 5% dextrose 0.45% saline, depending on plasma sodium), 100% of maintenance. Add potassium chloride 10 mmol 500 ml^{-1}, provided good urine output.

Hypovolaemia
- Consider bolus of isotonic fluid (20ml kg^{-1} 0.9% saline, colloid, blood) if child appears hypovolaemic.

Replacement fluids
(nasogastric losses, other on-going losses)
- Replace losses ml for ml with 0.9% saline + potassium chloride 10 mmol 500 ml^{-1}

Box 14.1 (*cont.*)

Neonates

Day 1 of life	60 ml kg^{-1} day^{-1}	10% dextrose
Day 2	90 ml kg^{-1} day^{-1}	5% dextrose 0.45% saline
Day 3	120 ml kg^{-1} day^{-1}	5% dextrose 0.45% saline
Day 4	150 ml kg^{-1} day^{-1}	5% dextrose 0.45% saline

Consider adding potassium chloride 10 mmol 500 ml^{-1} from day 2. Post surgery neonates do not need to be further restricted on day 1.

Monitoring

- Weigh all children prior to starting fluids, daily thereafter.
- Document an accurate daily fluid balance.
- Check electrolytes before starting intravenous fluids (except well children, elective surgery).
- Check electrolytes daily for the first 4 days of intravenous fluids, thereafter as clinically indicated.
- If electrolytes are abnormal, consider rechecking 6 hourly, definitely if sodium <130 mmol l^{-1}.

that any single type or rate of fluid administration will suit all children.

Intravenous fluids are prescribed in the peri-operative period with the same care as any drug (see Box 14.1). The child should be assessed clinically and the plasma sodium monitored at least daily during therapy. We use isotonic fluid initially, and our policy is to restrict fluids for those in intensive care or after major surgery. After the first few days, fluids are liberalised, the volume restriction relaxed, and free water may be introduced (5% dextrose in 0.45% saline). These decisions are dictated by clinical assessment or laboratory results, for instance when the child develops a post-surgery diuresis, post-operative oedema reduces, or if there is a high normal and rising plasma sodium.

'Desalination'

Acute hyponatraemia may still develop in situations where only isotonic fluids have been used, and has been reported for instance after craniofacial surgery where large volumes of fluids have been given. This may be due to a natriuresis from volume loading at the same time as there are high levels of ADH due to the stress response. Hypervolaemia during surgery should be avoided by close monitoring of fluid balance. Electrolytes should be monitored routinely where large volumes of fluid are given.

Neonates

Fluid requirement of neonates differs from older children. ADH levels are high in the first few days of life, and the maintenance requirement for water is low. Sodium requirements are also low and it is traditional to use 10% dextrose restricted to 50–60% of maintenance on day one of life. Electrolytes must be monitored carefully. Fluids are liberalised and sodium is added to maintenance fluids after a few days when the post-natal diuresis has occurred. Isotonic fluids should be used peri-operatively, and to replace abnormal losses such as gastrointestinal drainage post-operatively. It is important to monitor blood glucose. Premature neonates may have high insensible losses due to evaporation, and may require relatively higher volumes of maintenance fluids.

The need for dextrose in intravenous fluids

Most children maintain their blood glucose during surgery, and isotonic fluids can be used without added dextrose. However, some children may be vulnerable to hypoglycaemia during surgery and blood sugar should be checked routinely, particularly in the following cases:

- Neonates
- Prolonged surgery in infants
- Children with sepsis
- High dextrose requirements pre-operatively
- Receiving total parenteral nutrition (TPN)

Infants and children undergoing prolonged surgery or who have been starved for a long time may undergo lipolysis and become ketotic in theatre. The use of isotonic solutions containing 5% dextrose during surgery is associated with hyperglycaemia, but a number of European companies now produce isotonic solutions containing 1% dextrose that are effective in preventing both intra-operative hypoglycaemia and lipolysis. If such dextrose-containing solutions are used during surgery they must only be used for 'maintenance' and not be used to deliver a fluid bolus; a second bag of isotonic fluid without dextrose should be used for fluid boluses.

In the post-operative period children require a source of added dextrose to maintain normoglycaemia and prevent ketosis. Children under 6 years require a concentration of dextrose of at least $50\,\text{mg}\,\text{ml}^{-1}$ (i.e. at least 5% dextrose in isotonic saline) (see Box 14.1).

Hyperchloraemic acidosis

Solutions such as 0.9% saline contain a non-physiological concentration of chloride, whilst Hartmann's, Ringer's lactate and PlasmaLyte 148 have an electrolyte composition closer to that of plasma. These 'balanced salt solutions' contain lactate or acetate, which are more stable than bicarbonate but are metabolised to bicarbonate, to provide electrical neutrality (Table 14.1). Solutions containing 0.9% saline are more likely to be associated with hyperchloraemic acidosis in children and adults, and for this reason, balanced salt solutions are preferred in the peri-operative period. The physiological significance of hyperchloraemia is not clear, but a base-deficit solely due to hyperchloraemia does not require correction with fluid boluses.

Currently, solutions containing 5% dextrose in balanced salt solution are not readily available in the UK, so 5% dextrose 0.9% saline is generally used for maintenance for post-operative patients and other patients at risk of hyponatraemia. Hyperchloraemic acidosis was not seen in a small study published by Neville in 2010 where this solution was used post-operatively, but the ideal maintenance fluid remains a balanced salt solution +/− added dextrose. Hartmann's and Ringer's lactate are suitable as resuscitation fluids in the peri-operative period, or for maintenance in older children. They contain a relatively low concentration of sodium $(131\,\text{mmol}\,\text{l}^{-1})$, so should be used cautiously for large volume resuscitation, for instance in neurosurgical patients who are particularly at risk from hyponatraemia.

Intravenous fluids – guidance from the NPSA

The National Patient Safety Agency in England issued a Patient Safety Alert (PSA 22) in 2007 to warn of the risk of hyponatraemia when administering intravenous infusions to children. The PSA included a number of important recommendations that form the basis of recommended peri-operative fluid prescription (see Box 14.1):

- 4% dextrose in 0.18% saline should be removed from all ward areas and should only be used in specialist situations, for instance to treat children with diabetes insipidus, or in the management of acute hypernatraemia.
- Oral fluids should be used in preference to intravenous infusions where possible.
- Fluid deficits and fluid resuscitation should be managed with isotonic fluids only (correction of fluid deficit in hypernatraemic dehydration is a special situation – see below).
- The volume of maintenance fluids should be given according to the formula recommended by Holliday and Segar (Box 14.1), but may be restricted in the immediate post-operative period and in situations where ADH is likely to be increased (see above).
- The sodium content of maintenance fluids should be prescribed according to the clinical situation. Healthy children may tolerate hypotonic maintenance fluids (5% dextrose 0.45% saline) in the absence of an ADH drive, but children with the following conditions should **only** receive isotonic maintenance fluids:
  - Children who are peri- or post-operative
  - Plasma sodium at the lower normal reference range and definitely if less than $135\,\text{mmol}\,\text{l}^{-1}$
  - Intravascular volume depletion
  - Hypotension
  - CNS infection
  - Head injury
  - Bronchiolitis
  - Sepsis
  - Excessive gastric or diarrhoeal losses
  - Salt-wasting syndromes
  - Chronic conditions such as diabetes, cystic fibrosis and pituitary disease
- Fluid losses should be monitored accurately and replaced with the appropriate fluid (isotonic saline for nasogastric losses).
- Fluid therapy should be monitored accurately by daily weights and by measuring plasma urea and electrolytes at baseline and at least once a day thereafter (more frequently if necessary), ideally using the same analytical method. Urinary

osmolality and electrolytes should be measured in high-risk cases.

- Acute symptomatic hyponatraemia is a clinical emergency and should be managed in the PICU.

Management of acute hyponatraemic encephalopathy

It is important to respond appropriately to low plasma sodium. Mild hyponatraemia (sodium 131–135 mmol l^{-1}) can be managed by fluid restriction and stopping any hypotonic fluid intake.

Acute hyponatraemia is a medical emergency and should be suspected in any child receiving intravenous fluids who develops headache, vomiting, lethargy, nausea, altered level of consciousness, seizures or apnoea. Symptomatic hyponatraemic encephalopathy should be treated with bolus doses of hypertonic saline (3%) in order to control symptoms (stop seizures) and achieve a rise in plasma sodium of 5–6 mmol l^{-1} in the first 1–2 hours. There is a risk of over-correction if an infusion of hypertonic saline is used. Simple fluid restriction or isotonic fluids do not have a role in the emergency situation.

Moritz suggests the following treatment regimen for the management of acute hyponatraemic encephalopathy:

- 3% saline bolus, 2 ml kg^{-1} over 10 minutes (maximum 100 ml).
- Repeat bolus 1–2 times if symptoms persist.
- Recheck plasma sodium after second bolus or 2 hours.
- Stop therapy in the following circumstances:
  - Patient is symptom-free (awake, alert, responding to commands, resolution of nausea and headache).
  - A rise in plasma sodium of 5–6 mmol l^{-1} is achieved.
  - There is an acute rise in plasma sodium of 10 mmol l^{-1} in the first 5 hours.
- Do not exceed a correction of plasma sodium of 15–20 mmol l^{-1} in 48 hours.
- Avoid normo- or hypernatraemia in the first 48 hours.

Crystalloids versus colloids

The benefit of crystalloids versus colloids is a subject of debate in paediatric practice. Historically 4.5% albumin has been used in neonates and in resuscitation of children with sepsis. It has the advantage that it persists in the intravascular compartment, but in the UK it is expensive and as a blood product it cannot be guaranteed to be free of infection. A randomised controlled study of saline versus albumin in adults did not confirm safety concerns, but suggested greater benefit for saline in patients with head injury and albumin in patients with sepsis. Albumin is widely used in the United States.

Gelatins are derived from bovine collagen and are available suspended in saline or balanced salt solution (Table 14.1). They are effective plasma volume expanders and remain in the intravascular compartment for 2–3 hours. Gelatins are inexpensive, do not have an effect on renal function and cause coagulation problems only through dilution of coagulations factors, but they cause a higher incidence of anaphylactic reactions compared with other synthetic colloids. There is no maximum daily dose defined and they are widely used in the UK.

Hydroxyethyl starch solutions (HES) are derived from maize or potato starch and are also available suspended in saline or balanced salt solution. They are classified according to concentration, molecular weight and molar substitution. First-generation HES solutions were shown to be effective in volume expansion, but are broken down slowly, possibly leading to significant adverse effects. These included coagulopathy due to acquired von Willebrand syndrome with reduced fVIII activity and impaired platelet function, renal impairment due to deposits in renal tubules, and pruritis due to deposits in the reticuloendothelial system. Newer third-generation 6% HES 130/0.4 has a more favourable side effect profile, and safety studies in children are under way. It is approved for use in children at a maximum daily dose of 50 ml kg^{-1}. HES solutions are widely used in continental Europe.

Transfusion of blood and blood components

Red cells should be transfused where the principal fluid lost is blood. Healthy children have a high cardiac output and effective tissue oxygen delivery, and outside the immediate neonatal period, a haemoglobin concentration of 7 g dl^{-1} is well tolerated. Appropriate triggers for transfusion in other circumstances are shown in Table 14.2

All blood in the UK is leucodepleted to reduce the risk of variant Creutzfelt–Jacob disease (vCJD)

Table 14.2 General principles – transfusion triggers in children

Transfusion trigger	Haemoglobin concentration (g dl^{-1})
Anaemia in the first 12 hours of life	12
Acutely ill child	7
Cyanotic heart disease	10–12
Early severe sepsis	10

Table 14.3 Blood component therapy in children

Component	Volume
Red cell concentrate	4 ml kg^{-1} packed cells raises the haemoglobin by 1 g dl^{-1}
Platelet concentrate	Child < 5 kg: 10–20 ml kg^{-1} Child >15 kg: One standard pool
Fresh frozen plasma	10–20 ml kg^{-1}
Cryoprecipitate	Child <15 kg: 5ml kg^{-1} Child 15–30 kg: 5 units Child >30 kg: 10 units

transmission. Irradiation of red cells removes any remaining competent white cells and is required for immune-deficient patients including those with DiGeorge syndrome (22q11 deletion). Irradiation damages the plasma membrane of donor red cells and increases plasma potassium, so blood that is irradiated must be fresh (within 5 days of donation) and used within 24 hours of irradiation. Cytomegalovirus (CMV) negative blood should be given to babies under 1.5 kg and CMV negative patients with immune deficiency. Plasma should be screened for atypical maternal antibodies in the first four months of life – theoretically a maternal sample should be tested, but in practice the infant's serum is screened directly.

The volume of packed red cells required for a top-up transfusion can be calculated using the formula shown in Table 14.3; a target haemoglobin should be chosen so as to minimise donor exposure. Intra-operative cell salvage is cost-effective in many situations. Children are susceptible to hypothermia and to hyperkalaemia from infusing large volumes of cold blood; all blood should be warmed, particularly if a large volume transfusion is considered.

Recommended volumes of blood components are shown in Table 14.3. Infants undergoing cardiac surgery undergo the equivalent of an exchange transfusion and benefit from antifibrinolytic agents (tranexamic acid or aprotinin), cryoprecipitate and platelets.

In the UK, fresh frozen plasma (FFP) for children born after 1989 is obtained from US volunteer donors to reduce the risk of transmission of vCJD. Imported FFP is treated with methylene blue and white light to ensure virus inactivation. Cryoprecipitate is sourced from the UK and exposes the patient to multiple donors. Virally inactivated fibrinogen concentrate is available in some centres in Europe.

Routine peri-operative fluids – a practical approach

Minor surgery

Our policy is that children receive food, cow's milk or formula up to 6 hours pre-operatively, breast milk up to 4 hours and free clear fluids up to 2 hours pre-operatively. Children should not have a fasting deficit, but unfortunately it is common that starvation times are exceeded. It is usual practice to give a fluid bolus of 10–20 ml kg^{-1} Hartmann's to maintain blood pressure and reduce the need for early feeding, which may also reduce the incidence of post-operative nausea and vomiting. Intravenous fluids should not be continued post-operatively.

Major surgery

An initial fluid bolus of 10–20 ml kg^{-1} Hartmann's is given, with subsequent fluid boluses of 20 ml kg^{-1} Hartmann's, colloid or blood determined by clinical assessment (heart rate, capillary refill, blood pressure, core–peripheral temperature difference, base excess, urine output and haematocrit) and estimation of fluid losses (observation of surgical field, weighing swabs), remembering that the total blood volume is 80 ml kg^{-1}. As in adult practice, excessive fluid volume will lead to post-operative weight gain and oedema and should be avoided. Clinical signs are notoriously unreliable, and invasive monitoring is required if significant fluid shifts are expected. A variety of cardiac output monitors have been validated for use in children (oesophageal Doppler, LidCo®). Monitors used to assess end organ perfusion such as near-infrared spectroscopy (NIRS) or central venous oxygen saturation monitoring (target $S_{cv}O_2 > 70\%$) may also be useful. Cardiac output monitoring should be considered for major surgery involving large fluid shifts, or for children with limited cardiac reserve.

Emergency surgery

Children presenting for emergency surgery may be significantly dehydrated or hypovolaemic and require careful clinical assessment and replacement of fluid deficits before surgery. A similar approach of fluid bolus of $10–20\,ml\,kg^{-1}$ may be used, with careful monitoring of electrolytes and haemoglobin, and assessment of response before further fluid boluses are given.

Post-operative fluids

Isotonic maintenance fluids are required if oral fluids are precluded (Box 14.1); additional replacement fluid may be required to replace ongoing losses from wound drains or gastrointestinal losses ml for ml, or as a bolus of $10–20\,ml\,kg^{-1}$ to correct hypovolaemia. Potassium may be added to maintenance fluids on the second day, and electrolytes and fluid balance must be carefully monitored as described above. Hypotonic fluids may be tolerated once the ADH response has subsided, but are best avoided in the first 24 hours after surgery, and definitely if the plasma sodium is $<135\,mmol\,l^{-1}$.

Our policy is to give volume for maintenance fluids according to the Holliday and Segar formula, initially restricting to 50–70% if the patient is oedematous, or after major surgery or in critical care. Fluids may also need to be restricted if the child is oliguric, for instance owing to acute tubular necrosis (after pre-renal causes of renal impairment have been excluded), or in end-stage renal failure.

Fluid management in special situations
Shock

Shock occurs when perfusion does not meet the metabolic demands of the tissues, for instance because of hypovolaemia or sepsis.

- The clinical signs of shock in a child include tachycardia, cool peripheries, delayed capillary refill and weak pulses. Signs of decompensated shock include hypotension, mottling and confusion.
- Management is according to standard advanced life support algorithms ('ABC'); high flow oxygen should be given and a bolus of isotonic fluid 20 ml kg^{-1}, repeated if necessary after reassessment.
- The airway should be secured if more than $60\,ml\,kg^{-1}$ of resuscitation fluid is required.
- Aggressive fluid resuscitation improves outcomes in septic shock.
- Care should be taken when large volumes of crystalloid are administered to children with pre-existing anaemia (for instance shock in children with malaria).

Dehydration

Dehydration occurs when fluid is lost from all fluid compartments, often over a prolonged period of time, most commonly due to gastrointestinal causes.

- Dehydration is classified as mild (loss of 5% body weight), moderate (loss of 10% body weight), or severe (loss of 15% body weight), and may be described by clinical symptoms (see Table 14.4).
- Children with severe dehydration may be shocked and an initial bolus of $10–20\,ml\,kg^{-1}$ 0.9% saline should be considered.
- Caution is required in children with long-standing dehydration or severe malnutrition as fluid boluses may cause pulmonary oedema. The remaining fluid deficit should be corrected over 12–72 hours.
- Mild dehydration should be managed with oral rehydration solution if possible.

The relative balance between sodium and water loss may result in hypernatraemic, isonatraemic (most common) or hyponatraemic dehydration. Isotonic fluids should be used if plasma sodium is normal or low; hypotonic fluids may be used in hypernatraemic dehydration. Sodium correction should be slow where dehydration has occurred over a long period of time and where adaptive changes have occurred. Rapid correction of long-standing hyponatraemia may result in osmotic demyelination syndrome (quadriplegia and locked-in state) or in the case of hypernatraemia, may result in cerebral oedema.

Pyloric stenosis

If long-standing, pyloric stenosis results in a characteristic pattern of dehydration with hypochloraemic hypokalemic metabolic alkalosis. There may not be

Table 14.4 Clinical signs of dehydration

Degree of dehydration	Mild	Moderate	Severe
Weight loss	5%	10%	15%
Volume of deficit	$50\,ml\,kg^{-1}$	$100\,ml\,kg^{-1}$	$150\,ml\,kg^{-1}$
Clinical state	Not unwell	Apathetic	Usually shocked, unwell
Pulse	Normal	Tachycardia	Tachycardia
Capillary refill	<2 s	2–4 s	>4 s
Anterior fontanelle	Normal	Normal	Sunken
Tears	Present	Decreased	Absent
Eyes	Normal	Sunken	Deeply sunken
Mucous membrane	Normal	Dry	Parched
Skin	Normal	Reduced	Turgor doughy
Mental state	Normal	Lethargic	Unresponsive
Blood pressure	Normal	Normal	Reduced
Urine specific gravity	>1.020	>1.020	Oliguric or anuric

any electrolyte changes if diagnosed early (first few weeks of life). The plasma sodium may be normal, high or low.

- If the baby is shocked they should receive a bolus of $20\,ml\,kg^{-1}$ isotonic fluid.
- Mild dehydration may be corrected with intravenous fluid given over 6–12 hours, but severe dehydration should be corrected over 36–72 hours.
- The fluid deficit should be estimated (a record of body weight may be available), and given in addition to maintenance.
- The choice of fluid (5% dextrose in 0.9% saline or 5% dextrose in 0.45% saline) depends on plasma sodium. Potassium should be added once the baby is passing urine, and fluid balance and electrolytes must be monitored.
- If there is a significant metabolic alkalosis the baby will be at risk of post-operative apnoeas and should only undergo surgery when the metabolic alkalosis is corrected (bicarbonate $<26\,mmol\,l^{-1}$ and chloride $>90\,mmol\,l^{-1}$).

Diabetic ketoacidosis

- Dehydration due to the osmotic diuresis in diabetic ketoacidosis (DKA) has developed over a period of many weeks and must not be corrected rapidly. Water moves from the intracellular to the extracellular fluid compartment as part of the physiological adaptation, and rapid rehydration, especially when plasma sodium is allowed to fall, will result in cerebral oedema, the leading cause of death in children with DKA. Shock is rare, but if it occurs, a fluid bolus will be required, but should be limited to $7.5{-}10\,ml\,kg^{-1}$.
- The fluid deficit should be replaced over a minimum of 48 hours with isotonic fluid only.
- The blood sugar should be reduced slowly using an infusion of insulin with glucose introduced as it falls.
- Children with severe DKA should be monitored closely in intensive care.

For further guidance see http://www.strs.nhs.uk/resources/pdf/guidelines/DKAmarch08.pdf.

Neurosurgery

Neurosurgical patients are susceptible to a variety of conditions that affect sodium balance and in which fluid management requires special consideration (see Table 14.5):

- Diabetes insipidus (DI)
- Syndrome of inappropriate ADH (SIADH)
- Cerebral salt wasting (CSW)

Table 14.5 Disorders of sodium and water balance in neurosurgery

Condition	Description	Clinical picture	Treatment
Central diabetes insipidus	Deficiency of ADH, due to e.g. • Craniopharyngioma • Langerhans' cell histiocytosis • Head injury • Hypoxic brain injury	Polyuria, polydipsia. Normal plasma osmolality is maintained provided child able to drink water (often in large volumes!). Suspect in neurosurgical patient who develops urine output of $>5\,\mathrm{ml\,kg^{-1}\,h^{-1}}$. Severe hypernatraemic dehydration if access to hypotonic fluid restricted.	Desmopressin (DDAVP).
Syndrome of inappropriate ADH (SIADH)	High ADH after e.g. • Neurosurgery • Head injury • Cerebral haemorrhage • Meningitis • Carbamazepine	Oedema, weight gain. Hyponatraemia with inappropriately high urine osmolality in presence of low plasma osmolality.	Fluid restriction. Isotonic fluids only. Treat with 3% saline bolus if seizures/coma.
Cerebral salt wasting	Release of naturetic peptides after e.g. • Neurosurgery • Head injury • Cerebral haemorrhage • Meningitis	Naturesis and diuresis leading to hyponatraemia and contraction of extracellular fluid volume, weight loss, elevated urea and haemotocrit.	Bolus of isotonic fluid to replace deficit of sodium and water.

Major haemorrhage

Major haemorrhage has been defined as the loss of one circulating volume within a 24 hour period, 50% of the circulating blood volume within 3 hours, or blood loss of $2\,\mathrm{ml\,kg^{-1}\,min^{-1}}$ (150 ml minute^{-1} in an adult). It is essential to recognise early and institute appropriate interventions. Situations associated with massive haemorrhage in children include:

- Trauma
- Neurosurgery, craniofacial surgery, cardiac surgery, hepatic surgery, spinal surgery, ENT surgery (post-tonsillectomy), arterio-venous malformations, tumours, gastrointestinal haemorrhage
- Coagulopathies (haemophilia A, von Willebrand's disease)
- Acquired coagulopathy (post-cardiac surgery, ECMO, secondary to major haemorrhage)

Infants are particularly susceptible to major haemorrhage as they have low levels of vitamin K dependent factors and fibrinogen in the first few months of life. All newborn infants require vitamin K prophylaxis to prevent haemorrhagic disease of the newborn. Platelets are present in normal numbers at birth, and reach adult reactivity at 2 weeks of age. Coagulation screening tests are prolonged in normal infants up to the age of 6 months, which is reflected in values for the normal ranges.

The treatment priorities in major haemorrhage are to:

- Maintain the circulating blood volume and haemoglobin concentration to achieve adequate tissue oxygen delivery;
- Arrest the primary cause of bleeding;
- Correct coagulation defects;
- Correct the metabolic consequences of massive haemorrhage.

Close liaison with the haematologist and transfusion laboratory is essential, and effective team working will improve outcomes. The principles of management in children are the same as in adults; volume losses should be assessed if possible and two large-bore cannulae should be in place at minimum (size depends on the size of the child), with central venous access depending on the clinical situation (internal jugular or femoral). Intraosseous access may be used short term in cases of unexpected major haemorrhage in accident and emergency, avoiding proximal limb fractures.

Transfusion endpoints in major haemorrhage

Volume replacement should be guided by clinical endpoints such as heart rate, blood pressure, central venous pressure, capillary refill, acid–base status and lactate, aiming for a mean arterial pressure at the low end of normal. Target haemoglobin should be the same as in adults, higher in infants with cyanotic heart disease, or to avoid exposure to an additional donor. Laboratory and near-patient testing to guide transfusion is essential (haemoglobin, haematocrit, potassium, ionised calcium and coagulation). Unintended over-transfusion of red cells is common in small infants.

The volume of blood required depends on the child's circulating blood volume. Suggested transfusion volumes for red cells and clotting factors are shown in Table 14.3. Adult blood packs should be ordered in situations of major haemorrhage.

Coagulopathy in major haemorrhage is generally not significant until at least one circulating volume has been replaced, provided adequate tissue perfusion is maintained. The target minimum platelet count is 75×10^9 dl^{-1} (100×10^9 dl^{-1} in multiple trauma or head injured patients), fibrinogen >1 g l^{-1} and activated prothrombin time and activated partial thromboplastin time less than 1.5 times the normal for age.

The first line treatment of coagulopathy is with FFP, which may be given empirically after one blood volume loss if coagulation tests are not available. If the fibrinogen remains low, cryoprecipitate may be used as an alternative and will usually be needed with platelets once two blood volume losses have occurred.

Metabolic consequences of major haemorrhage in children

Large volume transfusions at rates exceeding 3 ml kg^{-1} min^{-1} for red cells and 1.5–2 ml kg^{-1} min^{-1} for FFP may be associated with a number of adverse events in children. These include:

- Low ionised calcium (<1 mmol l^{-1}). This is due to citrate toxicity and results in myocardial dysfunction. It should be corrected with calcium chloride 5–10 mg kg^{-1} by slow intravenous infusion via a central line.
- Hyperkalaemia due to high extracellular potassium in old stored blood or irradiated blood. Neonates and small infants are particularly vulnerable, and cardiac arrest has been reported. If the serum potassium is >7.5 mmol l^{-1} this constitutes a medical emergency, and treatment with 10% calcium gluconate 0.5 ml kg^{-1} and nebulised salbutamol or dextrose +/− insulin will be required.
- Hypomagnesaemia. This is due to citrate toxicity and results in ventricular arrhythmias. Hypomagnesaemia is treated with intravenous magnesium 25–50 mg kg^{-1} (maximum 2g).
- Hypothermia, metabolic acidosis, lactic acidosis. All blood should be warmed as this also helps to reduce the potassium level in the donor serum.

Key points

- Iatrogenic hyponatraemia is common in children who are acutely unwell.
- Oral fluids should be encouraged, and intravenous fluids used only if required.
- It is safest to use only isotonic fluid in the peri-operative period.
- No single fluid prescription or rate is correct for all children.
- Intravenous fluids require daily clinical and laboratory monitoring, with fluid prescriptions modified according to requirements. Hypotonic fluids should not be administered if the plasma sodium is less than 135 mmol l^{-1}.
- Hyponatremia, hypernatraemia, dehydration, shock and major haemorrhage are all special circumstances that require appropriate responses and close monitoring.

Further reading

Arieff AL, Ayus JC, Fraser CL. Hyponatraemia and death or permanent neurological damage in healthy children. *Br Med J* 1992;**304**:1218–22.

Holiday MA, Segar WE. The maintenance need for water in parenteral fluid therapy. *Pediatrics* 1957;**19**:823–32.

Moritz ML, Ayus JC. Intravenous fluid management for the acutely ill child. *Curr Opin Ped* 2011;**23**:186–93.

National Patient Safety Agency. Patient Safety Alert 22. Reducing the risk of hyponatraemia when administering intravenous infusions to children. 2007 http://www.nrls.npsa.nhs.uk/resources/?EntryId45=59809 (accessed 22 January 2012).

Neville KA, Sandeman DJ, Rubinstein A *et al*. Prevention of hyponatraemia during maintenance intravenous fluid administration: a prospective randomized study of fluid type versus fluid rate. *J Ped* 2010;**156**:313–319.

Sauden S. Is the use of colloids for fluid replacement harmless in children? *Curr Opin Anaes* 2010;**23**: 363–7.

Walker IA. Water, electrolytes and the kidney. In: Bingham R, Lloyd Thomas A, Sury M, eds. *Hatch and Sumner's Textbook of Paediatric Anaesthesia*, 3rd edition. Hodder Arnold. 2009; 57–77.

Chapter

15

Total intravenous anaesthesia (TIVA) in children

Vaithianadan Mani and Neil Morton

Introduction

Providing anaesthesia solely using intravenous agents has gained popularity because:

(1) There are new anaesthetic and analgesic drugs with favourable pharmacokinetic and pharmacodynamic properties.

(2) There is a better understanding of pharmacokinetics of these drugs in children, resulting in newer models capable of targeting either plasma or effect-site in order to achieve the desired clinical effect.

(3) There are new drug infusion devices with in-built pharmacokinetic models appropriate for use in children.

(4) Induction and equilibration between plasma and effect-site is rapid and independent of alveolar ventilation.

(5) There is improved quality of emergence from anaesthesia and smoother recovery.

(6) There is no risk of environmental pollution.

The most commonly used drugs for TIVA include propofol, the short-acting synthetic opioids such as remifentanil, dexmedetomidine, ketamine and midazolam. They can be administered using simple manual infusion schemes or by a target controlled infusion method (TCI). With TCI, a microprocessor-controlled infusion pump incorporating a pharmacokinetic model with age-appropriate parameters calculates the bolus dose and infusion rate to achieve a user-defined plasma or effect-site drug concentration.

Indications/uses for TIVA in children are:

- Children undergoing frequent repeated anaesthesia (e.g. radiation therapy);

- Brief radiological or painful procedures where rapid recovery is needed (e.g. MRI, bone marrow aspiration, gastrointestinal endoscopy);

- During major surgery to control the stress response;

- During neurosurgical procedures to assist with control of intracranial pressure and for cerebral metabolic protection;

- During spinal instrumentation surgery – for providing controlled hypotension and when there is a need for evoked motor and auditory brain potentials or an intra-operative wake up test;

- During airway procedures (e.g. bronchoscopy);

- Children at risk of malignant hyperthermia;

- Children with an increased risk of post-operative nausea and vomiting and during middle ear surgery.

Caution is needed in young children as pharmacokinetic data are incomplete and it is difficult to estimate blood concentration in real-time, so some experience is necessary to avoid awareness, pain and adverse effects.

Pharmacokinetics

Pharmacokinetics (PK) describe 'what the body does to the drug'. A PK model can be used to predict the blood or effect-site concentration profile of a drug after a bolus dose or an infusion. The behaviour of most drugs used for TIVA can be described either by two or three compartment models. Each model is described by:

- The compartments and their volumes
- The rate of transfer between compartments
- The rate of drug elimination

Core Topics in Paediatric Anaesthesia, ed. Ian James and Isabeau Walker. Published by Cambridge University Press. © 2013 Cambridge University Press.

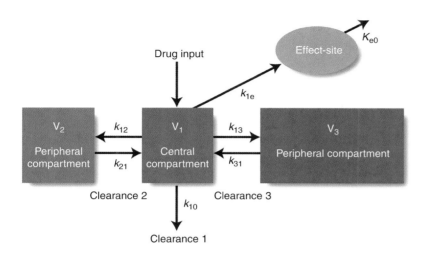

Figure 15.1 Three-compartment model (see text for details).

The drug is delivered and eliminated from a central compartment V_1 and distributes to and redistributes from two peripheral compartments, V_2 and V_3 (Figure 15.1). The compartment V_2 represents well-perfused organs and tissues (the fast compartment) while V_3 represents the vessel-poor (slow) compartment, mainly fat. A drug that is highly lipid-soluble or highly protein-bound will have a large volume of distribution. It should be noted that V_1 includes blood volume, but may be far larger than blood volume for these drugs.

The rate of transfer between compartments and elimination can be described using rate constants. By convention, k_{10} means rate constant for elimination, whereas k_{12}, k_{21}, k_{13} and k_{31} are used to denote the rate constants for drug transfer between V_1 and V_2, V_2 and V_1, V_1 and V_3, and V_3 and V_1 respectively.

Elimination by metabolism in the liver and excretion via the kidneys is assessed by the clearance (Cl), which is the volume of blood from which the drug is eliminated per unit of time. The time required for the blood concentration of a drug to decrease by 50% is its elimination half-life ($t_{1/2}$). The context-sensitive half-time (CSHT) is a helpful concept. When a drug is administered by infusion, it distributes from the central compartment to all the peripheral compartments. Once the infusion is stopped, the drug has to distribute back from the peripheral compartment into the central compartment and is then eliminated. The half-time of the decrease in drug concentration is therefore related to the *duration* of the infusion for most drugs (except remifentanil).

For an individual drug in an individual patient, CSHTs can be determined by graphing the elimination half-lives against the duration of the infusion. The CSHT graph will eventually become parallel to the time (x) axis. At that time, the infusion has become context-*in*sensitive. This pattern is observed for nearly all intravenous anaesthetics. The exception is remifentanil whose half-time becomes context-insensitive almost immediately after initiation of the infusion because its elimination is rapid and complete. Fentanyl has a short CSHT when given by infusion for a short time but this greatly increases as the duration of the infusion increases. Alfentanil's CSHT becomes constant after approximately 90 minutes of infusion.

Prolongation of the elimination of a drug reflects either an increase in the volume of distribution or a reduction in clearance, or both, and is evident in neonates and infants, and patients with liver or renal dysfunction. Propofol has a larger volume of distribution and higher clearance in children than in adults.

Concept of effect-site

The clinical effect of a drug depends on the concentration at the effect-site. After administration of a drug, there is usually a delay in clinical effect as the drug has to reach the effect-site from V_1. The rate of equilibration between blood and effect-site depends on several factors. These include the factors that influence the rate of delivery of the drug to the effect-site, such as cardiac output and cerebral blood flow, and the pharmacological properties of the drug, such as those that determine the rate of transfer of the drug across the blood–brain barrier (lipid solubility, degree of ionisation).

The time course of plasma/effect-site equilibration can be mathematically described by a rate constant typically referred to as the k_{e0}. This term k_{e0} should strictly be used to describe the rate of removal of drug from the effect-site, but the effect-site is usually regarded as a volume-less additional compartment, so that there is no need for separate constants describing the rate constants for movement into and out of the effect compartment.

Pharmacokinetic/pharmacodynamic modelling (PK-PD)

Pharmacodynamics (PD) can be thought of as 'what the drug does to the body', or its clinical effect. It is not possible for us to measure directly the concentration of the drug at the effect-site. However, the time course of the changes in the effect-site concentration can be estimated from measures of clinical effect (PD effect) such as evoked EEG parameters, bispectral index (BIS), and auditory evoked potentials (AEP). So, when the blood concentration in a group of subjects is known, then PD measurements can be used to estimate the k_{e0}. This is the basis of pharmacokinetic/pharmacodynamic modelling (PK/PD), in which PK and PD parameters from a study population are used to derive the k_{e0} for that particular population, and which may be applied to a similar population. The $t_{1/2} k_{e0}$ (which is $0.693/k_{e0}$) is sometimes used to express this rate constant. As k_{e0} increases, $t_{1/2} k_{e0}$ decreases and equilibration between blood and effect-site is quicker. Recently, age-related k_{e0} values have been derived for children.

The immature neonate, the critically ill child or the child with major organ failure needs considerably smaller doses of intravenous anaesthetic agents, and particular care is needed in children receiving vasodilator medication and in those with some types of congenital heart disease, as hypotension is a significant risk.

Principles of infusion schemes
Manual infusion

When drugs are administered at a fixed infusion rate, the blood concentrations take a very long time to reach a plateau or steady state. For a fixed infusion rate, it takes 5 half-lives to reach a steady state concentration (98% of the target) in the blood. To achieve steady state conditions more rapidly, a bolus dose or loading infusion may be administered. There are suitable manual infusion schemes for children.

Target controlled infusion

TCI is a microprocessor-controlled infusion program that aims to achieve a user-defined drug concentration in blood or at the effect-site, using a real-time multicompartmental PK model to calculate the bolus dose and infusion rates. The basic components of a TCI system are a user interface, a computer or one or more microprocessors, and an infusion device. The microprocessor controls the appearance of the user interface, implements the PK model, accepts data input and instruction from the user, performs the necessary mathematical calculations, controls and monitors the infusion device, and implements warning systems to alert the user to any problems. Audible and visible warning systems are essential features. Typical infusion devices that are used for TCI are capable of infusion rates up to $1200 \, \mathrm{ml \, h^{-1}}$ with an accuracy of up to $0.1 \, \mathrm{ml \, h^{-1}}$.

Blood targeted TCI

When blood targeted TCI is chosen, one needs to choose the desired PK model, and input the selected drug, its concentration and the patient's age and weight. The microprocessor then calculates the bolus required which is rapidly infused to fill the central compartment quickly. Once the target blood concentration is reached, the system stops the rapid infusion, and commences a stepwise-reducing infusion rate to replace drug that is lost by elimination and intercompartmental transfer (Figure 15.2). To deepen the level of anaesthesia, a bolus dose is given and the infusion rate is recalculated to maintain a higher target blood concentration. To lighten the level of anaesthesia, the system stops the infusion and waits until the calculated new lower target concentration is reached. The rate at which the blood concentration falls depends on the rate of elimination and the intercompartmental gradients of drug concentration.

Effect-site targeted TCI

The problem with blood TCI is that there is a relatively long delay before the concentration at the effect-site equilibrates with the blood concentration. With effect-site targeting, the TCI system calculates the blood concentration to bring about the user-defined effect-site concentration as rapidly as possible

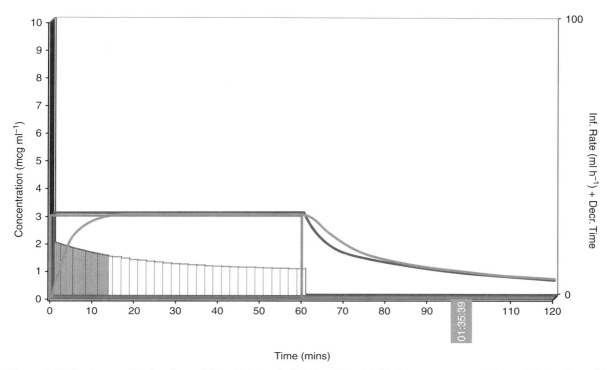

Figure 15.2 Blood targeted infusion of propofol in a child using the Paedfusor PK model. This diagram represents a 60 minute infusion of propofol where the blood target concentration (orange line) has been set at 3 mcg ml^{-1} and then the infusion is switched off (blood target 0). The red line represents the predicted blood concentration while the green line represents the effect-site concentration, which correlates with depth of sedation or anaesthesia. The effect-site concentration lags behind the blood concentration, and it takes around 10 minutes to reach an effect-site concentration equal to the target. The context-sensitive half-time is represented by the time it takes for the blood concentration to drop from 3 mcg ml^{-1} to 1.5 mcg ml^{-1}, which is in this case after 60 minutes of infusion approximately 20 minutes. Inf, infusion. See plate section for colour version.

(Figure 15.3). The system calculates the optimal peak blood concentration that will cause a sufficient blood to effect-site concentration gradient to produce the most rapid increase in effect-site concentration (analogous to the overpressure effect with volatile agents) but without an overshoot of the targeted effect-site concentration. This results in a relatively large loading infusion or bolus dose with a high peak blood concentration. While healthy children may be able to tolerate this higher peak blood concentration, it may cause cardiovascular instability with hypotension and bradycardia in children who are ill.

Drugs used for TIVA
Propofol
Manual propofol infusion

The simple '10–8–6' scheme devised by Roberts for propofol infusion in adults, is very effective in maintaining a propofol target blood concentration of 3 mcg ml^{-1}, which in most adults produces a state of anaesthesia. This scheme involves a loading dose of around 1 mg kg^{-1} of propofol followed by an infusion of 10 mg kg^{-1} h^{-1} for 10 minutes, then 8 mg kg^{-1} h^{-1} for 10 minutes and 6 mg kg^{-1} h^{-1} thereafter. When this regimen is used in children, however, a sub-therapeutic blood concentration of propofol is achieved. This low concentration is because of the larger V_1 and increased clearance of propofol in children when compared to adults. Using the Paedfusor data, it has been found that in order to achieve a blood concentration of 3 mcg ml^{-1} in children, the dosing of propofol infusion in children is approximately twice that in adults (a '19–15–12' regimen). Recent studies have shown that the target concentrations to produce anaesthesia are approximately the same as in adults.

The other simple manual infusion scheme to obtain a propofol blood target concentration of 3 mcg ml^{-1} was devised by Macfarlan, and validated

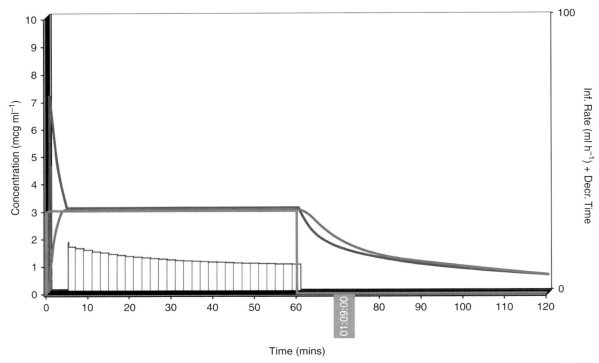

Figure 15.3 Effect-site targeted infusion of propofol in a child using the Paedfusor PK model. This diagram represents a 60 minute infusion of propofol where the effect-site target concentration (orange line) has been set at 3 mcg ml^{-1} and then the infusion is switched off (blood target 0). As in Figure 15.2, the red line represents the predicted blood concentration while the green line represents the effect-site concentration, which correlates with depth of sedation or anaesthesia. Although the effect-site concentration still lags behind the blood concentration, it takes only around 3 minutes to reach an effect-site concentration equal to the target. This is because a larger bolus is given to increase the blood concentration quickly to a higher peak which drives the propofol along a concentration gradient into the effect-site much more quickly. Thus induction of anaesthesia will be quicker but at the expense of potential adverse effects related to the higher peak blood concentration such as hypotension and bradycardia. See plate section for colour version.

by Engelhardt, using the Kataria dataset in children aged 1–6 years. In the Macfarlan model, anaesthesia is induced with a bolus dose of 2.5 mg kg^{-1} and then maintained with a propofol infusion regimen (commenced within 1 min of the propofol bolus) of:

- 15 mg kg^{-1} h^{-1} for the first 15 min
- 13 mg kg^{-1} h^{-1} for the next 15 min
- 11 mg kg^{-1} h^{-1} from 30 to 60 min
- 10 mg kg^{-1} h^{-1} from 1 to 2 hours, and
- 9 mg kg^{-1} h^{-1} from 2 to 4 hours

This results in a near steady state blood concentration of 3 mcg ml^{-1}.

Propofol TCI

Blood concentration targeting using propofol in children can be achieved using the Paedfusor dataset (that incorporates the Marsh model), or the Kataria model. The Paedfusor model makes an allowance for the steady increase in elimination clearance in younger children, particularly below 30 kg in weight. The validated lower age and weight limits for each model also differ, being age 1 year and 5 kg for the Paedfusor system, and 3 years and 15 kg for the Kataria system.

Effect-site targeting is possible now in paediatrics. If a typical adult k_{e0} of 0.26 min^{-1} is used, onset is slow despite a large bolus induction dose. Munoz et al. found the median k_{e0} values for the Paedfusor and Kataria models for children aged 3–11 years were 0.91 min^{-1} and 0.41 min^{-1} respectively. Jeleazcov et al. have recently derived age-related k_{e0} values, but these have yet to be evaluated clinically. Using their formula in paediatric computer simulations, a more rapid attainment of the target effect-site concentration is seen for a lower bolus dose of propofol in young children and this should improve the onset of clinical anaesthesia and cardiovascular stability.

Propofol related infusion syndrome (PRIS)

Propofol infusion is a safe anaesthetic technique but it is important to be aware of PRIS when using propofol by infusion in children. This was originally reported following its use for sedation in paediatric intensive care, and is defined as the occurrence of bradycardia, associated with lipaemic plasma, fatty liver enlargement, metabolic acidosis with negative base excess of more than 10 mmol l^{-1}, rhabdomyolysis or myoglobinuria. Risk factors for developing PRIS are:

- Airway infection;
- Severe head injury;
- Propofol sedation at more than 5 mg kg h^{-1} for more than 48 hours;
- Increased catecholamine and glucocorticoid serum levels;
- Low energy supply.

The pathophysiology behind PRIS is possibly an impairment of oxidation of fatty acids at mitochondrial level, leading to accumulation of free fatty acids and cytolysis of cardiac and skeletal muscle. Caution is required in children with disorders of fat or carbohydrate metabolism. Treatment for PRIS is to stop propofol, and institute cardiac pacing, inotropic support, carbohydrate substitution and haemofiltration. Extracorporeal life support may be required.

Propofol and lipid sparing techniques

Propofol 1% is a solution of 1 mg ml^{-1} propofol in an emulsion containing 0.1 g ml^{-1} lipid. Propofol 2% solutions are preferred, especially for longer duration anaesthesia as this halves the lipid load to the child. The disadvantage of propofol 2% is severe injection pain, which is best ameliorated by administering lidocaine 0.2 mg kg^{-1} and a short-acting opioid such as alfentanil 10–20 mcg kg^{-1} or remifentanil 0.5 mcg kg^{-1} immediately prior to injection of the propofol.

The use of adjuncts may also help to reduce the propofol dose. Opioids, especially remifentanil, have been extensively studied and found to reduce the dose of propofol for producing unconsciousness when used in TCI. Alpha$_2$ agonists, such as clonidine and dexmedetomidine, have also been shown to reduce the dose of propofol required to produce unconsciousness and also to maintain anaesthesia. Regional anaesthesia reduces the dose of propofol required for the maintenance of anaesthesia. Propofol and lipid-sparing techniques are important for safety of this technique in children and help to smooth and shorten recovery time.

Opioids for TIVA

Short-acting opioids used for TIVA are remifentanil, alfentanil, sufentanil and fentanyl. Appropriate postoperative analgesia must be planned for, especially when ultra-short-acting opioids such as remifentanil are used. Some suggested doses for opioids when used for TIVA are summarised in Table 15.1.

Recent evidence suggests that infants and younger children outside the neonatal period are more resistant to the effects of remifentanil, even when combined with propofol. Spontaneous respiration can be maintained at doses adequate to suppress somatic responses to painful procedures. The large interindividual variation in respiratory depressant effects necessitates individualised dose titration. The drug dose is more linearly related to variation in the respiratory rhythm and respiratory rate than to minute volume or end-tidal carbon dioxide. Apnoeic episodes are less likely when respiratory depressant drugs are administered slowly, as this allows time for the ETCO$_2$ level to rise to a new apnoeic threshold. The maximum dose of remifentanil tolerated by children breathing spontaneously under anaesthesia varies widely (between 0.05 and 0.3 mcg kg^{-1} min^{-1}). A dose of 0.05 mcg kg^{-1} min^{-1} will allow spontaneous respiration in more than 90% of children; a dose of 0.3 mcg kg^{-1} min^{-1} will prevent spontaneous respiration in 90% of children. Younger children, especially those less than 3 years old, maintain spontaneous respiration with a higher dose of remifentanil, up to 0.35 mcg kg^{-1} min^{-1}, in contrast to the lower doses tolerated in adults. The dose required to produce significant respiratory depression in children of the same age and weight is highly variable, despite the predictable plasma half-life of remifentanil. This variation may be due to an intrinsic difference in receptor sensitivity.

Dexmedetomidine

Dexmedetomidine is a highly selective alpha$_2$ agonist, which has sedative anxiolytic and analgesic properties. It does not produce respiratory depression and provides stable haemodynamics when given as a continuous infusion, except in children who are hypovolaemic or have heart block (Table 15.1).

Table 15.1 Commonly used doses for TIVA in children

Drug	Loading dose	Maintenance infusion	Notes
Propofol (Roberts)	1 mg kg^{-1}	13 mg kg^{-1} h^{-1} for 10 min, then 11 mg kg^{-1} h^{-1} for 10 min, then 9 mg kg^{-1} h^{-1} thereafter	Concurrently with alfentanil infusion
Propofol (Macfarlan)	2.5 mg kg^{-1}	15 mg kg^{-1} h^{-1} for the first 15 min, 13 mg kg^{-1} h^{-1} for the next 15 min, 11 mg kg^{-1} h^{-1} from 30 to 60 min, 10 mg kg^{-1} h^{-1} from 1 to 2 hours, 9 mg kg^{-1} h^{-1} from 2 to 4 hours	Achieves blood concentration of around 3 mcg ml^{-1}
Alfentanil	10–50 mcg kg^{-1}	1–5 mcg kg^{-1} min^{-1}	Results in blood concentration of 50–200 ng ml^{-1}
Remifentanil	0.5 mcg kg^{-1} min^{-1} for 3 minutes	0.25 mcg kg^{-1} min^{-1}	Produces blood concentrations of 6–9 ng ml^{-1}
Remifentanil	0.5–1.0 mcg kg^{-1} over 1 minute	0.1–0.5 mcg kg^{-1} min^{-1}	Produces blood concentrations of 5–10 ng ml^{-1}
Sufentanil	0.1–0.5 mcg kg^{-1}	0.005–0.01 mcg kg^{-1} min^{-1}	Results in blood concentration of 0.2 ng ml^{-1}
Sufentanil	1–5 mcg kg^{-1}	0.01–0.05 mcg kg^{-1} min^{-1}	Results in blood concentration of 0.6–3.0 ng ml^{-1}
Fentanyl	1–10 mcg kg^{-1}	0.1–0.2 mcg kg^{-1} min^{-1}	
Ketamine	2 mg kg^{-1}	11 mg kg^{-1} h^{-1} for first 20 min, then 7 mg kg^{-1} h^{-1} for next 20 min, 5 mg kg^{-1} h^{-1} for the next 20 min, 4 mg kg^{-1} h^{-1} for the next hour, then at 3.5 mg kg^{-1} h^{-1}	Produces blood concentration of 3 mg l^{-1}
Ketamine (Anaesthetic dose when administered with N$_2$O or midazolam)	2 mg kg^{-1}	7 mg kg^{-1} h^{-1} for first 20 min, then 5 mg kg^{-1} h^{-1} for next 20 min, 4 mg kg^{-1} h^{-1} for the next 20 min, 3 mg kg^{-1} h^{-1} from then on	Produces blood concentration of 2–2.2 mg l^{-1}
Midazolam	0.05–0.1 mg kg^{-1}	0.1–0.3 mg kg^{-1} h^{-1}	
Dexmedetomidine (sedation for non-invasive procedures)	0.5–1 mcg kg^{-1} over 10 min	0.5–1 mcg kg^{-1} h^{-1}	
Dexmedetomidine (sedation for invasive procedures)	1–2 mcg kg^{-1} over 10 min	1–2 mcg kg^{-1} h^{-1}	

Ketamine

Ketamine can be used in a simple basic manual regimen to produce dissociative sedation and analgesia as a loading dose of 1 mg kg^{-1} and a maintenance infusion of 0.1 mg kg^{-1} h^{-1}, with additional boluses of 1–2 mg kg^{-1} and increases in maintenance rate to 0.2 mg kg^{-1} h^{-1}. However, to achieve anaesthetic target blood concentrations higher loading doses and infusion rates are needed (Table 15.1). Although there are TCI PK models for adults, there is no described PK model for children. In their simulator study using PK parameters from published studies, Dallimore suggested an infusion regimen aiming to attain a plasma concentration of 3 mg l^{-1}. They suggested that a lower rate of infusion could be employed when ketamine is used along with nitrous oxide and/or midazolam. The large clearance and hence short context-sensitive half-time for infusions under 2 hours of racemic ketamine infusion in children makes ketamine a good choice as a sedative or anaesthetic agent for shorter duration procedures. In a study on sedation in the emergency department using racemic ketamine, Dallimore found that smaller bolus doses and repeated top-ups resulted in faster recovery. In children aged 12, 6 and 2 years, they suggested that a dosing regimen of 0.275, 0.3 and 0.35 mg kg^{-1} respectively, followed by an infusion of 2.75, 3 and 3.5 mg kg^{-1} h^{-1} for 15 minutes, gives a more even sedation level and rapid recovery (20 minutes to being awake).

Midazolam

Slow bolus dosing of up to 0.1 mg kg^{-1} midazolam followed by an infusion rate of 0.1 mg kg^{-1} h^{-1} provides baseline sedation, with adjustments and additional bolus doses often needed. Caution is required with bolus dosing in neonates and infants and in the critically ill as hypotension may occur and the depth of sedation achieved with midazolam is tremendously variable (Table 15.1).

Drug interactions

PK interactions

Most commonly described interactions for intravenous agents are those between propofol and various opioid agents. Both fentanyl and alfentanil increase the volume of V_1 and clearance of propofol, while propofol and midazolam inhibit the metabolism of alfentanil by competing for the same cytochrome P_{450} enzyme isoform CYP_{3A4}. Also, a higher concentration

of propofol alters its own metabolism by causing changes in cardiac output and hepatic blood flow. Alfentanil concentrations are also significantly higher when it is infused with propofol than when it is infused alone. Propofol and opioid clearances tend to be reduced after cardiopulmonary bypass. Although all these PK interactions should be borne in mind, it is seldom necessary to alter the target concentrations. It is the synergism arising from PD interactions among anaesthetic agents that requires a decrease of target concentration.

PD interactions

In practice, the effect-site concentration of propofol required to produce and maintain unconsciousness is reduced by concurrent administration of an opioid. In one study a remifentanil concentration of 4 ng ml^{-1} was found to reduce the propofol target concentration for loss of response to verbal command from 2.9 mcg ml^{-1} to 2.2 mcg ml^{-1}. This reduced propofol dose improves haemodynamic stability.

Key points

- TIVA is becoming more popular in paediatric anaesthesia and open-TCI pumps with appropriate paediatric software are now available.
- TCI propofol is possible down to age 1 year.
- Blood targeted propofol infusions may be replaced by effect-site targeted infusions as age-appropriate software is introduced.
- Techniques should be used where possible to limit the propofol and lipid dose, and 2% propofol solutions are recommended.
- Injection pain is preventable using pre-injection of lidocaine and an opioid.

Further reading

Absalom A, Struys M. *An Overview of TCI and TIVA*. Academic Press. 2005.

Absalom A, Amutike D, Lal A, White M, Kenny GN. Accuracy of the 'Paedfusor' in children undergoing cardiac surgery or catheterization. *Br J Anaes* 2003;**91**(4): 507–13.

Absalom A, Kenny G. 'Paedfusor' pharmacokinetic data set. *Br J Anaes* 2005;**95**(1):110.

Anderson BJ. Pediatric models for adult target-controlled infusion pumps. *Paed Anaes* 2009;**20**(3):223–32.

Jeleazcov C, Ihmsen H, Schmidt J *et al*. Pharmacodynamic modelling of the bispectral index response to propofol-based anaesthesia during

general surgery in children. *Br J Anaes* 2008;**100**(4):509–16.

Kam PC, Cardone D. Propofol infusion syndrome. *Anaesthesia* 2007;**62** (7):690–701.

Lerman J, Johr M. Inhalational anesthesia vs total intravenous anesthesia (TIVA) for pediatric anesthesia. *Paed Anaes* 2009;**19** (5):521–34.

Mani V, Morton NS. Overview of total intravenous anesthesia in children. *Paed Anaes* 2009;**20**(3):211–22.

Marsh B, White M, Morton N, Kenny GN. Pharmacokinetic model driven infusion of propofol in children. *Br J Anaes* 1991;**67**(1):41–8.

Munoz HR, Cortinez LI, Ibacache ME, Altermatt FR. Estimation of the plasma effect-site equilibration rate constant (ke0) of propofol in children using the time to peak effect: comparison with adults. *Anesthesiology* 2004;**101**(6): 1269–74.

Munoz HR, Cortinez LI, Ibacache ME, Leon PJ. Effect site concentrations of propofol producing hypnosis in children and adults: comparison using the bispectral index. *Acta Anaesthesiol Scand* 2006;**50**(7): 882–7.

Tirel O, Wodey E, Harris R, Bansard JY, Ecoffey C, Senhadji L. Variation of bispectral index under TIVA with propofol in a paediatric population. *Br J Anaes* 2008;**100**(1):82–7.

Varveris DA, Morton NS. Target controlled infusion of propofol for induction and maintenance of anaesthesia using the Paedfusor: an open pilot study. *Paed Anaes* 2002;**12**(7):589–93.

Regional anaesthesia in children

Naveen Raj and Steve Roberts

Introduction

Regional anaesthesia is an important aspect of paediatric anaesthesia and should be considered for all suitable cases. The benefits of excellent analgesia need to be balanced against the potential risks; where possible the most appropriate and peripheral technique should be used. Peripheral nerve blocks (PNB) should only be performed by those with the correct training, equipment and assistance. It is essential that the signs and management of local anaesthesia toxicity are understood by those performing and assisting with PNB.

In the United Kingdom the bulk of paediatric PNBs are performed under general anaesthesia (GA). In the rare circumstance where blocks are performed awake (e.g. minor surgery on older cooperative children) then age-specific pre-operative information, a quiet theatre environment and reassurance are essential to minimise the child's and carer's anxiety.

As with adults the use of landmarks and peripheral nerve stimulation (PNS) for nerve location predominate, although ultrasound imaging is increasingly used. No matter what technology is used a thorough understanding of the anatomy involved and the surgery being performed is essential.

The nerve blocks to be discussed are listed in Table 16.1.

General points

For all blocks, a thorough history and examination is mandatory to identify any contraindications to regional anaesthesia (see Table 16.2) along with appropriate preparation of the child and carers.

- *History*: allergies, previous regional/general anaesthesia, co-morbidities, current medications.

Table 16.1 Common regional blocks

Head and neck	Auriculotemporal Greater auricular Superficial cervical plexus
Upper limb blocks	Supraclavicular Axilla Forearm Ring block
Truncal blocks	Paravertebral Rectus sheath Transversus abdominis (TAP) Ilioinguinal/iliohypogastric Penile
Lower limb blocks	Lateral femoral cutaneous nerve Femoral Fascia iliaca Lumbar plexus Sciatic proximal and distal Ankle Metatarsal and ring blocks
Central blocks	Caudal – single shot

- *Planned procedure*: to determine the most suitable block, and whether a catheter technique would be beneficial for continued pain relief in the post-operative period.
- *Examination*: of the operative site and potential puncture site, to exclude local infection.
- *Weight*: to calculate maximum dose of local anaesthetic (LA).
- *Consent*: to explain potential advantages, side effects, complications and alternative methods of pain relief if the block fails. General complications include failure, nerve damage, LA toxicity, haematoma, infection and anaphylaxis.

Core Topics in Paediatric Anaesthesia, ed. Ian James and Isabeau Walker. Published by Cambridge University Press. © 2013 Cambridge University Press.

Table 16.2 General contraindications to regional anaesthesia

Absolute contraindications	Relative contraindications
Lesions (infective) at the site of injection	Neuromuscular disorders
History of allergy to LA	Risk of compartment syndrome especially following trauma (discuss with surgeon)
Lack of consent	Systemic infection (catheter techniques) Bleeding disorders (the use of ultrasound can avoid inadvertent damage to blood vessels)

- *Pre-operatively*: where a GA can be avoided the patient can be prepared by a play specialist if necessary and age-suitable distraction provided. Prior to coming to theatre topical anaesthesia can be applied to the proposed puncture site. In these circumstances parental presence can be reassuring. Administration of paracetamol and a NSAID to supplement the block should be considered.
- *Anaesthetic room*: A trained assistant should be present, along with accessibility of resuscitation equipment and drugs, including 20% Intralipid. Prior to performing the block the airway and IV access should be established, and full monitoring instituted.
- *Equipment*: An insulated short bevelled needle with extension tubing, gauze swabs, antiseptic solution, sterile gloves, sterile drapes, syringe, LA, a PNS (for mixed nerves) and/or an ultrasound machine (with high frequency probe, sterile gel and probe cover).
- *Procedure*: For those children not having a GA the skin should be infiltrated with lidocaine first; the administration of Entonox can smooth proceedings.
- *Asepsis*: Single-shot techniques require a basic sterile technique, but those involving catheters should have a full aseptic technique.

Technique

- As the regional needles are quite blunt it is useful to nick the skin first with a hypodermic needle. This ensures that the fascial planes are appreciated as the short bevelled needle is advanced.
- If a PNS is used an initial current of 2 mA is set; as the needle is advanced and the relevant motor response elicited the current is decreased to 0.5 mA.

- After initial aspiration, 1 ml of LA is injected, abolishing the motor response. The injection is made slowly with frequent aspiration to exclude a bloody tap.
- Usually a long-acting LA is appropriate, providing analgesia for 6–12 hours. If prolonged analgesia is required the insertion of a catheter should be considered.
- To minimise the risk of dislodgement the catheter should be tunnelled 3–4 cm subcutaneously. The use of a drop of Indermil® tissue glue over the puncture site limits the leak; this prevents the LA escaping and causing the dressing to lift off and the catheter to fall out.
- Run the infusion intra-operatively as this may highlight any occlusion issues.

Post-operative

In the recovery area a failed block can be difficult to differentiate from emergence delirium; if in doubt pain should be assumed and treated promptly with either 0.25–0.5 mg kg^{-1} of ketamine or 0.5 mcg kg^{-1} of fentanyl. This achieves quick control and the need for morphine can then be considered. Carers and patient should be advised to protect the anaesthetised area; this should include warning of decreased sensation (especially temperature) and motor weakness. Upper limbs should be kept in a sling. Where lower limb blockade is used, ensure means of ambulation and discharge are in place.

Local anaesthetics

Levobupivacaine is the LA of choice owing to its longer duration of action, and low cardio/neurotoxicity. As the blocks usually accompany a GA, concentrations of 0.125 to 0.25% are adequate. Ropivacaine is preferred in some centres as it may cause less profound motor block. Lidocaine is indicated for

Table 16.3 Local anaesthetics

LA	Single-shot block (mg kg^{-1})	PNB catheter infusions (mg kg^{-1} h^{-1})	Maximum dose per 4 hours (mg kg^{-1})
L-bupivacaine	2	0.125–0.4	2.0
Ropivacaine	3	0.4	1.6
Lidocaine	4	NA	NA

infiltration prior to block performance in awake children. (See Table 16.3.)

Neonates and infants are at greater risk of LA toxicity because of lower protein binding, and the immature blood–brain barrier and liver. Consideration should be given to halving LA doses in these patients and limiting LA infusions to 48 hours.

Local anaesthetic toxicity

Prevention is preferable:

- Never exceed the maximum dose of LA (see Table 16.3);
- Always aspirate before injection;
- Use ultrasound to observe the injection (note that this is not infallible);
- Maintain a high level of suspicion.

Systemic toxicity results in depression of both the central nervous and cardiovascular systems with readily recognisable symptoms and signs, increasing in severity from somnolence through to convulsion and cardiac arrhythmia (see Table 16.4). However, as most children receive regional anaesthesia under GA, the earlier warning signs may be masked, and thus the first manifestation of a problem may be cardiovascular collapse.

In the event of toxicity, management should follow an established protocol such as that in Box 16.1. Arrhythmias may be refractory, and resuscitation may be very prolonged.

Specific blocks
Head and neck
Ear surgery
Auriculotemporal nerve
This nerve supplies the superior two-thirds of the anterior surface of the ear, the external auditory canal and the temporal region of the forehead. It is blocked

Table 16.4 Signs of local anaesthesia toxicity

Restlessness or agitation, followed by slurred speech or loss of consciousness
Muscle twitching, which may progress to seizures
Respiratory depression
Bradycardia, heart block, hypotension
Ventricular tachyarrhythmias, progressing to cardiac arrest

by subcutaneous infiltration of LA in front of the tragus behind the superficial temporal artery.

Great auricular nerve and lesser occipital nerve
These nerves from the cervical plexus supply the posterior surface of the ear, the lower third of the anterior surface and variable area over the angle of the mandible. They can be blocked either by a superficial cervical plexus block (see below) or by subcutaneous local anaesthetic infiltration from the angle of the mandible to the mastoid process. This is used for pinnaplasty and mastoidectomy.

Neck surgery
Superficial cervical plexus
This blocks the anterior primary rami of the upper four cervical nerves and leads to reduced sensation over the anterolateral area of the neck up to the level of T2 dermatome. The head is turned away from the side to be blocked and the posterior border of the sternocleidomastoid muscle is identified. Under aseptic conditions a fine needle is introduced at the midpoint of this posterior border and advanced 0.5–2 cm caudally along the border; LA is injected as the needle is withdrawn. It is then directed cephaloid and same procedure repeated. As the external jugular vein crosses the sternocleidomastoid muscle in this area, caution must be taken to avoid intravascular injection.

Box 16.1   Management of LA toxicity

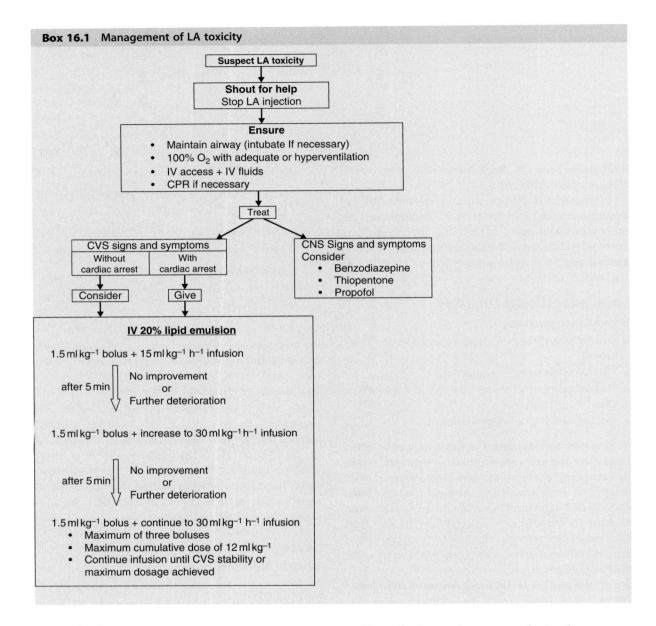

Upper limb

Brachial plexus anatomy

The anterior primary rami of C5 to T1 form the brachial plexus. They emerge from the intervertebral foramina sandwiched between the scalenus anterior and medius muscles enclosed within a fascial sheath. The roots come together to form the trunks (C5 and C6 unite to form the superior trunk, C7 forms the middle trunk, and the C8 and T1 roots unite to form the lower trunk).

From the interscalene groove the trunks pass over the first rib supero-posterior to the subclavian artery. At the lateral border of the first rib the trunks divide into anterior and posterior divisions. The anterior divisions of the upper and middle trunks join to become the *lateral cord*, the anterior division of the lower trunk continues as the *medial cord*. The posterior divisions of the three trunks join to form the *posterior cord*. The cords are named according to their position in relation to the axillary artery; they divide into the nerves that supply the arm.

- Lateral cord: becomes the *Lateral root of median nerve, and Musculocutaneous nerve*
- Medial cord: becomes the *Medial root of median nerve, Ulnar nerve, and Medial Cutaneous nerves of arm and forearm*
- Posterior cord: becomes the *Axillary and Radial nerves.*

Supraclavicular block

The brachial plexus at this point is in close proximity to the subclavian artery and pleura. For this reason a block at this level should only be performed by the experienced, and arguably only with ultrasound. Classically it is said that this approach can miss the lower nerve roots. However, using ultrasound this poor LA distribution can be observed and corrected. Specific relative contraindications include previous neck surgery and contralateral pneumothorax.

When performed with ultrasound the whole upper limb can be anaesthetised with the exception of the shoulder.

Ultrasound technique

The patient lies supine with a roll between the shoulders and the head turned to the opposite side to the intended surgery; this allows adequate room for needle manipulation. Ensure that you, the ultrasound machine and equipment are positioned ergonomically.

A linear probe of appropriate size footprint is placed parallel to the clavicle. The three main structures to identify are the pleura, and the subclavian and dorsal scapular arteries. The brachial plexus is seen as a group of hypo-echoic (black) bubbles posterior and slightly superficial to the subclavian artery (Figure 16.1). The dorsal scapular artery often passes through the brachial plexus, so always scout the area for vessels using the colour Doppler. The needle is inserted using an in-plane (IP) technique, travelling in a posterolateral to anteromedial direction. The tip of the needle is aimed between the bubbles where the subclavian artery and pleura come together. LA injection is monitored and appropriate needle manipulation made to ensure uniform spread.

Specific complications include pneumothorax, phrenic and recurrent laryngeal nerve blockade, and Horner's syndrome.

Axillary block

The three main branches of the brachial plexus lie in close association to the axillary artery. In the supine child the three main branches are commonly

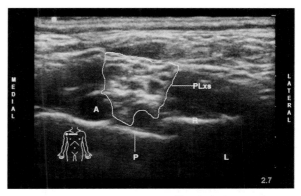

Figure 16.1 Ultrasound appearance of brachial plexus in the supraclavicular region (Plxs); subclavian artery (A), pleura (P), lung (L), rib (R).

positioned with the median and musculocutaneous nerves superior, the ulnar nerve inferior, and the radial nerve posterior to the artery. Note that the musculocutaneous and axillary nerves leave the 'sheath' at the level of the coracoid process, hence the absence of block in this nerve in up to 50% of blocks. This block is appropriate for hand and forearm surgery.

PNS technique

This is essentially the same as in adults. The child's arm is abducted and externally rotated. The primary landmark is the axillary artery; this is palpated against the humerus. The needle is inserted superior to the artery aiming towards the midpoint of the clavicle at a 45° angle. As it is inserted, nerve stimulation causing hand twitch is sought; a current of 0.5 mA is appropriate. A maximum of $0.5 \, \mathrm{ml \, kg^{-1}}$ of 0.25% levobupivacaine is injected.

Ultrasound technique

With a linear probe held transverse across the upper arm at the level of insertion of the pectoralis major muscle an IP needling technique can be elegantly employed to block the four main nerves individually (Figure 16.2). The musculocutaneous nerve is easily identified within the coracobrachialis muscle thus ensuring analgesia for the lateral forearm. The musculocutaneous nerve is oval in shape changing to a triangular shape distally. As the arrangement of the nerves in the axilla is very variable the most reliable way of identifying them is to follow their path distally with the ultrasound. Block the deepest nerve structures

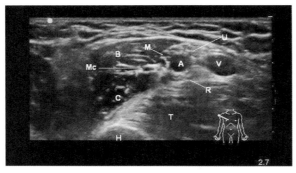

Figure 16.2 Ultrasound appearance of the brachial plexus in the axillary region showing axillary artery (A), axillary vein (V), median nerve (M), ulnar nerve (U), radial nerve (R), triceps (T), humerus (H) and the musculocutaneous nerve (Mc) between the biceps (B) and coracobrachialis (C).

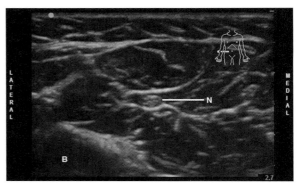

Figure 16.3 Ultrasound appearance of the median nerve (N) in the mid-forearm; bone shadow (B).

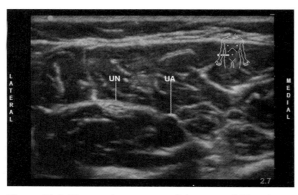

Figure 16.4 Ultrasound appearance of ulnar nerve (UN) in the mid-forearm; ulnar artery (UA).

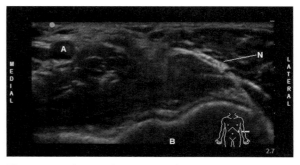

Figure 16.5 Ultrasound appearance of the radial nerve (N) in the elbow joint; brachial artery (A), humerus (B).

first in case air artefact obscures the view. Each nerve can be blocked with as little as 1–2 ml.

Forearm

The three nerves can be blocked individually anywhere along their path within the forearm. They can be employed for hand surgery or as rescue blocks for failed upper limb blocks.

Ultrasound technique

Either an out of plane (OOP) or IP needling technique is suitable.

The median nerve is most easily blocked mid-forearm where it sits between the deep and superficial flexor muscles. The probe is placed in a transverse plane (TP) mid-forearm (Figure 16.3). At this point there is little vasculature to hit and few tendons to confuse with the nerve.

The ulnar nerve is best blocked in the proximal third of the forearm as the associated artery does not join the nerve till further down. By placing the probe at the midpoint of the ulnar aspect of the forearm the ulnar nerve can be imaged lying on the flexor carpi ulnaris muscle (Figure 16.4).

The radial nerve is blocked preferably at the elbow at the position of a traditional landmark approach (between the tendons of biceps brachii and brachioradialis). The probe is placed transversely over the groove between the tendons. The division of the radial nerve into superficial and deep branches can be imaged at this point; an accompanying artery is present and must be avoided (Figure 16.5).

Ring blocks

This simple block is used for operations on the fingers e.g. nail bed repair. The digital nerves are branches of the median and ulna nerves ventrally and the ulna and radial nerves dorsally. Each digit is supplied by four nerves in the 2, 5, 7 and 10 o'clock positions in relation to the phalanx.

The needle is inserted medially and laterally to the extensor tendon. The needle is passed subcutaneously down both the medial and lateral aspects of the phalanx.

The needle is inserted as far as the volar skin before being slowly withdrawn as LA is injected.

In the awake patient this is a painful block to perform, therefore topical anaesthesia should be placed around the base of the finger. **Vasoconstrictors must not be used**.

Truncal blocks

The intercostal nerves are the anterior primary rami of the spinal nerves T1–T11. Those typically supplying the thoracic wall are T4–T6. The upper thoracic nerves (T1–T3) additionally join the brachial plexus and the lower five thoracic nerves (T5–T12) supply the abdominal wall.

Thoracic paravertebral block

The aim of this block is to inject LA into the wedge-shaped paravertebral space found either side of the vertebral column. The base is formed by the posterolateral part of the vertebral body, the disc and the intervertebral foramina with its contents, the anterolateral boundary by the parietal pleura and the posterior wall by the superior-costotransverse ligament.

Empyema and tumour occupying the space are contraindications. It may not be possible to find the space easily in children with kyphoscoliosis, or be successful in children with a history of previous thoracotomy.

Indications

Thoracotomies and upper abdominal procedures. Although commonly done unilaterally, bilateral paravertebral blocks have been described and both single shot and catheter techniques are used. A catheter can be placed by the surgeon under direct vision during thoracotomy.

Landmark technique

The anaesthetised child is placed in the lateral decubitus position with the knees bent up and the side to be blocked uppermost. For thoracotomies the needle is inserted at the level of T6 and for upper abdominal procedures at the level of T10.

An 18G Tuohy epidural needle is inserted lateral to the lower border of the spinous process. The distance is equivalent to the distance between two adjacent spinous processes.

Alternatively, the predicted lateral distance (in millimetres) to needle insertion is 10.2 + (0.12 × weight in kilograms), and the skin to space depth is 21.2 + (0.53 × weight in kilograms). The needle is advanced slowly in a perpendicular direction to contact the transverse process of the vertebrae below and the depth noted. The needle should not be advanced beyond 2–4 cm as this increases the risk of pleural puncture. If the transverse process is not contacted at this depth then it should be withdrawn and redirected either caudad or cephalad.

A loss of resistance syringe filled with saline is attached to the needle, which is then walked off the superior aspect of the transverse process. As it pierces the costotransverse ligament there is a sudden loss of resistance (usually at a depth of 1–1.5 cm), though it is less definite than that felt with an epidural.

A dose of $0.5\,\mathrm{ml\,kg^{-1}}$ LA is used. A catheter can be inserted following the injection although this may need some manipulation. If the catheter feeds in easily, entry of the catheter into the pleural space should be suspected.

Ultrasound technique

Ultrasound can be used prior to the landmark technique to assess depth to the transverse process and pleura. Alternatively, full ultrasound guidance is possible, placing a linear probe in TP on the appropriate rib and using an IP needling technique. The rib is imaged as a hyperechoic line with acoustic shadowing underneath. The probe is moved slightly caudally into the intercostal space. The transverse process is identified, deep to the paraspinal muscles, as a hyperechoic convex line. The following can be imaged lateral to the transverse process (from superficial to deep): the external intercostal muscle, the internal intercostal membrane and then the pleura which appears as a hyperechoic line with characteristic lung shadow underneath. The paravertebral space appears adjacent to the transverse process as a wedge shaped hypoechoic area with the base to the side of the process and the internal intercostal membrane and the hyperechoic pleura forming the superior and inferior borders respectively. The apex of the space continues laterally with the intercostal space (see Figure 16.6). Under aseptic precautions a 22G regional block needle or an 18G Tuohy with the bevel facing up is inserted from the lateral edge of the probe and directed medially. The aim is to penetrate the internal intercostal membrane at the apex of the space so that

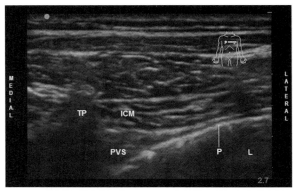

Figure 16.6 Ultrasound appearance of the paravertebral region; transverse process (TP), intercostal muscle (ICM), paravertebral space (PVS), pleura (P), lung (L).

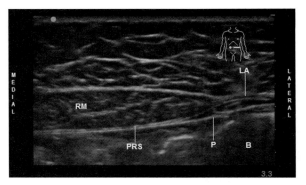

Figure 16.7 Ultrasound appearance of the rectus muscle (RM); posterior rectus sheath (PRS), linea alba (LA), peritoneum (P), bowel (B).

when LA is injected the space is seen to widen with the anterior displacement of the pleura.

Complications

Pneumothorax, contralateral paravertebral spread, epidural spread and dural tap.

Rectus sheath block

The rectus sheath is formed from the aponeuroses of the transverse abdominal muscles and has an anterior and posterior wall. The sheath encloses the rectus muscle and fuses in the midline to form the linea alba. The rectus muscle is adherent to the anterior sheath at the level of the xiphisternum, the umbilicus and midway between these two points. The anterior cutaneous branches of the lower 5 thoracic nerve can be blocked.

Indications

Pyloromyotomy, umbilical hernia, duodenal atresia repair.

Landmark technique

A 22G regional block needle attached to a syringe containing LA is inserted perpendicularly through the skin at the apex of the bulge of the rectus muscle, 2–3 cm lateral to the midline, just above the umbilicus. The anterior sheath is identified by moving the needle back and forth until a scratching sensation is felt; a pop is felt as the needle passes through the sheath. The needle is advanced through the muscle with continued movement of the needle until a scratching is again felt (this indicates the posterior sheath). If there is swelling in the region or resistance

to injection then it is not sited correctly. The technique is then repeated on the other side. Local anaesthetic 0.3–0.5 ml kg^{-1} is injected on each side.

Ultrasound technique

A high frequency linear probe is placed in TP above the umbilicus. The linea alba is identified and the probe moved laterally to appreciate the rectus muscle enclosed in its sheath which appears as a hyperechoic line above and below the muscle (Figure 16.7). The peritoneum with the bowel underneath can be seen beneath the posterior sheath. The inferior epigastric vessels can be identified with colour Doppler. As the probe is moved laterally the lateral abdominal muscles are imaged. A 22G regional block needle is inserted IP and advanced through the anterior sheath and the rectus muscle to reach the plane between the muscle and posterior sheath. After aspiration 0.5 ml LA is injected to ensure the muscle splits from the posterior sheath. The rest of the LA is then injected (0.1–0.2 ml kg^{-1} per side). Placing the probe longitudinally allows assessment of spread. The procedure is then repeated on the opposite side.

Transversus abdominis plane block (TAP)

The lateral abdominal wall is made up of the external oblique, internal oblique and transversus abdominis muscles (Figure 16.8); it is between these inner two muscles that the anterior primary rami of the lower six thoracic and the first lumbar nerve pass.

Indications

It can be performed unilaterally, e.g. open appendicectomy, or bilaterally, e.g. for laparoscopic operations. It must be remembered that it does not

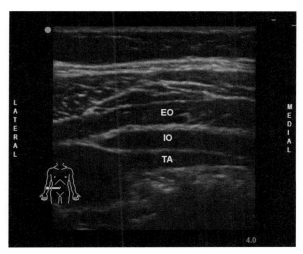

Figure 16.8 Ultrasound appearance of transversus abdominis block region; external oblique muscle (EO), internal oblique muscle (IO), transversus abdominis muscle (TA).

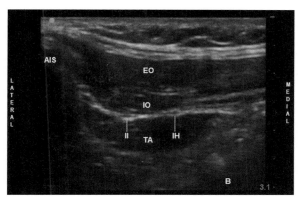

Figure 16.9 Ultrasound appearance of the ilioinguinal region; anterior iliac spine (AIS), external oblique muscle (EO), internal oblique muscle (IO), transversus abdominis muscle (TA), bowel underneath the peritoneum (B), ilioinguinal (II) and iliohypogastric (IH) nerves.

provide visceral analgesia. The ultrasound and landmark techniques have been much debated; the former has a more anterior injection site and is generally only suitable for infra-umbilical surgery. Here we have only discussed the ultrasound technique.

Ultrasound technique

A linear multifrequency probe of appropriate footprint is placed in TP on the lateral abdominal wall halfway between the costal margin and the iliac crest. All three layers of muscles and the peritoneum can be imaged. A 22G regional block needle is inserted IP in an anterior–posterior direction to reach the plane just posterior to midaxillary line. A small volume of LA is injected to confirm correct placement of the needle, seen as splitting of the two muscle layers; a total of $0.5 \, \text{ml} \, \text{kg}^{-1}$ is injected. If there is difficulty in entering the correct plane, carefully insert the needle tip into the internal oblique muscle; as the needle is then slowly withdrawn have an assistant inject saline.

Ilioinguinal and iliohypogastric nerve block

The iliohypogastric nerve supplies the gluteal region and the skin over symphysis pubis. The ilioinguinal nerve supplies the area of skin beneath that supplied by the iliohypogastric nerve and the anterior scrotum. There is much anatomical variation of nerve position between the abdominal wall muscles; this has resulted in many techniques none of which has a success rate greater than 70–80%.

Indications

Inguinal hernia repair, hydrocoele.

Landmark technique

Draw an imaginary line from the anterior superior iliac spine (ASIS) to the umbilicus; 2.5 mm medial from the ASIS on this line insert the needle perpendicular to the skin. A single pop is felt as the internal oblique is traversed. Owing to variation in the formation of aponeuroses a second pop can lead to intraperitoneal injection or femoral nerve block. Depth of injection is independent of age or size. A volume of 0.3 to $0.5 \, \text{ml} \, \text{kg}^{-1}$ is injected.

Ultrasound technique

A linear probe is positioned on the same line described above, with the lateral aspect of the probe resting on the ASIS. The probe is arced around the ASIS to define the muscle layers (external oblique, internal oblique and transversus abdominis); the nerves are seen as small hypoechoic ellipses between the innermost two muscles (Figure 16.9). Deep to the muscle the peritoneum and bowel can be identified. In expert hands a significantly smaller volume of $0.075 \, \text{ml} \, \text{kg}^{-1}$ is used with an impressive 95% success rate.

Complications

Femoral nerve block may be an unintended complication (seen in up to 10% of cases).

161

Penile block

This block is primarily used for circumcisions, although it may be used for distal hypospadias repair after discussion with the surgeon. There are two simple ways of performing this block. The first is to inject subcutaneously around the base of the penis. The second approach requires injection into the sub-pubic space; this space is divided into left and right by the suspensory ligament. It is within this space that the dorsal penile nerves pass. It should be remembered that the vessels travel in the midline. The penis is gently pulled caudally so that the skin is taut; the needle is then carefully placed under the skin in the midline just below the pubic symphysis. Once through the skin the needle is redirected from the perpendicular so that it points laterally (10°), and slightly cephalad; it is then advanced until a 'pop' is felt (this is Scarpa's fascia). The depth of the fascia is independent of age and weight (generally 8–30 mm). After aspiration $0.1\,\mathrm{ml\,kg^{-1}}$ of LA is injected; the process is then repeated for the other side. **Vasoconstrictors should not be used**.

Lower limb blocks

The nerve supply to the lower limb is derived from the lumbosacral plexus.

Lateral femoral cutaneous nerve

This is a purely sensory nerve arising from the dorsal divisions of L2 and L3. The nerve emerges from the lateral border of the psoas muscle and then runs down and lateral across the iliac fossa before passing beneath the inguinal ligament just medial to the ASIS. It divides into an anterior branch supplying the anterolateral thigh and a posterior branch supplying the lateral area from the greater trochanter to the mid-thigh region.

Indications

Slipped upper femoral epiphysis (used in conjunction with a femoral block).

Landmark technique

A 22G regional block is introduced perpendicular to the skin at a point 1 cm inferior and medial to the ASIS. The needle is advanced until a pop or a give is felt as it pierces the fascia lata. LA is injected and the needle is withdrawn and directed first medially and then laterally in a fan like manner and the process repeated. A dose of $0.3\,\mathrm{ml\,kg^{-1}}$ is required for the block.

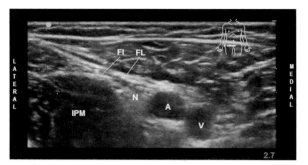

Figure 16.10 Ultrasound appearance of the femoral nerve block area; fascia lata (FL), fascia iliaca (FI), femoral nerve (N), femoral artery (A), femoral vein (V), iliopsoas muscle (IPM).

Femoral nerve block

This is the largest branch of the lumbar plexus arising from the dorsal divisions of the second to fourth lumbar nerves. It emerges from the lower border of the psoas muscle and runs between the psoas and the iliacus muscle and passes underneath the inguinal ligament into the femoral triangle. At the level of the inguinal ligament it lies deep to fascia lata and iliaca in a groove between the iliacus and the psoas muscle and is separated from the femoral vessels which lie in a separate fascial compartment medial to the nerve. It supplies the anterior compartment of the thigh.

Indications

Femoral fracture.

Landmark technique

A 22G needle attached to a PNS (set at 1.5 mA) is inserted immediately lateral to the femoral artery at the inguinal crease. The needle is aimed at a 45° angle cephalad. Usually two pops are felt as it passes through the fascia lata and iliaca. A patellar twitch indicating quadriceps femoris muscle stimulation is sought. Continued femoral nerve stimulation with reduction in current strength to 0.5 mA indicates correct position of the needle and $0.3\,\mathrm{ml\,kg^{-1}}$ of LA is injected.

Ultrasound technique

A linear multifrequency transducer is placed on the inguinal crease. The femoral vein and artery are identified. The nerve is found lateral to the femoral artery in a triangular hyperechoic area (Figure 16.10). The regional block needle is inserted OOP/IP (from lateral to medial). Often more than two pops are felt as this needle pierces the fascias; ensure the LA is deposited under the fascia iliaca and not in the iliacus muscle deep to the nerve. The increased contrast between the LA and the nerve allows the latter to be better imaged. The nerve should be surrounded with LA without exceeding toxic doses; remember if you want to try to get the lateral cutaneous nerve a large volume will be needed.

Fascia iliaca block

The fascia iliaca block is a useful block for above-knee surgery as it blocks the femoral (100%), lateral femoral cutaneous nerve (90%) and obturator nerve (75%) with a single injection. It is more successful than the 3 in 1 block. The nerves lie in a compartment which is bound superficially by the fascia iliaca (investing the iliacus muscle), superiorly by the iliac crest, and posteriorly by the psoas muscle.

Landmark technique

A line is drawn along the inguinal ligament from the ASIS to the pubic tubercle and divided into thirds. A regional block needle is inserted perpendicular to the skin 0.5 to 1 cm inferior to the junction of the outer and middle thirds of the ligament. As the needle is advanced under the skin two pops are felt as it pierces the fascia lata and fascia iliaca. A volume of $0.5\,\mathrm{ml\,kg^{-1}}$ is required to block all three nerves and application of pressure distal to the injection site is recommended during the injection.

Ultrasound technique

A linear probe is placed in a longitudinal plane just medial to the ASIS. The iliacus muscle is identified and the probe moved cephalad following the muscle as it passes over the pelvic brim. The needle is inserted IP from caudad to cephalad so the tip is positioned beneath the fascia iliaca. The LA is injected and the fascia lifted off the muscle, the needle can then be carefully advanced further and the fascial plane dissected open further. A large volume of LA $(0.5–0.7\,\mathrm{ml\,kg^{-1}})$ is needed to get the required spread (Figure 16.11).

Psoas compartment block

This is a paravertebral block which blocks the lumbar plexus that innervates the lower abdomen and upper leg. The lumbar plexus is formed by the ventral rami of the first four lumbar nerves and lies in the junction of the anterior two-thirds and posterior third of the psoas muscle, anterior to the transverse process of the lumbar vertebrae.

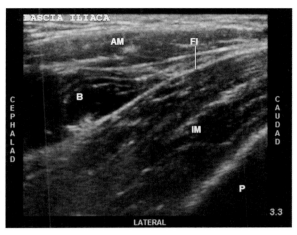

Figure 16.11 Ultrasound appearance of fasciailiaca block areas; abdominal muscles (AM), fascia iliaca (FI), bowel beneath peritoneum (B), iliacus muscle (IM), pelvis (P).

Indications

It is indicated for procedures requiring blockade of femoral, lateral femoral cutaneous and obturator nerves and in combination with a sciatic nerve block will provide analgesia for the entire lower limb.

There are numerous approaches to this block; only the author's preference is described.

Landmark technique

The anaesthetised child is placed in the lateral position as for an epidural with the side to be blocked uppermost. The lumbar spines are noted and a line is drawn parallel to these to pass through the posterior iliac spine on the side to be blocked. A second line is drawn to pass through the highest points of both the iliac crests and this usually passes over the transverse process of the fourth lumbar vertebrae. A 50–100 mm (depending on age) regional block needle attached to a nerve stimulator set at 1.5 mA is inserted perpendicular to the skin at the intersection between these two lines. This is advanced slowly looking for contractions of the quadriceps femoris muscle. As the needle is advanced it is very common to hit the transverse process; if so the needle is withdrawn slightly and walked off caudally. The needle should not be advanced more than 2 cm beyond the transverse process (this increases the risk to retroperitoneal structures). Once the movement of the patella is seen the current strength is reduced to 0.5 mA and with continued stimulation $0.5\,\mathrm{ml\,kg^{-1}}$ of LA is injected. If flexion of the hip is observed the needle is too deep, and if stimulation of the hamstring is seen the needle has been inserted in a more caudal and medial site. A catheter can be placed if required for continuous post-operative analgesia.

Loss of resistance to saline can also be used, as close to the vertebral body the main part of the psoas muscle is separated from the accessory posterior part by a thin fascia within which lies the root of the lumbar plexus.

Ultrasound can be used to identify the depth from the skin to the transverse process and psoas muscle.

Complications

These include damage to retroperitoneal vital structures and dural spread similar to other paravertebral blocks.

Sciatic nerve blocks

The sciatic nerve has tibial and common peroneal components. It enters the gluteal region from the pelvis through the greater sciatic foramen, and runs down between the ischial tuberosity and the greater trochanter of the femur. It usually divides at the apex of the popliteal fossa, though this can occur anywhere along the course of the nerve. As it exits the gluteal region it is usually accompanied by the posterior cutaneous nerve of the thigh on its medial side.

The nerve supplies the skin on the posterior part of the thigh, hamstring and biceps femoris muscles and most of the leg below the knee joint except for the area supplied by the saphenous nerve.

Popliteal block

Indications

When used with a saphenous or femoral nerve block it can be used for any operation below the knee, e.g. club foot surgery.

Landmark technique

The child lies prone or in the recovery position (with the operative side uppermost). The popliteal fossa is bordered superiorly by the biceps femoris tendon laterally, and semimembranosus and semitendinosus tendons medially. A triangle is formed by the popliteal crease; the triangle is divided into medial and lateral halves. A 22G block needle attached to a peripheral nerve stimulator set at 1–2 mA is inserted perpendicular to the skin at a point 1 cm lateral to the dividing line and 2 cm proximal to the popliteal crease. As it is advanced, inversion of the foot is sought as this requires stimulation of both tibial and

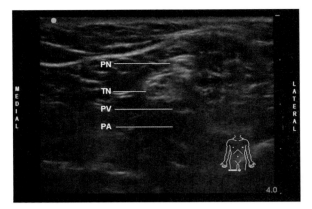

Figure 16.12 Ultrasound appearance of popliteal area for sciatic nerve block; peroneal (PN) and tibial (TN) components of sciatic nerve, popliteal vein (PV), popliteal artery (PA).

peroneal component. The current is reduced to 0.5 mA to confirm the proximity of the nerves and $0.5–0.7\,\mathrm{ml\,kg^{-1}}$ of LA is injected.

Ultrasound technique

The child is placed in the lateral position with the leg to be blocked on the top and straight. The linear multifrequency probe is placed slightly superior to the popliteal crease. The popliteal vessels are identified over the femoral bone. The tibial branch of the sciatic nerve is usually found slightly superior and lateral to the popliteal vein. Once identified continue scanning proximally along the nerve to find the common peroneal nerve which appears to join the tibial to form the sciatic nerve. Measure the depth to the nerve at this point as this is probably the best site for injection (Figure 16.12). Using an IP technique a 22G regional block needle is inserted into the lateral side of the thigh at the depth previously measured. The needle which is flushed and attached to LA syringe is advanced deep to the nerve until a subtle give is felt and half the LA is injected. The injection normally makes the visualisation of the nerve better. The needle is then withdrawn and directed superficial to the nerve where the rest of the LA is injected.

If it is difficult to identify the nerve above the popliteal crease, tilting the probe caudad or cephaloid may help. Also dorsiflexion and plantar flexion of the foot will produce the 'seesaw sign' where the tibial and peroneal components slide against one another and help with their identification. In cerebral palsy patients, nerve identification may be challenging owing to muscle fibrosis obscuring the nerve. The branching of the sciatic can occur more proximally and so scanning the nerve through its entire course is advised.

Infragluteal block

Landmark technique

The sciatic nerve is targeted in the groove where it lies between the ischial tuberosity and the greater trochanter of the femur. With child lying supine the leg is held flexed 90° at both the hip and knee joint. At the level of the gluteal crease the ischial tuberosity, the greater trochanter of femur, and the groove in the middle of the two are identified. With the usual precautions of safety and sterility a 50–100 mm regional block needle attached to a nerve stimulator set at 1–2 mA is introduced perpendicular to the skin and advanced in the horizontal plane until dorsiflexion/ plantar flexion of the foot is observed. The position of the needle is adjusted for continued stimulation of the nerve when the nerve stimulator is reduced to 0.5 mA and 0.5 ml kg^{-1} of LA injected.

Ankle block

The foot is supplied by the terminal branches of the femoral and sciatic nerves. The tibial branch of the sciatic nerve divides into a posterior tibial and sural nerve in the leg.

The posterior tibial nerve lies on the medial side of the Achilles tendon posterior to the posterior tibial artery and supplies the heel, the skin of the sole of the foot and the deep structures of the foot. It is blocked at the level of the medial malleolus. The needle is inserted into the subcutaneous tissue posterior to the tibial arterial pulsation and LA injected. As it is the only motor nerve to the foot a nerve stimulator can be used.

The sural nerve receives a branch from the common peroneal nerve and passes lateral to the Achilles tendon behind the lateral malleolus to supply the lateral border of foot up to the tip of little toe. It is blocked by subcutaneous infiltration behind the lateral malleolus.

The deep peroneal nerve passes beneath the external retinaculum midway between the lateral and medial malleolus to lie lateral to the dorsalis pedis artery. The deep peroneal nerve is blocked at the mid foot immediately lateral to the dorsalis pedis artery. A 23-gauge needle is inserted at 90° and advanced until bone is contacted. It is then withdrawn slightly and the anaesthetic injected.

The saphenous nerve, which is the terminal branch of the femoral nerve, runs downwards in front of the saphenous veins anterior to the medial malleolus and supplies the medial border up to the base of the great toe. The superficial peroneal nerve pierces the deep fascia in the lower part of the leg and runs in the superficial fascia over the dorsum of foot and supplies skin over most of the dorsum of the foot except the cleft between the first and second toes which is supplied by the deep peroneal nerve, and the medial and lateral borders of the foot. The saphenous nerve and superficial peroneal nerves can be blocked by a field block by a single insertion point at the mid point of the line joining the two malleoli. A 23G needle is inserted at this point and advanced subcutaneously towards the medial malleoli. LA is injected as the needle is withdrawn and then the needle is advanced towards the lateral malleoli and the procedure repeated. Care should be taken not to puncture the anterior tibial artery.

Digital nerve block

The toes are supplied by the digital nerves which are the terminal branches of the tibial nerve.

Ring block

As for fingers.

Metatarsal block

The metatarsal block is a more proximal block which involves the introduction of the needle on the dorsal surface of the foot on either side of the junction of the metatarsal head and the shaft of the targeted toe. The needle is advanced between the bones until the pressure of the needle is felt under the skin on the plantar surface of the foot. The LA is then injected while the needle is withdrawn.

Vasoconstrictors are contraindicated for these blocks. Care should also be taken not to inject a large volume as the pressure may compromise the blood supply to the digits.

Caudal block

The single-shot caudal is very popular owing to its simplicity and general reliability. The indications are broad; in infants any operation below the umbilicus may be appropriate, although in older children thoracic spread is unreliable.

Contraindications are as for any central block. Specific contraindications are the presence of cutaneous stigmata of spinal dysraphism e.g. sacral pit, or anorectal malformations. In these circumstances the spine should be cleared by ultrasound, and if necessary MRI, prior to caudal.

The sacrum is made up of five cartilaginous vertebrae that eventually ossify and fuse in adulthood. This causes the hiatus to become increasingly narrow and in some cases obliterated so hindering needle placement. The posterior arch of the fifth and occasionally the fourth vertebra fails to fuse: this is the sacral hiatus. This area is covered by the sacrococcygeal membrane.

At birth the dural sac is low at the S3/4 vertebral level; by 3 years of age it has ascended to the S2 vertebral level.

The child is positioned in the lateral position with the knees drawn up towards the chest. The sacral hiatus is palpated in the midline; it forms the apex of a triangle formed by it and the two posterior superior iliac crests. For neonates a 24G needle is used, 22G thereafter; for the occasional older child where a caudal is appropriate a 20G needle is used.

The needle is introduced perpendicular to the skin just below the upper limit of the hiatus. Gently advance the needle until resistance is felt, the needle is then redirected at a 45–60° angle; a pop may be felt at this point and if a cannula is used it can be advanced over the needle (if a needle is used then it should not be advanced more than a few millimetres). Simple measures are then employed to ensure correct placement (aspiration and opening the needle to air). A reliable method in infants under 2 years of age is the use of ultrasound (Figure 16.13) to identify an injection of saline ($<0.1 \, \mathrm{ml \, kg^{-1}}$). The LA can then be injected, usually 0.25% levobupivacaine. If a greater volume and extent is required then 0.125% levobupivacaine can be used. Generally speaking, $0.5 \, \mathrm{ml \, kg^{-1}}$ is used to cover the sacral roots, and $1 \, \mathrm{ml \, kg^{-1}}$ for

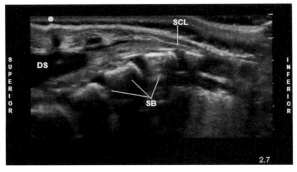

Figure 16.13 Ultrasound appearance of caudal space; sacrococcygeal ligament (SCL), dural sac (DS), sacral bone (SB).

high lumbar roots. To monitor the gross spread of LA ultrasound is reliable and allows the anaesthetist to aim for mid-thoracic spread if the case requires it. In those over 6 months of age the analgesia can be prolonged by the addition of $0.5 \, \mathrm{mg \, kg^{-1}}$ **preservative-free** ketamine.

Complications

Specific complications include dural tap, total spinal blockade, intravascular/intraosseous injection and perforation of the rectum.

Key points

- Regional anaesthesia is an important component of paediatric anaesthesia and should be considered for all suitable cases.
- Neonates and infants are at greater risk of LA toxicity, owing to their lower protein binding and the immature blood–brain barrier.
- Cardiac arrhythmias and circulatory collapse may be refractory to treatment, and resuscitation should be prolonged.

Further reading

Brown DL. *Atlas of Regional Anesthesia*, 2nd edition. Saunders. 1999. http://www.nysora.com/regional_anesthesia/sub-specialties/pediatric_anesthesia/index.1.html

Hadzic A. *Textbook of Regional Anesthesia and Acute Pain Management*. McGraw-Hill Professional. 2006.

Harmon D, Frizelle H, Sandhu N, Colreavy F, Griffin M. *Peri-operative Diagnostic and Interventional Ultrasound*. Elsevier. 2007.

Peutrell JM, Mather SJ. *Regional Anaesthesia in Babies and Children*. Oxford University Press. 1996.

Sedation for procedures in children

Mike R. J. Sury

Introduction

Trends in healthcare provision within large populations have centralised services so that it has become possible to devote expensive anaesthesia resources to meet the demand of medical and radiological procedures. Sedation techniques should be part of the armamentarium of anaesthetists. This chapter describes practical and recommended sedation techniques for common procedures.

Background knowledge

Definitions

Table 17.1 lists widely accepted ASA definitions of sedation; alternative descriptions are also listed in

Table 17.2. Conscious sedation is a term that remains in use, at least within the United Kingdom, which focuses on the ability to respond to the verbal command. It is especially important amongst dentists who need to use sedation outside a hospital setting. Ideally a conscious sedation drug technique should have a margin of safety wide enough to make loss of consciousness unlikely.

The problem with moderate sedation

In moderate sedation, the child will be easily rousable and therefore needs to show some degree of cooperation. Failure is common. Moderate sedation requires patience and skill, and the time investment may be worthwhile if the failure rate is low.

Table 17.1 American Society of Anesthesiologists (ASA) levels of sedation

	Conscious state	Respiratory depression
Minimal sedation	• Awake and calm • Normal response to verbal commands • Cognitive function and coordination may be impaired	• None
Moderate sedation	• Sleepy • Responds purposefully to verbal commands or light tactile stimulation • Reflex withdrawal from a painful stimulus is not a purposeful response	• Detected • Intervention rarely necessary
Deep sedation	• Asleep • Cannot be easily roused • Responds purposefully to repeated or painful stimulation	• Common • Intervention often necessary • Cardiovascular function is usually maintained
Anaesthesia	• Asleep • Unrousable	• Usual • Routine airway intervention • Cardiovascular depression common

Core Topics in Paediatric Anaesthesia, ed. Ian James and Isabeau Walker. Published by Cambridge University Press. © 2013 Cambridge University Press.

Table 17.2 Alternative definitions of sedation

	Conscious state	Respiratory and circulatory intervention
Conscious sedation	• Sleepy • Opens mouth to verbal commands (see 'Dental procedures')	• Rarely necessary with basic techniques • To be expected with advanced techniques
Safe sleep	• Asleep • Rousability not tested	• Rarely necessary
Ketamine	• Eyes open • Unresponsive • Immobile	• 1% brief apnoea and/or laryngospasm
Minimal anaesthesia	• Asleep with short-acting drug/s • Not easily roused or briefly unrousable • Rapid recovery when drug delivery stops	• Routine airway intervention • Cardiovascular depression common but intervention unnecessary

When moderate sedation becomes deep

If a child will not cooperate, the dose of sedation can be increased but this risks deep sedation. It is in general not possible to be certain what dose can cause deep sedation. Nitrous oxide alone is the exception – 50% nitrous oxide does not cause an unrousable state in otherwise normal children. Sedation therefore should be considered to be unpredictable; the level can vary between conscious and deep depending on the dose and the stimulation of the procedure. Techniques combining opioid and benzodiazepine are notorious for causing delayed respiratory depression after the pain of a procedure has subsided.

Pushing the boundaries – specialist sedation techniques

Potent drugs, such as propofol and sevoflurane, can be used to achieve moderate sedation, and these advanced techniques, developed for dental procedures, can be applied by anaesthetists in medical hospital practice. For anaesthetists, the boundary between sedation and anaesthesia need not be clear. In other words, if the facilities and personnel can deliver anaesthesia, the sedation level achieved is not important provided the child is safe, comfortable and recovers quickly. This ideal can be achieved using short-acting potent drugs, and these specialist techniques – which cause a state that fluctuates between sedation and anaesthesia – are valuable and are described in this chapter. They have been called minimal anaesthesia, and this may be a more appropriate term depending upon the circumstances.

Common procedures

Sedation is specific to the type of procedure. Some require immobility, others require analgesia. Sedation techniques for four common procedures are described below. The procedures are:

- Painless imaging (e.g. magnetic resonance imaging)
- Painful procedures (e.g. suture of laceration, manipulation of a fracture)
- Gastrointestinal endoscopy (e.g. gastroscopy and colonoscopy)
- Dental procedures

Patient preparation
Assessment

- Is the child capable of cooperation?

Moderate sedation is unlikely to be successful in toddlers and infants. Anxious patients will need to be motivated to tolerate moderate sedation. Children with behavioural disorders and learning difficulties are less likely to cooperate.

- Are there factors that change airway management?

Assess the physical status and understand what the procedure entails. The child may need tracheal intubation.

Fasting

- Is the child fasted?

Fasting is recommended for any technique in which verbal contact may be lost. Fasting is not needed for minimal sedation, nitrous oxide alone or moderate sedation using 'wide margin of safety' techniques. Hungry, thirsty children are less likely to cooperate under moderate sedation.

Gaining consent and assent

- Do the parents know what the procedure involves, the proposed sedation, the alternatives to sedation, and the risks and benefits?

Obtain written informed consent.

- Will play preparation help the child?

Much may be gained by spending time preparing a child psychologically.

- Does the child know what they will experience, what they should do and how they will cope?

Gaining a child's trust and assent is invaluable in many situations. Parents can provide reassurance and help during the procedure.

- Are many procedures planned?

If conscious sedation is practical for the child, then the time investment in gaining the child's cooperation could save repeated anaesthesia.

Common scenarios
Painless imaging

MRI and similar imaging techniques need the child to keep sufficiently still in a confined noisy space.

Some children will lie still, others will not. Within a busy radiology department there will need to be an efficient selection process and a sedation strategy (see Figure 17.1).

Patient selection for sedation

Infants less than 3 months old may sleep peacefully after a feed, and this can be attempted if the scan is not urgent. Feed the infant 30 minutes before the scan and wrap them up warmly. If this fails, sedation or anaesthesia has to be delayed for at least 6 hours (4 hours for breast milk).

Older children usually fall into two categories: those who will lie still without any sedation and those who need sedation deeper than moderate sedation. Remember that intravenous gadolinium may be necessary – decide if it is necessary and when the cannula will be inserted.

It is possible to select children who can be calmed by behavioural techniques, and some play specialists are remarkably successful. If the scan is not urgent this allows time for the child to get used to what is expected of them. It may take several sessions, and the principle of encouragement and reward helps. Enlist the services of a play specialist. If this is not possible or practical, use sedation or anaesthesia to put the child to sleep.

Safe sleep versus minimal anaesthesia

If an anaesthesia service is available the level of sedation is not important; it is the success and complication rates that dictate the technique. Short-acting potent drugs such as propofol or sevoflurane are standard techniques for the anaesthetist, and probably

Figure 17.1 Sedation strategy for MRI.

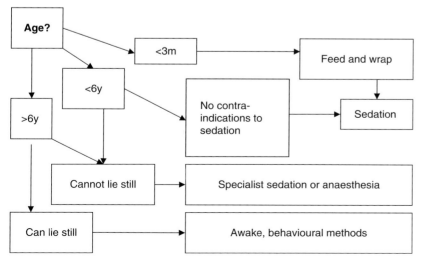

there is no need to use low doses of either in order to try to sedate a child. In the majority of cases anaesthetic doses are recommended to achieve sleep and immobility. Where these doses are not advisable then sedation doses could be considered. An example might be in a child with cardiomyopathy (low-dose propofol is useful) or an infant with poor venous access (sevoflurane delivered by nasal cannulae could be considered) – but these situations are rare.

Minimal anaesthesia

Propofol infusion has the advantage of almost 100% success rate and rapid pleasant recovery; the disadvantage is the need for IV access. An artificial airway is unnecessary for the majority of children who have normal airway anatomy.

- If an airway device is used, the dose of propofol may need to be higher to reduce the chance of awakening.
- Remote capnography monitoring of the breathing is essential (use nasal speculae).
- Use a propofol infusion (bolus dose $2–3\,\mathrm{mg\,kg}^{-1}$ followed by $10\,\mathrm{mg\,kg}^{-1}\,\mathrm{h}^{-1}$).

Occasionally propofol does not immobilise the child and the addition of ketamine, or an opioid or midazolam, is necessary; use low doses that maintain spontaneous breathing. Sevoflurane inhalational anaesthesia has obvious advantages in children who fear needles and those in whom venous access is difficult. Once anaesthesia is induced it can be converted to a propofol technique if necessary. Propofol has the advantage of being associated with less crying in recovery (sevoflurane may cause delirium in up to 30%). Delirium may be treated by subanaesthetic (or sedative) doses of propofol in recovery ($0.5–1\,\mathrm{mg\,kg}^{-1}$).

Moderate/deep sedation ('safe sleep')

If non-anaesthetists provide a service, the level of sedation is important and the technique should ideally be limited to moderate sedation. However, testing the level of sedation is counter-productive for scanning, and therefore the true level of sedation will be unknown. Whatever level of sedation is achieved, the term 'safe sleep' has been used for this scenario. In the author's hospital a list of contra-indications for sedation has been helpful and may have prevented any respiratory complications of sedation (Table 17.3).

The following sedation methods could be considered.

- Chloral hydrate. Use $100\,\mathrm{mg\,kg}^{-1}$ (maximum dose 1 g) orally. Limited to children less than 15 kg. Sleep begins within 10 minutes in most cases and lasts for up to 60 minutes. Vomiting is common. Intravenous cannulation and top-up with midazolam is necessary in 5–10% of children. Expect a failure rate of 5%.
- Midazolam. Intravenous doses should be titrated to effect. Start with $25–50\,\mathrm{mcg\,kg}^{-1}$ and increase to a maximum of 6 mg, 10 mg and 7.5 mg for children aged 1 m to 6 yr, 6–12 yr and 12–18 yr respectively.

Dexmedetomidine, given intravenously in high doses, is also effective at achieving moderate sedation for imaging, but it is not yet available in the UK.

Painful procedures

Some painful procedures, in emergency departments and in hospital wards, can be managed using moderate sedation. Manipulation of a fracture or the suturing of a wound are common examples.

- Local anaesthetic should be used whenever possible. In addition the following may be required.

Minimal sedation is appropriate in cooperative children and can be achieved with:

- Nitrous oxide. In a maximum concentration of 50% in oxygen it should be 'self-administered' by the patient.
- Midazolam (oral or intranasal).
  - ○ Oral midazolam ($0.5\,\mathrm{mg\,kg}^{-1}$) is an effective anxiolytic within 30 minutes.
  - ○ Nasal midazolam ($0.2\,\mathrm{mg\,kg}^{-1}$) has an onset as fast as the intravenous route (nasal drops are painful, atomised midazolam much less so). The buccal route is also useful.

When these are not effective two techniques can be considered:

- Ketamine. This type of sedation is unique and is called 'dissociative'. Children are immobile, calm, unreactive to pain yet their eyes may remain open. Airway and breathing reflexes are usually maintained. Ketamine is not considered to be conscious sedation, yet appreciable airway and respiratory effects

Table 17.3 Common contraindications to sedation

System	Details
Airway obstruction (actual or potential)	• Snoring or stridor • Blocked nose • Small mandible • Large tongue
Apnoeic spells	• Related to brain damage or previous drug treatment
Respiratory disease	• SpO_2 less than 94% in air • High respiratory rate • Oxygen treatment • Unable to cough or cry
High intracranial pressure	• Drowsiness • Headache • Vomiting
Epilepsy	• Major neurological or neuromuscular disease • Rectal diazepam within the last 24 hours or used more frequently than once in 2 weeks • Previous adverse reaction to sedation • Requiring resuscitation within the past month • Cyanosis more frequent than once per day • Convulsion less than 4 hours before sedation • Failure to regain full consciousness and mobility after a recent convulsion
Risk of pulmonary aspiration of gastric contents	• Abdominal distension • Appreciable volumes draining from NG tube • Vomiting
Severe metabolic, liver or renal disease	• Requiring IV fluids or dextrose • Jaundice or abdominal distension • Requiring peritoneal or haemodialysis

are uncommon at recommended doses. It can be administered by the intravenous or intramuscular routes. Expect a low incidence of laryngospasm caused by airway secretions. Recovery is usual within 90 minutes.

- o IV, 2 mg kg^{-1}; give additional doses of 1 mg kg^{-1} if necessary.
- o IM, 5–10 mg kg^{-1}.

• Midazolam (IV) with or without fentanyl (IV) is an effective conscious sedation technique but is less reliable than ketamine, and respiratory interventions are more likely. Titrate both drugs carefully; a starting dose of midazolam is 25–50 mcg kg^{-1}. The effect of fentanyl may outlast the pain, so that once the procedure is over, the fentanyl may cause respiratory depression. A starting dose of fentanyl is 0.25–0.5 mcg kg^{-1}.

• When these techniques are unsuitable or ineffective, a specialist technique or anaesthesia should be used.

• A combination of propofol and opioid such as fentanyl, alfentanil or remifentanil is effective and suitable for short procedures. Lumbar puncture and bone marrow aspirate procedures, so common in oncology departments, can be achieved under short-acting anaesthesia using propofol (2–3 mg kg^{-1}) and remifentanil (1 mcg kg^{-1}). Apnoea almost always occurs with remifentanil and a short period of assisted ventilation is necessary. Delivered via indwelling central venous catheters (common in oncology patients) this technique allows fast recovery – children can eat and drink within a few minutes afterwards. Post-operative analgesia other than local anaesthesia is not usually necessary.

Dental procedures

The mouth shuts during sleep. Consequently, provided a mouth prop is not used, the conscious level can be checked by an open mouth. Dental treatment can be exquisitely painful; always use local anaesthesia (LA) when possible. Effective LA reduces the need for sedation.

In the UK, dental conscious sedation is divided into basic and advanced (formerly standard and alternative). Standard conscious sedation requires the cooperation of the child and involves one of two techniques.

- Nitrous oxide is administered via a nasal mask in concentrations up to 70%. Usually only 30% is necessary because higher concentrations cause dysphoria.
- Midazolam, titrated intravenously, is recommended for anxious adolescent children and young people. A starting dose is 25–50 mcg kg^{-1}.

Both techniques are successful and safe. If they are not suitable or sufficient, either an advanced sedation technique or anaesthesia should be considered. The specialist techniques themselves involve the use of combinations of potent drugs and there may be a risk of unintended deep sedation, depending on the drugs and their doses. Specialist techniques should only be used by specially trained teams and are only safe in fully equipped facilities.

Endoscopy

Some adults can swallow an endoscope or accept the indignity and discomfort of colonoscopy without any sedation. Colonoscopy is uncomfortable but not usually painful except when the colon is stretched, often during biopsy of the terminal ileum. Children, however, almost always require sedation and many prefer anaesthesia. Propofol sedation or anaesthesia, without tracheal intubation, is being used widely, but almost certainly the level of sedation is not conscious.

Moderate sedation

Nevertheless, endoscopy is possible under moderate sedation in many children using intravenous midazolam, and an opioid is sometimes necessary. Both drugs should be titrated carefully. In summary, two techniques are recommended:

- Midazolam IV for upper gastrointestinal endoscopy. A starting dose is 25–50 mcg kg^{-1}.
- Midazolam combined with fentanyl (or equivalent opioid, both IV) for lower gastrointestinal endoscopy. A starting dose of fentanyl is 0.25–0.5 mcg kg^{-1}.

Minimal anaesthesia

Place the patient on their side. Place monitoring. Put on nasal speculae incorporating oxygen delivery and capnography (see Figure 17.2).

Use propofol – induce sedation/anaesthesia with 1–2 mg kg^{-1}.

- Gastroscopy
  - Insert a mouth gag to protect the endoscope.
  - Test the depth of anaesthesia by inserting a suction catheter into the pharynx.
  - Give 1–2 mg kg^{-1}, more if there is too much movement.
  - Some gag reflex should be preserved but not enough to make the procedure difficult.
  - Insert the gastroscope. Insert a soft suction catheter to remove pharyngeal secretions (this prevents laryngospasm – see Figure 17.2).

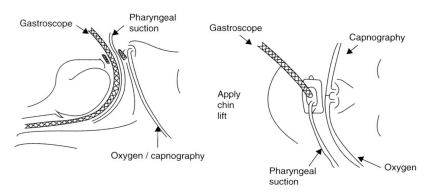

Figure 17.2 Position of suction tubing during gastroscopy.

- o It may be necessary to perform a jaw thrust to maintain the airway.
- o Inject further boluses of propofol as required $(1 \, \text{mg} \, \text{kg}^{-1})$.
- o Total dose is usually 3–$4 \, \text{mg} \, \text{kg}^{-1}$ for a 10 minute procedure.
- o Duodenoscopy often causes retching.
- Colonoscopy
  - o This is uncomfortable but not usually painful.
  - o Maintain anaesthesia with propofol $10 \, \text{mg} \, \text{kg}^{-1} \, \text{h}^{-1}$.
  - o Further boluses may be necessary.
  - o Colonic distension is painful and boluses of remifentanil may be necessary $(0.25$–$0.5 \, \text{mcg} \, \text{kg}^{-1})$.

- o Entering the terminal ileum is usually the most stimulating part of the procedure.
- o Over 45 minutes of colonoscopy time, 8–$9 \, \text{mg} \, \text{kg}^{-1}$ is the common dose required.

Key points

- Sedation can be effective in common scenarios.
- Standard fasting protocols should be applied for any technique in which verbal contact may be lost.
- Practitioners should be trained and ready to prevent or manage complications of potent drugs.

Further reading

Two UK guidelines are recent. The SIGN guideline concentrates on safe moderate sedation techniques. NICE guideline 112 covers all types of effective sedation including specialist techniques and recommends a framework of training to use them safely.

National Institute for Clinical Excellence. *Sedation for Diagnostic and Therapeutic Procedures in* *Children and Young People*. 2010. http://guidance.nice.org.uk/CG112.

Scottish Intercollegiate GN. SIGN Guideline 58: Safe sedation of children undergoing diagnostic and therapeutic procedures. *Paed Anaes* 2008;**18**(1):11–12.

Chapter 18

Peri-operative analgesia in children

Glyn Williams

Introduction

The effective and safe management of pain in children of all ages requires significant background knowledge on the part of their caregivers. Numerous factors can influence the success of analgesic treatment:

- Developmental age has a profound effect on both the processing of nociceptive information and the response to analgesia.
- The pharmacology of all drugs is age- and size-dependent, requiring appropriate dosage adjustments.
- Communication with the very young or those with developmental delay can influence the ability to assess pain and monitor the response to treatment.

Pain perception

Nociceptive pathways are present from birth, and even the most premature infant is born with the capacity to detect and respond to painful stimulation. During fetal, neonatal and infant life the nervous system is continually evolving. This allows structural and functional changes to occur continuously in response to the child's needs as it grows and develops. The pain pathways mirror these changes, with different components developing along differing time frames. The structural components required to perceive pain are present from early fetal life although pathways involved in modifying pain perception are still developing during infancy. The expression of the many molecules and receptors involved in the pain pathways vary in their number, type and distribution between early life and adulthood.

These structural and functional changes will affect both the immediate and short-term responses to pain and analgesic effect in infancy. Conversely, pain or analgesic treatment at this time may also predispose to persistent or long-term changes affecting the function of the somatosensory system in later life.

Peri-operative pain management

Successful pain management is based on the formulation of a sensible analgesic plan for each individual patient. It is best to take a practical and pragmatic approach dependent on the patient, the type of surgery and the resources available. The primary aims are to:

- Recognise pain in children;
- Prevent pain where it is predictable;
- Minimise moderate and severe pain safely in all children;
- Bring pain rapidly under control;
- Continue pain control after discharge from hospital.

Analgesic plan

An analgesic plan should be devised for each individual patient. The plan will depend on a number of factors (Table 18.1). The plan should be discussed with the patient, parents and staff to confirm acceptability, consider preferences, answer questions and take into account previous experiences.

The plan should allow treatment to be titrated to effect and also include provision for the rapid control of breakthrough pain and the identification and treatment of side effects. In established paediatric centres with a high level of resources, a dedicated paediatric pain service is the standard of care. Where this is not available, significant improvements in pain management can be made by the establishment of clinical

Core Topics in Paediatric Anaesthesia, ed. Ian James and Isabeau Walker. Published by Cambridge University Press. © 2013 Cambridge University Press.

routines and protocols for the treatment and assessment of post-operative pain and a network of interested medical and nursing staff to provide ongoing education.

Pain assessment

Appropriate clinical assessment of pain improves both the safety and efficacy of pain management in children. It allows for the prompt administration of analgesia and is an effective method of monitoring treatment. Effective pain assessment involves regular clinical monitoring of the child by trained staff allied with the use of an appropriate pain-scoring tool.

Pain is subjective in nature, and the use of self-reporting pain tools is generally regarded as the gold standard measure. This requires a certain degree of both cognitive and physical development. In younger, especially non-verbal, children, or those with cognitive or communication difficulties, other approaches are necessary, and tools using behavioural and/or physiological measures have been developed. Tools for routine clinical use should be practical, valid for the clinical setting and age range of the patients and be acceptable to staff, patients and parents.

Self-reporting tools

Linear visual analogue scores are generally accepted as appropriate in children older than 7 to 8 years.

Table 18.1 Factors to consider in designing an analgesic plan

The pain	Type, severity, location, onset, duration
The patient	Age, development, medical history, drug history and ongoing treatment, cognitive ability
The setting	Home, hospital, available staff and resources
The techniques/ drugs available	Pharmacology, resources, safety, routes of administration

'Child-friendly' adaptations of these scores have been designed for younger patients and have been used down to ages as low as 4, e.g. a face-type scale (Figure 18.1). At these younger ages the scales may not be truly linear and are not directly interchangeable or numerically comparable with other scales.

Behavioural and physiological measures

Using pain-related behaviours, such as crying, facial expression, body posture and restlessness, is considered to be one of the most reliable indirect methods of pain assessment. These form the basis of the many validated pain assessment scores available, for example the FLACC pain measurement tool (Figure 18.2). It is important to remember, however, that these behaviours are affected by a number of factors:

- Age of the child;
- Other factors such as hunger, distress, anxiety;
- Concurrent drug treatment;
- Individual interpretation by the healthcare workers using the tools.

Physiological measures such as heart rate and blood pressure, and hormonal responses, have also been used to assess pain either on their own or in conjunction with behavioural observations, but they lack both sensitivity and specificity, and this approach is of limited value.

Multimodal analgesia

Multimodal or balanced analgesia involves the simultaneous use of a number of analgesic interventions to achieve optimal pain management. Analgesics acting independently and synchronously on pain mechanisms at different points on the pain pathway are likely to be more effective than a single drug. Potentially, this also minimises the doses of drugs used, thereby reducing side effects and possibly accelerating

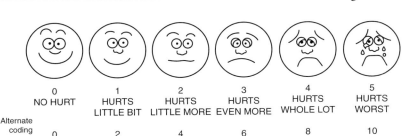

| 0 NO HURT | 1 HURTS LITTLE BIT | 2 HURTS LITTLE MORE | 3 HURTS EVEN MORE | 4 HURTS WHOLE LOT | 5 HURTS WORST |

Alternate coding 0   2   4   6   8   10

Figure 18.1 Wong–Baker Faces pain rating scale. Originally published in Whaley & Wong's *Nursing Care of Infants and Children*. © Elsevier Inc. Reproduced with permission.

Categories	Scoring		
	0	**1**	**2**
Face	No particular expression or smile	Occasional grimace or frown, withdrawn, disinterested	Frequent to constant frown, clenched jaw, quivering chin
Legs	Normal position or relaxed	Uneasy, restless, tense	Kicking, or legs drawn up
Activity	Lying quietly, normal position, moves easily	Squirming, shifting back and forth, tense	Arched, rigid, or jerking
Cry	No cry (awake or asleep)	Moans or whimpers, occasional complaint	Crying steadily, screams or sobs, frequent complaints
Consolability	Content, relaxed	Reassured by occasional touching, hugging, or being talked to, distractable	Difficult to console or comfort

Each of the five categories (F) Face; (L) Legs; (A) Activity; (C) Cry; (C) Consolability is scored from 0–2, which results in a total score between zero and ten.

Figure 18.2 FLACC behavioural scale © 2002, The Regents of the University of Michigan. All rights reserved. Used with permission.

recovery. Multimodal analgesia also allows for the use of non-pharmacological pain control strategies, such as comfort measures and psychological techniques, where possible.

Using a multimodal approach, effective pain management is achievable for most cases, and the technique can be adapted for day cases, major cases, the critically ill child, or the very young. In current practice, most analgesic techniques in children are based on differing combinations of four main classes of analgesics:

- Paracetamol
- Non-steroidal anti-inflammatory drugs (NSAIDs)
- Opioids
- Local anaesthetics

Unless there is a contraindication to do so, a local/regional analgesic technique should be used in all cases (see also Chapter 16). For many minor and day-case procedures this may allow opioids to be omitted, particularly if used in combination with paracetamol and NSAIDs.

Routes of administration

Analgesic drugs can be given by a variety of routes and the choice of route can have a significant impact on the efficacy of pain management. The choice(s) must be acceptable to the patient, parents and staff. For example, intramuscular injection is painful and is relatively contraindicated despite clinical effectiveness. Poor compliance with this technique, which was disliked by both staff and children, was a major factor that led to the early reports highlighting the undertreatment of pain in children. Where possible, prescriptions should allow for more than one choice of route.

The routes in common use are:

Oral: This is generally the preferred route but is not always achievable at all times in the peri-operative period due to the child being 'nil by mouth' for some of this time. For most commonly used analgesics, many different formulations are available in terms of flavour and liquids or tablets to allow for the varied tastes of children.

Rectal: This is a useful and convenient alternative when the oral route is unavailable. However, the rectal absorption of many drugs is slow, erratic and unreliable. Rectal administration can also be unpleasant or unacceptable to some patients although its use under general anaesthesia is usually more palatable if discussed prior to surgery.

Intravenous: This allows for rapid onset and high efficacy, and is the preferred route intra-operatively, provided suitable formulations are available. Post-operative use will be dependent on the availability of trained staff and suitable resources and monitoring. Securing intravenous access is easily done under general anaesthesia but may prove problematic at other times.

Subcutaneous: This allows for continuous and intermittent infusion of low volumes of drugs and subcutaneous access is often easier to establish compared with intravenous access. Provided tissue perfusion is good, absorption seems to be predictable and rapid, but the pharmacokinetics of subcutaneous analgesics in children have not been well studied.

Epidural: This provides extensive and profound analgesia at the site of surgical insult with little systemic effect and the option of long-term infusion. It requires a skilled anaesthetist, and trained staff with adequate resources and monitoring for subsequent management. Epidurals are inserted under general anaesthesia in the majority of children and have a good safety profile.

Transdermal and *Transmucosal:* Lipid-soluble drugs can be rapidly absorbed in small volumes from highly vascular sites. This allows a potentially rapid onset and high efficacy without the need for painful access. Intranasal diamorphine has been used with success in the emergency room and for painful procedures. Significant opioid-related side effects are still common. Absorption via the transdermal route is slower but newer technologies in delivery systems are improving this. Topical application of local anaesthetics is frequently used for minor painful procedures.

Inhalation: Nitrous oxide/oxygen (Entonox) inhalation has been successfully used for the management of brief painful procedures in children. Acceptability is often good but trained staff with specialist equipment and a suitable environment are required.

Analgesic drugs and techniques

Pain intensity and duration in the peri-operative period are usually predictable, and planning analgesic requirements is relatively straightforward. Many combinations of drugs and techniques are possible. Potent analgesic combinations are usually required initially, with a gradual reduction over time as healing occurs, and pain finally being managed by simple, readily available analgesics. Opioids, paracetamol and NSAIDs are usually administered regularly as part of a multimodal strategy. Local anaesthesia can be used in the form of a 'single-shot' technique at the time of surgery or as a post-operative infusion either centrally or peripherally. Other agents such as NMDA antagonists (ketamine) and α_2-adrenergic agonists (clonidine) can be added to supplement the multimodal strategy and/or prolong the effect of local anaesthetics.

Recommended doses of commonly used analgesics are given in Table 18.2.

Paracetamol

Paracetamol is the most widely prescribed drug in paediatric hospitals and has become the mainstay base analgesic for almost all procedures. The analgesic potency is low and it is effective against mild pain. In combination with NSAIDs and weak opioids it has been shown to be effective for moderate pain, and it has an opioid-sparing effect when used in tandem with the more potent opioids.

Paracetamol has a mainly central mode of action, producing both analgesic and antipyretic effects. It has been shown to inhibit prostaglandin synthesis in the hypothalamus, reduce hyperalgesia mediated by substance P, and reduce nitric oxide generation involved in spinal hyperalgesia induced by substance P or NMDA.

The oral bioavailability of paracetamol is very good as it is rapidly absorbed from the small bowel. Rectal absorption is slow and incomplete, except in neonates. If paracetamol is given rectally at the start of a short procedure (<1 hour) it is unlikely to reach therapeutic plasma levels by the time the child wakes in the recovery room. Thus, if possible, paracetamol should be given orally pre-operatively or intravenously. Intravenous paracetamol may have a higher analgesic potency than both the oral and rectal preparations, as uptake into the cerebrospinal fluid (CSF) is greater and faster following intravenous administration than via the other routes. Regular rather than an 'as required' post-operative prescription has been shown to provide better analgesia.

Non-steroidal anti-inflammatory drugs

NSAIDs act mainly peripherally by inhibiting prostaglandin synthesis and thus reducing inflammation, although central effects have also been postulated involving the opioid, serotonin and nitric oxide pathways. They are highly efficacious in their own right in the treatment of mild to moderate pain in children.

Table 18.2 Commonly used analgesic drugs in children

Drug	Dose	Comments
Paracetamol	**Neonates:** **IV:** 10 mg kg^{-1} 6 hourly **Max dose:** 10 mg kg^{-1} 6 hourly **Max dose:** 40 mg kg^{-1} d^{-1} **Oral/rectal**: Loading dose: 20 mg kg^{-1} Then: 10–15 mg kg^{-1} 6 hourly **Max daily dose:** Term neonate 60 mg kg^{-1} d^{-1} Preterm 45 mg kg^{-1} d^{-1}	**Mild analgesic and antipyretic drug** Rectal route less reliable than IV or oral routes.
	Others: **IV:** 15 mg kg^{-1} 6 hourly **Max daily dose:** 60 mg kg^{-1} d^{-1} (Max 1 g 6 hourly) **Oral:** Loading dose: 20 mg kg^{-1} Then: 15–20 mg kg^{-1} 6 hourly **Max daily dose:** 90 mg kg^{-1} d^{-1} **Rectal: Loading dose:** 30–40 mg kg^{-1} Then: 20 mg kg^{-1} 6 hourly **Max daily dose:** 90 mg kg^{-1} d^{-1}	Consider reverting to 60 mg kg^{-1} d^{-1} after 5 days to reduce accumulation/adverse effects.
Diclofenac	**Oral/rectal:** 1 mg kg^{-1} 8 hourly **Max dose:** 50 mg **Max daily dose:** 3 mg kg^{-1} d^{-1}	**NSAID** (use one only). Not neonates or infants <6 mths. Caution in asthma or renal impairment, history of GI bleed, low platelet count.
Ibuprofen	**Oral: 1–3 mths:** 5 mg kg^{-1} 6–8 hourly **Max daily dose:** 20 mg kg^{-1} d^{-1} **Oral: >3 mths:** 5–10 mg kg^{-1} 6–8 hourly **Max dose:** 400 mg **Max daily dose:** 30 mg kg^{-1} d^{-1}	**NSAID** (use one only). Not neonates (<1 month or <5 kg). Caution in asthma or renal impairment, history of GI bleed, low platelet count.
Tramadol	**Oral/IV:** 1 mg kg^{-1} 4–6 hourly	**Moderate potency opioid/5HT antagonist** Moderate to severe pain.
Codeine	**Oral/rectal:** 1 mg kg^{-1} 4–6 hourly	**Moderate potency opioid** Not recommended for IV use
Oxycodone	**Oral:** 0.2 mg kg^{-1} 6 hourly	**Moderate potency opioid**
Morphine	**Oral:** <1 year 100 mcg kg^{-1} 4–6 hourly ≥1 year 200–400 mcg kg^{-1} 4 hourly **IV:** Neonate 25–50 mcg kg^{-1} >1 month 25–100 mcg kg^{-1}	**Moderate/strong potency opioid** Monitor respiratory rate. Intravenous dosage interval is 4 hourly when given by bolus doses but can be used as a continuous or PCA/NCA infusion – titrate to effect.
Fentanyl	**IV**: 0.5–1 mcg kg^{-1}	**Strong potency opioid** Monitor respiratory rate. Bolus doses usually used intra-operatively. Can be used as a continuous or nurse-controlled/patient-controlled infusion – titrate to effect.
Diamorphine	**Intranasal:** 0.05–0.1 mg kg^{-1}	**Strong potency opioid** Monitor respiratory rate.

Table 18.2 (cont.)

Drug	Dose	Comments
Clonidine	**Oral/IV:** 1–2 mcg kg^{-1} 6–8 hourly **Caudal:** 1–2 mcg kg^{-1} +/− local anaesthetic	α_2-adrenergic agonist
Ketamine	**Oral:** 0.5–1 mg kg^{-1} 6 hourly **IV:** 0.1 mg kg^{-1} 6 hourly **Caudal:** 0.25–1 mg kg^{-1} +/− local anaesthetic	NMDA receptor antagonist Use preservative-free preparation via epidural route

They have a reported opioid-sparing effect of 30–40% when used in combination with opioids, and they also reduce opioid-related adverse affects as well as facilitating more rapid weaning of opioid infusions. They have also been shown to be highly effective in combination with a local or regional nerve block. Combination with paracetamol produces better analgesia than either drug alone.

There are limitations to their use in paediatric populations. In the UK ibuprofen is now available in over-the-counter formulations for ages 3 months and above, and it is used in children down to 1 month in the hospital setting. At present diclofenac and other NSAIDs are not recommended for children less than 6 months of age. Care should also be taken in those patients who are asthmatic or have a known aspirin or NSAID allergy, and those with hypovolaemia, dehydration, renal impairment, coagulopathy or where there is a significant risk of haemorrhage. A careful history of previous use of NSAIDs should be taken in every case. Different NSAIDs have different side-effect profiles, and the relative risks associated with each of the contraindications given will differ between drugs. In the UK the Committee on the Safety of Medicines has classified ibuprofen and diclofenac as having the best side-effects profile.

Rectal and oral bioavailability are both good, though again for short cases they are best given orally pre-operatively. There is a higher than expected dose requirement in children if scaled by body weight from adult doses. Other routes of administration are available, such as intravenous and topical, although their use in children so far has been limited.

Opioids

Opioids remain the mainstay of analgesic treatment for the majority of all but minor surgical procedures. The choice of which opioid to use will depend on the patient's medical history, the type of surgery, drug availability, any locally devised protocols and, often, individual anaesthetic preference. The pharmacology of these agents changes during early life, and these changes are not consistent between different drugs. When using a particular opioid in neonates and infants it is important to understand the pharmacology of that particular drug in those age groups to ensure both efficacy and safety.

Morphine remains the most commonly used opioid. Morphine clearance is decreased and the elimination half-life is increased in neonates compared with infants and older children. Also in neonates the glucuronidation pathways, the main metabolic pathways for morphine, are still developing, slowing morphine metabolism and giving a relatively increased production of morphine-6-glucuronide, an active metabolite of morphine. These differences may to some extent account for the increased efficacy of morphine seen clinically in neonates.

Codeine, another popular opioid in neonates and infants, works via metabolism to morphine. The cytochrome P-450 enzyme, CYP2D6, responsible for this conversion shows markedly reduced activity at these ages compared with that seen in older children and adults. Thus it may be that little or no morphine is produced from a dose of codeine. In addition the CYP2D6 enzyme demonstrates genetic polymorphism, and the ability of individuals of all ages to convert codeine to morphine varies considerably. This may explain codeine's good safety profile in young children but may also suggest that the analgesic efficacy is questionable.

Tramadol has a dual mode of action. It is an agonist at mu receptors but also works by enhancing descending inhibition via the serotinergic and noradrenergic systems. In children it has been shown to be efficacious for mild to moderate pain with a good safety profile. Oxycodone is similar in structure to codeine, although the analgesic effect is via the parent molecule rather than its metabolites. It has also been shown to be effective for treatment of mild to moderate pain in children.

Opioid infusions

The requirements for opioid infusion analgesia include:

- Clear protocols for infusion rates and the detection and treatment of side effects;
- Staff educated in the use of opioid infusion techniques;
- Appropriate monitoring;
- A safe nursing environment.

If all these factors are in place then opioid infusions can be effectively and safely used in even the most premature neonate.

Continuous infusion: Morphine at infusion rates of 10–40 mcg kg^{-1}h^{-1} will effectively manage most post-operative pain. Lower infusion rates (5–15 mcg kg^{-1}h^{-1}) should be used in neonates. Fentanyl (0.5–2 mcg kg^{-1}h^{-1}) has been shown to be a useful alternative to morphine. Infusion analgesia can be comparable with the more flexible nurse-controlled and patient-controlled analgesia (NCA and PCA) techniques, but changes in rate alter plasma levels slowly in comparison with methods that include supplemental boluses.

Nurse-controlled analgesia: This effectively increases the flexibility of a continuous infusion by combining a moderate background infusion with the ability to give two to three extra demand-led boluses per hour. Efficacy is improved by the use of reliable pain assessment.

Patient-controlled analgesia: In children a small background infusion (4 mcg kg^{-1}h^{-1}) has been shown to improve night-time sleep patterns without increasing side effects. Aside from this, traditional adult PCA settings are used. With the right supervision and monitoring, PCA can be used in children as young as 5 years.

Suggested NCA and PCA infusion protocols are shown in Table 18.3. Opioid-related side effects such as nausea and vomiting, itching, sedation and respiratory depression can occur in a dose-dependent fashion. Sedation scoring and monitoring of the respiratory rate should be undertaken in all patients receiving an opioid infusion. Oxygen and opioid antagonists must be easily accessible in case of

Table 18.3 NCA/PCA infusion protocols, GOSH Pain Control Service

Up to 50 kg: morphine 1 mg kg^{-1} or fentanyl 25 mcg kg^{-1} in 50 ml 5% glucose or 0.9% saline

	Background (ml h^{-1})	Bolus (ml)	Lockout (mins)
PCA	0 or 0.2	0.5 or 1	5 or 10
NCA	0, 0.2, 0.5 or 1	0.5 or 1	20 or 30

>50 kg: morphine 50 mg or fentanyl 1250 mcg in 50 ml 5% glucose or 0.9% saline

	Background (ml h^{-1})	Bolus (ml)	Lockout (mins)
PCA	0	1 or 2	5 or 10
NCA	0, 0.2, 0.5 or 1	1	20 or 30

emergency, and antiemetics and antipruritics should be available if required. The subcutaneous route remains an alternative to intravenous administration but it should not be used in hypovolaemic patients.

Local anaesthetics

A technique of nerve blockade is appropriate for nearly all surgical procedures and forms an important component of a balanced analgesic technique. It allows site-specific analgesia, demonstrates a lack of sedative and respiratory side effects and reduces the systemic analgesic requirements.

Many techniques of nerve blockade have been described in children although only a small number are common, and they are generally simple, safe and effective (Table 18.4). Traditionally insertion has been guided by anatomical landmarks but newer methods such as ultrasound and electrical surface mapping have added to the efficacy and safety. (See also Chapter 16.)

Bupivacaine has mainly been the local anaesthetic of choice in paediatric practice. It has been extensively studied, and safe dosing guidelines have been established which have greatly reduced the incidence of systemic toxicity. Neonates demonstrate decreased clearance, increased half-life and decreased protein binding of local anaesthetic agents. Therefore, at this age, there is a risk of systemic toxicity and dosing schedules have to be adjusted. Ropivacaine and levobupivacaine have been introduced into

Table 18.4 Some commonly used nerve blocks in children

Block	Procedure
Wound infiltration	Most surgical wounds
Ilioinguinal nerve	Inguinal hernia Orchidopexy
Penile dorsal nerve	Circumcision
Rectus sheath block	Umbilical hernia repair Laparoscopic insertion site
Axillary brachial plexus block	Hand surgery
Infraorbital nerve block	Cleft palate
Femoral/sciatic nerve Fascia iliaca compartment block	Surgery to thigh/femur
Intercostal nerve	Thoracotomy
Paravertebral block	Thoracotomy Abdominal surgery
Epidural (caudal, lumbar or thoracic)	Abdominal/genito-urinary surgery Orthopaedics/spinal surgery Thoracotomy Cardiac surgery

paediatric practice and have demonstrated both efficacy and safety.

'Single-shot' techniques: Single-shot central blocks (epidural/caudal), regional or local blocks can be used to provide excellent intra-operative and early post-operative analgesia. They decrease the use of other analgesics and the incidence of side effects, and potentially avoid the use of opioids. The analgesic plan, however, must allow for sufficient analgesia to be in use when the effect of the block wears off.

Caudal analgesia remains popular owing to its versatility and simplicity. Adjuncts are often added to extend the spread and duration of the block. Ketamine and clonidine have been shown to be effective with a low incidence of side effects at low doses (see Table 18.2). Concern has been expressed about both drugs, however, in relation to their effects on the developing nervous system and the incidence of side effects in neonates and infants. As a consequence their use by this route has been questioned in these age groups. Caudal opioids are associated with an increased incidence of side effects and are not now commonly used.

Infusion techniques: Continuous local anaesthetic infusions can be used to extend the duration of nerve blockade for days into the post-operative period. Accumulation of local anaesthetic is a factor in children, and potential toxicity can limit the duration and efficacy of an infusion. Local infection at the insertion site and catheter occlusion or dislodgement can also occur, especially in smaller children.

Lumbar and thoracic epidural infusions are well established in children for severe acute pain. Efficacy and post-operative respiratory benefits have been demonstrated in children, but the relative benefits and risks in comparison with other techniques have not been well studied.

Generally insertion is performed under general anaesthesia, and most practitioners use a continuous loss of resistance to saline technique. There is now increased use of ultrasound-guided insertion to attempt to improve the success and safety of the technique. Shorter (5 cm) 18G and 19G Toughy needles are available for use in children along with the standard 8 cm 16G and 18G ones. The catheter size varies according to needle size (23G with 19G needle and 21G with 18G needle). The 23G catheter has been reported as having a high incidence of displacement. As with adults at least 3 cm should be left in the epidural space to decrease the risk of the catheter falling out. Epidural infusions in children are prone to leaking but are often effective in spite of this.

Opioids and clonidine have been used as adjuncts with the local anaesthetic to improve efficacy and limit local anaesthetic usage. Some common infusion regimens are given in Table 18.5. Clear established protocols for the management of epidural infusions must be in place along with trained staff, appropriate monitoring and a safe environment. Treatment protocols for side effects should also be used and if opioids are added then urinary catheterisation is recommended.

Continuous infusion techniques for intrapleural, paravertebral, brachial plexus block, sciatic nerve block, fascia iliaca compartment block and popliteal block have all been reported in children.

Clonidine

Clonidine is an α_2-adrenergic agonist that has a wide range of uses in children. It can be used as part of a multimodal strategy for peri-operative pain by the oral, intravenous and epidural routes, and it is often

Table 18.5 Drug doses and infusion rates for epidural analgesia

Drug	Initial dose	Infusion	Rate
Levobupivacaine	0.25% 0.5–0.75 ml kg^{-1}	0.125%	0.1–0.4 ml kg^{-1} h^{-1} (Max 15 ml h^{-1})*
Ropivacaine	0.2% 0.5–0.75 ml kg^{-1}	0.2%	0.1–0.4 ml kg^{-1} h^{-1} (Max 15 ml h^{-1})*
Levobupivacaine + Morphine	0.25% 0.5–0.75 ml kg^{-1}	0.125% + Morphine 0.001%	0.1–0.4 ml kg^{-1} h^{-1} (Max 15 ml h^{-1})*
Levobupivacaine + Fentanyl	0.25% 0.5–0.75 ml kg^{-1}	0.125% + Fentanyl 1–2 g ml^{-1}	0.1–0.4 ml kg^{-1} h^{-1} (Max 15 ml h^{-1})*
Ropivacaine + Fentanyl	0.2% 0.5–0.75 ml kg^{-1}	0.2% + Fentanyl 1–2 mcg ml^{-1}	0.1–0.4 ml kg^{-1} h^{-1} (Max 15 ml h^{-1})*

* Maximum infusion rate in neonates 0.2 ml h^{-1}

used as an adjunct to local anaesthetics. It is also used for premedication owing to its sedative properties.

Ketamine

Ketamine is a NMDA receptor antagonist. It has analgesic properties in its own right at lower doses than those used for anaesthesia. It also prevents the induction of central sensitisation and wind-up and the development of opioid tolerance. Efficacy has been shown in children when combined with opioids, or with local anaesthetics and when used as part of a multimodal strategy. At the low doses used for analgesia the potential psychomimetic effects of ketamine are rare. It has also been used successfully for premedication.

Post-operative nausea and vomiting (PONV)

Nausea and vomiting are commonly seen postoperatively in children. The causes are multifactorial with analgesia potentially involved, especially opioids. Pain can also be a factor, however, and adequate analgesia has been shown to reduce the incidence of PONV.

Other risk factors are increasing age (greater than 3 years), a history of PONV or motion sickness, the duration and type of surgery, and the use of volatile anaesthetics. The effect of nitrous oxide on PONV has not been proven in children. Owing to the complexity of the pathogenesis of PONV, it is postulated that

a multimodal-type strategy for treatment may give better outcomes. Ondansetron and dexamethasone are the most commonly used drugs peri-operatively, and combination therapy has been shown to be superior to either drug on its own. Acustimulation using the P6 acupuncture point has been shown to be as effective as using antiemetics.

Key points

- Nociceptive pathways are present from birth, and even the most premature infant is born with the capacity to detect and respond to painful stimulation.
- Developmental age has a profound effect on both the processing of nociceptive information and the response to analgesia.
- It is essential to know the pharmacology of analgesic drugs at all ages.
- An analgesic plan is required in all cases and the plan should be flexible, sufficient and safe.
- Adopting a multimodal approach to treatment provides optimal pain management.
- Regular pain assessment improves the safety and efficacy of pain management in children.
- Complex pain management requires the use of clear protocols for infusion rates and the detection and treatment of side effects. It also requires educated staff, appropriate monitoring and a safe nursing environment.

Further reading

Howard RF. Complex pain management. In Bingham R, Lloyd-Thomas A, Sury M, eds. *Hatch & Sumner's Textbook* *of Paediatric Anaesthesia*, 3rd edition. Hodder Arnold. 2008; 407–23.

Howard RF *et al*. Good practice in post-operative and procedural pain management. *Ped Anaes* 2008:**18**; Suppl 1.

Lonnqvist P-A, Morton NS. Post-operative analgesia in infants and children. *Br J Anaes* 2005:**95**;59–68.

Chapter

19

Prevention and treatment of post-operative nausea and vomiting in children

Alison S. Carr

Introduction

Nausea and vomiting are very common after surgery. Vomiting is defined as the forceful expulsion of gastric contents through the mouth. It has a definite endpoint and is easy to measure. Nausea is defined as an unpleasant sensation associated with awareness of the urge to vomit. Nausea is harder to quantify in studies of post-operative nausea and vomiting in children, especially in young children.

Preventing post-operative nausea and vomiting is very important in paediatric anaesthesia. Post-operative vomiting is still twice as frequent in children as in adults. It is the commonest cause of unanticipated hospital admission after surgery and a cause of parental dissatisfaction. With anaesthetic techniques common in the late 1980s, up to 80% of patients reported post-operative vomiting after high-risk surgical procedures. While in some studies post-operative vomiting in children still reaches 40%, identifying risk factors for post-operative vomiting and tailoring the anaesthetic to the patient and the surgery with the appropriate use of antiemetics should allow the incidence of post-operative vomiting to be less than 10%.

The frequency of post-operative vomiting is also an important consideration. Often when the incidence of post-operative vomiting is high, the frequency of vomiting for an individual child may also be high. In some studies of post-operative vomiting, children have vomited as many as 10 times in the first 24 hours post-operatively. Appropriate antiemetics prescribed on an individual basis are essential for a child in these circumstances.

The incidence of post-operative nausea and vomiting is reported in a number of ways in the literature. In some publications nausea and vomiting are reported together, in others separately, and other publications report nausea or vomiting. Although children experience nausea, small children do not consistently report this, and consequently studies on emesis in children frequently describe and report vomiting rather than nausea and vomiting. In this chapter, for consistency, I will describe factors affecting post-operative vomiting (POV) rather than nausea and vomiting.

The duration over which the incidence of POV is measured is also important. POV within the first 6 hours of surgery is defined as early POV. POV occurring in the 6–24 hour period is defined as late POV. Studies on POV should report the incidence of vomiting for the first 24 hours after surgery. In studies reporting only recovery room data the actual incidence of POV will be underestimated.

Preventing POV requires an understanding of the factors influencing it. Knowing factors responsible for increasing POV allows you to tailor the anaesthetic appropriately to the child to reduce the incidence of POV. It is also important to know when it is appropriate to use antiemetics to prevent POV and which antiemetics are effective in children. The converse is also true: it is just as important to recognise where antiemetics are not needed in preventing POV, as otherwise their use will unnecessarily increase cost and may cause needless adverse drug reactions.

Why does post-operative nausea and vomiting occur?

Nausea and vomiting are the body's important defence mechanisms against toxin ingestion. Vomiting involves the coordination of gastrointestinal, respiratory and abdominal muscles. This action is controlled by the emetic centre situated in the lateral reticular formation close to the tractus

Core Topics in Paediatric Anaesthesia, ed. Ian James and Isabeau Walker. Published by Cambridge University Press. © 2013 Cambridge University Press.

solitarius in the brain stem. If this area is stimulated electrically, vomiting is produced. Likewise if the emetic centre is ablated, chemically induced vomiting such as after apomorphine does not occur. In spite of this, there are no known anaesthetic drugs that act directly on the emetic centre. Stimuli from other parts of the nervous system may affect the emetic centre, inducing nausea and vomiting. These include afferent nerves from the pharynx and gastrointestinal system and nerves from higher centres such as the visual centre, the vestibular branch of the eighth cranial nerve and the chemoreceptor trigger zone (CTZ) in the area postrema. The CTZ is very vascular and there is no effective blood–brain barrier; consequently chemicals in the blood or cerebrospinal fluid may stimulate it to induce nausea and vomiting. The area postrema has many dopamine, 5-hydroxytryptamine and opioid receptors. The nucleus tractus solitarius is rich in cholinergic receptors and enkephalins. The cholinergic receptors are thought likely to transmit impulses to the emetic centre to induce vomiting. Some of the antiemetic drugs are thought to act by blocking the receptors aforementioned.

What factors affect the incidence of post-operative vomiting?

Factors affecting the incidence of POV may be conveniently divided into patient factors, anaesthetic factors and surgical factors.

Patient factors

Several patient factors affect the incidence of POV in children: age, previous POV, motion sickness and gender. The contributions of factors such as pre-operative anxiety, obesity and smoking have not been proven in children.

The incidence of POV is lowest in infants. Children under 3 years old rarely vomit unless there are additional risk factors. The incidence of POV rises by 0.2–0.8% per year from age 3 years up to adolescence.

Children who have experienced POV previously are more likely to vomit after future surgery. This is more likely if the previous vomiting episodes were associated with surgery at low risk of inducing vomiting. While not yet fully developed specifically for children, several risk scoring systems for POV in adults include previous POV as a risk factor.

Large studies of adults have identified motion sickness as a strong predictor of POV. There is a paucity of literature in children, but small studies have shown motion sickness to be a risk factor for POV.

The female gender is a high risk factor for POV in girls who have reached puberty. Adolescent and adult females have two to four times the risk of POV compared with males, but there is no increase in risk of POV in pre-pubertal girls compared with boys.

Anaesthetic factors

There are a number of anaesthetic factors that have been described as associated with increased POV in children. Not all the anaesthetic risk factors for POV in adults are risk factors in children.

A large meta-analysis comparing volatile agents to propofol for maintenance anaesthesia showed volatile anaesthetics to be far more emetogenic, particularly when the anaesthetic was of long duration. Volatile anaesthetic agents may contribute to early POV, particularly in high-risk children. Volatile anaesthetic agents may increase the risk of vomiting in children when compared with intravenous propofol, but the benefits of intravenous anaesthesia seem less than in adults. A hypothesis proposed for this was the use of the Mapleson F breathing system in children. Sevoflurane has been shown to produce small concentrations of formaldehyde in the circle system at low flow rates that may produce emesis for up to 24 hours. Using the Mapleson F circuit avoids its production and may consequently reduce the emetic effects of sevoflurane in children.

Unlike the adult data, there is no compelling evidence in children on the benefits of avoiding nitrous oxide for reducing POV. Several mixed adult and paediatric studies indicate that nitrous oxide avoidance may reduce vomiting but not nausea after surgery. Studies in children on the efficacy of nitrous oxide in increasing POV show mixed results. There is no evidence to date that avoiding nitrous oxide even for procedures associated with high risk of POV confers any benefit in reducing POV risk.

While it is considered that all peri-operative opioids increase the risk of POV in children, evidence from the paediatric literature is less compelling than that in adults. While many studies show peri-operative morphine to increase POV after a range of surgical procedures including strabismus surgery, adenotonsillectomy and dental surgery, other studies show little difference in POV risk where opioids are used peri-operatively.

- Tracheal intubation has been shown to be associated with increased POV in children. It may be that this is due to the relationship between tracheal intubation and long anaesthetics rather than to intubation directly.
- The use of anticholinesterase drugs for antagonism of neuromuscular blockade in mixed adult/paediatric studies has also been associated with increased POV.
- The use of peri-operative fluids may affect the incidence of POV in children. Superhydration ($30\,\mathrm{ml\,kg^{-1}\,h^{-1}}$ of IV Hartmann's solution intra-operatively) has been shown to halve the incidence of POV in children when compared with those receiving IV Hartmanns solution $10\,\mathrm{ml\,kg^{-1}\,h^{-1}}$. Post-operatively, children are less likely to vomit if they are given oral fluids on demand rather than mandatory oral fluids, as forcing children to drink who do not wish to is associated with increased POV.

Surgical factors

There is clear evidence that strabismus surgery and adenotonsillectomy are associated with increased POV. Evidence for other surgical procedures increasing the risk of POV is more controversial. It is often hard to unravel true from surrogate risk factors such as longer duration of anaesthesia and the use of peri-operative opioids in certain surgical procedures, as both are associated with increased risk of POV.

The incidence of POV has been reported as high as 87% in studies after strabismus surgery and 89% after adenotonsillectomy. Some of the high incidence in POV may have been due to the use of peri-operative opioids in the past. In strabismus surgery, the avoidance of opioids and administration of routine antiemetics now sees the incidence of POV in children as low as 5–10%. Likewise a study without antiemetics in adenotonsillectomy where peri-operative opioids were avoided and non-steroidals prescribed showed POV incidence in children to be only 11%.

- Opioids are often required for children undergoing adenotonsillectomy and the avoidance of opioids is not recommended.

- Otoplasty has been associated with high POV in the past, but this can be reduced if local anaesthesia is used prior to the start of surgery and the ear is not packed at the end of the procedure.
- Groin surgery, in particular orchidopexy, was associated with an increased risk of POV. It is likely that the cause was peri-operative opioid administration rather than a direct effect of surgery.
- Emergency surgery such as appendicectomy has been associated with a raised POV risk in some studies. The general condition of the child and the use of peri-operative opioids may be contributory factors.

Which antiemetics are effective in children for preventing and reducing POV?

Many studies have looked at the efficacy of different antiemetics for preventing POV in children. In comparison there is very little evidence on how children with established POV should be treated.

$5HT_3$ antagonists

There is a great body of evidence showing $5HT_3$ antagonists to be effective antiemetics in children. Several $5HT_3$ antagonists have been studied in children: ondansetron, granisetron, dolasetron and topisetron; however, the bulk of evidence relates to the use of ondansetron. In the UK, ondansetron is licensed for use in children and young people (age 2–18 years) for reducing POV. The product licence is for ondansetron $0.1\,\mathrm{mg\,kg^{-1}}$ up to a maximum of 4 mg. No other $5HT_3$ antagonists are licensed in the UK for POV prevention after surgery.

Ondansetron is a very effective antiemetic in children and has been selected as the first-line drug for reducing POV in children in a dose of 0.1–$0.15\,\mathrm{mg}$ $\mathrm{kg^{-1}}$ up to a maximum total dose of 4 mg. Ondansetron produces a dose-related response in reducing POV in dose ranges from 0.05 to $3.0\,\mathrm{mg\,kg^{-1}}$. The product licence for ondansetron states that the dose of $0.15\,\mathrm{mg\,kg^{-1}}$ is more effective than $0.1\,\mathrm{mg.kg^{-1}}$, and studies have shown that the higher dose range is associated with a smaller number-needed-to-treat (NNT) to prevent early and late POV. A smaller dose of ondansetron ($0.05\,\mathrm{mg\,kg^{-1}}$) used alone is much less effective in preventing POV in children. Ondansetron $0.15\,\mathrm{mg\,kg^{-1}}$ may be used as a single agent to prevent early and late POV.

Ondansetron may be administered orally or intravenously and is equally effective in preventing POV via either route. Ondansetron has a good safety profile, with adverse effects being mild and rare in children.

There is currently no evidence demonstrating a benefit of timing the dose of ondansetron in children with respect to time of surgery: ondansetron may be given before induction, at induction, intra-operatively or immediately post-operatively.

Dexamethasone

Dexamethasone is an effective antiemetic in children alone or in combination with ondansetron. Both ondansetron and dexamethasone significantly reduce total POV and early POV. Dexamethasone is more effective than ondansetron at reducing late POV.

A systematic review on the efficacy of dexamethasone for POV in adults and children included seven paediatric studies. The systematic review showed that dexamethasone $1.0–1.5\,\mathrm{mg\,kg^{-1}}$ had a NNT of 10 in preventing early POV and a NNT of 3.2 in preventing late POV when compared with placebo (see Henzi et al., 2000).

Care should be taken when injecting dexamethasone intravenously in the awake child: dexamethasone may cause perineal warmth that may be disturbing and is minimised by slow injection. Dexamethasone may also induce insomnia when administered in the late evening. To date there is no evidence for any detrimental effects on the immune system in children or in increasing wound infection rates. Dexamethasone does not increase blood sugars in children without diabetes.

There have recently been several case reports of dexamethasone precipitating acute tumour lysis syndrome when administered to prevent POV in susceptible children. Tumour lysis syndrome is a potentially lethal condition that may occur in children with haematological malignancies after treatment with cytotoxic drugs. Dexamethasone has caused tumour lysis in patients with newly diagnosed acute leukaemia and non-Hodgkin's lymphoma and should be avoided in children likely to have these susceptible cancers where acute tumour lysis syndrome may potentially be induced.

Ondansetron and dexamethasone are both effective antiemetics for preventing POV in children. There is evidence that the combination of ondansetron and dexamethasone is more effective for preventing POV than using either of the drugs alone. Reports of studies measuring POV in children after strabismus surgery have shown the combination of intravenous ondansetron $0.05\,\mathrm{mg\,kg^{-1}}$ and dexamethasone $0.15\,\mathrm{mg\,kg^{-1}}$ to be more effective than ondansetron $0.15\,\mathrm{mg\,kg^{-1}}$ alone or dexamethasone $0.15\,\mathrm{mg\,kg^{-1}}$ alone. The incidence of vomiting in the groups receiving ondansetron and dexamethasone was less than 10%, excellent results for high-risk surgery. This combination of intravenous ondansetron $0.05\,\mathrm{mg\,kg^{-1}}$ and dexamethasone $0.15\,\mathrm{mg\,kg^{-1}}$ has been selected as most appropriate for prophylaxis against POV in high-risk circumstances by the Association of Paediatric Anaesthetists guidelines group.

Other antiemetics

There is poor evidence of the efficacy of other antiemetics in reliably preventing or reducing POV. Ondansetron compares very effectively for preventing POV in children with other antiemetics: metoclopramide and droperidol are less clinically effective than ondansetron. Metoclopramide in doses of $0.25\,\mathrm{mg\,kg^{-1}}$ or less does not reliably reduce POV in children. Its use is associated with extrapyramidal effects that are more common in children and occur within the therapeutic doses recommended for preventing POV. There is also no evidence yet of the efficacy of prochlorperazine or cyclizine in reducing POV in children. Dimenhydrinate, the theoclate salt of diphenhydramine, is widely used in North America as an antiemetic in children since it is inexpensive and considered effective. From the literature there is evidence to support the use of dimenhydrinate as prophylaxis in children for surgical procedures with moderate or high risk of vomiting, excluding adenotonsillectomy.

Are any non-pharmacological treatments for POV effective in children?

Although a number of different non-pharmacological methods have been reported as methods of preventing or treating POV in children, further studies are required to report on the effectiveness of these methods, with the exception of stimulation of the P6 acupuncture point in children.

The P6 acupuncture point is on the inner aspect of the wrist, between the tendons of palmaris longus and flexor carpi radialis, two to three of the child's fingerbreadths proximal to the proximal wrist fold. It may be stimulated by acupressure, acupuncture or electrical/laser stimulation in children. Acupuncture is more effective than acupressure and electrical stimulation in preventing POV after a high-risk surgery such as strabismus surgery or adenotonsillectomy, and may be as effective as antiemetic drugs in children. Where acceptable, acupuncture may be considered as an alternative treatment to antiemetic drugs for surgery associated with a high risk of POV.

Which antiemetic regimen should be prescribed for children at increased risk of POV?

For the purposes of selecting appropriate antiemetics for prevention of POV, children may be divided into those at increased risk of POV and those at high risk of POV.

Children at increased risk of POV

As described earlier, patient factors, surgical factors and anaesthetic factors may result in a child being at increased risk of POV. In such cases children should receive IV ondansetron 0.15 mg kg^{-1} at induction of anaesthesia.

Children at high risk of POV

All children undergoing strabismus surgery or adenotonsillectomy should be considered at high risk of POV. Children who have previously experienced POV having received IV ondansetron to prevent POV should also be considered high risk. All children at high risk of POV should receive IV ondansetron 0.05 mg kg^{-1} and IV dexamethasone 0.15 mg kg^{-1} at induction of anaesthesia.

A case example illustrates how to approach anaesthesia in children at high risk of POV.

Anna was a 6-year-old girl scheduled for adeno-tonsillectomy. She had been anaesthetised when she was 3 years old for suturing of a laceration on her lip and had not experienced any POV. She did not suffer from motion sickness and had no other relevant anaesthetic history.

Ametop was applied topically to the skin of both hands and an intravenous cannula was inserted. Anna was anaesthetised with intravenous propofol and fentanyl (1 mcg kg^{-1} at induction and a further 1 mcg kg^{-1} during surgery in divided doses), and breathed isoflurane in nitrous oxide and oxygen administered via a laryngeal mask airway.

Although there were no patient factors increasing Anna's risk factors for POV, adeno-tonsillectomy is considered to pose a high risk of POV. Consequently Anna received antiemetics at induction of anaesthesia prophylactically: IV ondansetron 0.05 mg kg^{-1} and dexamethasone 0.15 mg kg^{-1}. She also received suppositories rectally of paracetamol and diclofenac. In theatre 20 ml kg^{-1} IV Hartmanns solution was given.

In recovery, Anna received a small dose of IV fentanyl for mild discomfort and on the ward received regular paracetamol and ibuprofen orally 6 hourly. When Anna wished to drink she took sips of water first and then progressed to eating and drinking as she desired. Anna did not experience any POV and made an uneventful recovery.

In this case:
- The type of surgery placed Anna at high risk of POV, so IV ondansetron 0.05 mg kg^{-1} and dexamethasone 0.15 mg kg^{-1} was administered at induction of anaesthesia.
- As patient factors lowered Anna's risk of POV, an inhalational anaesthetic technique was selected rather than intravenous anaesthesia.
- Non-steroidal anti-inflammatory drugs were prescribed regularly, reducing the requirements for peri-operative opioid drugs. Fentanyl, a shorter-acting opioid drug, was administered as an alternative to morphine.
- Intravenous fluids were administered intra-operatively and oral fluids were given only when Anna wished to drink.

Which antiemetic regimen should be prescribed for children for established POV?

There are very few studies on which to base any recommendations for established POV in children. Based on the efficacy of antiemetics in children, IV ondansetron

Toby was an 8-year-old boy scheduled for a circumcision. He experienced POV when he underwent dental extractions several years ago. He also suffers from motion sickness.

Ametop was applied topically to the skin of both hands and an intravenous cannula was inserted. Toby was anaesthetised with intravenous propofol and breathed isoflurane in nitrous oxide and oxygen administered via a laryngeal mask airway.

Patient factors placed Toby at increased risk of POV since he had experienced POV previously from surgery not associated with a high risk of POV and suffered from motion sickness. Consequently Toby received an antiemetic at induction of anaesthesia prophylactically: IV ondansetron 0.15 mg kg^{-1}. He also received suppositories rectally of paracetamol and diclofenac and a penile block for analgesia. In theatre 20 ml kg^{-1} IV Hartmanns solution was given.

In recovery, Toby vomited on emergence from anaesthesia and IV dexamethasone 0.15 mg kg^{-1} was administered. When Toby was fully awake he requested a drink of water that he kept down. Toby did not experience any more POV and was discharged from hospital in the afternoon. His mother was contacted the following day and confirmed that Toby had not suffered any further episodes of POV.

In this case:
- Patient factors placed Toby at increased risk of POV; consequently IV ondansetron 0.15 mg kg^{-1} was administered at induction of anaesthesia.
- An inhalational anaesthetic technique was selected rather than intravenous anaesthesia as although Toby was at increased risk of POV, the type of surgery was not associated with an increased POV risk.
- Non-steroidal anti-inflammatory drugs were prescribed regularly and a penile block used, allowing peri-operative opioids to be avoided.
- Intravenous fluids were administered intraoperatively.
- In spite of these measures taken to reduce risk of POV, Toby vomited in recovery. Since he had already received IV ondansetron within 6 hours, he was given IV dexamethasone 0.15 mg kg^{-1} slowly.
- Oral fluids were given at Toby's request rather than electively post-operatively.
- If Toby requires any further anaesthetics he should be considered at high risk of POV and treated accordingly.

(a)

(b)

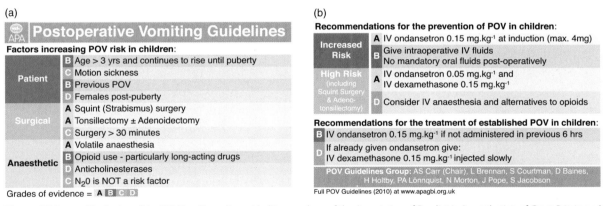

Figure 19.1 a and b, Copies of the POV 'credit card' provided to members of the Association of Paediatric Anaesthetists of Great Britain and Ireland, summarising factors increasing POV risk in children and recommendations for prevention and treatment of POV in children. See plate section for colour version.

0.15 mg kg^{-1} should be administered to children who have not previously received ondansetron within the past 6 hours. Where children have experienced POV after receiving ondansetron within the past 6 hours, a second class of antiemetic should be prescribed, for example IV dexamethasone 0.15 mg kg^{-1}.

A case example illustrates how to approach anaesthesia in children at increased risk of POV who vomit post-operatively.

Factors affecting risk of POV in children and the antiemetic recipes for preventing and treating POV are summarised in Figure 19.1.

Key points

- Patient factors, anaesthetic factors and surgical factors cause children to be at risk of POV.
- Children may be categorised into those at increased risk of POV and those at high risk of POV.

- The anaesthetic should be tailored towards the risk posed for POV and, where indicated, appropriate antiemetics administered IV at induction.
- Children should be followed up for 24 hours post-operatively for POV, and any POV experienced should be documented in the hospital notes to inform future anaesthetics.

Further reading

Association of Paediatric Anaesthetists of Great Britain and Ireland. *Guidelines on the Prevention of Post-operative Vomiting in Children.* http://www.apagbi.org.uk/sites/default/files/APA_Guidelines_on_the_Prevention_of_Post-operative_Vomiting_in_Children.pdf

Figueredo ED, Canosa LG. Ondansetron in the prophylaxis of post-operative vomiting: a meta-analysis. *J Clin Anes* 1998;**10**(3): 211–21.

Gan TJ, Meyer T, Apfel CC *et al.* Consensus guidelines for managing post-operative nausea and vomiting. *Anes Analg* 2003;**97**:62–71.

Henzi I, Walder B, Tramer MR. Dexamethasone for the prevention of post-operative nausea and vomiting: a quantitative systematic review. *Anes Analg* 2000;**90**(1):186–94.

Watcha MF, White PF. Post-operative nausea and vomiting: its etiology, treatment and prevention. *Anesthesiology* 1992;**77**:162–84.

Acknowledgements

Since 2006, I have chaired the guidelines group on post-operative vomiting for the Association of Paediatric Anaesthetists of Great Britain and Ireland. Following a systematic appraisal of the literature, the group presented a comprehensive report on the prevention and treatment of post-operative vomiting in children and guidelines on the appropriate use of antiemetics for the prevention and treatment of vomiting in children. I would like to acknowledge members of this group who have helped to identify important information on post-operative vomiting, much of which I have presented in this chapter.

Chapter

20

Anaesthesia for general paediatric and neonatal surgery

Mark Thomas

Introduction

Children presenting for general paediatric surgery range in age and complexity from the extreme premature infant undergoing laparotomy for necrotising enterocolitis, to the healthy term neonate undergoing hernia repair, or the older child undergoing appendicectomy or excision of extensive neuroblastoma. Many patients presenting for repair of congenital defects are born prematurely, which leads to additional challenges. Specific issues related to the premature infant are discussed in Chapter 9. In this chapter we shall consider common neonatal surgical conditions and provide an overview of general surgery in children beyond the neonatal period.

Neonatal surgery

General considerations

The most common general surgical conditions presenting in the newborn period are:

- Inguinal hernia
- Oesophageal atresia (OA), with or without tracheo-oesophageal fistula (TOF)
- Intestinal atresias, including anorectal anomalies
- Malrotation of the intestines
- Hirschsprung's disease
- Congenital diaphragmatic hernia (CDH)
- Exomphalos and gastroschisis
- Necrotising enterocolitis (NEC)

Anaesthetic techniques must be tailored to the specific surgical condition, but most of the key principles of management are similar and require a thorough knowledge of the anatomical, physiological and pharmacological differences between older children and this vulnerable group of patients. Anatomical and physiological differences are discussed in detail in Chapter 1.

The following differences are of particular importance in the context of anaesthesia for neonatal general surgery:

- Oxygen consumption is twice that of the adult, being $7 \, \text{ml} \, \text{kg}^{-1} \, \text{h}^{-1}$ compared with $3.5 \, \text{ml} \, \text{kg}^{-1} \, \text{h}^{-1}$ for adults. Hypoxia develops very quickly if alveolar ventilation is compromised.

- The intercostal muscles are poorly developed and contribute very little to the mechanics of respiration in the neonatal period. Diaphragmatic breathing is important in the neonate, but many surgical conditions in the neonatal period result in abdominal distension, which may compromise ventilation significantly.

- Neonates have limited ability to maintain body temperature, are less well insulated and lose body heat readily. Normothermia must be maintained by attention to ambient temperature and humidity, the warming of all fluids and active warming strategies whenever possible.

- The response to hypoxaemia is temperature-dependent in neonates: peripheral chemoreceptors initiate hyperventilation if the baby is normothermic, but if the baby is cold, hypoxaemia may result in hypoventilation and apnoeas.

- The haemoglobin in neonates may be as high as $20 \, \text{g} \, \text{dl}^{-1}$, but is mainly fetal haemoglobin, which is characterised by relatively poor tissue oxygen delivery. A higher trigger for transfusion is required for neonates who have not been transfused previously (Hb $10–12 \, \text{g} \, \text{dl}^{-1}$).

- All neonates are at risk of post-operative apnoea, and this risk is greater in the premature neonate

Core Topics in Paediatric Anaesthesia, ed. Ian James and Isabeau Walker. Published by Cambridge University Press. © 2013 Cambridge University Press.

and in the presence of anaemia (Hb less than $10\,\mathrm{g}\,\mathrm{dl}^{-1}$). The risk of post-operative apnoeas in ex-premature infants is low by 50–60 weeks post-conceptional age.

- Vitamin K-dependent clotting factors are very low at birth. Vitamin K (1 mg IM) should be given before surgery if it has not been given at delivery.
- Nociceptive pathways develop within the first trimester and are particularly vulnerable to maladaptive changes that could have life-long consequences for the newborn. Adequate analgesia must be provided.
- Hypoglycaemia is a risk, especially in very premature babies. Blood glucose should be monitored closely and regularly, and glucose-containing fluids given as required.

Most neonatal surgery is for repair of congenital defects, and many of these infants also have congenital heart disease (CHD). For some lesions, such as TOF, exomphalos or anorectal anomalies, CHD may be present in around 50% of cases. Cardiac lesions are often diagnosed antenatally. The presence of cyanosis should alert the vigilant doctor to the possibility of undiagnosed CHD, although many cardiac defects are acyanotic. Neonatal surgery should be undertaken in specialist centres, and it should be standard practice for echocardiography to be undertaken pre-operatively. Surgery is not usually postponed in the presence of a cardiac lesion, but it is important to understand the cardiac physiology to best manage the baby in the peri-operative period (see Chapter 33). Occasionally, prostacyclin infusion may be required to maintain patency of the ductus arteriosus. In lesions associated with very poor pulmonary blood flow such as severe tetralogy of Fallot, it may be necessary to undertake a systemic to pulmonary artery shunt prior to the general surgical procedure. Close communication is required with the cardiologists to determine which lesion takes surgical priority.

Blood needs to be cross-matched for most surgery in the neonatal period. Coagulation may be disordered in neonates with NEC, and platelets and other blood products may be necessary.

Anaesthesia

For elective cases, breast-fed babies need only be fasted for 3–4 hours whereas for babies receiving formula milk, the usual 6 hours should apply. Clear fluids may be given up to 2 hours pre-operatively.

Almost all neonatal surgery is best managed by tracheal intubation and ventilation as these babies have limited respiratory reserve and airway obstruction is common. The size 1 laryngeal mask can be used for short cases but is easily displaced, making it less reliable than in older children.

The minimum alveolar concentration (MAC) for all the volatile agents is slightly higher in neonates than adults, increasing with age to reach a maximum at 1–6 months of age before declining over the rest of life. The neonatal myocardium is particularly sensitive to the depressant and vagotonic effects of volatile agents, and it may be advisable to administer atropine $20\,\mathrm{mcg}\,\mathrm{kg}^{-1}$ to prevent hypotension and bradycardia. It is common to use sevoflurane for induction and then either sevoflurane or isoflurane for maintenance. Desflurane is gaining in popularity for this group of patients. A balanced technique using fentanyl will enable a lower dose of volatile agent to be given, although high-dose techniques will increase the likelihood of needing post-operative ventilation. Recent evidence that volatile agents may have a detrimental effect on the developing brain has led many practitioners to consider more opioid-based techniques when post-operative ventilation is already inevitable.

Some anaesthetists advocate the use of spinal anaesthesia for surgical procedures such as inguinal hernia repair to avoid the disadvantages of general anaesthesia, but the surgery must be completed within 1 hour if a spinal is used. Multi-centre studies are in progress to determine whether one or other technique is preferable in terms of post-operative apnoea and neurological development.

Venous capacitance is relatively low in neonates and arterial blood pressure will fall in the face of a small drop in circulating volume. For most major cases an arterial line is well worth the time invested.

Finally, maintaining normothermia is a challenge in these cases. Overhead heaters should be used during induction and siting of lines, and fluid warmers and forced air warming mattresses should all be used. Despite meticulous care it is not always possible to prevent heat loss.

Post-operative analgesia

After major surgery this may be achieved by IV nurse-controlled morphine. Morphine increases the risk of post-operative apnoea in neonates who are not ventilated; unventilated neonates should be managed in a high-dependency area with oxygen saturation and apnoea monitoring. It is our practice to use slow IV boluses of morphine $10 \, \text{mcg} \, \text{kg}^{-1}$ for neonates with a 20–30 minute lockout, and to avoid a background infusion.

Ibuprofen is not licensed for use below 3 months of age. There are limited data on the safety of intravenous paracetamol in neonates, and the following 24-hour dose limits for paracetamol should not be exceeded:

- Premature neonates, 28–32 weeks post-menstrual age, $45 \, \text{mg} \, \text{kg}^{-1}$
- 32 weeks post-menstrual age to 3 months, $60 \, \text{mg} \, \text{kg}^{-1}$

Epidurals work well in neonates and may avoid the requirement for post-operative ventilation. Neonates have lower levels of plasma binding proteins (in particular alpha-1 glycoprotein), and higher free plasma levels of local analgesic are possible. Our preference is to use plain 0.125% levobupivacaine, up to $0.3 \, \text{ml} \, \text{kg}^{-1} \, \text{h}^{-1}$.

Specific neonatal conditions

Oesophageal atresia (OA) and tracheo-oesophageal fistula (TOF)

There are several variants of this condition (Figure 20.1). The most common is the combination of oesophageal atresia with a distal tracheo-oesophageal fistula (Type C), which accounts for more than 90% of cases. Antenatal ultrasound may identify polyhydramnios, or associated anomalies. Many babies present with choking on the first feed and failure to pass a nasogastric (NG)

tube. The diagnosis is confirmed by chest X-ray, which shows the NG tube coiled in the proximal oesophageal pouch (Figure 20.2). H-type fistulae can present in the older child as chronic overspill and aspiration. These children may develop chronic lung disease with low lung compliance and high oxygen requirement. Congenital heart disease is seen in up to 40% of these patients, most commonly VSD and tetralogy of Fallot. VACTERL association occurs when TOF is associated with Vertebral, Anorectal, Cardiac, Renal or Radial and Limb defects (TE = Tracheo-Esophageal fistula). Babies born preterm, with low birth weight or cardiac abnormalities are at higher risk of peri-operative morbidity and mortality.

Children with TOF/OA require a Replogle suction catheter in the blind oesophageal pouch pre-operatively to help prevent pooling and overspill of secretions. This is a double-barrelled oesophageal tube that is kept on continuous low-level suction.

Inadvertent ventilation of the gastrointestinal tract may occur if the baby requires respiratory support pre-operatively. This will result in bowel distension and further respiratory compromise. The requirement for pre-operative ventilation is an indication for urgent surgery to close the fistula.

A gentle gas induction is commonly used, avoiding the use of nitrous oxide. Gentle lung ventilation should be used to avoid distension of the stomach or gastrointestinal tract, which will make ventilation progressively more difficult. Preferential lung ventilation may be achieved prior to intubation by gentle epigastric pressure by the assistant. Our practice is to place the tracheal tube into the right or left main bronchus, with the bevel of the tracheal tube facing anteriorly. The tube is then withdrawn until

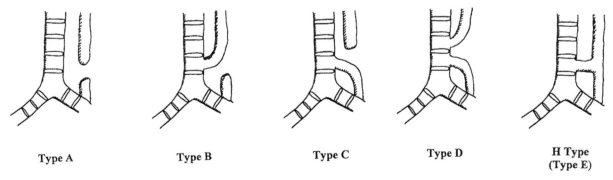

| Type A | Type B | Type C | Type D | H Type (Type E) |

Figure 20.1 Gross's classification of oesophageal atresia and tracheo-oesophageal fistula. (From Gross, RE. *The Surgery of Infancy and Childhood*. Philadelphia, PA: WB Saunders; figure by M. Thomas.)

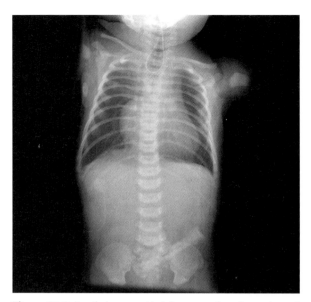

Figure 20.2 A coiled nasogastric tube suggestive of oesophageal atresia in a neonate with Down syndrome. (With thanks to Dr Frank Galliard, http://radiopaedia.org, reproduced with permission.)

bilateral air entry is obtained. The fistula is usually in the posterior wall of the trachea, close to the carina, and this technique ensures that the tube is as distal as possible and less likely to result in ventilation of the fistula. Some surgeons perform a rigid bronchoscopy under anaesthesia prior to intubation to assess the size and location of the fistula and to exclude a proximal fistula. Babies with a large fistula may have problems with ventilation at induction. If gastric distension occurs, disconnect the tracheal tube and apply gentle pressure to decompress the stomach via the tracheal tube. Whilst tempting, emergency surgical decompression of the stomach via a gastrostomy will not be useful in this situation, as the gastrostomy will offer a route of low resistance and will be ventilated in preference to the lungs. This is a particular concern in premature babies where lung compliance may be reduced. Some centres advocate the use of a Fogarty catheter to block the fistula if large, but this is not the practice at our institution.

Surgical access is through a right thoracotomy with the baby on their side and the right arm above the head. If pre-operative echo has confirmed a right-sided aortic arch then some surgeons may opt for a left thoracotomy, but this is unusual. The right lung is retracted. Gentle ventilation should be used until the fistula can be ligated. At the time of ligation, it is

prudent to gently hand ventilate to establish that it is not the right main bronchus or trachea that is about to be tied off. Close cooperation is required with the surgeon if the child is small or unstable and has frequent desaturations. Intermittent re-ventilation of the compressed lung may be required.

After successful ligation of the fistula a primary oesophageal anastomosis is usually performed, provided the oesophageal gap is small. A transanastomotic tube (TAT) is placed by the surgeon; it must not be removed post-operatively and must be clearly labelled. In long gap oesophageal atresia a feeding gastrostomy is placed at the time of fistula ligation, and delayed oesophageal anastomosis is completed some weeks later. In this situation, the blind end of the oesophageal pouch is brought out into the neck to form an oesophagostomy to facilitate drainage and prevent constant oral drooling and the need for long-term suction.

Some of these babies can be extubated at the end of the procedure, but most babies in our institution are ventilated and sedated post-operatively. Babies who have an oesophageal anastomosis under tension are electively paralysed and ventilated for 5 days post-operatively. It is better to err on the side of caution rather than risk disruption of the freshly sutured trachea should re-intubation be necessary.

Babies commonly develop a characteristic barking 'TOF cough' after TOF repair, and gastro-oesophageal reflux is common, probably owing to oesophageal dysmotility. Some infants develop tracheomalacia which may require aortopexy if clinical symptoms are severe. Oesophageal stricture may occur and some of these babies will present with dysphagia as they progress to a more solid diet. Repeated oesophageal dilation will often be necessary.

Bowel obstruction

Obstruction may occur at any point along the gastrointestinal tract either as a result of complete atresia or as a result of stenosis. Proximal obstruction will present with vomiting whereas distal obstruction is more likely to declare itself as abdominal distension and the failure to pass stools. Imperforate anus should be evident by external examination. Obstruction can be intraluminal as in the case of meconium ileus or functional as in the case of the aganglionic distal bowel of Hirschsprung's disease. Extrinsic compression can also occur, for example as a result of fibrous bands.

Duodenal atresia occurs in approximately 1 in 6000 births. Around 40% of these children have trisomy 21, and may therefore have an associated cardiac anomaly. There may be complete atresia or an intraluminal web that will need excising. Presentation is with either bilious or non-bilious vomiting, depending on whether the obstruction is distal or proximal to the ampulla of Vater.

Jejuno-ileal atresias are rarely (<1%) associated with chromosomal abnormalities, but there may be multiple atresias. The baby presents with vomiting. Good outcomes can be obtained with excision and primary anastomosis.

Malrotation, a congenital failure of the normal rotation and fixation of the intestines, may result in *volvulus,* a life-threatening disorder in which the intestines and mesentery twist upon themselves. The bowel may become ischaemic within a matter of hours owing to compromise of blood flow in the superior mesenteric artery. These infants present with bilious vomiting, abdominal distension and obvious pain. Fluid may be sequestered into the obstructed bowel, which can lead to significant intravascular hypovolaemia and shock. Such infants require resuscitation with considerable volumes of intravenous fluid and inotropic support. Time is of the essence as delay in surgery can lead to extensive and irreversible ischaemia of the bowel.

Meconium ileus is an intraluminal obstruction due to the presence of tenacious thick meconium. Twenty per cent of neonates with cystic fibrosis (CF) present in this way, and these children tend to develop more severe disease. All babies presenting with meconium ileus should have a sweat test. If rehydration or bowel washouts fail to clear the obstruction then a laparotomy and stoma formation will be needed.

Hirschsprung's disease is due to aganglionosis, usually of distal bowel. It may present in later childhood as constipation or obstruction but the most common clinical presentation is a term newborn who is unable to pass meconium. Surgery involves a 'pull-through' anastomosis of normal bowel to the rectum. Serial bowel biopsies are taken at the time of surgery to establish the line of demarcation between abnormal and normally innervated bowel. Occasionally an interim stoma is formed.

Imperforate anus should be obvious on clinical examination at birth. A superficial covering membrane may be amenable to a primary anoplasty but more commonly an interim stoma is formed and a formal anoplasty performed at a later date.

Anaesthetic management

Babies presenting with small bowel obstruction and vomiting are at risk of aspiration during induction. A modified rapid sequence induction should be performed, with ventilation of the baby in the presence of cricoid pressure, and use of non-depolarising relaxants such as atracurium. It is common to ask the parents to leave the anaesthetic room prior to neonatal rapid sequence induction since this can be stressful for everyone and parental presence is of little benefit to children of this age.

An epidural can be performed by an experienced clinician but more commonly local infiltration up to a maximum of 0.8 ml kg^{-1} of 0.25% levobupivacaine and a nurse-controlled (NCA) morphine infusion are employed. Babies undergoing laparotomy for bowel obstruction may require a large volume of intravascular fluid, sometimes in excess of 80 ml kg^{-1} during a 2–3 hour case. The baby should be monitored clinically and haematocrit, blood gases, lactate and blood sugar checked regularly. The baby must be kept warm.

Congenital diaphragmatic hernia

This condition is rare, affecting 1 in 5000 live births. The diaphragmatic hernia is almost always on the left-hand side and antenatal diagnosis is usual. Clinically, CDH presents as respiratory distress in the newborn. An X-ray confirms that bowel and sometimes other abdominal viscera are present in the hemithorax (Figure 20.3). The current theory is that the underlying defect in CDH is a failure of the lung to develop, which leaves a space for the abdominal contents to migrate cranially and thus prevent formation of the diaphragm on the affected side. The mediastinum can be pushed across the midline, and there may also be impaired growth of the contralateral lung. The degree of respiratory distress reflects the adequacy of lung tissue. Babies presenting with severe respiratory distress may require high-frequency oscillatory ventilation or extracorporeal membrane oxygenation (ECMO). The pulmonary vasculature is also underdeveloped so pulmonary vascular resistance is high and pulmonary hypertension is common. Inhaled nitric oxide may be needed in the newborn period. Surgical closure should only be entertained once

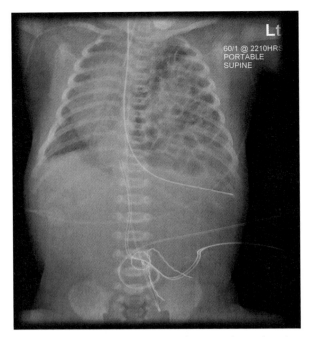

Figure 20.3 Left-sided congenital diaphragmatic hernia: bowel can be seen herniating into the left hemithorax with displacement of the cardiac silhouette to the right. (With thanks to Dr Frank Galliard, http://radiopaedia.org, reproduced with permission.)

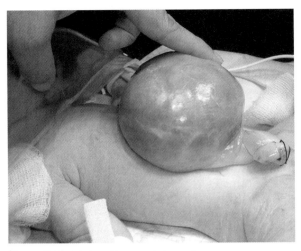

Figure 20.4 A baby with exomphalos major.

the child is stable on conventional ventilation and preferably off inotropic support.

More than 95% of CDH are posterolateral (Bochdalek), almost all on the left. Approximately 2% of hernias are retrosternal (Morgagni). Primary closure of a large hernia may not be possible and a patch is commonly needed to close the diaphragm. Less commonly, a patch may also be needed to close the anterior abdominal wall since it is underdeveloped and scaphoid as a result of not having contained the normal viscera. The underlying aetiology is primarily that of lung hypoplasia, and reduction of CDH does not usually make these babies better in the short term. Indeed, handling of the immature lung may lead to increased pulmonary hypertension and right to left shunting through the ductus arteriosus, and further hypoxia. Close cooperation is required between the neonatologists and the surgeons to decide the optimal time for surgery.

Malrotation is a common association due to the migration of the abdominal contents into the chest. The surgeon electively 'derotates' the abdominal contents when replacing them in the abdominal cavity, fixing them in a more anatomically correct position, and widening the mesenteric base of the bowel to prevent later midgut volvulus (Ladd's procedure). An elective appendicectomy may also be done at this time since the appendix often lies in the left upper quadrant, which may result in appendicitis being missed in later life.

Exomphalos and gastroschisis

Exomphalos is very rare, occurring in approximately 1 in 10 000 live births. It is a periumbilical defect in the abdominal wall. The defect may involve only minor herniation of the bowel (exomphalos minor), or may be large, involving herniation of the bowel and entire abdominal contents, including the liver (exomphalos major). Exomphalos major is associated with poorly developed abdominal and thoracic cavities and pulmonary hypoplasia. The bowel in exomphalos is covered in a membranous sac, which reduces evaporative losses and allows semi-urgent repair (unless the sac ruptures) (Figure 20.4). More than 50% of children have other congenital defects including major cardiac abnormalities, most commonly VSD. Atresias of the intestine are common. Exomphalos is associated with Beckwith–Wiedemann syndrome in 10% of cases (macroglossia and persistent hypoglycaemia).

Gastroschisis is not as rare as exomphalos (approx. 1 in 5000 live births) and presents with herniation of bowel through a defect in the abdominal wall, lateral to the umbilicus (Figure 20.5). The bowel wall is

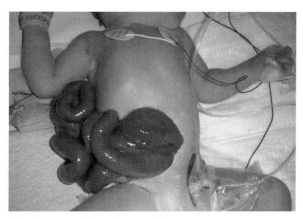

Figure 20.5 A baby with gastroschisis.

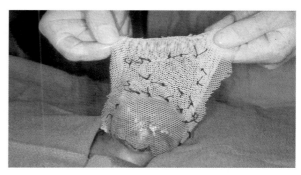

Figure 20.6 Management of gastroschisis with silo with sequential tucks.

thickened and covered in fibrin 'peel' due to exposure to amniotic fluid *in utero*. Gastroschisis is associated with prematurity more commonly than exomphalos, but other congenital abnormalities are unusual. The defect should be repaired urgently as water and protein losses from the exposed bowel are high. The viscera should be wrapped in cling film to minimise these losses prior to surgery.

The peri-operative management for both exomphalos and gastroschisis is similar. A nasogastric tube should be placed to decompress the stomach. Nitrous oxide should be avoided in order to prevent bowel distension. Either a gas induction or a gentle intravenous induction followed by full muscle relaxation and ventilation should be used.

- In exomphalos minor the surgeon will attempt to reduce the herniated contents and close the defect in one operation.
- In exomphalos major and gastroschisis, single-stage closure may compromise diaphragmatic function or result in abdominal compartment syndrome, particularly in children with a scaphoid abdomen. The bowel is accommodated in a temporary silo (prolene mesh sac) sutured to the anterior abdominal wall. The surgeon and the anaesthetist need to work closely together as the decision to place a silo or to close the abdominal wall will be guided by clinical signs such as change in lung compliance and gas exchange. Full muscle relaxation is essential if chest/lung compliance is to be judged accurately. Some centres measure pressure in the abdominal cavity, for instance the intragastric or intravesical pressure, to guide decision-making.

Post-operatively these babies almost all require ventilation, particularly if primary closure has been done. An opioid-based analgesia regimen is entirely appropriate. Some surgeons may request muscle relaxation in the immediate post-operative period. Babies with an abdominal silo may be extubated early. The silo is suspended above the baby to allow the bowel to be reduced under gravity, and a series of silo 'tucks' are performed over the next few days in the NICU (see Figure 20.6). The baby is then taken back to theatre for formal closure of the abdominal wall. Gut motility is commonly impaired after reduction of gastroschisis, and TPN is usually required. The anaesthetist should take care to preserve veins that may be used for access for peripheral TPN.

Necrotising enterocolitis

This is the most common emergency operation in the neonatal period, particularly in premature infants, and continues to be a cause of significant morbidity and mortality. Inflammation of the bowel leads to ischaemia and perforation and may necessitate removal of a large portion of the intestine. The exact aetiology is unclear, but may relate to poor regional blood flow in the premature bowel. An infective cause has also been sought. The distal ileum near the ileocaecal valve is commonly affected, and free air or gas within the bowel wall may be seen on X-ray. Clotting and platelets are frequently deranged and should be normalised prior to surgery, which may require transfusion of fresh frozen plasma, cryoprecipitate and platelets. It should be noted that the prothrombin time (PT) and activated partial thromboplastin time (APTT) in neonates are generally higher than for adults, so neonatal reference ranges should be used.

In particular, APTT in neonates may be as high as 55 seconds for several weeks after birth.

These babies are often extremely premature, and many weigh less than 1 kg. They frequently require inotropic support and should all have invasive arterial monitoring and preferably central venous access. In very high-risk cases, an emergency abdominal drain may need to be inserted in the NICU.

Older children

Pyloric stenosis

This is due to hypertrophy of the pyloric sphincter, and leads to gastric outlet obstruction. It occurs in approximately 1 in 500 live births. It classically presents with projectile vomiting in the immediate post-neonatal period, but only rarely after the age of 6 months. These babies develop metabolic alkalosis with hypochloraemia as a result of losing hydrochloric acid from the gastric contents. Untreated, they can become severely dehydrated. Renal compensation includes excretion of bicarbonate ions along with sodium. As vomiting continues, renal compensation switches from sodium excretion to excretion of potassium and hydrogen, further worsening the initial alkalosis and causing hypokalaemia with possible hyponatraemia. This is a medical rather than surgical emergency.

- The child needs careful rehydration with 0.45% saline with 5% dextrose at 1.5 times the normal maintenance rate.
- If the baby is hyponatraemic, the deficit should be made up with 0.9% saline until the sodium is in the normal range.
- A bolus of 0.9% saline may be required if the baby is shocked.
- Additional potassium may be needed as guided by capillary or venous gas levels.
- These babies should only be considered for surgery when rehydrated and with a serum chloride level of greater than 100 mmol l^{-1} and serum bicarbonate less than 28 mmol l^{-1}. The baby is at risk of post-operative apnoeas if surgery is performed before the metabolic alkalosis is resolved.

An umbilical approach is usually used nowadays, although the classic Ramstedt's procedure or laparoscopic approach are also used. The pylorus is incised down to the mucosa. The surgeon may ask for air to be introduced via the nasogastric tube to look for a leak in the mucosal layer. Fentanyl 1–2 mcg kg^{-1} IV, local infiltration and paracetamol usually provide sufficient analgesia. Saturation and respiratory rate should be monitored post-operatively.

Inguinal hernia repair

Inguinal hernias are common in children, occurring in approximately 3% of the paediatric population. This incidence rises to approximately 30% in babies born prematurely. Repair of obstructed hernias is undertaken as an emergency and babies should be treated as if they have a potentially full stomach. Effective analgesia for a unilateral repair undertaken as an open procedure is provided by a unilateral ilioinguinal/iliohypogastric nerve block. Analgesia for bilateral repair may be provided by bilateral blocks or a caudal using 1.0 ml kg^{-1} of 0.25% levobupivacaine.

Acute appendicitis

This is still relatively common in Western society, and is the most common indication for emergency surgery in children. The peak incidence is at 10–12 years of age with a 7% chance of developing the disease during a lifetime. A child younger than 6 years with symptoms for more than 48 hours is more likely to have perforated appendicitis. Urgent surgery is required since peritonitis and sepsis will ensue if left untreated.

- Pre-operative rehydration is essential and these children will often come to the anaesthetic room with intravenous fluid running.
- A rapid sequence induction should be used.
- A nasogastric tube should be placed in the unlikely event that one is not present already.
- The operation may be performed open or, more commonly, laparoscopically.
- A reliable analgesic regimen consists of 1–2 mcg kg^{-1} of fentanyl followed by a loading dose of 50–100 mcg kg^{-1} of morphine and regular paracetamol with a NSAID.
- NCA or PCA should be used for an open procedure.

In the presence of a high white count and/or fever most anaesthetists would shy away from siting an epidural for these emergency cases. Local analgesic infiltration or TAP block may be used, provided contamination of the wound is avoided.

Intussusception

This usually occurs in children aged from 6 months to 2 years, but can occur in the neonatal period. In this condition the bowel 'telescopes' in on itself, and the resultant wall oedema causes obstruction. Children usually present with abdominal pain and a palpable mass. They may have rectal bleeding as a result of mucosal sloughing, the so-called 'currant jelly stool', and they may require fluid resuscitation and occasionally blood transfusion. The internal herniation can be reduced with a combination of air and saline or contrast enema in the X-ray department in up to 75% of cases, but if this fails then surgical reduction is necessary. Ninety per cent have no identifiable lead point for the apex but a Meckel's diverticulum or polyp should always be sought at laparotomy or laparoscopy.

Nissen fundoplication

Gastro-oesophageal reflux disease (GORD) is common in children with neurodevelopmental problems, particularly cerebral palsy, CDH and TOF/OA, although reflux may also occur in healthy children. It may be associated with failure to thrive, oesophagitis, oesophageal stricture and chronic lung disease due to recurrent aspiration. Some infants may have life-threatening aspiration episodes. GORD should be confirmed, for instance by a 24-hour pH probe. If GORD is unresponsive to medical therapy, the child may require Nissen fundoplication. In this operation, the fundus is wrapped around the lower oesophagus to reinforce the lower oesophageal sphincter. A laparoscopic approach is often preferred, although there is significant soft tissue dissection, and NCA morphine infusion will be required post-operatively. An epidural is usually reserved for open cases, particularly for children with chronic lung disease.

Laparoscopic surgery

An increasing number of procedures are carried out laparoscopically, including Nissen's fundoplication, appendicectomy, colectomy and pyloromyotomy, as well as primary surgical procedures during the neonatal period.

Anaesthesia considerations for laparoscopic surgery are as follows:

- *Increased intra-abdominal pressure.* A cuffed or snug-fitting tracheal tube should be used to facilitate ventilation in the face of possible reduced respiratory compliance.
- *The insufflation gas.* This is almost always carbon dioxide; systemic absorption can rapidly lead to high arterial partial pressure of carbon dioxide, P_aCO_2. This should be monitored regularly, with either arterial sampling or using a transcutaneous CO_2 monitor. It may be necessary to deflate the abdomen periodically to enable CO_2 to be cleared, or sometimes to convert to an open procedure, particularly in small children with poor lung function such as those with CDH.
- *Cardiovascular consequences.* Increased intra-abdominal pressure may reduce venous return and may also stimulate vagal reflexes because of peritoneal stretching. This may be relevant in neonates and children with CHD, such as those with a single ventricle circulation who are dependent on venous return for adequate pulmonary blood flow and cardiac output.
- *Temperature.* The insufflation gas is cold. Body temperature needs to be monitored and the child should be kept warm, in the usual ways.
- *Gas embolism.* This should be considered if there is a sudden drop in the end-tidal carbon dioxide level.
- *Inadvertent gastric perforation.* Insertion of a nasogastric tube to deflate the stomach prior to insertion of the trocar will help reduce this risk. Nitrous oxide must not be used.

Abdominal tumours

General surgery is an important component of multidisciplinary care of children with solid tumours. The common tumours presenting to general surgeons are shown in Table 20.1.

Neuroblastoma

Neuroblastoma is one of the most common abdominal tumours in children. It usually presents around 2 years of age and is rare after the age of 10 years. Neuroblastoma arises from cells of the sympathetic nervous system, commonly in the adrenal gland, although paraspinal, thoracic, pelvic and cervical primaries may occur. Children usually present with

Table 20.1 Abdominal tumours in children

	Number of cases	Percentage total of all cases of malignancy registered
Neuroblastoma	250	6
Wilms' tumour	247	5
Soft tissue tumours	294	6
Germ cell tumours	164	4
Hepatoblastoma	55	1

From UK National Registry of Childhood Cancers 2006–2008
http://www.ccrg.ox.ac.uk/datasets/registrations.shtml)

Wilms' tumour

Wilms' tumour (nephroblastoma) has a similar incidence to neuroblastoma, but much better prognosis. Children usually present with a large painless abdominal mass, although they may present with pain, occasionally requiring fluid resuscitation, if there is bleeding into the tumour. Tumours may be bilateral, and there may be pulmonary metastases, or in some cases, extension of the tumour into the inferior vena cava (IVC). Five to ten per cent of children have acquired von Willebrand's disease, and may require treatment with desmopressin (DDAVP) or cryoprecipitate prior to surgery. There is an association between Wilms' tumour and Beckwith–Wiedemann syndrome. Hypertension is uncommon, and is due to compression of the renal artery causing elevated renin levels. It is unusual to need to use specific antihypertensive agents pre-operatively or intra-operatively in these children.

In contrast to neuroblastoma, 90% of children with Wilms' tumour have a good prognosis, with 5-year survival around 85%. In the USA, surgery may be undertaken before chemotherapy, but in Europe the preference is for treatment with several cycles of chemotherapy using agents such as vincristine, actinomycin-D and doxorubicin, followed by nephrectomy (or heminephrectomy in bilateral Wilms'), and radiotherapy in high-risk cases. Children with residual tumour in the IVC after chemotherapy may require surgery on bypass. Children who relapse and receive high-dose chemotherapy and/or radiotherapy may be susceptible to late adverse effects of treatment, particularly second neoplasms and cardiomyopathy.

Anaesthesia and surgery for children with abdominal tumours

Children with abdominal tumours may present for diagnostic and staging procedures such as CT and/or MRI, bone marrow and trephine, or in some cases, tumour biopsy. Most children require line insertion for chemotherapy. Neuroblastoma cells take up $I^{123/131}$-meta-iodobenzylguanidine (MIBG), which is the basis of MIBG scans to identify primary tumour and metastatic disease in neuroblastoma.

Surgery for tumour excision can be long and difficult, and there is the potential for high fluid requirements and major blood loss. Neuroblastoma commonly encases major vessels such as the aorta and

non-specific symptoms of fever, weight loss, fatigue and bone pain. An abdominal primary is present in two-thirds of cases. Metastases to the liver, lymph nodes, bone and bone marrow are common at presentation. Urinary catecholamines (vanillylmandelic acid (VMA) or homovanillic acid (HVA)) are raised in 90%, but unlike phaeochromocytoma, persistent hypertension is uncommon. Children with orbital secondaries may present with bilateral 'black eyes', and growth of a paraspinal tumour may present with neurological symptoms due to cord compression. There is an associated paraneoplastic syndrome associated with random eye movements and myoclonic jerks, which may not resolve as the tumour is treated. Children less than 18 months may be asymptomatic, and present with an incidental finding of thoracic neuroblastoma.

Prognosis depends on age at presentation, tumour biology and tumour spread; the overall survival is only around 65% at 5 years from presentation, although low-, intermediate- and high-risk groups can be identified. Neuroblastoma is chemosensitive, and most children undergo several cycles of chemotherapy pre-operatively, using agents such as cyclophosphamide, doxorubicin, carboplatin and etoposide, followed by surgical excision of residual tumour. Children with high-risk disease may undergo radiotherapy, myeloablative chemotherapy with stem-cell rescue, or immunotherapy (see Chapter 37). Infants younger than 6 months may present with a small primary, with metastatic spread to the skin, liver and bone marrow. This distinct condition is associated with spontaneous resolution without treatment (stage 4S disease).

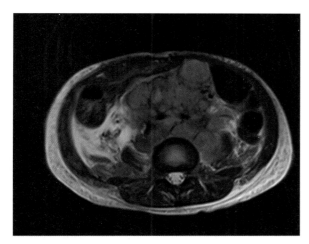

Figure 20.7 Extensive pelvic neuroblastoma encasing the iliac arteries.

IVC, and Wilms' tumours may be very vascular, particularly if the child has not received prior chemotherapy. Pre-operative imaging should be reviewed (see Figure 20.7). If the child has received pre-operative chemotherapy with anthracyclines such as doxorubicin, a recent echocardiogram should be reviewed.

Children usually have a tunnelled central line prior to surgery. Intravenous access suitable for rapid transfusion is necessary, and children should be cross-matched with at least two units prior to theatre. Bleeding may occur from the IVC, so IV access in the upper body is required. Invasive monitoring should be used. Serial arterial blood gases will help guide fluid and blood replacement. Appropriate warming is required and a urinary catheter should be inserted before laparotomy to allow for accurate measurement of urine output. If possible an epidural should be sited for intra- and post-operative use, although this is contraindicated in children with paraspinal neuroblastoma or coagulopathy. If all goes well, most children do not require post-operative ventilation and can be cared for in the high-dependency area of the ward post-operatively. Fluid balance should be observed closely, and laboratory blood results reviewed (full blood count, electrolytes). If an epidural has not been used, children over 5 years will usually manage with a patient-controlled analgesia pump, although a background infusion may be required for the first post-operative night.

Key points

- Neonates have particular physiological and pharmacological requirements.
- Post-operative apnoea is a risk in neonates; many of these patients will require post-operative ventilatory support.
- Congenital abnormalities requiring general surgery are often associated with cardiac and other pathologies.
- Major surgery is an important component of multidisciplinary care for children with neuroblastoma and Wilms' tumour.
- Multimodal analgesia should always be provided.

Further reading

Irish M, Grewal H. Pediatric intussusception surgery. Medscape reference April 2011 http://emedicine.medscape.com/article/937730 (accessed 6 August 2012)

Tobias JD. Preoperative blood pressure management of children with catecholamine-secreting tumors: time for a change. *Ped Anes* 2005;**15**:537–540.

Whyte SD, Ansermino JM. Anesthetic considerations in the management of Wilms' tumor. *Ped Anes* 2006;**16**: 504–13.

Anaesthesia for otorhinolaryngology in children

Adrian R. Lloyd-Thomas

Introduction

Procedures such as myringotomy with ventilation tubes (grommets), adenoidectomy and tonsillectomy are commonly required in children. Assessment and management of congenital and acquired airway problems, from infancy to the older child, is also frequently necessary. Many of these procedures require the surgeon and anaesthetist to share the airway, so the potential for complications is great. Considerable anaesthetic skill and preparation is needed to ensure patient safety.

Adenotonsillectomy, myringotomy and grommets

Persistent middle ear effusions (glue ear) and recurrent otitis media are common in infants from the age of 3–6 months up to the age of 6 years, while adenoidectomy and tonsillectomy are the most commonly undertaken surgical procedures in children.

Pre-operative assessment

Standard pre-operative assessment should be undertaken but with particular emphasis on:

- The airway;
- Co-morbidities such as sickle cell disease or bleeding abnormalities;
- Associated syndromes, such as CHARGE (Coloboma, Heart, choanal Atresia, Retardation, Genitourinary, Ear) association;
- Medication history.

Some children presenting for adenotonsillectomy may have obstructive sleep apnoea syndrome (OSAS). Assessment by overnight oximetry can be used to assign a McGill Oximetry Score (MOS) (Table 21.1);

patients with a score of MOS4 are at high risk of post-operative respiratory complications and may require post-operative care in a high-dependency (HDU) or paediatric intensive care (PICU) environment. Formal sleep studies (polysomnography) may be needed if simple assessment is unclear. Rarely, hypoxia due to OSAS may lead to pulmonary vasoconstriction, right ventricular hypertrophy and right heart failure, necessitating therapy with diuretics and airway support (continuous positive airway support, CPAP) before surgery.

Anaesthesia management

Children undergoing ENT surgery rarely require pre-operative sedation; it should be avoided in all patients with OSAS. When intravenous induction is planned, topical anaesthetic cream is applied. Children with sickle cell disease will require pre-operative preparation according to local guidelines, including intravenous hydration and operation early in the day.

Routine monitoring should be established prior to induction. A standard approach to induction is employed. If using inhalational induction in OSAS, the airway may be difficult to maintain and obstruction will occur at light planes of anaesthesia. Application of CPAP, keeping the mouth slightly open, will help to maintain the airway until anaesthesia is sufficiently deep to permit insertion of an oral airway.

After obtaining intravenous access the airway may be managed by insertion of a laryngeal mask airway (LMA) or tracheal intubation. An LMA may compromise surgical access in patients undergoing adenotonsillectomy for OSAS, especially those under 3 years of age, and tracheal intubation is preferred. Tracheal intubation may be facilitated by neuromuscular block. The position and function of the LMA or

Core Topics in Paediatric Anaesthesia, ed. Ian James and Isabeau Walker. Published by Cambridge University Press. © 2013 Cambridge University Press.

Table 21.1 McGill Oximetry Score for pre-operative classification of OSAS

Clusters of overnight desaturations			Severity of OSAS	McGill Oximetry Score (MOS)
<90%	<85%	<80%		
<3	0	0	Normal/inconclusive for OSA	1
≥3	≤3	0	Mild OSA	2
≥3	>3	≤3	Moderate OSA	3
≥3	>3	>3	Severe OSA	4

Adapted from Nixon GM *et al.*, *Pediatrics* 2004;**113**;e19–e25.

tracheal tube should be monitored throughout surgery as obstruction or displacement by the surgical gag may occur. The blood volume should be calculated ($75\,ml\,kg^{-1}$) and losses careful monitored. Direct vision unipolar suction diathermy for adenoidectomy and low energy bipolar diathermy dissection for tonsillectomy minimise blood loss.

Post-operative nausea and vomiting (PONV) can be minimised by 5HT receptor block, for example ondansetron ($50–150\,mcg\,kg^{-1}$, max 8 mg) and dexamethasone ($150\,mcg\,kg^{-1}$, max 8 mg). In patients scored as MOS4, the dose of dexamethasone should be increased to $300\,mcg\,kg^{-1}$ (max 10 mg), not to treat PONV, but to reduce post-operative upper airway oedema. Dehydration may contribute to PONV; intra-operative intravenous rehydration should be given in all except the shortest procedures.

Multimodal analgesia is essential in all ENT surgery. Paracetamol ($15\,mg\,kg^{-1}$ IV, max 1g) is commonly combined with an NSAID (e.g. diclofenac $1\,mg\,kg^{-1}$, max 50 mg). Peak analgesia from paracetamol, even when given intravenously, occurs between 1 and 2 hours after administration. For short operations, oral paracetamol premedication ($20\,mg\,kg^{-1}$ 1 hour pre-op) may afford maximum post-operative analgesia at the time of recovery.

NSAIDs should be avoided in those with bleeding disorders and in those with poorly controlled asthma on maximal medical therapy. Do NSAIDs increase the risk of post-tonsillectomy haemorrhage? Data suggest that 2% of patients may require re-operation if they receive an NSAID, but those not given an NSAID have a higher re-admission risk for PONV and failure to eat. Post-tonsillectomy bleeding is multifactorial; the incidence varies significantly with experience and surgical technique (blunt dissection and ties lowest risk, unipolar dissection highest risk). It is our practice to give NSAIDs unless there is a specific contraindication.

Sensible use of opioids is vital in ENT anaesthesia. Myringotomy and insertion of ventilation tubes is more painful than is commonly thought. Intra-operative opioids (fentanyl $0.5–1\,mcg\,kg^{-1}$) should be given. Opioid administration in adenotonsillectomy should be guided by the degree of obstruction at pre-operative assessment. The choice of opioid should be determined by local experience and preference. Our practice is to use fentanyl $1–2\,mcg\,kg^{-1}$ and/or morphine $50–100\,mcg\,kg^{-1}$, depending on the clinical condition of the child. Those with minimal or no OSAS, in whom the indication for tonsillectomy is recurrent infection, should receive liberal intra-operative opioids as the dissection of scarred tonsils is very painful. By contrast those with OSAS, especially those with a MOS4 score, have a significantly increased respiratory sensitivity to opioids and should be given minimal intra- and post-operative narcotics. Dexamethasone has opioid-sparing properties, and its use facilitates the use of minimal opioids in those with OSAS.

The risk of post-operative respiratory morbidity is reduced by employing a technique of anaesthesia that allows early awakening and rapid return of laryngeal reflexes. In those with severe OSAS a nasopharyngeal airway may be placed under direct vision at the end of surgery. Keeping this in for the first post-operative night helps to bypass upper airway oedema consequent upon surgery. This is particularly helpful in children with sickle cell disease. Intravenous access must be left in place in case of immediate post-operative bleeding.

Post-operative care

Regular analgesia with paracetamol and an NSAID is supplemented by codeine $1\,mg\,kg^{-1}$ 6 hourly as required. Patients with severe OSAS must not be sent home to take codeine regularly; if they are rapid acetylators they are at risk of respiratory depression. Tramadol is an alternative, although it may be associated with an increased incidence of nausea and vomiting. It is currently licensed for children over the age of 12 years (dose 1–2 mg kg^{-1} 4–6 hourly, maximum single dose 100 mg, maximum daily dose 400 mg).

Bleeding following tonsillectomy may occur within a few hours of surgery (primary) or at 7–10 days post-operatively (secondary).

Early signs of important blood loss include:

- Pallor
- Slow capillary refill (>1 second)
- Tachycardia

Restlessness, confusion and hypotension are late signs and suggest significant blood loss. Large amounts of blood may be swallowed, leading to an underestimate of losses. A full blood count, clotting screen and blood cross-match should be performed. Although a return to theatre must not be delayed, resuscitation using crystalloid, colloid or blood must be achieved before induction of anaesthesia, as cardiovascular collapse may occur with the onset of anaesthesia in a hypovolaemic child.

Aside from hypovolaemia, anaesthesia is problematic because the child may have a stomach full of blood. Moreover, active bleeding may make laryngoscopy and intubation difficult. There is little agreement on the safest technique of anaesthesia for a bleeding tonsil; the anaesthetist should adopt an approach with which they are comfortable, cognisant of the potential hazards. A rapid sequence induction with pre-oxygenation and cricoid pressure is advocated by some, whilst others prefer an inhalational induction with sevoflurane in oxygen, starting in a head down, lateral position. If using inhalational induction, a laryngoscope blade can be gently introduced after the child is anaesthetised to check for bleeding, after which the child should be moved to the supine position, suxamethonium may be given and cricoid pressure applied until the trachea is intubated. Facemask ventilation should be avoided as it may precipitate regurgitation of blood from the stomach.

During the operation further fluid and blood should be given as required; near patient testing can help guide transfusion requirements. Before termination of anaesthesia, a wide bore orogastric tube should be passed in an attempt to empty the stomach. Extubation should be in a lateral, head down position with the child wide awake.

Diagnostic and therapeutic endoscopy

Diagnostic and therapeutic microlaryngoscopy and bronchoscopy (MLB) is central to paediatric ENT surgery. MLB may involve the use of a suspension laryngoscope and operating microscope or more commonly a Storz ventilating bronchoscope (Figure 21.1) through which is passed a Hopkins rod telescope.

Diagnostic endoscopy

MLB is performed in children with mild to moderate airway obstruction.

Optimal anaesthesia for MLB requires an understanding of the likely pathology and the underlying medical condition (see Table 22.1). Many common abnormalities of the paediatric airway are dynamic (e.g. laryngomalacia, tracheomalacia and vocal cord palsy). In order to make a diagnosis the surgeon needs a still larynx, unobstructed by a tracheal tube, with spontaneous respiration preserved. The depth of anaesthesia may need to be varied rapidly, as accurate assessments of dynamic pathology need the patient to be almost awake – yet not prone to laryngeal spasm.

Pre-operative preparation

Signs of upper airway obstruction include:

- Stridor
- Sternal depression
- Indrawing of the supraclavicular, intercostal and subdiaphragmatic areas

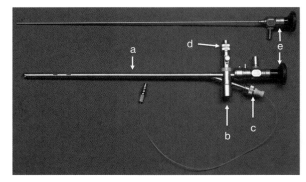

Figure 21.1 Storz ventilating bronchoscope and Hopkins rod. (a) Centre channel, through which Hopkins rod can be passed; (b) port for anaesthetic gas flow; (c) suction channel; (d) light source attachment; (e) Hopkins rod. The lower image shows the bronchoscope with the Hopkins rod inserted.

They are evident when the airway is reduced by 70%, especially in the compliant chest wall of infancy.

Inspiratory stridor indicates obstruction at or above the larynx whilst *hoarseness* suggests vocal cord involvement.

Biphasic stridor (inspiratory and expiratory) is heard with obstruction above or below the vocal cords.

Expiratory stridor alone is a symptom of intrathoracic obstruction.

The history and examination will direct appropriate pre-operative investigations which may include chest X-ray, lateral neck X-ray, barium swallow and echocardiography. Previous tracheal intubation may have given rise to airway pathology such as cricoarytenoid fixation, subglottic stenosis (SGS) or tracheal stenosis, while surgery may have resulted in injury (e.g. recurrent laryngeal nerve palsy during ligation of a patent ductus arteriosus). Where possible a full medical summary should be obtained.

If possible patients should be premedicated with an anticholinergic agent. By controlling secretions the incidence of coughing, breath-holding and laryngospasm is reduced.

Anaesthesia

Preservation of spontaneous respiration is an important principle during induction and maintenance of anaesthesia in children with airway obstruction. Muscle relaxants should be avoided until it is clear that reliable manual inflation of the lungs is possible.

Inhalational anaesthesia

Inhalational induction using sevoflurane in 100% O_2 is the method of choice. Once consciousness is lost CPAP is often needed to maintain the airway and improve gas exchange. Where there is significant airway obstruction, minute ventilation will be reduced and induction of anaesthesia will be prolonged. It may take several minutes to achieve a sufficient depth of anaesthesia to permit laryngoscopy; loss of tone in the abdominal musculature is a good clinical sign. Whilst induction is in progress, intravenous access is obtained and a decision on the use of neuromuscular relaxants is made. Short-acting relaxants enable application of topical anaesthesia without causing laryngeal spasm. If mask ventilation is difficult relaxants should not be given; instead anaesthesia should be deepened until it is possible to view the larynx. Lidocaine ($3-5\,mg\,kg^{-1}$, max

160 mg) is sprayed onto the glottis, vallecula and trachea. If relaxants are not used the risk of laryngeal spasm is high and careful assessment of the depth of anaesthesia is vital before attempting to administer the lidocaine.

Spontaneous respiration is re-established, a nasopharyngeal airway is passed into the posterior pharyngeal space and anaesthesia is maintained by insufflation of 100% oxygen and sevoflurane. The use of 100% oxygen ensures that the oxygen reserves are as high as possible in all patients, even the premature where the risks of hypoxia are significant. Close monitoring is essential to detect hypoxia and hypoventilation or excessively light anaesthesia. At the end of the examination anaesthesia is stopped, 100% oxygen is continued and the larynx is observed until the patient is virtually awake.

TIVA

An alternative approach is to use TIVA, employing a combination of propofol ($200-400\,mcg\,kg^{-1}\,min^{-1}$) with remifentanil ($0.05-0.1\,mcg\,kg^{-1}\,min^{-1}$) by infusion, or propofol and alfentanil by intermittent injection.

In older children, over about 2 years of age, TIVA results in a better recovery than with volatile agents, but should not be attempted where there is doubt as to the ability to maintain the airway satisfactorily following induction.

On induction (propofol $1-2\,mg\,kg^{-1}$ with alfentanil $5-10\,mcg\,kg^{-1}$) apnoea will result allowing laryngoscopy and application of topical anaesthesia. Manual ventilation with 100% oxygen should be undertaken before laryngoscopy. Thereafter, spontaneous ventilation is allowed to recommence and anaesthesia is maintained by the intermittent injection of propofol and alfentanil (propofol $10-20\,mg\,kg^{-1}\,h^{-1}$ and alfentanil $20-30\,mcg\,kg^{-1}\,h^{-1}$). The degree of stimulus varies substantially throughout the examination, and titration to clinical response demands very close attention by the anaesthetist. Excessive administration can result in intermittent gasping respiration due to the opioid, and the associated laryngeal movement can be distracting to the surgeon.

Oxygenation is maintained in an identical manner to the volatile technique using 100% oxygen and a nasopharyngeal airway. Employing TIVA means that the maintenance of anaesthesia is independent of the airway, which is an advantage where intermittent obstruction by the surgeon can otherwise lead to light anaesthesia.

Diagnostic bronchoscopy

The majority of diagnostic ENT bronchoscopies are now undertaken using just the Hopkins rod, and anaesthesia continues as described above. On occasion a full bronchoscopic examination is needed.

A Storz ventilating bronchoscope will be used. A side arm allows attachment of an anaesthetic T-piece for administration of 100% oxygen with or without volatile agent (see Figure 21.1). Once the Hopkins rod is in place a closed system exists, allowing ventilation to occur in the annular space between the telescope and the surrounding bronchoscope. A 'spaghetti' suction catheter can also be passed through another side arm on the instrument. Resistance is high in the smaller bronchoscopes, significantly increasing the work of breathing, particularly for infants. Furthermore, resistance increases with the length of the instrument – at a 3 l min^{-1} flow rate the resistance of a 30 cm 3.5 bronchoscope is four times that of a 20 cm model. Assisted ventilation may be needed, especially for infants. Resistance to expiration is high, and air trapping can occur unless a long expiratory phase is employed. It may be necessary to remove the telescope temporarily and allow unobstructed ventilation through the empty bronchoscope.

Fibre-optic endoscopy can be used in the diagnosis of upper airway obstruction, more commonly by respiratory physicians or interventional radiologists. Anaesthesia is best conducted with an LMA or facemask using a bronchoscopic swivel mount, which has a small self-sealing hole through which is passed the fibrescope. A diagnostic bronchogram may be performed at the same time (see Chapter 36).

Loss of airway during diagnostic investigation

On occasion the loss of tone associated with the onset of anaesthesia may result in airway decompensation, requiring CPAP to preserve respiration. This manoeuvre may be insufficient, especially in patients with SGS who may be very difficult to intubate. Cole-pattern shouldered neonatal tracheal tubes are more rigid than the smallest 2.0 tracheal tube and are easier to pass in patients with Grade II and III SGS.

Specific conditions identified by diagnostic endoscopy or bronchoscopy

Laryngomalacia

This is the commonest cause of stridor in infancy. Stridor is often present within a few days of birth, but it rarely requires immediate intervention. Referral is usually made to a specialist centre. Infants may have inspiratory stridor with marked sternal recession and tracheal tug. Feeding difficulties are common in more severe cases. The airway obstruction is due to collapse of the supraglottic structures on inspiration. The natural history of the condition is to resolve within the first 2 years, but in severe cases with marked stridor, recession and faltering growth due to feeding difficulties, surgery to divide the aryepiglottic folds or remove excess arytenoid mucosa is usually successful. This is usually performed after airway examination under spontaneous ventilation with anaesthetic gas delivered either via a nasopharyngeal airway or via the suspension laryngoscope.

Tracheomalacia and tracheobronchomalacia

These conditions cause collapse of the airway on expiration. Symptoms may be intermittent and include expiratory wheeze, stridor and severe episodes of cyanosis and reflex apnoeas sometimes called 'dying spells'. The presentation is usually during the first year of life. It may be due to underlying deficiency or weakness of the tracheal rings, caused by extrinsic compression commonly from a vascular anomaly, or seen in babies after repair of tracheo-oesophageal fistula. Diagnosis is made by bronchoscopy and/or bronchogram with spontaneous ventilation maintained. The level of PEEP required to maintain airway patency can be measured during the bronchogram.

- In the acute situation, airway management is not usually difficult and positive pressure ventilation stabilises the child.
- Surgical options depend on the aetiology of the problem and include correction of the vascular anomaly, aortopexy or, occasionally, airway stenting.
- In the case of cartilaginous weakness, prolonged positive pressure airway support may be needed, sometimes via a tracheostomy.

Vocal cord palsies

These may be present from birth or develop after thoracic surgery or neurological injury. Unilateral cord palsy often causes relatively mild symptoms of

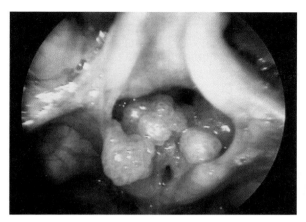

Figure 21.2 Laryngeal papillomas causing partial airway obstruction (with thanks to Dr S. Bew). See plate section for colour version.

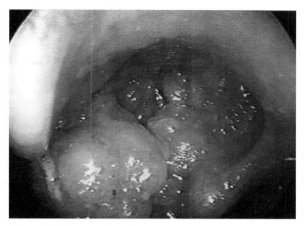

Figure 21.3 Laryngeal papillomas causing severe airway obstruction (with thanks to Dr S. Bew). See plate section for colour version.

stridor and a whispery cry, but may be a cause of failed extubation after cardiac surgery. Bilateral cord palsy will cause much more severe symptoms of stridor with marked sternal recession and tracheal tug. If acute intervention is required the application of PEEP during induction acts as a dynamic splint to maintain a wider airway. Treatment options depend on the severity of symptoms; tracheostomy may be required for bilateral vocal cord palsy.

Therapeutic endoscopy

A wide range of therapeutic operations is performed on the airway, often in patients with significant airway obstruction. Maintenance of anaesthesia by volatile agents or TIVA, as described above, is indicated. Paracetamol and a NSAID should be given as analgesia.

On occasion the CO_2 laser is used with the aid of an operating microscope. Tracheo-bronchial lesions may be treated with the potassium titanyl phosphate (KTP) laser, using a fibre-optic cable inserted through the side arm of the ventilating broncho-scope. The inspired oxygen concentration should be reduced when employing the KTP laser, as fire in the airway is a particular risk. Laser surgery should only be undertaken in properly equipped theatres, and all staff should wear appropriate eye protection. When viral papillomas are to be lasered, high volume theatre scavenging is important, as vaporised viral particles may be released, and theatre staff should wear masks.

Specific conditions treated by therapeutic endoscopy

Laryngeal papillomas

These are benign proliferations of squamous epithelium usually caused by the human papilloma virus types 6 and 11. The usual site is the larynx, but they can occur anywhere in the tracheobronchial tree (see Figures 21.2, 21.3). The onset of symptoms is often very slow with progressive dyspnoea sometimes treated as asthma, and hoarse voice or aphonia. These children may require anaesthesia as a planned procedure for airway investigation or for surgery, but may present acutely with severe respiratory distress and stridor with an airway almost completely obstructed by florid cauliflower-like growths.

- Anaesthesia should be induced by gas induction and deepened with spontaneous ventilation until laryngoscopy and airway examination is tolerated.
- It will take a long time to attain a suitable depth of anaesthesia.
- Topical lidocaine is applied as the treatment is by surgical debulking usually with spontaneous ventilation without intubation to reduce the chance of seeding papilloma further down the airway.
- Anaesthesia is maintained with gas delivery either via a nasopharyngeal airway or via a connector on the surgical suspension laryngoscope. Adjuvant treatments such as intralesional injections of the antiviral cidofovir are sometimes used.

The condition is recurrent in some cases, requiring numerous procedures over the years to maintain an airway. In future, countries where the quadrivalent human papilloma virus vaccine is given to prevent cervical cancer could see a significant reduction in the incidence of laryngeal papillomatosis.

Cysts

Congenital supraglottic cysts are uncommon, but may present with stridor from birth sometimes requiring immediate intervention. Although at times very large, they are fluid-filled and compressible and can sometimes be pushed aside by a tube with a stylet allowing intubation. Occasionally the whole larynx is obscured and the cyst may need aspiration under direct laryngoscopy to reveal the larynx. The cysts are then marsupialised to prevent recurrence.

Subglottic cysts are usually seen in infants who have been intubated as a neonate. They probably result from subglottic trauma, although the period of intubation does not need to be prolonged. These infants may present with biphasic stridor or audible harsh breathing sounds and respiratory distress several months after discharge from the neonatal unit. Subglottic cysts can be excised using a laser or sickle knife. The history and presenting symptoms do not distinguish subglottic cysts, which can be decompressed to restore the airway, and a fixed subglottic stenosis, which may require a tracheostomy (see below).

Post-anaesthesia care

Meticulous observation in the post-anaesthesia care unit (PACU) is essential following diagnostic or therapeutic endoscopy. Airway oedema as a result of intervention or instrumentation is common, and children may develop respiratory distress with stridor on recovery. All patients undergoing therapeutic endoscopy and those in whom instrumentation may have been difficult should receive dexamethasone (250 mcg kg^{-1} initial dose, thereafter 100 mcg kg^{-1} 8 hourly).

Stridor in the PACU may also require nebulised adrenaline (1:1000, 5 ml). The ECG should be monitored during administration of nebulised adrenaline, which should be stopped temporarily if the heart rate is >190 beats per minute.

Airway emergencies

The management of paediatric airway emergencies is part of the role of the paediatric anaesthetist.

Acute airway emergencies

The most common infective conditions are acute viral laryngotracheobronchitis (croup), acute epiglottitis and bacterial tracheitis.

Epiglottitis

The incidence of this condition fell steeply in 1992 after the introduction of routine vaccination against *Haemophilus influenzae* type b. However, the disease is still seen in unvaccinated children, in cases of vaccine failure or when other organisms cause epiglottitis. Epiglottitis presents with rapidly progressive fever, dysphagia, drooling, tachypnoea and stridor, typically in children between 1 and 6 years of age. Classically these children adopt a tripod posture, leaning forward on their hands to maintain their airway. The swollen epiglottis can be seen on a lateral neck X-ray, but the diagnosis is clinical and time should not be wasted on investigations that do not influence management. Experienced anaesthetic and ENT help should be sought.

- The child is toxic and unwell, and should be kept in a comfortable position with oxygen delivered as tolerated, which is often more effective with the parent holding the mask.
- A pulse oximeter is usually well tolerated, but avoid cannulation as crying will increase the respiratory distress.
- Nebulised adrenaline may buy time as preparations are made for intubation.
- Anaesthesia should be by gas induction with the child in the sitting position.
- Spontaneous ventilation should be maintained as anaesthesia is deepened. Be patient; it may take many minutes for anaesthesia to deepen and it will feel a lot longer while you are holding the mask.

The larynx may be very difficult to identify with all supraglottic structures red, swollen and distorted (see Figure 21.4). The movement of secretions or a bubble of gas from the larynx may help. Intubate with a tube smaller than expected for age. Once the airway is secured, ceftriaxone or cefuroxime 50 mg kg^{-1} should be given if antibiotic treatment has not yet started. The child should remain intubated on PICU until a leak develops round the tube.

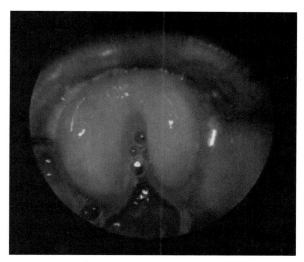

Figure 21.4 Endoscopic view of the epiglottis in epiglottitis. (Reprinted from Hammer J. Acquired upper airway obstruction. *Paed Resp Rev* 2004;**5**:29, with permission from Elsevier.) See plate section for colour version.

Croup or laryngotracheobronchitis

This is an upper respiratory infection usually caused by the parainfluenza virus.

- Symptoms are slower in onset than in epiglottitis and are characterised by a barking cough.
- The subglottis is narrowed by swelling, which can be seen on an AP neck X-ray as a loss of the normal shouldered appearance of the air column giving the appearance of an inverted V known as the steeple sign (see Figure 21.5).
- Mild croup is common in the winter affecting 3% of children under the age of 6, but only 2% of these require hospital admission. Most respond to medical treatment with inhaled budesonide or intravenous dexamethasone and nebulised adrenaline.
- Humidification of inspired gases is also widely used, although of doubtful efficacy.
- A small number of children do not respond to medical treatment and gradually deteriorate, becoming exhausted and requiring intubation.

Although there will be inflammation of the supraglottic tissues and excess secretions, the laryngoscopy is not usually difficult, although a smaller than expected for age tracheal tube will be needed.

Bacterial tracheitis or pseudomembranous croup

In some centres this is now a more common cause of PICU admission than croup.

- The initial presentation is often similar to croup, but the child is toxic and rapidly deteriorates with cough, fever and stridor. An AP neck X-ray may also show the steeple sign.
- The most common organism is *Staphylococcus aureus,* which causes inflammation and thick mucopurulent secretions (see Figure 21.6).
- The tracheal tube may become obstructed by secretions or sloughing of the tracheal epithelium, and the child will require frequent suctioning or occasionally rigid bronchoscopy to remove the pseudomembranes.
- The course on PICU may be complicated by sepsis and pneumonia, and the duration of intubation is usually longer than in croup.

Retropharyngeal abscess

This is caused by lymphatic spread of infection from sinuses, teeth or middle ear into the space between the posterior pharyngeal wall and the prevertebral fascia. It is mainly seen in young children and presents with fever, sore throat, neck pain and swelling with limitation of movement and drooling.

- These children are usually stable enough for a CT scan, and larger fluid collections will require surgical drainage.
- Stridor is not often a major feature but the intubation can be very difficult with copious secretions and tissues distorted by the bulging pharyngeal wall.
- Attempts to pass a tube or bougie can rupture the abscess with the risk of airway soiling and the laryngeal view becoming obscured by purulent secretions.

Removal of an inhaled foreign body

Inhalation of a foreign body usually occurs between the age of 1 and 3 years; it is more common in males. The episode is often witnessed; an episode of choking is usually followed by a bout of coughing. Hoarseness and/or stridor suggest that the foreign body is impacted in the larynx, whereas passage into the trachea or main bronchi may cause wheeze or

(a)

(b)

(c)

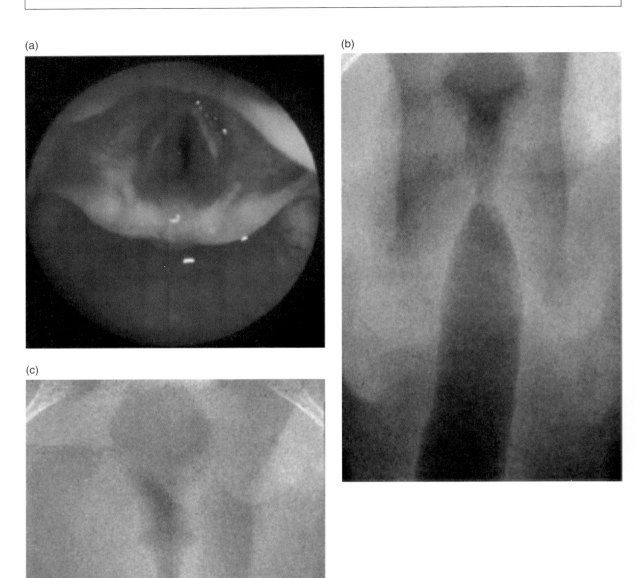

Figure 21.5 Endoscopic view of the larynx in croup (a). Radiological presentation of subglottic oedema in viral croup (b), compared with normal (c). Reprinted from Hammer J. Acquired upper airway obstruction. *Paed Resp Rev* 2004;**5**:26, with permission from Elsevier. See plate section for colour version of (a).

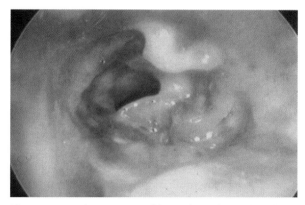

Figure 21.6 Endoscopic view of the trachea in bacterial tracheitis. See plate section for colour version.

unilaterally reduced breath sounds. Rarely, an object causes a complete glottic or subglottic obstruction, which is rapidly fatal. Partial obstruction is caused by objects lodged in or around the laryngeal inlet. The initial choking or coughing episode is followed by biphasic stridor and a change in the voice or cry, which may become hoarse. An object with sharp edges may cause pain on swallowing causing infants to drool. Most children will present immediately with marked respiratory distress.

If it is radio-opaque the foreign body may be seen on chest X-ray (CXR), but the majority are radiolucent. Inspiration and expiration films are required as hyperinflation may be seen on the affected side but a normal CXR does not exclude the diagnosis. In later presentations, collapse and consolidation may be seen distal to the obstruction.

The approach to anaesthesia is as for diagnostic bronchoscopy. Atropine premedication, gaseous induction using oxygen and an inhalational agent, with topical anaesthesia are satisfactory. If there is respiratory distress urgent bronchoscopy is indicated, otherwise the procedure should wait for an appropriate starvation period. A smooth technique using deep anaesthesia and avoiding coughing is essential. Intubation should be avoided if the foreign body is in or near the larynx, while IPPV is best avoided if the foreign body is in the trachea or creating ball-valve obstruction.

A 30 cm ventilating bronchoscope with Hopkins rod and grasping forceps is used. Application of topical adrenaline (1:10 000) to the area of impaction is useful to reduce oedema and facilitate removal. Ventilation may need to be gently assisted if the bronchoscope is in a main bronchus for a prolonged period. Side holes in the Storz bronchoscope assist proximal ventilation.

Once the object is firmly grasped in the forceps, the whole instrument is slowly removed from the airway under vision, ensuring that the foreign body does not fall out of the forceps. Once the bronchoscope has been removed anaesthesia is maintained by mask, while awaiting re-insertion of the bronchoscope to confirm full removal. When withdrawing the bronchoscope with the foreign body, the danger is loss of the object either in the trachea or larynx which may cause total obstruction to ventilation. Should this occur the bronchoscope should be reinserted to push the object into the distal airway so that satisfactory ventilation can be re-established.

Choanal atresia

Choanal atresia is a membranous or bony occlusion of the posterior nares with an incidence of 1:8000 births. It may be unilateral, when presentation is often delayed. Bilateral obstruction causes acute respiratory distress in neonates as they are obligate nasal breathers. An oral airway and an orogastric tube should be inserted and taped to the face, while surgery is undertaken within 24 hours. Other anomalies are common (e.g. CHARGE syndrome) and thorough pre-operative assessment including echocardiography is needed.

In choanal atresia, surgery involves dividing the membrane; where there is bony occlusion a passageway is drilled. In the latter case, bleeding can be significant despite intra-operative use of topical adrenaline, and a pre-operative request for group and save serum should be made. Standard techniques for neonatal anaesthesia should be employed, using a muscle relaxant, tracheal intubation (RAE tracheal tube), IPPV and analgesia (paracetamol/codeine). A throat pack is not used, as it obstructs the surgical view. Patency of the new nasal passageway is ensured by the insertion of nasopharyngeal stents fashioned from standard tracheal tubes. These require regular suctioning and are left *in situ* for 8 weeks. Re-stenosis is common (20%), and patients may return for further surgical correction.

Anaesthesia for tracheostomy

Tracheostomy is indicated for congenital or acquired airway obstruction, to facilitate long-term respiratory support or in the presence of a neurological abnormality. Children should receive anticholinergic premedication and receive an inhalational induction with sevoflurane in oxygen. Intravenous access is obtained and full monitoring applied. Relaxants should be avoided unless reliable manual IPPV can be achieved. Some patients (e.g. those with Pierre Robin syndrome) may be impossible to intubate. In these patients anaesthesia is maintained using oxygen, a volatile agent and spontaneous respiration, while the airway is maintained using an LMA or facemask. On rare occasions it is impossible to maintain the airway, the patient is awoken and the tracheostomy performed under local anaesthesia.

A secure airway allows the use of muscle relaxants, IPPV and a volatile agent. Respiratory obstruction may occur during surgery, and hand ventilation permits early detection. The patient is positioned with the head extended using a sandbag under the shoulders; strapping is passed around the chin and secured to the operating table thereby stabilising the head. Infiltration with lidocaine 1% and 1:200 000 adrenaline is made and the trachea identified by dissection. The second and third tracheal rings are identified and two stay sutures are inserted, one on either side of the planned tracheal incision. These sutures are taped to the chest at the end of the operation and are not removed until the first tube change at 1 week. They are vital for the patient's post-operative safety; if the tracheostomy tube falls out these sutures are used to pull the trachea to the surface to facilitate tube re-insertion.

Before the tracheal incision is made 100% oxygen is given and the proposed tracheostomy tube and connector is checked. Standard tracheostomy tubes (Portex, Shiley or Bivona) with 15 mm connectors are used. Once the trachea has been incised, the tracheal tube is withdrawn into the upper trachea and the tracheostomy tube is placed. The anaesthesia circuit is connected and ventilation is checked (auscultation of the chest, end-tidal CO_2) to confirm correct placement. At the end of surgery the head is taken out of extension and tracheostomy tapes are passed around the neck to secure the tube.

Post-operatively a CXR is taken to confirm correct tube placement and to exclude a pneumothorax. Warmed humidified air/oxygen, using elephant tubing and tracheostomy mask, is given to neonates and infants; cold humidity is used for older children. This is combined with regular sterile suctioning with saline irrigation (1–2 ml) to ensure that crusting and blockage do not occur. A spare tracheostomy tube, tapes and dilators are kept with the patient. Humidification can usually stop after the first tube change and a 'Swedish nose' is used instead.

Open operations on the larynx
Subglottic stenosis

This may be congenital, but more often develops post-intubation and can occur at any age after even a brief period of intubation. Children may present with biphasic stridor, dyspnoea on exertion and croupy cough, or after failed extubation in the PICU. In some patients the symptoms and signs may be very subtle. An infant who is not yet mobile may show only minimal subcostal recession, and rather than stridor, have soft biphasic respiratory sounds.

- It is important to maintain spontaneous ventilation while the airway is assessed under anaesthesia as it may be extremely difficult to ventilate through a very narrow airway, and the high pressures cause gastric distension.
- If intubation is required either to secure a safe airway or for a tracheostomy it can be very difficult to pass a tube. It may be possible to pass a straight 5 Fr bougie and corkscrew in a size 2 tracheal tube, but at times even this is too big. A Cole tube is more rigid and may be useful in this situation.
- Repeated attempts to pass a tube will rapidly lead to oedema and worsening obstruction. A tracheostomy should be performed whilst spontaneous ventilation and facemask anaesthesia is still possible.

Definitive treatment of SGS is by anterior cricoid split, laryngotracheal reconstruction or cricotracheal resection.

Anterior cricoid split

This operation is used in children with SGS, often those unable to be extubated in the PICU but who are otherwise well with no pulmonary disease. Positioning of the head is the same as for a tracheostomy; the trachea is dissected after which the cricoid cartilage, first and second tracheal rings are divided in the midline anteriorly. Anaesthesia with tracheal intubation, a muscle relaxant, opioid and IPPV by hand is appropriate. Following the split a nasotracheal tube of a larger size is passed with the tube tip positioned just distal to the lowest divided ring; this acts as a tracheal stent for 5–10 days.

Patients are cared for in the PICU where meticulous attention to the tracheal tube is needed. Blockage or accidental extubation are very hazardous, as attempts at re-intubation can result in the bevel being pushed through the anterior tracheal wall, creating a false passage. Should extubation occur, nasotracheal re-intubation should not be attempted in the PICU as the angle of tracheal tube passing through the larynx from the nose encourages anterior perforation through the surgical division. The airway should be supported with a mask, oxygenation ensured and oro-tracheal intubation should be attempted. Afterwards the patient can be returned to theatre for nasotracheal intubation in controlled circumstances. At 5–10 days extubation is attempted using steroid cover.

Laryngotracheal reconstruction

This may be performed as a single-stage or two-stage procedure with a tracheostomy. It involves a similar approach to the cricoid split, but opens the larynx anteriorly and posteriorly if required. Harvested rib cartilage is interposed into the anterior and posterior split thereby increasing the diameter of the airway. If performed as a single-stage procedure, with no covering tracheostomy, the anaesthetic and PICU considerations are the same as those for the cricoid split, including the caveat regarding re-intubation. If a posterior graft is needed, a sterile cuffed flexometallic tracheal tube or cut-down RAE tube is placed by the surgeon in the trachea distal to the graft site; ventilation is continued in this manner until just before the anterior graft is ready to be placed. At this point a larger nasotracheal tube is passed with the tip positioned just below the graft site by the surgeon under direct vision. Wet neurosurgical patties can be used to pack around this tube to create a seal for IPPV.

The patient is returned to the PICU for care as described above. Patients tolerate nasotracheal tubes well and after the first 24–48 hours only minimal sedation is needed.

Laryngotracheal reconstruction is also performed as a two-stage procedure, the first stage being a tracheostomy. At the second stage, anaesthesia is induced through the pre-existing tracheostomy; maintenance is with an opioid, muscle relaxant and volatile agent. Intravenous fluids are given and continued post-operatively, and a nasogastric tube is passed.

To manage the airway, a cuffed flexometallic tracheal tube or cut-down RAE tracheal tube is inserted through the tracheostome, after which the anaesthetist should check for equal ventilation. The tube is secured by surgical suture just below the tracheostome. Care is needed during the operation as surgical manipulation can move the tube resulting in extubation or bronchial intubation; the cuff can also be pierced by surgical suturing. Should this happen the surgeon will need to assist with tube positioning, and wet neurosurgical patties will create a seal if the cuff ruptures.

A stent is placed in the trachea to support the grafts, after which the anterior larynx is closed. The flexometallic tube is removed after careful tracheal suctioning, a tracheostomy tube is re-inserted and the patient is awoken to be returned to the ENT ward. Humidified oxygen is given via a tracheostomy mask. A CXR is required to exclude a pneumothorax which may occur as a result of the rib harvest. Analgesia is with paracetamol, an NSAID and morphine PCA/NCA. A local anaesthetic infusion (72 hours) through an epidural catheter placed in the site of rib harvest can afford useful pain relief.

Cricotracheal resection

Short segment tracheal resection can be performed for Grade III and IV SGS. The patient will already have a tracheostomy and the approach to anaesthesia is the same as the two-stage laryngotracheal reconstruction. A segment of trachea is excised and a new cricotracheal anastomosis is made. Difficulties with the temporary cuffed flexometallic tube are even more likely in this operation. More complex slide tracheoplasties are used for patients with long segment tracheal stenosis; these require cardiopulmonary bypass and are highly specialised operations.

Non-airway ENT surgery

Middle ear surgery

Exploration of the middle ear requires the anaesthetist to consider:

- Control of bleeding
- Preservation of the facial nerve
- Avoidance of graft displacement

Table 21.2 Strategies to minimise blood loss during middle ear surgery

Strategy	Method		Comment
Smooth induction of anaesthesia avoiding tachycardia or hypertension	Calm, relaxed patient	Sedative premedication if required	Avoid anticholinergic medication
	Avoid coughing or straining on intubation	Establish TIVA before intubation	Use remifentanil to facilitate intubation, 0.5–1 mcg kg^{-1} over 1 min: Propofol loading dose 1 mg kg^{-1}
		Use topical laryngeal anaesthesia	
Keep the venous pressure low	Patient positioning	Head up tilt of 15–20° Avoid excessive head turning	May obstruct the contralateral internal jugular
	IPPV	Normocapnia Slow respiratory rate No PEEP	Long expiratory time
Aim for a systolic blood pressure of 80 mmHg	Analgesia	Infiltration with lidocaine and adrenaline 1:200 000	
	Anaesthesia (TIVA)	Remifentanil 0.1–0.5 mcg kg^{-1} min^{-1} Propofol 2% Target control or Manual control 13/11/9 mg kg^{-1} h^{-1}	Titrate to desired blood pressure Propofol manual control dose reduction steps at 10 min intervals until 9 mg kg^{-1} h^{-1} maintenance

Procedures include

- Mastoidectomy
- Myringoplasty
- Cochlea implantation

Minimising blood loss

Bleeding can be of arterial origin secondary to a hyperdynamic circulation with a high cardiac output, hypertension and tachycardia. Control of heart rate and cardiac output will minimise this loss. Venous ooze secondary to raised internal jugular venous pressure may be caused by poor patient positioning, partial airway obstruction during spontaneous respiration, abdominal compression, or raised mean intra-thoracic pressure with IPPV or positive end-expiratory pressure (PEEP).

Strategies to minimise blood loss during middle ear surgery are presented in Table 21.2. These involve controlled hypotension which may be defined as a reduction of systolic blood pressure to 80 to 90 mmHg, a reduction of mean arterial pressure (MAP) to 50 to 65 mmHg or a 30% reduction of baseline MAP. Total intravenous anaesthesia has revolutionised anaesthesia for middle ear surgery. The blood pressure cuff should be sited on the arm opposite to the operation to avoid interference with

readings by surgical activity. The remifentanil infusion is stopped 15 minutes before the end of surgery and a long-acting opioid, paracetamol and NSAID are given. A post-operative antiemetic (e.g. cyclizine 1 mg kg^{-1}, max 25 mg) should be prescribed as PONV can be problematic after middle ear surgery.

Preservation of the facial nerve

The tympanic segment of the facial nerve is at risk during middle ear surgery; facial nerve monitoring is used, based upon electromyography, and requires neuromuscular function. Neuromuscular blockers are thus avoided.

Avoiding graft displacement

Nitrous oxide (N_2O), being more soluble than nitrogen, diffuses in and out of body cavities more quickly than nitrogen. When the middle ear has been closed by a myringoplasty, termination of N_2O will result in a negative pressure being applied to the graft. Using TIVA or avoiding N_2O is ideal.

Surgery for congenital ear defects

Children with congenital defects of the external ear present for the insertion of osseo-integrated temporal screws for an artificial pinna or bone anchored hearing aid; reconstructive surgery to form an external ear is also undertaken (see Chapter 28). These defects are associated with Treacher–Collins and Goldenhar syndromes, both of which present difficulty for tracheal intubation. Anaesthesia for these operations can usually be managed using a flexible LMA which obviates the need for intubation. It is essential to be satisfied with the performance of the LMA with the head in the position for operation, before surgery commences.

Head and neck tumours

Extensive dissection may be required in some head and neck masses. Anaesthesia management includes potentially difficult intubation, appropriate monitoring, compensation for heat loss, and preparation for rapid transfusion if needed, as in any major surgical intervention.

Key points

- Extreme vigilance is essential during procedures on the airway.
- Diagnostic microlaryngoscopy and bronchoscopy requires spontaneous ventilation to be maintained. This necessitates good topical anaesthesia of the larynx.
- Post-operative vomiting occurs commonly during ENT surgery and antiemetics should be administered in all cases.
- TIVA is the most appropriate mode of anaesthesia for middle ear surgery.

The compromised paediatric airway

Stephanie Bew

Introduction

The airway anatomy and respiratory physiology of children predisposes them to airway compromise. Managing such situations can be very challenging and stressful for all involved. Anaesthetists may be required to provide anaesthesia for elective surgery in a child with a known difficult airway, for diagnostic airway examination, or to establish a definitive airway in a child in an emergency situation. This chapter will concentrate on the management of the child who presents with acute airway compromise or a 'difficult airway'.

The paediatric airway

There are numerous causes of airway compromise in children, but the most frequent causes are infections or congenital abnormalities (see Table 22.1). Infections present acutely, often in children with no underlying health problems. Children with a known difficult airway may present for planned investigation or surgery, but may also present acutely with symptoms exacerbated by respiratory infection. Congenital abnormalities associated with a hypoplastic mandible are typically associated with difficult intubation, those with midface hypoplasia with difficult bag-mask ventilation, and those with macroglossia with difficult bag-mask ventilation and difficult intubation.

Fortunately, unexpected airway difficulties are rare, although maintaining the airway in a normal neonate or infant under anaesthesia can occasionally prove a challenge for the inexperienced practitioner; the prominent occiput tends to cause neck flexion, and the tongue is relatively large. Both these factors contribute to airway obstruction as pharyngeal tone is lost. Simple techniques such as chin lift (avoiding compression of the structures of the floor of the mouth), application of continuous positive airway pressure (CPAP), and insertion of a Guedel airway (if the child is adequately anaesthetised) are the mainstay of the paediatric anaesthetist. The laryngeal mask airway has an important role in managing the difficult airway in children of all ages.

The upper airway mucosa is loosely adherent to the submucosa in infants and prone to oedema, except over the vocal cords and laryngeal surface of the epiglottis. Laryngeal oedema from repeated intubation attempts may convert the difficult intubation into an impossible intubation. The diameter of the airway at the cricoid in neonates is only 4–5 mm, and even 1 mm of oedema, for instance from an infective cause, results in significant reduction in cross-sectional area and an increase in resistance (Poiseuille's law). The cartilaginous structures of the chest wall are compliant in infants and young children, and increased respiratory effort causes sternal and subcostal recession with decreased mechanical efficiency. The metabolic rate and oxygen consumption are high, the functional residual capacity is relatively small and the diaphragm has fewer fatigue-resistant fibres; respiratory reserve is limited. The infant with severe respiratory infection is easily exhausted, and airway obstruction leads to rapid desaturation.

In some cases the progression to severe airway compromise is rapid and immediate intervention is required. In other children problems may develop over a period of days or weeks, or the child may present for elective surgery unrelated to the airway. In any situation it is important to assess the airway carefully, to formulate a clear plan, and have an alternative plan should the first one fail.

Core Topics in Paediatric Anaesthesia, ed. Ian James and Isabeau Walker. Published by Cambridge University Press. © 2013 Cambridge University Press.

Table 22.1 Common causes of upper airway obstruction in children

Congenital		Acquired	
Choanal atresia		*Infections*	Croup (laryngotracheobronchitis)
			Epiglottitis
			Bacterial tracheitis
Craniofacial malformations	Pierre Robin syndrome		Quinsy
	Treacher–Collins syndrome		Ludwig's angina
	Goldenhar syndrome		Diphtheria
	Mid-facial hypoplasia		
Macroglossia	Down syndrome	*Physical obstruction*	Foreign body
	Beckwith–Wiedemann		Adenotonsillar hypertrophy
	Mucopolysaccharidoses		Trauma
			Thermal or chemical burns
Larynx	Laryngomalacia		Post-intubation oedema
	Laryngeal web		Post-operative oedema
	Laryngeal cleft		Angio-oedema
	Vocal cord palsy		Acquired laryngeal or subglottic stenosis
	Subglottic stenosis		Rheumatoid arthritis
	Haemangioma		Tumours
			Cysts
Tracheal	Tracheomalacia		Lymph nodes
	Tracheal stenosis		
	Vascular rings	*Neurogenic*	Depressed consciousness
			Nerve palsy

Assessment of the airway

The diagnosis of a narrow or compromised airway may be obvious, for instance in a child with a named congenital condition, or a child who presents with loud stridor or marked respiratory distress. Sometimes the signs may be very subtle, and it is easy to underestimate the degree of airway compromise. This is particularly the case where there is a slowly worsening fixed (rather then dynamic) narrowing when there is often minimal stridor and little sign of increased work of breathing at rest. An example of this is the child with subglottic stenosis, or airway complications of caustic ingestion.

The Mallampati score is not useful in young infants due to poor cooperation, and there are no standard measurements for thyromental distance to predict difficult laryngoscopy. Assessment of the airway requires a careful clinical history and examination to obtain an indication of the likely cause and whether the problem is supraglottic, glottic, subglottic or lower down the respiratory tract. Investigations are rarely helpful or appropriate in the acute situation, but may have a role in the stable child.

History

In addition to the normal anaesthetic history, questions should be targeted at airway problems. Is this a previously normal airway?

Ask about

- Previous airway problems or airway surgery;
- Previous episodes of intubation and ventilation, especially for ex-premature infants. Even very short periods of intubation can lead to the development of subglottic stenosis or cysts that may not cause symptoms until several months after discharge from the neonatal unit;
- Previous cardiac surgery or repair of a tracheoesophageal fistula; this makes vocal cord palsy or tracheomalacia more likely;
- Previous respiratory problems such as asthma, especially if atypical or not responding to treatment.

Have the parents heard stridor or other respiratory noise?

- Is the noise constant or intermittent, what are the effects of positioning or exertion? Is it getting worse or better?

Ask about the onset and duration of the problem:

- Are there any exacerbating or relieving factors?
- Has there been any response to treatment?

Has there been a witnessed coughing or choking episode suggestive of an inhaled or swallowed foreign body?

Is the child's voice or cry normal or has it changed, becoming weak, hoarse or even aphonic suggesting laryngeal pathology?

Assess the respiratory reserve:

- What is the exercise tolerance compared with other children? In infants, is the baby too breathless to feed or is nasogastric feeding necessary?

Ask about the airway when the child is asleep:

- Does the child snore? Are there episodes of obstruction suggesting sleep apnoea or do they adopt abnormal postures to maintain the airway during sleep? Children who obstruct their airways during sleep will almost certainly obstruct on induction of anaesthesia.

Look at the child

Look at the child's general appearance:

- Expected size for age? If small are they an ex-premature infant or is faltering growth due to chronic airway obstruction? If obese beware of more rapid desaturation.
- Nasogastric tube present?

Look at the child's position:

- Are they maintaining a tripod position or extended neck to maintain the best airway?
- Do they have torticollis? This may suggest neck pain associated with retropharyngeal abscess.

Look at the pattern of breathing:

- Signs of exhaustion
- Apnoeas
- Prolonged expiration suggesting laryngeal or subglottic narrowing
- Mouth breather? The nasal airway may be completely obstructed by hypertrophied adenoidal tissue. Do not include the use of a nasopharyngeal airway or a nasal intubation in your airway management plan.
- Drooling suggests pain or inability to swallow due to epiglottitis, laryngeal foreign body or retropharyngeal abscess.

Look for signs of increased work of breathing, tracheal tug, sternal recession, subcostal recession, head bobbing, nasal flaring, grunting, tachypnoea.

Are there signs of hypoxaemia or hypercapnia such as tachycardia, pallor, peripheral or central cyanosis, agitation and confusion?

Listen

Listen to the breathing and any other respiratory noise. Is this typical of what the parents hear? The noise often indicates the site of airway narrowing, but the volume of the stridor does not relate to the severity of obstruction. A child with a critically obstructed airway may be almost silent.

- Stridor
  - Inspiratory stridor is classically associated with a narrowing above the cords;
  - Expiratory stridor is associated with narrowing below the vocal cords, or an intrathoracic problem;
  - Biphasic stridor is associated with narrowing at or just below the cords.
- Stertor
  - Obstruction at the tongue base
- Croupy cough
  - Subglottic pathology
- Hoarse cry or breathy voice
  - Vocal cord pathology

Examine

Is the child likely to present a difficult laryngoscopy or difficult facemask ventilation?

- Syndrome associated with a difficult airway
- Retrognathia or micrognathia – remember to look in profile
- Abnormalities of the external ears are often associated with micrognathia
- Neck swelling
- Mouth opening
- Examine the tongue and teeth and neck movement

Examine the chest for lung pathology. If present, is there a problem that could be treated? Decreased respiratory reserve will cause extremely rapid desaturation during anaesthesia.

- Chronic lung disease, common in ex-premature infants
- Chest infection
- Asthma

Is the child feverish? Increased metabolic rate and oxygen consumption may exacerbate the rapid rate of desaturation during anaesthesia.

Remember to assess vascular access, as this may be very difficult in the ex-premature infant.

Monitor

Pulse oximetry is well tolerated and allows continuous monitoring of heart rate as well as oxygen saturation. In the acute situation, the respiratory rate must be checked frequently. Increased rate suggests increased work of breathing; marked decrease in rate suggests exhaustion. Frequent documentation of these observations will highlight the trends and allow rapid recognition of deterioration which may require urgent intervention to secure the airway.

Investigations

Investigations and imaging are often inappropriate in the acute situation. Attempts to take a sample for blood gas analysis or site a cannula may cause agitation and crying, increase turbulent airflow, worsen respiratory distress and occasionally precipitate complete airway obstruction. In a stable child anteroposterior (AP) and lateral soft tissue neck X-rays may be helpful in diagnosis, for example in croup or retropharyngeal abscess. In children with a chronic problem, MRI and CT scans or barium swallow to look for tracheal compression may be helpful. Increasingly, ENT surgeons are using awake nasendoscopy in children. These investigations may give detailed information about the size and site of narrowing. Children with obstructed breathing during sleep may have a sleep study or overnight oximetry recording.

Management: acute airway compromise

In acute airway compromise, medical management will sometimes resolve the problem or avoid the need for immediate intubation. The use of inhaled or intravenous steroids and nebulised adrenaline in the treatment of croup reduces the duration of illness and the need for intubation (dexamethasone 600 mcg kg^{-1} PO (max 8 mg), or nebulised budesonide 2 mg; nebulised adrenaline 0.5 ml kg^{-1} 1:1000 solution (max 5 ml)). These treatments may also 'buy time' and stabilise the child whilst preparations are made to secure the airway. Occasionally, inhaling a helium–oxygen mixture (heliox, usually 21% O_2 in helium) is helpful in reducing work of breathing and preventing exhaustion, and may allow time for steroids to work.

Planning management of acute airway problems

On the basis of your assessment decide what difficulties you anticipate and how you will manage these with the skills and equipment available. If you need more help call early. Two experienced anaesthetists are often needed along with a skilled anaesthetic assistant and a surgeon capable of performing a tracheostomy. Decide if you need to move to an anaesthetic room or theatre to secure the airway. Is it safe to move? How will you get there and who accompanies the child?

Prepare your plan and the contingency plans; these may need to change in the light of changing circumstances. Prepare the child and parents for the type of induction and airway management. Consider giving oral atropine 20–30 mcg kg^{-1}, although this requires over an hour to be effective. Parents need to know what problems you anticipate, what to expect in the anaesthetic room, and how they can help their child. The possibility of tracheostomy may need to be discussed, also the need for intensive care. Having decided what equipment you require, you must check personally that it is all working and that you have the appropriate sizes. Good communication is essential, and this may involve the child, the parents, anaesthetist, anaesthetic assistant, theatre nurses, surgeons and PICU. Everyone needs to know the plan and who is taking the lead, particularly if there are two anaesthetists.

Only rarely in paediatrics is the airway secured awake, either by fibre-optic intubation or tracheostomy under local anaesthetic. In most acute cases with the exact pathology and degree of narrowing unknown, anaesthesia should be induced with inhalation of sevoflurane in oxygen. Each case needs individual assessment of whether to insert a cannula before induction or whether this would cause distress and worsening of symptoms. Similarly the application of full monitoring prior to induction may not be appropriate, but pulse oximetry is generally well tolerated. If the child is adopting a particular position to maintain the best airway, anaesthesia should be induced in this position. Consider giving atropine 20 mcg kg^{-1} IV after intravenous access is obtained.

The basic principle is to maintain spontaneous ventilation and deepen anaesthesia until direct laryngoscopy is tolerated. Apnoea may occur particularly during induction with sevoflurane, but resist the temptation to assist ventilation. Ensure an unobstructed upper airway and wait with the mask applied for the resumption of spontaneous ventilation. Airway obstruction may worsen as anaesthesia is deepened. At a light plane of anaesthesia even a firm jaw thrust may not be tolerated. Maintain the best airway you can with gentle opening manoeuvres, and apply continuous positive airway pressure (CPAP) via the facemask. Putting the child in the lateral position may improve the airway, allowing you to deepen anaesthesia. In children with adenotonsillar hypertrophy, application of jaw thrust to maintain mouth-opening works better than chin lift. Try an oropharyngeal airway if anaesthesia is deep enough, or if the nasal airway is patent, a well-lubricated nasopharyngeal airway may be gently inserted at a lighter plane. Assess the effect of each manoeuvre as you proceed. The diameter of the airway is increased in the lateral position, and this or even semi-prone may get a better airway. CPAP is almost always helpful, acting as a dynamic splint to increase the airway diameter, reduce atelectasis and reduce thoracoabdominal asynchrony. Aim for 5–10 cm of CPAP, but beware that too much pressure can cause gastric distension. If this does occur the stomach is easily deflated with oral or nasogastric passage of a suction catheter. Sometimes you need two hands to maintain the airway and get a good mask seal and a second anaesthetist to apply CPAP. Consider whether an LMA would provide a better airway to deepen anaesthesia.

Be prepared to wait a long time to achieve the required depth of anaesthesia, particularly when the airway is extremely narrow and there is little gas moving with each breath. If in doubt wait a little longer. Check for small central pupils and a settled regular respiratory pattern and no response to a firm jaw thrust. Assess the view on direct laryngoscopy.

If the child is having a diagnostic airway examination rather than immediate intubation, anaesthetise the larynx with lidocaine spray 3 mg kg^{-1} and maintain spontaneous ventilation while the surgeon proceeds with the examination.

If you need to intubate and you have a good view, intubate under deep inhalational anaesthesia remembering that you may need a much smaller tracheal tube than expected for age. If you do not get a good view or cannot pass a tube at the first attempt, return to the mask airway and maintain spontaneous respiration. Think carefully about how you will proceed.

There are three common scenarios:

- A second attempt at direct laryngoscopy is likely to succeed. Consider a different laryngoscope such as a McCoy or use a bougie, stylet or smaller tube. In many compromised airways a direct laryngoscopic view is possible but the tissues are swollen and distorted and the airway narrow. An appropriately sized bougie is often the most useful piece of equipment in these circumstances.
- Further attempts at direct laryngoscopy are unlikely to succeed as you cannot obtain a 'line of sight' view. The larynx may be normal, but mandibular or tongue base abnormality prevents a view and intubation is only possible with equipment allowing you to 'see round the corner'. Previously this required a flexible fibre-optic laryngoscope, but a wide range of rigid indirect laryngoscopes and optical stylets are now available for use in these situations. The choice of technique depends on the equipment available and the skills and experience of the anaesthetist. If a flexible fibre-optic laryngoscope is used, anaesthesia and oxygenation can either be maintained with a circuit attached to a short tracheal tube used as a nasopharyngeal airway, or alternatively an LMA can be used to maintain the airway and to act as a conduit for fibre-optic intubation using a guidewire and airway exchange catheter (see below).
- Intubation is not possible. There may be a mass obstructing the airway, unrecognisable anatomy or the airway is too narrow for smallest tube. Repeated attempts at laryngoscopy and intubation will cause oedema and bleeding. Maintain spontaneous ventilation and consider the following options:

- o Secure the airway with an LMA
- o Wake the child up. This may not be possible in the child with acute airway compromise but should always be considered.
- o Secure the airway with a rigid bronchoscope, for the surgeon to remove a mass or aspirate a cyst under spontaneous respiration; or
- o Proceed to a surgical airway under facemask anaesthesia.

Effective decision-making is crucial. Repeated attempts at laryngoscopy and intubation will cause oedema and bleeding. The airway may already be narrow and inflamed, and the situation can rapidly spiral out of control. In a normal infant who is pre-oxygenated the saturations will fall to 90% in about 90 seconds if the airway is completely obstructed. This time is greatly reduced in children with compromised airways, especially if the child is toxic or has pre-existing lung disease.

Elective intubation of the child with a known difficult airway

In the elective intubation of a child with a known difficult airway the same detailed assessment is required as for acute airway compromise. There is a wide spectrum of difficulty, from easy mask airway but difficult laryngoscopy, to airways in which every aspect of management is challenging. Previous anaesthetic records may be helpful, but must not be relied on as the airway may change as the child grows. There should be time for an informed discussion with the parents and child about anticipated difficulties and strategies for managing these, which may include planned tracheostomy or the possibility of waking the child up if the airway cannot be safely managed. Parents often have very useful information about previous anaesthetic experiences.

Many of the known difficult airways in children are associated with mandibular abnormalities as part of a well-recognised syndrome such as Pierre Robin complex. In general, it is not difficult to maintain oxygenation after induction of anaesthesia, and there is time for controlled intubation using flexible fibre-optic or rigid indirect laryngoscopy. In some children, maintaining oxygenation may be very difficult and other co-morbidity can make airway management very challenging. For instance, children with mucopolysaccharidoses may have limited oxygen reserve, cardiac valve disease, an unstable neck and copious airway secretions, as well as having very difficult mask airways and laryngoscopy. These children need an approach similar to the child with acute airway compromise. Two experienced anaesthetists should be present.

Techniques for difficult intubation in children

A range of 'non-conventional' laryngoscopes is now available for paediatric use. They can be broadly categorised as bladed devices, optical bougies and conduits:

- The Glidescope videolaryngoscope has a blade curved through 60° and requires the tracheal tube to be mounted on a curved stylet.
- The Storz videolaryngoscope uses a conventional blade with a video camera.
- Bonfils and Brambrink are optical stylets with the tracheal tube mounted directly on the stylet.
- Devices such as the Airtraq use a system of prisms with the tube inserted through an integral conduit.

As with any new piece of airway equipment it is important to be familiar with the device itself and the indications for its use, and to build up practical experience. These devices have a place in the management of the elective difficult intubation but all require a different technique from that of direct laryngoscopy. In general the view of the larynx is obtained easily, but manipulating the tracheal tube into position has a longer learning curve.

Technique for fibre-optic intubation in children via the LMA

Acceptance of an awake fibre-optic procedure is possible in an older child, particularly if there have been previous airway difficulties. However, in general, fibre-optic techniques in children require the child to be anaesthetised, with anaesthesia maintained via a facemask, nasopharyngeal airway or, if possible, an LMA, a technique which will be described below.

If you have a small enough fibre-optic scope, the tracheal tube can be mounted directly onto a fibre-optic scope, and the child intubated using the LMA as a conduit. This leaves you with both a LMA and the tube *in situ*. The technique described allows you to maintain oxygenation and anaesthesia during intubation, allows for removal of the LMA before intubation, and allows for easy tube change if the initial tube selected is the wrong size. It is also suitable if your fibre-optic scope is too big to have the tube mounted directly.

Equipment

(See Figures 22.1–22.3.)

- Fibre-optic scope
- LMA. This technique was originally described using the classic LMA (cLMA), which is made from silicone so that the fibre-optic scope usually passes smoothly between the epiglottic bars and the bars do not need to be removed. If a disposable LMA is used (made from polyvinyl chloride) you may encounter resistance passing the fibre-optic scope through the epiglottic bars and it is better to remove them before starting. It is essential to check meticulously that any bars that are removed are identified and disposed of well away from the equipment trolley.
- Angle piece with suction port
- J-tipped guidewire
- 8 Fr paediatric airway exchange catheter
- Tracheal tube

Remember to check the equipment before starting; in particular make sure your guidewire fits through the suction port and is long enough for your fibre-optic scope.

- Anaesthetise patient and maintain spontaneous breathing. Insert appropriate size LMA as usual.
- Maintain anaesthesia and oxygenation via the LMA. Pass the fibre-optic scope through the port on the angle piece and into the LMA. The larynx is usually easily visualised or the scope can be manipulated past the epiglottis to get a view. If the epiglottis is completely obscuring the view it may be helpful to start again after repositioning the LMA. Once the scope is positioned above the larynx, apply topical lidocaine 1% via the suction

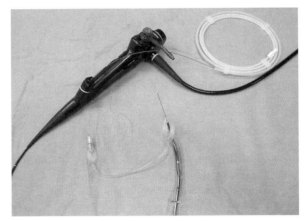

Figure 22.2 Fibre-optic scope with wire passing through suction port and laryngeal mask.

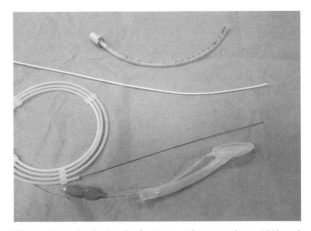

Figure 22.3 Guidewire, Cook airway exchange catheter, LMA and tracheal tube.

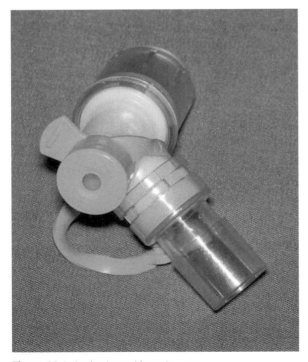

Figure 22.1 Angle piece with suction port.

port either using an epidural catheter inserted through the port or a 5 ml syringe with 4 ml of air and 1 ml of lidocaine to spray the larynx. Maximum dose 3 mg kg^{-1}. Alternatively, a muscle relaxant may be administered and ventilation maintained via the LMA.

- The J-tipped guidewire is now passed through the suction port and into the distal trachea, and the fibre-optic scope is removed.
- The airway exchange catheter is railroaded over the guidewire. Remove the wire to leave the airway exchange catheter in place through the LMA. It is easier to intubate over the stiff airway exchange catheter, as inserting the tube over the guidewire alone usually results in oesophageal intubation.
- A capnograph can be attached to the airway exchange catheter to check for CO_2.
- Remove the LMA leaving the airway exchange catheter in place; again you can check for CO_2.
- The tracheal tube can now be inserted over the airway exchange catheter and the position checked in the usual way.

If the patient has been given muscle relaxant, ventilation can be maintained via the LMA throughout the procedure.

Extubation and continuing care of children with airway compromise

A child undergoing a difficult intubation requires a plan for extubation. Many children will need to remain intubated on the intensive care unit for a period of time while airway oedema and infection resolve, and they may require a further airway examination under anaesthesia before extubation. Some will require tracheostomy either permanently or until surgery or natural growth ensures a safe airway. More rarely the child may be extubated after a surgical procedure to improve the airway, such as excision of a cyst. Stridor and partial airway obstruction can be worse during emergence than on induction. A nasopharyngeal airway inserted prior to waking can help maintain the airway until muscle tone has returned, and PEEP applied with a facemask is useful.

- Adrenaline nebulisers using standard 1:1000 adrenaline at a dose of 0.5 ml kg^{-1} up to a maximum of 5 ml can be helpful to get through the initial phase.

- Heliox may reduce the work of breathing and prevent the onset of exhaustion and hypercapnia. The helium/oxygen mixture has a low density and reduces resistance by reducing turbulent flow.
- Dexamethasone 200–500 mg kg^{-1} IV may be used to reduce oedema. It is best administered intra-operatively with four doses 6 hourly post-operatively.

Occasionally if oxygenation and intubation have been very difficult, it may be prudent to pass a guidewire through the tube into the trachea and leave this taped in place after extubation. If emergency re-intubation is required, a small airway exchange catheter can be passed over the wire and a tube railroaded over.

Difficult airways in children are uncommon, and elective intubations of children with known difficult airways are important opportunities for teaching and mutual sharing of experience for anaesthetists, anaesthetic assistants and theatre staff. It is important to document findings, with a clear description of how any difficulties were managed. Parents also need to be informed as the child may present subsequently at a time and place where the anaesthetic records are not available. Documentation also aids decision-making about the risks and benefits of future procedures.

Difficult airway guidelines and 'Cannot intubate, cannot ventilate'

The Association of Paediatric Anaesthetists of Great Britain and Ireland and the Difficult Airway Society have recently published a series of algorithms for difficult airways in children: difficult mask ventilation in a child 1–8 years of age; unanticipated difficult intubation; and cannot intubate and cannot ventilate (see http://www.apagbi.org.uk/publications/apa-guidelines and Figures 22.4–22.6). In children with compromised airways, oxygenation is often difficult but it is rarely impossible. If the situation does deteriorate to 'can't intubate, can't oxygenate', hypoxia and bradycardia will rapidly ensue and a transtracheal airway must be achieved immediately. In a small infant the options are very limited and there is little evidence in the literature to guide practice.

Cricothyroidotomy as a rescue technique is very rarely required in children, and surgical tracheostomy may be a safer option. However, paediatric ENT support is not available in every hospital where children are anaesthetised, and occasionally an anaesthetist

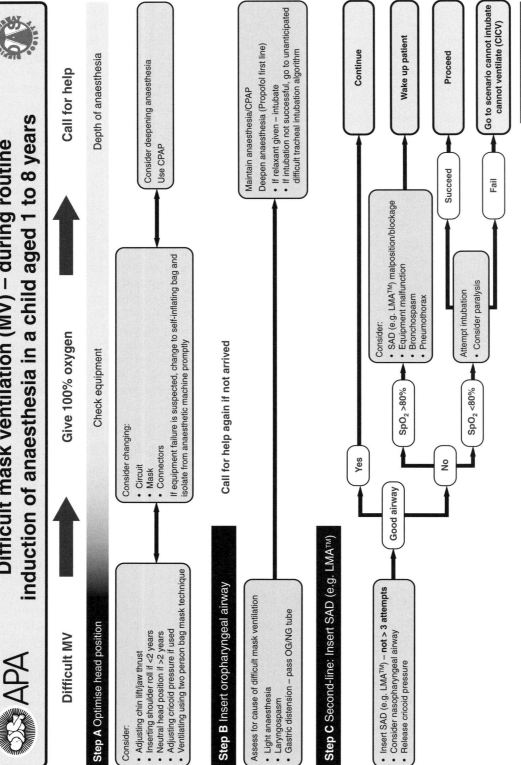

Difficult mask ventilation (MV) – during routine induction of anaesthesia in a child aged 1 to 8 years

Difficult MV → Give 100% oxygen → Call for help

Optimise head position | Check equipment | Depth of anaesthesia

Step A Optimise head position

Consider:
- Adjusting chin lift/jaw thrust
- Inserting shoulder roll if <2 years
- Neutral head position if >2 years
- Adjusting cricoid pressure if used
- Ventilating using two person bag mask technique

Consider changing:
- Circuit
- Mask
- Connectors

If equipment failure is suspected, change to self-inflating bag and isolate from anaesthetic machine promptly

Consider deepening anaesthesia
Use CPAP

Step B Insert oropharyngeal airway

Assess for cause of difficult mask ventilation
- Light anaesthesia
- Laryngospasm
- Gastric distension – pass OG/NG tube

Call for help again if not arrived

Maintain anaesthesia/CPAP
Deepen anaesthesia (Propofol first line)
- If relaxant given – intubate
- If intubation not successful, go to unanticipated difficult tracheal intubation algorithm

Step C Second-line: Insert SAD (e.g. LMA™)

- Insert SAD (e.g. LMA™) – **not > 3 attempts**
- Consider nasopharyngeal airway
- Release cricoid pressure

Good airway → Yes → Continue

Good airway → No

No → SpO₂ >80%

Consider:
- SAD (e.g. LMA™) malposition/blockage
- Equipment malfunction
- Bronchospasm
- Pneumothorax

SpO₂ >80% → Wake up patient

No → SpO₂ <80%

Attempt intubation
- Consider paralysis

SpO₂ <80% → Succeed → Proceed

Fail → Go to scenario cannot intubate cannot ventilate (CICV)

SAD = supraglottic airway device

Figure 22.4 APA Difficult mask ventilation algorithm. (Reproduced with permission of the Association of Paediatric Anaesthetists of Great Britain and Ireland.)

APA Unanticipated difficult tracheal intubation – during routine induction of anaesthesia in a child aged 1 to 8 years

Difficult direct laryngoscopy → Give 100% oxygen and maintain anaesthesia → Call for help

Step A Initial tracheal intubation plan when mask ventilation is satisfactory   Ensure: Oxygenation, anaesthesia, CPAP, management of gastric distension with OG/NG tube

Direct laryngoscopy – **not > 4 attempts**
Check:
• Neck flexion and head extension
• Laryngoscopy technique
• External laryngeal manipulation – remove or adjust
• Vocal cords open and immobile (adequate paralysis)
If poor view – consider bougie, straight blade laryngoscope* and/or smaller ETT

→ **Succeed** → Tracheal intubation → Verify ETT position
• Capnography
• Visual if possible
• Ausculation
If ETT too small consider using throat pack and tie to ETT
If in doubt, take ETT out

Failed intubation with good oxygenation

Step B Secondary tracheal intubation plan

Call for help again if not arrived

• Insert SAD (e.g. LMA™) – **not > 3 attempts**
• Oxygenate and ventilate
• Consider increasing size of SAD (e.g. LMA™) once if ventilation inadequate

→ **Succeed** →
• Consider modifying anaesthesia and surgery plan
• Assess safety of proceeding with surgery using a SAD (e.g. LMA™)

→ **Unsafe** → Postpone surgery Wake up patient

→ **Safe** → Proceed with surgery

→ **Safe** → • **Consider 1 attempt** at FOI via SAD (e.g. LMA™) → Verify intubation, leave SAD (e.g. LMA™) in place and proceed with surgery → **Succeed** → Proceed with surgery

Failed oxygenation e.g. SpO$_2$ <90% with FiO$_2$ 1.0

• Convert to face mask
• Optimise head position
• Oxygenate and ventilate
• Ventilate using two person bag mask technique, CPAP and oro/nasopharyngeal airway
• Manage gastric distension with OG/NG tube
• Reverse non-depolarising relaxant

→ **Succeed** → Failed intubation via SAD (e.g. LMA™) → Postpone surgery Wake up patient

→ Failed ventilation and oxygenation → Go to scenario cannot intubate cannot ventilate (CICV)

Following intubation attempts, consider • Trauma to the airway • Extubation in a controlled setting

*Consider using indirect laryngoscope if experienced in their use   SAD = supraglottic airway device

Figure 22.5 APA Unanticipated difficult tracheal intubation algorithm. ETT, endotracheal tube. (Reproduced with permission of the Association of Paediatric Anaesthetists of Great Britain and Ireland.)

Cannot intubate and cannot ventilate (CICV) in a paralysed anaesthetised child aged 1 to 8 years

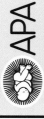

Failed intubation inadequate ventilation → **Give 100% oxygen** → **Call for help**

Step A Continue to attempt oxygenation and ventilation

- FiO$_2$ 1.0
- Optimise head position and chin lift/jaw thrust
- Insert oropharyngeal airway or SAD (e.g. LMA™)
- Ventilate using two person bag mask technique
- Manage gastric distension with an OG/NG tubet

Step B Attempt wake up if maintaining SpO$_2$ >80%

If rocuronium or vecuronium used, consider suggamadex (16mg/kg) for full reversal

Prepare for rescue techniques in case child deteriorates

Step C Airway rescue techniques for CICV (SpO$_2$ <80% and falling) and/or heart rate decreasing

Call for help again if not arrived

Call for specialist ENT assistance

- ENT available → Consider:
  - Surgical tracheostomy
  - Rigid bronchoscopy + ventilate / jet ventilation (pressure limited)

- ENT not available → Percutaneous cannula cricothyroidotomy / transtracheal jet ventilation (pressure limited)
  - Succeed → Continue jet ventilation set to lowest delivery pressure until wake up or definitive airway established
  - Fail → Perform surgical cricothyroidotomy / transtracheal and insertion of ETT / tracheostomy tube*
    - Consider passive O$_2$ insufflation while preparing

Cannula cricothyroidotomy

- Extend the neck (shoulder roll)
- Stabilise larynx with non-dominant hand
- Access the cricoithyroidotomy membrane with a dedicated 14/16 gauge cannula
- Aim in a caudad direction
- Confirm position by air aspiration using a syringe with saline
- Connect to either:
  - adjustable pressure limiting device, set to lowest delivery pressure

  or

  - 4Bar O$_2$ source with a flowmeter (match flow l/min to child's age) and Y connector
- Cautiously increase inflation pressure/flow rate to achieve adequate chest expansion
  Wait for full expiration before next inflation
- Maintain upper airway patency to aid expiration

SAD = supraglottic airway device

*Note: Cricothyroidotomy techniques can have serious complications and training is required – only use in life-threatening situations and convert to a definitive airway as soon as possible

Figure 22.6 APA Cannot intubate and cannot ventilate algorithm. (Reproduced with permission of the Association of Paediatric Anaesthetists of Great Britain and Ireland.)

may need to achieve a transtracheal airway for a child *in extremis*.

In the small infant, the cartilages of the larynx are difficult to palpate and identify even with neck extension, and the cricothyroid membrane measures only 2.6×3 mm. A 16 gauge jet ventilation catheter or intravenous catheter can be inserted between the tracheal rings if the cricothyroid membrane cannot be identified. The length of the trachea is only 5 cm, and the cannula should only be inserted a couple of centimetres at most and fixed securely. Oxygenation can be achieved by jet ventilation, but only if a device with adjustable pressure and flow is available. Start at low pressure (0.4 bar) and slowly increase to see the chest rise. Exhalation has to occur through the natural airway so the rate of jetting may need to be very slow. Alternatively a T-piece circuit can be used to provide oxygenation and ventilation at a low rate. The T-piece can be connected directly to the 15 mm fitting on a jet ventilation catheter or to the connector from a 3 mm tracheal tube which fits into the hub of a 16G intravenous cannula.

In the older child, cannula cricothyroidotomy or a percutaneous cricothyroidotomy may be performed as in an adult, the latter allowing insertion of a small tracheostomy tube. Several manufacturers make devices in paediatric sizes. Spontaneous or positive pressure ventilation is possible through these tubes.

A recent audit of major complications of airway management in the UK (NAP4) found that cricothyroidotomy by anaesthetists was associated with a high rate of failure even in adult patients. In children the need for an emergency transtracheal airway was reported to NAP4 on four occasions. An attempt at needle cricothyroidotomy in an older child was unsuccessful but surgical tracheostomy was successful in three, and it might be better to consider a surgical tracheostomy as a first option.

Key points

- Airway compromise in children is a rare but challenging problem. It is important to get appropriate help early.
- Careful assessment, contingency planning, thorough preparation and good communication are essential.
- Maintain spontaneous ventilation until the airway is secured.
- Maintain skills and experience through shared management of elective cases, practice scenarios and airway skills training using manikins.
- Detailed documentation, discussion and debrief afterwards are essential.

Further reading

Adewale L. Anatomy and assessment of the pediatric airway. *Ped Anes* 2009;**19**:(suppl 1):1–8.

Black AE. Management of the difficult airway. In: Bingham R, Lloyd-Thomas A, Sury M, eds. *Hatch and Sumner's Textbook of Paediatric Anaesthesia* 3rd edition. Hodder Arnold. 2008. 315–329.

Bruce IA, Rothera MP. Upper airway obstruction in children. *Ped Anes* 2009;**19**:(suppl 1): 88–99.

Cote CJ, Hartnick CJ. Pediatric transtracheal and cricothyrotomy airway devices for emergency use: which are appropriate for infants and children? *Ped Anes* 2009;**19**:(suppl 1): 66–76.

Jenkins IA, Saunders M. Infections of the airway. *Ped Anes* 2009;**19**: (suppl 1):118–30.

Royal College of Anaesthetists and the Difficult Airway Society. *4th National Audit Project: Major Complications of Airway Management in the United Kingdom. Report and Findings.* Chapter 21: Children. March 2011.

Chapter

23

Anaesthesia for cleft lip and palate surgery in children

Agnes Watson

Introduction

Successful administration of anaesthesia for cleft lip and palate surgery requires an understanding of the cleft condition, associated abnormalities and the surgery involved. Close cooperation with the surgeon is vital to manage the child's airway during and after surgery. The aim is to provide balanced anaesthesia and optimum analgesia so a child starts feeding and is able to return to normal activities as soon as possible after surgery.

Incidence, type of cleft and embryology

Cleft lip and palate is a common congenital abnormality with an incidence of 1 in 700 live births, with just over 1000 affected children born in the UK each year. It encompasses two distinct conditions, cleft lip with or without cleft palate, and isolated cleft palate.

The embryological abnormality is a failure of fusion of the five facial prominences that form the facial structures, occurring at 4–8 weeks of fetal life. The medial nasal process and lateral maxillary process fuse to form the upper lip and front of the mouth. The embryonic palatal shelves fuse to form the palate – the primary palate anterior to the incisive foramen and the secondary palate posterior to this.

Cleft lip with or without cleft palate

Cleft lip with or without cleft palate has an incidence of 1 in 1000 live births, and accounts for 60% of all clefts; 25% are unilateral cleft lip, 25% unilateral cleft lip and palate, 10% bilateral cleft lip and palate. The abnormality is more often left-sided and has a male preponderance. It is more common in Chinese people than Caucasians and less common in the African-Caribbean population. The aetiology is both genetic and environmental. A cleft lip with or without cleft palate in a first-degree relative increases the risk of a cleft to 3–4%. Environmental factors that have been implicated are maternal diabetes, alcohol, folic acid deficiency and drugs, including phenytoin, corticosteroids and diazepam.

The condition varies from a small notch in the lip caused by a defect in the muscle of the upper lip, called a microform cleft lip, to a wide bilateral cleft lip and palate. Cleft lip is termed complete if it goes to the nasal sill and incomplete if not. A scheme for surgical classification is shown in Figure 23.1.

Isolated cleft palate

Isolated cleft palate is less common, with an incidence of 1 in 2000 live births. It accounts for 40% of clefts and has a female preponderance. The genetic risk of recurrence depends on the risk of recurrence of any associated syndrome.

The cleft may be of the soft palate or extend into the hard palate (Figure 23.1). A submucous cleft palate is a defect in the musculature of the soft palate; the palate may look normal or there may be a bifid uvula or central lucency of the soft palate. A submucous cleft may present with speech abnormality or nasal regurgitation of food.

Associated abnormalities

In a review of 1000 children with clefts of the lip, palate or both, Shprintzen found that half had associated congenital abnormalities, with 22% having recognised syndromes, sequences or associations (see Further reading). Isolated cleft palate is more likely to be associated with other congenital abnormalities, and this should be borne in mind during anaesthetic assessment. Infants with clefts are more likely to be

Core Topics in Paediatric Anaesthesia, ed. Ian James and Isabeau Walker. Published by Cambridge University Press. © 2013 Cambridge University Press.

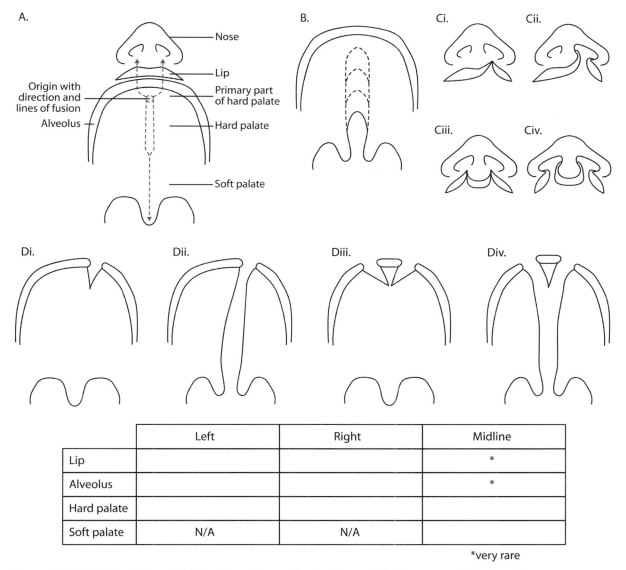

Figure 23.1 Surgical classification of cleft lip with or without cleft palate. Diagnostic findings are recorded in the grid.
Key:
A = Normal anatomy of nose, lip and alveolus and hard and soft palate with the lines of fusion emanating from the incisive foramen.
B = Differing extent of isolated cleft palate.
C = Cleft lip variants: Ci = Left unilateral incomplete cleft lip; Cii = Left unilateral complete cleft lip; Ciii = Bilateral incomplete cleft lip;
Civ = Bilateral complete cleft lip.
D = Cleft palate variants: Di = Cleft unilateral cleft of alveolus and primary hard palate; Dii = Left unilateral cleft of alveolus, hard and soft palate; Diii = Bilateral cleft of alveolus and primary hard palate; Div = Bilateral cleft of alveolus, hard and soft palate.
(Reprinted from Demircioglu M, Kangesu L, Ismail A *et al*. Increasing accuracy of antenatal ultrasound diagnosis of cleft lip with or without cleft palate, in cases referred to the North Thames London Region. *Ultrasound in Obstetrics and Gynaecology* 2008;**31**:649 copyright ISUOG, with permission from John Wiley and Sons.)

born preterm with low birth weight. Up to 150 different congenital syndromes have been associated with clefts, and some of the more commonly occurring syndromes are listed in Table 23.1. Syndromes causing mandibular hypoplasia (micrognathia) result in airway problems, and those with associated cardiac defects are of particular relevance to the anaesthetist. Reviews of children with clefts have quoted an

Table 23.1 Common syndromes associated with cleft lip and/or palate

Name of syndrome (Affected chromosome)	Clinical features
Velocardiofacial syndrome (22q11.2) (DiGeorge syndrome)	Isolated cleft palate or submucous cleft, cardiac defects, defective thymic development, learning disability, characteristic facial appearance
Pierre Robin sequence	Cleft palate, micrognathia and glossoptosis
Stickler (12q13.11–q13.2, 1p21, 6p21.3)	Collagen disorder, micrognathia, eye abnormalities, hearing loss, joint problems, characteristic facial appearance
Van der Woude (1q32–q41)	Cleft lip, lower lip pits, missing teeth. Autosomal dominant
Treacher Collins (5q32–q33.1)	Micrognathia, ear abnormalities, deafness, abnormal lower eyelids
Hemifacial microsomia (Goldenhar) (14q32)	Vertebral and cardiac abnormalities
Down (trisomy 21)	Macroglossia, cardiac defects, atlanto-axial instability, learning disability
Edwards (trisomy 18)	Cardiac defects, micrognathia, renal malformations. Often fatal in infancy
Patau (trisomy 13)	Mental retardation, microcephaly, micrognathia, cardiac defects. Often fatal in infancy
Ectrodactyly ectodermal dysplasia and clefting syndrome (7q11.2–q21.3, 3q27)	Disordered temperature control with hypohidrosis, malnutrition, respiratory tract infections

incidence of congenital heart disease from 3.7% to 15%, much higher than that in the general population.

Pierre Robin sequence

Approximately one-third of children with isolated cleft palate have Pierre Robin sequence. The combination of cleft palate, micrognathia and glossoptosis (posterior displacement of the tongue) can cause severe upper airway obstruction. Prone positioning or insertion of a nasopharyngeal airway may help, but if these interventions are not successful, a minority will require tracheostomy. There are often associated feeding difficulties and sometimes nasogastric feeding will be required. Airway problems resolve with age as mandibular growth occurs.

Velocardiofacial syndrome

Velocardiofacial syndrome (VCFS) is the syndrome most commonly associated with clefts. Children may present with isolated cleft palate or submucous cleft palate causing velopharyngeal incompetence and hypernasal speech. There is a wide spectrum of associated abnormalities, including cardiac defects (interrupted aortic arch, truncus arteriosus, tetralogy of Fallot or pulmonary atresia with VSD), typical facial characteristics of a broad nose and long face, hypotonia in infancy, defective thymic development and

learning disabilities. VCFS is caused by a microdeletion on chromosome 22, which usually occurs as a new mutation although in some cases there is autosomal dominant inheritance.

Multidisciplinary care – the cleft team

The care of the child with a cleft requires a multidisciplinary approach from a team ideally involving specialist cleft nurses, plastic, maxillofacial and ENT surgeons, orthodontists, speech therapists, dieticians, paediatricians, geneticists and clinical psychology. In the UK resources have now been concentrated into 12 cleft centres following a review of services in 1998 by the Clinical Standards Advisory Group (CSAG). The goals of treatment are normal speech and hearing, minimal facial disfigurement and normal dentition to enable the baby to develop into a confident child who becomes a socially integrated adult.

About 60% of babies with cleft lip are diagnosed by the 20 week anomaly scan, and support from the cleft team can be arranged at this stage. In other cases, diagnosis and referral are made after birth. Paediatricians are advised to make a visual inspection of the palate to exclude cleft palate rather than digital examination. After diagnosis, assessment of feeding, facial appearance, speech, hearing and dentition is necessary to plan treatment.

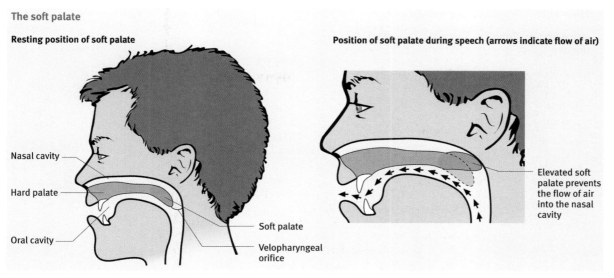

The soft palate

Resting position of soft palate

Nasal cavity

Hard palate

Oral cavity

Soft palate

Velopharyngeal orifice

Position of soft palate during speech (arrows indicate flow of air)

Elevated soft palate prevents the flow of air into the nasal cavity

Figure 23.2 The position of the soft palate at rest and during speech. (Reprinted from Mosahebi A. Kangesu L. Cleft lip and palate. *Surgery (Oxford)* 2006;**24**:34–37, with permission from Elsevier.) See plate section for colour version.

Feeding difficulties are common for babies with cleft palate as they will not be able to suck effectively; the baby will have to work hard to feed and will be slow to put on weight. Mothers are advised to use a special feeding bottle or to use a spoon to feed the baby. Nasogastric feeding is sometimes necessary if oral feeding is unsuccessful, or if the baby presents for surgery with severe failure to thrive. Babies may also have uncoordinated swallowing and problems with reflux of milk. Most infants with isolated cleft lip are able to breast-feed successfully.

Hearing assessment is important in older infants as the Eustachian tube does not open properly. Secretory otitis media is common, and grommets may be required at the time of cleft palate surgery. Orthodontic surgery is required to repair alveolar defects to improve cosmetic appearance and facilitate normal eruption of secondary teeth.

Expert surgical care is the cornerstone of successful management. Repair of cleft lip is undertaken at approximately 3 months of age, and involves correction of the lip and nasal deformity (flattened alar margin and loss of nasal tip prominence on the cleft side and a displaced septum). Closure of the palate before the age of 12 months is recommended for optimum speech development. Late repair in older children or adults produces poor results. The aim of surgery is to close the cleft palate and ensure good function of the soft palate, without

affecting normal maxillary growth. If the palate is short or does not function properly, air escapes through the velopharyngeal orifice during speech (termed velopharyngeal incompetence, VPI), which impairs phonation and causes hypernasal speech. The function of the normal soft palate is shown in Figure 23.2.

Depending on the type of cleft, the child may require one procedure or multiple operations from infancy to early adulthood. The surgical procedures and the typical age at surgery in the North Thames Cleft Network are described in Table 23.2. Ongoing support for the family by the cleft team is essential, and in the UK there are also national groups such as the Cleft Lip and Palate Association (CLAPA) who have played an important role in the design of patient-centred services.

Primary repair of lip and palate

The quality of primary surgery is thought to determine the outcome of speech and facial growth. The practice in the North Thames Cleft Network is to undertake primary repair of cleft lip, nose and anterior palate (if required) at 3 months, and primary repair of the palate at 9 months. Closure of the lip and palate during the neonatal period has been advocated by some but adds additional risk and appears to confer no surgical benefit.

Table 23.2 Timing of surgery by the North Thames Cleft Network

Age at surgery	Potential surgical procedures
3 months	Primary cleft lip and nose repair and anterior palate
9 months	Primary cleft palate repair +/− grommets
1 year	Second stage lip repair for bilateral cleft lip
3 years onwards	Lip +/− nose revision
3 years onwards	Secondary speech surgery – re-explore palate, buccinator flaps, pharyngoplasty, autologous fat transfer
Any age	Repair of palatal fistula
Any age	Primary repair of submucous palate
9–10 years	Alveolar bone graft
17–20 years	Maxillary osteotomy
17–20 years	Rhinoplasty

Repair of the lip involves repositioning of the orbicularis and perioral muscles and correction of the nasal deformity. Our practice includes mobilisation of the periosteum of the septum, called a vomerine flap, to cover the defect in the anterior part of the hard palate, if present.

Closure of the palate is performed using an operating microscope to dissect the soft palate muscles and realign them transversely to the back of the soft palate (Figure 23.3). Lateral releasing incisions through the mucosa may be performed to reduce tension on the midline repair. Grommets may be inserted at the same time as palatal surgery, if required.

Pre-operative assessment

Prior to surgery infants should be well, thriving and gaining weight. It is important to identify potential airway problems and other associated abnormalities. The rule of 10s advocated by Wilhelmsen and Musgrave in 1966 is a useful guide for infants having lip repair. The infant should be:

- Over 10 lbs (4.5 kg)
- Over 10 weeks old with a haemoglobin $> 10 \, \mathrm{g} \, \mathrm{dl}^{-1}$
- WCC $< 10 \times 10^9 \, \mathrm{dl}^{-1}$

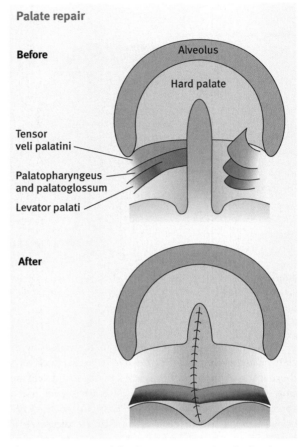

Palate repair

Before

Alveolus

Hard palate

Tensor veli palatini

Palatopharyngeus and palatoglossum

Levator palati

After

Figure 23.3 Primary cleft palate repair – muscles of soft palate are realigned transversely. (Reprinted from Mosahebi A. Kangesu L. Cleft lip and palate. *Surgery (Oxford)* 2006;**24**:34–37, with permission from Elsevier.) See plate section for colour version.

Assessment of weight gain, feeding difficulty and symptoms of oesophageal reflux is important. Infants with cleft palate often have chronic nasal discharge and reflux of milk through the nose, but this should be distinguished from an active upper respiratory tract infection. Infants who are unwell with mucopurulent nasal secretions or raised temperature are best postponed as they are at much higher risk of airway complications peri-operatively.

Airway assessment includes questioning regarding a history of obstructive symptoms and looking for micrognathia (best viewed in lateral profile). Severity of obstructive symptoms can be investigated with overnight oxygen saturation monitoring and polysomnography. Infants with severe micrognathia, most commonly associated with Pierre Robin sequence,

(a)

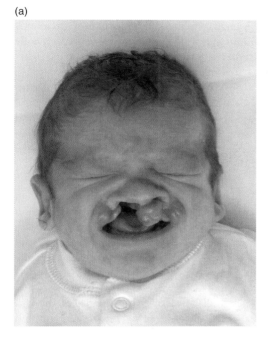

(b)

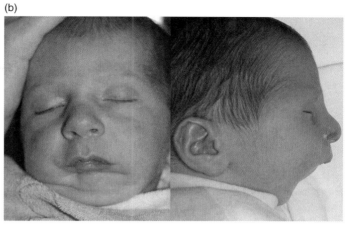

Figure 23.4 Factors predicting difficult intubation. (a) Wide bilateral cleft lip and palate with protruding premaxilla. (b) Micrognathia in an infant with Pierre Robin sequence. (Reprinted with permission from Sesenna E, Magri AS, Magnani C *et al.* Mandibular distraction in neonates: indications, techniques and results. *Ital J Ped* 2012;**38**:7, http://www.ijponline.net/content/pdf/1824-7288-38-7.pdf, accessed 15 August 2012.)

may have a nasopharyngeal airway *in situ* to relieve obstruction, but may have grown sufficiently so that an airway is no longer needed.

Infants with suspected cardiac abnormalities, such as those with low oxygen saturation readings or a heart murmur, require an echocardiogram and formal cardiology assessment. Healthy infants scheduled for simple lip repair do not require any routine blood tests. Those who are failing to thrive, clinically anaemic or having a bilateral lip repair or palate repair require baseline haemoglobin measurement.

Anaesthesia and airway management

Premedication in infants is not generally required. Inhalation induction of anaesthesia with sevoflurane in 100% oxygen is recommended to ensure good oxygenation and allow assessment of the airway while maintaining spontaneous ventilation. Infants with micrognathia may develop airway obstruction as they lose pharyngeal tone; this can usually be relieved by repositioning, use of continuous positive airway pressure, or insertion of a nasal or oral airway. It is an early indicator of the need for a nasopharyngeal airway post-operatively. After intravenous access is secured, a non-depolarising muscle relaxant can be administered after the ability to inflate the lungs

is confirmed. If there is difficulty, spontaneous breathing should be maintained.

The majority of infants will be easy to intubate. A preformed south facing tracheal tube fixed in the midline provides a stable airway and aids surgical access. Difficult laryngoscopy is seen in approximately 5–8% of cases. Factors that predict a grade 3 or 4 Cormack and Lehane view at laryngoscopy are a wide bilateral cleft with protruding premaxilla, or micrognathia in an infant under 6 months of age (Figures 23.4a and b). It is helpful that these factors are all readily identifiable pre-operatively. Children with Pierre Robin sequence generally become easier to intubate as they become older, but this is not the case for children with other syndromes such as Treacher Collins or hemifacial microsomia.

Should difficulty be encountered with intubation, a variety of aids can be employed. Simple manoeuvres such as pressure over the larynx, use of a gum elastic bougie or a stylet and a lateral approach with a straight bladed laryngoscope are usually effective. Both the left and right paraglossal approaches have been described to improve the view at laryngoscopy.

More advanced techniques depend on the equipment available and the experience of the anaesthetist. A fibre-optic scope can be used alone or using a laryngeal mask airway as a conduit. The tracheal tube may be railroaded over the scope or a guidewire placed via the suction channel. An airway exchange catheter is then railroaded over the guidewire and the tracheal tube passed over this (see Chapter 22)

It is rare that intubation is not possible (less than 1% of cases). In this situation, it may be wise to postpone surgery as the child may become easier to intubate with age and plans for difficult airway management can be made, including tracheostomy if necessary.

A throat pack is placed either by the anaesthetist or surgeon, which must be communicated to the theatre team and must be included with the nursing swab count.

Anaesthesia should be maintained with a volatile agent. Analgesia may be achieved with a variety of analgesic techniques such as intermittent boluses of fentanyl ($1-3 \, \mathrm{mcg \, kg^{-1}}$) or remifentanil infusion ($0.1-0.2 \, \mathrm{mcg \, kg^{-1} \, min^{-1}}$). Lateral releasing incisions are particularly painful. Effective analgesia will contribute to smooth anaesthesia and may avoid the need for further muscle relaxation.

During surgery, the infant is positioned with the head in a neutral position on a head ring. Ensuring correct tube length is crucial. The anaesthetist must be constantly alert to possible disconnection of the circuit near the patient end, and to accidental extubation. A mouth gag is inserted during cleft palate repair. The tracheal tube must be checked by hand ventilation or by assessing airway pressures when the gag is opened to make sure that the tube is not compressed. The gag time should be limited to 2 hours to avoid development of tongue oedema secondary to impaired perfusion.

Total anaesthetic and surgical time ranges from 90 minutes for a simple lip or palate repair to up to 3 hours for a bilateral lip repair. Pressure areas should be protected, the infant warmed and temperature monitored to avoid overheating. Blood loss is usually not significant, although there is often more bleeding associated with a vomerine flap repair or if lateral release incisions have been performed.

Extubation and post-operative airway management

Upper airway obstruction may occur in some infants after palate repair, particularly those with micrognathia or where the palate is long. It is due to obstruction of the nasopharyngeal airway by the oedematous palate, and is particularly problematic in young infants who are still obligate nose breathers.

The infant should be extubated when completely awake, after direct inspection and suction of the pharynx and documented removal of the throat pack. Signs of airway obstruction include sternal and subcostal recession, decreasing oxygen saturation and stertor. Residual anaesthetic effect, opioids and blood or secretions can contribute to upper airway obstruction. Other important causes to exclude are a swollen tongue, if the gag has been in place for a long time, or a retained throat pack.

The child should be managed with 100% oxygen, continuous positive airway pressure and/or insertion of a nasopharyngeal airway (NPA), taking care with the surgical repair. The NPA can be fashioned from a tracheal tube or a preformed nasal airway, usually 0.5 mm diameter smaller than that used to intubate the trachea. Tube length can be estimated by measuring from tip of the nostril to the tragus of the ear. If obstruction is not relieved by the NPA, reintubation may be required. In infants with micrognathia who are likely to develop airway obstruction postoperatively, it is better to place the NPA electively at the end of surgery while the child is still anaesthetised, particularly for those with Pierre Robin sequence. This minimises damage to the surgical repair and ensures the correct length of the NPA, that is, with the tip of the NPA just protruding from behind the soft palate. If the NPA is too short it will be ineffective; if it is too long it will irritate the larynx and the baby will not settle post-operatively owing to coughing.

Any baby that is dependent on a NPA needs to be monitored closely post-operatively, and the NPA needs to be suctioned regularly to make sure that it remains patent. Intravenous dexamethasone is useful to help to reduce surgical oedema (first dose $250 \, \mathrm{mcg \, kg^{-1}}$ IV; three further doses $100 \, \mathrm{mcg \, kg^{-1}}$ IV 8 hourly). Positioning the baby prone or sitting may help airway patency. Tongue sutures are seldom used. The NPA can usually be removed after 24 hours.

Analgesic management

Multimodal analgesia should be used so that the infant is comfortable but not over-sedated at extubation. There are a wide variety of analgesic techniques available and our current practice in the North Thames Cleft Network will be described.

Infants undergoing cleft lip repair are managed with infraorbital nerve blocks with bupivacaine, performed using an intra-oral approach. Blocks are performed prior to the start of surgery by the anaesthetist or the surgeon. The surgeon will also infiltrate the surgical field with local anaesthetic containing adrenaline 1 in 200 000 to reduce blood loss and aid surgery. Intravenous paracetamol is given intra-operatively, with regular paracetamol and ibuprofen PO post-operatively. The anterior palate is not anaesthetised by the infraorbital nerve block, and children who undergo vomerine flap repair at the same time as lip repair receive a loading dose of morphine towards at the end of surgery (50–100 mcg kg^{-1} IV). These children may also require oral morphine for breakthrough pain in the post-operative period, as for cleft palate repair below.

Cleft palate repair is a more painful procedure. All children receive a combination of IV paracetamol, rectal diclofenac and morphine administered towards the end of surgery (50–100 mcg kg^{-1} IV). Our practice is for the surgeon to infiltrate the palate with bupivacaine 0.25% and adrenaline 1:200 000, maximum 0.8 ml kg^{-1}, to provide pain relief and to reduce blood loss. Clonidine 1–2 mcg kg^{-1} IV is a useful adjunct to provide analgesia without respiratory depression for children older than 6 months undergoing cleft palate repair.

The use of a validated pain score such as FLACC allows objective assessment of pain in the post-operative period and guides analgesic use. If the infant does not settle with feed or comforting in the recovery room, increments of morphine (20 mcg kg^{-1} IV) are given. On the post-operative ward regular oral paracetamol and ibuprofen are given, with oral morphine for breakthrough pain as required (morphine 100 mcg kg^{-1} PO).

Peri-operative fluid management

It is our practice to administer an intra-operative fluid bolus of 20 ml kg^{-1} of Hartmann's solution to replace deficit and for maintenance requirements. Additional Hartmann's is given as required, but blood loss is usually small and transfusion is seldom required. Tranexamic acid (10 mg kg^{-1} IV) is useful for persistent bleeding, particularly following vomerine flap.

Infants are encouraged to feed post-operatively and after lip repair most will manage well. If a baby has required nasogastric feeding pre-operatively this should be continued post-operatively. Almost half the infants will require short-term intravenous fluid after palate repair until feeding is established.

Post-operative care

Post-operative bleeding after palate repair is rare but may require blood transfusion and return to theatre. Anaesthesia management is similar to that after bleeding tonsil – the infant will need fluid resuscitation, there will be blood in the airway, intubation may be difficult, residual anaesthesia must be taken into account, and there may be a full stomach due to swallowed blood.

Infants who undergo uncomplicated cleft lip surgery are usually discharged from hospital after one night, although term infants having lip repair without vomerine flap may be managed as a day case if there are no other concerns. A two-night stay is usual for infants having palate repair. Infants undergoing cleft lip repair require removal of sutures 5–7 days post-operatively, either under general anaesthesia or oral sedation, unless absorbable sutures have been used.

Primary repair of submucous cleft palate

Some children who develop hypernasal speech are diagnosed with submucous cleft palate and will require primary repair to realign the palatal musculature. This can become apparent after adenoidectomy and is commonly associated with VCFS. Submucous cleft repair is generally performed in older children, but the anaesthetic principles are the same as for primary repair of cleft palate in infancy.

Secondary cleft surgery

Children may present for a variety of secondary procedures in childhood (Table 23.2). Children for secondary procedures may become increasingly anxious about anaesthesia. Discussion about their concerns, giving choices around method of induction, and using different distraction and coping techniques can help. Sedative premedication with oral midazolam may be useful.

Secondary procedures on the lip and nose may be undertaken to improve cosmetic appearance. Anaesthetic technique is generally similar for primary lip repair although revisions in older children and adults can be performed using a laryngeal mask. Palate re-exploration may be undertaken to improve palatal length (and hence function) or to repair a palatal fistula. Principles are as for primary palate repair.

Alveolar bone graft is performed for children with a defect in the alveolus to provide a base for the eruption of the permanent teeth. Bone is taken from either the iliac crest or tibia. For details of anaesthesia for maxillofacial procedures please refer to Chapter 24.

Secondary speech surgery may be carried out after investigation by videofluoroscopy and nasal endoscopy performed by speech therapists. Children are usually over 3 years old. There are two operations that are commonly undertaken to improve the quality of speech and reduce velopharyngeal incompetence: buccinator flaps and pharyngoplasty.

Buccinator flaps

This operation increases the length of the palate by rotating buccinator myomucosal flaps from the inner cheek into the junction between the hard and soft palate. The donor sites on each cheek are closed directly. The trachea should be intubated with a pre-formed south-facing tracheal tube. Good pain relief is important with a combination of local anaesthetic infiltration, paracetamol, a NSAID and morphine. Intravenous clonidine is a useful adjunct. Post-operatively, regular simple analgesics are given with rescue analgesia provided by oral morphine.

This is a painful procedure, and some children are particularly reluctant to take oral fluids post-operatively. A nasogastric tube may be passed intra-operatively to provide a route for analgesia administration and post-operative feeding and fluid intake until the child is eating and drinking. After three weeks the muscle flaps have vascularised and the flap pedicles are divided under general anaesthesia.

Pharyngoplasty

A Hynes pharyngoplasty involves mobilising local flaps from the posterior wall of the nasopharynx to produce a ridge that can then oppose the end of the soft palate to provide palatal competence. For a sphincter pharyngoplasty local flaps are positioned lower down on the posterior pharyngeal wall. The name relates to the proposed sphincter action of the muscle in the flaps, helping to seal the velopharyngeal

orifice during speech. Another form of pharyngoplasty is that of a superiorly based posterior pharyngeal flap which is sutured onto the soft palate.

Conduct of anaesthesia is similar to primary palate repair and requires tracheal intubation. The procedure is painful, and multimodal analgesia should be used with care so as not to cause over-sedation with opioids. The operation, by its nature, produces a degree of upper airway obstruction particularly in the immediate recovery period. Close monitoring is required, including monitoring of oxygen saturation. Dexamethasone may reduce local oedema. The passage of a nasopharyngeal airway is contraindicated, as this will cause damage to the surgical site. Nasal intubation for future surgery is also contraindicated for the same reason.

Post-operative haemorrhage may occur as a complication of pharyngoplasty, owing to bleeding from the posterior pharynx. Particular care should be taken with children with VCFS who have more medial carotid arteries lying close to the pharyngeal flap donor site. Occasionally bleeding may necessitate transfusion and/or return to theatre. The child will need fluid resuscitation and careful induction of anaesthesia to avoid aspiration.

Obstructive sleep apnoea occurs more frequently after posterior pharyngeal flap surgery than other techniques, and may persist for up to 3 months post-operatively. Severe obstruction can be life-threatening and death has been reported in the literature. The child may require re-intubation and return to theatre to reverse the surgery.

Acknowledgements

I wish to thank Mr Loshan Kangesu for his advice regarding surgical management.

Key points

- There are two distinct cleft conditions: cleft lip with or without cleft palate, and isolated cleft palate.
- Of children with a cleft, 50% will have associated abnormalities, more commonly in those with isolated cleft palate; of particular importance are airway problems and cardiac defects.
- Depending on the type of cleft, children may require only one operation for correction or

several procedures throughout childhood. A multidisciplinary approach is essential.
- Most children will be easy to intubate for primary repair. Children under 6 months with micrognathia or a wide bilateral cleft may be more difficult to intubate.
- Cleft palate repair is managed with multimodal analgesia including opioids, taking care to avoid over-sedation.

- Upper airway obstruction following cleft palate repair should be anticipated. It is more common in infants with micrognathia and can be managed with a nasopharyngeal airway.
- Pharyngoplasty surgery may be complicated by post-operative upper airway obstruction and bleeding.

Further reading

Hatch DJ. Airway management in cleft lip and palate surgery. *Br J Anaes* 1996;**76**:755–6.

Mosahebi A, Kangesu L. Cleft lip and palate. *Surgery (Oxford)* 2006;**24**:33–37.

Shprintzen RJ, Siegel-Sadewitz VL, Amato J, Goldberg RB. Anomalies associated with cleft lip, cleft palate or both. *Am J Med Genet* 1985;**20**:585–596.

Simion C, Corcoran J, Iyer A, Suresh S. Post-operative pain control for primary cleft lip repair in infants: is there an advantage in performing peripheral nerve blocks? *Ped Anes* 2008;**18**:1060–5.

Sommerlad BC. Management of cleft lip and palate. *Curr Paediatr* 1994;**4**:189–95.

Xue FS, Zhang GH, Li P *et al.* The clinical observation of difficult laryngoscopy and difficult intubation in infants with cleft lip and palate. *Ped Anes* 2006;**16**:283–9.

Anaesthesia for dental and maxillofacial surgery in children

Lola Adewale

Introduction

Commonly performed dental and maxillofacial surgical procedures in children include:

- Dental extractions
- Dental restorations
- Dental exposure and bonding
- Alveolar bone grafts

These will all be considered in more detail below, together with the management of dentofacial infection and maxillofacial trauma in children. Although sedation and local anaesthetic techniques have been used successfully for dental procedures in children, there will always be a requirement for general anaesthesia for dental and maxillofacial surgery. Many of these procedures are performed as either day-case or outpatient procedures, although in some cases inpatient care may be required. The process of general anaesthesia involves pre-operative assessment, patient preparation, intra-operative management and post-operative care, including the provision of adequate analgesia.

Local anaesthetic techniques are often used to supplement post-operative analgesia and will be outlined at the end of this chapter.

General principles

Assessment of patients prior to general anaesthesia may occur during a separate hospital visit, although in many centres this takes place on the day of planned surgery.

- Parents and carers should be informed of the risks of general anaesthesia and offered alternative treatment where indicated. Written consent should also be taken for the procedure.
- Pre-operative assessment involves obtaining a comprehensive medical history, performing a physical examination and reviewing the results of appropriate clinical investigations.
- The involvement of play therapists and child psychologists may also be considered at this stage since, in some cases, such preparation may obviate the need for general anaesthesia.
- Management strategies for the uncooperative child should be clarified pre-operatively.
- In all cases the child should be adequately starved.
- Applying a topical local anaesthetic cream makes intravenous cannulation easier, and sedative oral pre-medication may also be indicated in some children.

The availability of anaesthetic and resuscitation equipment should comply with national guidelines, such as those published by the Association of Anaesthetists of Great Britain and Ireland. Similar guidelines exist for the use of peri-operative monitoring.

Induction of anaesthesia may be achieved using either the intravenous or inhalational method, with intravenous access obtained at the earliest possible opportunity. Intra-operatively, the main considerations are maintenance of the airway whilst allowing adequate surgical access. The potential presence of blood or debris in the pharynx should also be considered. The airway device employed is usually determined by the procedure to be performed and ranges from a nasal mask or laryngeal mask airway (LMA) to either an oral or nasal tracheal tube.

Throat packs are often indicated and must be removed at the end of the procedure, before the child's emergence from anaesthesia. Recent guidelines advise that both visual and documented evidence should be provided whenever a throat pack is inserted. A clearly established procedure should also be in place to ensure that the throat pack is always removed.

Core Topics in Paediatric Anaesthesia, ed. Ian James and Isabeau Walker. Published by Cambridge University Press. © 2013 Cambridge University Press.

Adequate peri-operative analgesia should always be administered, with antiemetic agents as indicated.

At the end of the procedure, suction to the oropharynx should be performed under direct vision where possible. The patient should then be placed in the left lateral position unless this is contraindicated. In the period immediately following general anaesthesia for dental or maxillofacial surgery, the child should be managed in the post-anaesthetic care unit by a designated member of staff who is trained in both basic and advanced paediatric resuscitation techniques. Supplemental oxygen should be administered until the child is fully awake.

Paediatric dental patients may suffer from conditions that have major anaesthetic implications, such as cardiac disease or epidermolysis bullosa. These will require appropriate modifications to the anaesthetic technique employed.

Antibacterial prophylaxis and chlorhexidine mouthwash are no longer recommended for the prevention of endocarditis in patients with cardiac disease.

The complications of general anaesthesia for dental and maxillofacial surgery may be minor or major. Minor complications include:

- Post-operative headache, nausea, retching and vomiting, with the latter occurring particularly in association with swallowed blood;
- Damage to teeth or soft tissues adjacent to the operative site;
- Injury to the neck as a result of intra-operative positioning;
- Post-operative cough and sore throat following tracheal intubation or as a result of irritation from the throat pack.

Major complications include complete respiratory obstruction from inhalation of foreign material or cardiac arrest secondary to arrhythmias. Isolated ventricular extrasystoles are known to be associated with dental extractions.

Dental extractions

When complete, the primary dentition consists of 20 teeth, whereas there are 32 permanent teeth. The most commonly used dental identification system divides the dental arch into four quadrants. All primary central incisors are designated tooth 'A' and followed posteriorly in alphabetical order so that all primary second molars are designated tooth 'E'. All permanent central incisors are designated tooth '1' and are followed posteriorly in numerical order to tooth '8', which is the third molar or 'wisdom tooth'.

Dental extractions are commonly required in children who suffer from dental caries or trauma, as well as those who undergo orthodontic treatment regimes. The main indications for general anaesthesia for dental extractions in children are:

- Contraindication to local anaesthesia
- Previous failure of local anaesthesia or sedation
- Lack of patient cooperation owing to immaturity, disability or language difficulties
- Presence of psychological disorders
- Diagnosis of advanced decay
- Requirement for multiple extractions

Recent guidance has recommended that all paediatric dental patients referred for general anaesthesia should be assessed by dental practitioners who are skilled and trained in the treatment of children.

Most dental extractions in children are performed as either day-case or outpatient procedures. The general principles of day-case anaesthesia should apply for both these patient groups; however, outpatient general anaesthesia requires additional consideration and meticulous patient selection. Conditions requiring special consideration include coagulation disorders or anticoagulant therapy, syndromes associated with increased anaesthetic risk, a family history of abnormal response to general anaesthesia, haemoglobinopathies and severe behavioural abnormalities.

Premedication with local anaesthetic cream may be useful when intravenous induction of anaesthesia is planned. Pre-operative oral analgesia is commonly prescribed (usually paracetamol and/or ibuprofen). Despite the risks of prolonging the recovery period, oral midazolam may also be required for some children. Physical intervention in the management of an uncooperative child is considered to be a major infringement of the individual's right to liberty. It is therefore important that the rules governing such an intervention are clearly understood by members of staff working in this area.

Induction of general anaesthesia is commonly achieved intravenously using propofol, or via the inhalational route using sevoflurane. Regardless of the method of induction, intravenous access should be considered in all cases and obtained at the earliest opportunity. Anaesthesia may then be maintained using sevoflurane or propofol. A nasal mask (Figure 24.1) is commonly employed to maintain the airway intra-operatively, but a laryngeal mask airway may facilitate the procedure in some circumstances. Tracheal intubation is sometimes performed for day-case or inpatient procedures, particularly in patients with special needs who may require extensive treatment.

Controversy exists over the ideal intra-operative position for a patient undergoing dental extractions.

- The supine position is the most familiar position for many anaesthetists. The advantages of this position are unimpeded venous return from the lower limbs with better maintenance of cardiac output and blood pressure. The disadvantages are an increase in the work of breathing during spontaneous ventilation, and the risk that fluid and solid debris may fall backwards into the oropharynx.
- The sitting position tends to be more familiar for many dentists. In this position blood or debris is generally thought to gravitate to the anterior part of the oral cavity, facilitating removal by suction apparatus and thus reducing contamination of the oropharynx and larynx. It is also thought that regurgitation and aspiration may be less common in this position. The main disadvantage during general anaesthesia and surgery is a decrease in venous return from the lower part of the body, potentially leading to a reduction in cardiac output.
- The reclining position has been suggested as a compromise.

During general anaesthesia in the sitting position, the postural reflexes controlling the position of the head are abolished, so the anaesthetist must support and fix the head during dental extractions. If the weight of the head is taken by the dental chair or trolley in a reclining position, less physical effort is required to maintain stability of the head and neck. This facilitates correct positioning of a nasal mask without impinging on the nares, as well as the application of a jaw thrust to maintain airway patency. A mouth gag or prop is generally positioned under direct vision, with the airway then protected using a carefully positioned throat pack. The latter discourages mouth breathing, thus allowing a nasal mask to be used for maintenance of anaesthesia. The use of efficient suctioning apparatus is also essential for protection of the airway intra-operatively.

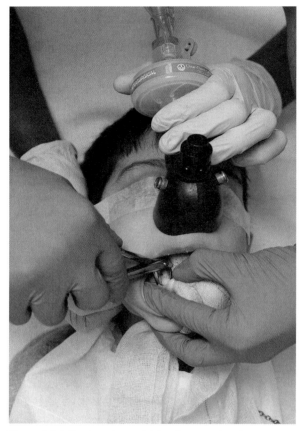

Figure 24.1 Nasal mask in a child undergoing dental extraction.

Common complications related to general anaesthesia for dental extractions include airway obstruction due to the position of the throat pack or mouth prop, or the presence of blood or debris. Dislocation of the temporomandibular joint may also occur.

Despite the fact that halothane is no longer used for dental general anaesthesia, cardiac arrhythmias may still occur intra-operatively and are thought to be related to high levels of circulating catecholamines and stimulation of the trigeminal nerve. The use of local anaesthetic agents containing adrenaline may also be a contributing factor. The latter are usually administered by the dental practitioner and may be injected into the buccal fold of the gum adjacent to the tooth to be treated. Lingual and mental nerve blocks may also be performed intra-orally to provide more extensive anaesthesia to the lower incisors. Infraorbital nerve blockade will anaesthetise the upper jaw.

Additional oral analgesia may be required prior to the patient being discharged home. Opioid analgesics and antiemetics are not routinely required following uncomplicated dental extractions.

Dental restorations

Restorative dental treatment is performed in children to limit or repair the damage caused by dental caries. Such procedures are often performed in children with special needs, who may require extensive treatment necessitating tracheal intubation via the nasal route. This provides unobstructed access to all four quadrants of the mouth and also facilitates the assessment of tooth alignment and occlusion.

Dental exposure and bonding

Palatal impaction of maxillary canine teeth is a problem that is frequently encountered in paediatric orthodontic clinical practice. A commonly adopted treatment strategy is surgical exposure of the impacted tooth, followed by bonding of an orthodontic bracket with a miniature gold chain attached to it. A rubber band will then be attached to the chain to institute a gentle eruptive pulling force on the impacted tooth.

In children, the surgery usually occurs under general anaesthesia, most commonly as a day-case procedure. The general principles of day-case general anaesthesia apply, with the additional considerations of managing the airway while allowing adequate surgical access.

Tracheal intubation is usually required, most commonly via the oral route, with the possibility of direct laryngoscopy being complicated by irregularly spaced dentition. A pre-formed south-facing oral tracheal tube (RAE tube) is useful. Flexible laryngeal masks have also been employed successfully for this procedure. A throat pack is required to protect the airway from soiling.

- Before commencing the procedure, the dental surgeon will usually infiltrate an adrenaline-containing local anaesthetic solution, which improves haemostasis and also contributes to post-operative analgesia.
- An adequate analgesic regimen is usually provided by paracetamol administered either pre-operatively via the oral route or intra-operatively via the intravenous route, together with a non-steroidal anti-inflammatory agent administered in the post-operative period.
- Opioid analgesics are rarely required, although antiemetic therapy may be indicated depending on the individual child concerned.

Alveolar bone grafts

Surgical repair of a cleft lip or palate in infancy does not usually involve correction of the alveolar cleft defect. This may result in residual oronasal fistulae with disruption of the maxillary alveolus. Alveolar cleft bone grafts unite the alveolar segments and help to prevent collapse and constriction of the dental arch. Support is then provided for teeth adjacent to the cleft and for those that will erupt into the area of the cleft. The graft also leads to closure of the oronasal fistula, augmentation of the alveolar ridge, and the creation of a solid foundation for the lip and alar base of the nose.

The alveolar cleft graft is usually performed as an inpatient procedure when the child is between the ages of 6 and 10 years. General anaesthesia is induced via either the intravenous or inhalation route, with tracheal intubation using an oral pre-formed south-facing (RAE) tube. Bone is then removed from the patient's iliac crest and placed in the alveolar cleft. The surgical procedure is associated with a small risk of bleeding and requires adequate intravenous access with the administration of intravenous fluids perioperatively.

- Remifentanil is useful to maintain haemodynamic stability, and if used, the administration of other intra-operative opioids is rarely required.
- Dexamethasone and ondansetron are usually administered, together with antibiotics as indicated.
- Post-operative analgesia is provided by intravenous paracetamol together with the administration of local anaesthetic solution to the donor site.
- Post-operative analgesia may be enhanced if a catheter is placed by the surgeon into the iliac wound site and used post-operatively for the intermittent or continuous administration of local anaesthetic solution.

Management of dentofacial infection

Dentofacial infection may be either acute or chronic. Acute infection usually presents as an emergency with pain, pyrexia and often a red, swollen face. Chronic infection may present as a buccal sinus or a mobile tooth. The management of dentofacial infection involves removal of the cause, together with local drainage and debridement intra-orally or extra-orally as required.

Dental abscesses are usually localised, but cellulitis and oedema may occur because of spread of infection via lymphatics and tissue planes. Limited mouth opening may be caused by pain or spasm (trismus) of the masseter or pterygoid muscles. Pus may also be present within the airway.

The anaesthetic considerations are as for dental extractions. Antisialagogue agents administered at induction are sometimes useful to control excessive secretions. If problems with the airway are anticipated, an anaesthetic technique that maintains spontaneous ventilation should be employed. It is usually possible to achieve adequate mouth opening after induction of anaesthesia; occasionally, however, fibre-optic tracheal intubation is required.

Maxillofacial trauma

Facial trauma in very young children is commonly the result of falls or accidents, but children may also be victims of assault or road traffic collisions. It is important to recognise and report any suspicion of non-accidental injury. Blunt trauma tends to cause greater damage to the soft tissues and supporting structures, whereas high-velocity or sharp injuries cause luxations and fractures of the teeth.

General anaesthesia is often required for the suturing of facial lacerations and the management of maxillofacial fractures. Consideration should be given to the possibility of associated injuries that may involve the head, neck, chest and spinal cord. There is also the potential for airway obstruction, aspiration of gastric contents and intra-oral haemorrhage.

Management of maxillofacial fractures may involve long surgical procedures that are sometimes associated with significant blood loss. There is also a risk of bradycardia due to the oculocardiac reflex. Fractures of the zygomatic arch are associated with limited mouth opening. Maxillary fractures are often even more serious and are associated with significant head injury (Table 24.1).

The reduction of nasal fractures is often a very quick procedure. A laryngeal mask airway is commonly used, but the risk of epistaxis may necessitate tracheal intubation together with the insertion of a throat pack.

Table 24.1 Classification of midfacial fractures

Fracture	Type of injury
Le Fort I	Fracture separating inferior portion of maxilla horizontally, extending from piriform aperture of nose to pterygoid maxillary suture area
Le Fort II	Fracture involving separation of maxilla and nasal complex from cranial base, zygomatic orbital rim area, and pterygoid maxillary suture area
Le Fort III	Complete separation of midface at level of naso-orbital ethmoid complex and zygomaticofrontal suture area. Fracture extends through orbits bilaterally

Local anaesthesia in paediatric dentistry

Local anaesthesia (LA) may be used to supplement general anaesthesia for dental and maxillofacial surgery in children. This is usually administered by the dental surgeon, the agents most commonly used being lidocaine 2% with adrenaline 1:80 000, or prilocaine 3% with felypressin (octapressin). The techniques for providing LA in children are similar to those used in adults. However, owing to the reduced bone density of the maxilla and mandible in children, there is more rapid diffusion and absorption of LA solution with a faster onset and shorter duration of block.

The upper teeth receive their sensory nerve supply from the superior alveolar (dental) nerves, which are branches of the maxillary division of the trigeminal nerve. The peripheral fibres of these nerves can be blocked effectively at the apical foramina of the tooth by injection of local anaesthetic into the sulcus adjacent to the tooth requiring anaesthesia. The infra-orbital nerve, a terminal branch of the maxillary nerve, can be blocked at the infra-orbital foramen which lies just below the inferior orbital margin, approximately halfway along its length. It can be reached from the upper labial sulcus opposite the canine tooth. The block will also include branches of the anterior superior alveolar nerve and will provide anaesthesia to the anterior maxilla and upper lip. The buccal and labial soft tissues are anaesthetised by LA infiltration to these areas. Anaesthesia of the hard and soft palate requires injection directly into the palate.

The lower teeth receive their sensory nerve supply from the inferior alveolar (dental) nerve, a branch of the mandibular division of the trigeminal nerve. This may be blocked before it enters the mandibular foramen on the medial aspect of the ramus, just behind the lingula, providing anaesthesia to the bone of the mandibular body and the pulps of the lower teeth on that side of the mouth. There may be incomplete anaesthesia of the central incisor as there may be some crossover supply from the contralateral inferior dental nerve. The mental nerve can be blocked at the mental foramen, providing anaesthesia to the soft tissues of the labial gingivae, the lower lip and chin. Diffusion of anaesthetic agent via the mental foramen will reach the incisive branch which supplies the pulps of the lower first premolar, canine and incisor teeth. There is some communication with the nerve supply on the opposite side. A periodontal ligament injection may be necessary in older children to achieve adequate anaesthesia of a single mandibular tooth.

As with any use of local anaesthetic agents, the possibility of LA toxicity due to accidental intravascular injection should be anticipated. Convulsions, cardiac arrhythmias and hypotension may occur. All members of staff should be aware of the management protocol for LA toxicity, including the availability of intravenous lipid emulsion solution (see also Chapter 16). Tachycardia and arrhythmias may also be associated with adrenaline-containing solutions. Hypersensitivity reactions to local anaesthetics are very rare, although allergic reactions to preservative agents have been described.

Key points

- Adequate pre-operative assessment and patient preparation is necessary, particularly prior to outpatient general anaesthesia.
- Management of the airway requires careful consideration and may present specific problems if the patient is managed in the sitting position.
- A throat pack is required for most procedures and must always be removed after the surgical procedure.
- Local anaesthetic techniques may contribute to the provision of adequate post-operative analgesia.

Further reading

Association of Anaesthetists of Great Britain and Ireland. *Recommendations for Standards of Monitoring during Anaesthesia and Recovery*, 4th edition. 2007.

Association of Paediatric Anaesthetists of Great Britain & Ireland. *Guidelines for the Management of Children Referred for Dental Extractions under General Anaesthesia*. 2011.

Nunn J, Foster M *et al.* British Society of Paediatric Dentistry: a policy document on consent and the use of physical intervention in the dental care of children. *Int J Paed Dentistry* 2008; **18**(Suppl. 1):39–46.

Ouaki J, Dadure C *et al.* continuous infusion of ropivacaine: an optimal post-operative analgesia regimen for iliac crest bone graft in children. *Ped Anes* 2009; **19**:887–91.

Robinson PD, Pitt Ford TR, McDonald F. *Local Anaesthesia in Dentistry*. Elsevier Science Ltd. 2003;31–80.

Royal College of Anaesthetists. *Standards & Guidelines for General Anaesthesia for Dentistry*. 1999.

Tochel C, Hosey M-T *et al.* Assessment of children prior to dental extractions under general anaesthesia in Scotland. *Br Dent J* 2004; **196**:629–33.

Chapter

25

Anaesthesia for craniofacial surgery in children

David de Beer

Introduction

Craniofacial surgery is concerned with the management of patients presenting with congenital or acquired conditions that affect the hard and soft tissues of the head and face. A broad spectrum of patients with a wide variety of craniofacial anomalies may present for surgery, ranging from infants and children with single suture craniosynostosis to syndromic children with complex multisutural craniofacial dysostoses, orbital dysostoses, encephalocoeles and craniofacial clefts (Figure 25.1). The surgery is complex and often protracted, and although the incidence of serious complications is fortunately very low the risk is never zero.

Successful peri-operative management of these patients depends on careful pre-operative assessment, meticulous intra-operative planning in collaboration with the surgical team, anticipation and prompt treatment of intra-operative complications and a high level of post-operative care. This is best achieved within the multidisciplinary setting of specialist craniofacial units.

Classification of craniosynostosis

Craniosynostosis results from the premature fusion of one or more of the major cranial sutures and occurs in approximately 1:2500 births. It can be divided into two groups, non-syndromic or syndromic synostosis. Non-syndromic (simple) synostosis is more common than its syndromic counterpart and typically involves the premature fusion of a single suture (sagittal, coronal, metopic and rarely unilateral lambdoid). Occasionally two sutures may be involved as in non-syndromic bicoronal synostosis. The resulting skull

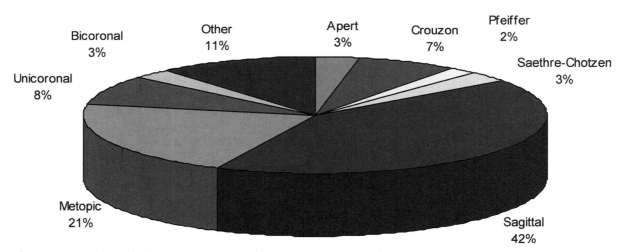

Figure 25.1 Distribution by diagnosis amongst 122 children undergoing cranial vault surgery (GOSH 2008–2009). See plate section for colour version.

Core Topics in Paediatric Anaesthesia, ed. Ian James and Isabeau Walker. Published by Cambridge University Press. © 2013 Cambridge University Press.

deformity depends on the suture involved and is primarily cosmetic in nature (Figure 25.2).

Syndromic (multisutural) craniosynostosis affects both the skull vault and facial skeleton. Involvement of the facial skeleton may result in functional problems such as raised intracranial pressure, upper airway obstruction secondary to midface hypoplasia, exorbitism, feeding difficulties and behavioural or psychological problems. There are a number of craniofacial-associated syndromes or dysostoses, the most common ones being:

- Crouzon syndrome
- Apert syndrome
- Pfeiffer syndrome
- Saethre–Chotzen syndrome
- Carpenter and Muenke syndromes (less frequently encountered).

Surgical procedures for these conditions can be classified according to the region of the craniofacial skeleton that they address as well as the degree of complexity (Table 25.1). The optimum timing for reconstructive surgery varies between different surgeons and craniofacial units. In order to achieve lasting results, definitive surgery should ideally be delayed until the period of maximum growth for the affected area is over. However, earlier surgical intervention may be required in order to treat an urgent functional problem such as raised intracranial pressure, exorbitism or airway obstruction. Consideration should also be given to the potential psychological impact that the deformity may have on an individual child. Waiting for the 'ideal' time to perform reconstructive surgery may not be acceptable to a child or their parents, thereby necessitating earlier treatment.

Table 25.1 Classification of craniofacial procedures

Major surgery

Cranial vault/ forehead

- Fronto-orbital remodelling for metopic and coronal synostosis
- Anterior–posterior shortening with barrel staving osteotomies (<6 months) or total calvarial remodelling for sagittal synostosis
- Posterior vault expansion for lambdoid synostosis

Subcranial/facial

- Le Fort osteotomies (commonly Le Fort I and III)
- Subcranial hypertelorism correction

Complex major surgery

Craniofacial

- Monobloc frontofacial advancement for anterior–posterior and vertical anomalies
- Frontofacial bipartition for three-dimensional anomalies of the skull, face and orbits
- Orbital box osteotomy for lateral or vertical orbital anomalies

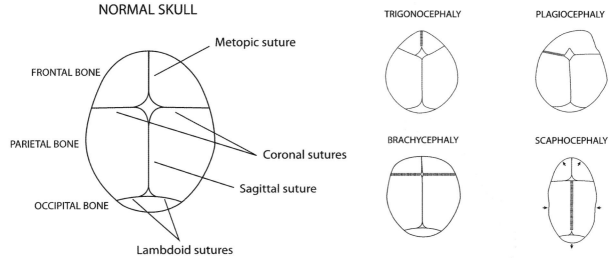

Figure 25.2 Skull deformity based on suture involved.

Pre-operative assessment

Two groups of patients present for craniofacial surgery: non-syndromic children with simple craniosynostosis and syndromic children with craniofacial dysostosis. A thorough pre-operative assessment is essential with particular emphasis being placed on a detailed airway assessment. Pre-operative investigations should be tailored to the patient's clinical status and the proposed surgical procedure. As a minimum, baseline haematological and biochemical tests should be performed. More specific investigations may need to be performed in patients with syndromic craniosynostosis, including sleep studies, visual evoked potentials (a pathological pattern may precede papilloedema or other signs of raised intracranial pressure) and ENT assessment. Blood should also be cross-matched; two units of packed red cells are usually adequate for major procedures while four to six units should be cross-matched for complex major procedures.

Airway assessment

Children with craniofacial dysostoses commonly have some degree of supraglottic airway obstruction secondary to maxillary hypoplasia. This ranges from mild nasal obstruction to severe obstructive sleep apnoea, which occurs in almost half of cases. In patients with moderate to severe symptoms, a pre-operative sleep study should be performed. Treatment of symptomatic airway obstruction may include the use of nasal prong airways, adenotonsillectomy, uvulopharyngo-palatoplasty, nasal continuous positive airway pressure (CPAP) or in the most severe cases tracheostomy pending monobloc frontofacial advancement.

It is important to recognise that a child's physical appearance may not necessarily be a good guide to predicting potential difficulty with laryngoscopy. Although children with maxillary hypoplasia may look abnormal they rarely present any difficulty at laryngoscopy. However, children who look relatively normal following corrective surgery may in fact be very difficult to intubate as a result of maxillary advancement and reduced temporomandibular joint movement. The presence of a rigid external distraction (RED) device (Figure 25.3) should also be noted as it may make laryngoscopy awkward if not impossible.

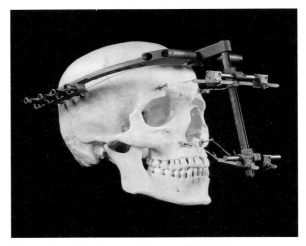

Figure 25.3 A rigid external distractor (RED) *in situ.*

Indications for tracheostomy

While a tracheostomy may be required in a minority of patients, it is best avoided if possible owing to the associated increased risk of surgical infection and potential difficulty with subsequent decannulation. The decision to perform a tracheostomy should be made on an individual patient basis following consultation among members of the surgical team, anaesthetist, parents and patient if appropriate.

Indications for a tracheostomy include:

- Severe and deteriorating upper airway obstruction, including life-threatening obstructive sleep apnoea;
- Patients less than 1 year of age undergoing frontofacial monobloc advancement;
- Children undergoing extensive facial osteotomies in whom re-intubation may be difficult.

When a decision is made to perform a tracheostomy, it is best done as a separate procedure at least 2 weeks prior to scheduled craniofacial surgery. This not only ensures a well-formed tracheostome at the time of definitive surgery but also avoids the potential problem of an occult pneumothorax resulting from the tracheostomy progressing to a tension pneumothorax with positive pressure ventilation. A minority of patients with a history of significant airway obstruction and obstructive sleep apnoea may present for surgery with a tracheostomy *in situ.*

Premedication

If intravenous induction of anaesthesia is planned, a topical anaesthetic cream should be applied pre-operatively to potential cannulation sites so as to ensure pain free cannulation. Patients who are anxious or those with significant behavioural problems may benefit from pre-operative psychological preparation with or without a sedative premedication. Extreme caution should be exercised when using sedative pre-medication in children with airway obstruction or raised intracranial pressure.

Antiembolism compression stockings (TEDS) should be considered in the older teenager undergoing prolonged complex major surgery.

Conduct of anaesthesia

Induction

Induction of anaesthesia may be achieved using either an inhalational or intravenous technique. The technique chosen will depend on the patient's, parents' and anaesthetist's preference as well as on the presence of potential airway or venous access difficulties. Prior to induction of anaesthesia, standard monitoring should be applied with a pulse oximeter being an absolute minimum.

Airway management

Following induction of anaesthesia, maintenance of a good airway may be challenging as a result of sub-optimal facemask seal secondary to facial asymmetry, maxillary hypoplasia or exorbitism. A soft-seal face-mask, rotated through 180° if necessary, with simple airway manoeuvres and adjuncts and a high fresh gas flow usually allows adequate mask ventilation. In addition, application of continuous pressure via the facemask helps to alleviate upper airway obstruction which is common in children with midface hypoplasia.

Once the ability to ventilate the patient has been confirmed, a muscle relaxant can be administered and the airway secured with a tracheal tube. Difficult laryngoscopy is unusual in patients with midface hypoplasia although children who have previously undergone corrective surgery may prove difficult to intubate. A full range of intubation equipment, including a laryngeal mask airway, should be readily available in theatre.

The choice of tracheal tube will depend on the type of surgery. A preformed south-facing RAE oro-tracheal tube is ideal for patients undergoing surgery in the supine 'head-up' tilt position. For those undergoing surgery in the prone position, a reinforced oral tracheal tube with secure facial strapping is more appropriate. Where intra-oral surgical access is required either a nasal or, more commonly, a reinforced oral tracheal tube secured with a circum-mandibular wire is used. A cuffed tracheal tube is frequently used in children over 6 years of age. Optimal tracheal tube position may best be achieved by initial endobronchial intubation followed by withdrawal of the tube until breath sounds are heard bilaterally. Patients presenting for surgery with a tracheostomy *in situ* should have the tracheostome intubated with a reinforced tube which is then sutured to the anterior chest wall.

Intravascular access

Adequate intravenous access is achieved by siting two large bore cannulae. This may be difficult in syndromic patients with syndactyly or other limb abnormalities. The long saphenous vein is a particularly useful vessel as it allows cannulation with a relatively wide bore cannula that is easily accessible intra-operatively. All children undergoing major cranio-facial surgery should have an arterial line placed to facilitate continuous arterial blood pressure monitoring and serial measurement of haemoglobin and blood gases. A femoral central venous line may be useful in patients undergoing more prolonged major surgery.

It is usual to provide antibiotic cover at induction, with anaerobic cover being important for intra-oral procedures. Local policies generally dictate the choice of antibiotics.

Maintenance

Maintenance of anaesthesia is achieved using a balanced technique involving a volatile inhalational agent such as isoflurane or sevoflurane delivered in a mixture of oxygen in air, with either fentanyl, up to 10 mcg kg^{-1}, or a remifentanil infusion for analgesia. A total intravenous technique using propofol may be considered in the older child. In addition to an intravenous opioid, multimodal analgesia includes pre-operative tumescent infiltration of a solution containing triamcinolone acetate, lidocaine, levobupivacaine, hyaluronidase and adrenaline $(7 \, \text{ml kg}^{-1})$ and the administration of intravenous paracetamol. Intravenous morphine up to $100 \, \text{mcg kg}^{-1}$ is titrated towards the end of surgery, particularly if remifentanil has been used intra-operatively.

Intra-operative monitoring and patient positioning

Standard monitoring includes oxygen saturation, end-tidal carbon dioxide, ECG, invasive blood pressure, central and peripheral temperature and peripheral nerve function. Measurement of central venous pressure may be useful in patients undergoing prolonged major or complex major surgery. Maintenance of normothermia is essential and may be achieved using a forced air-warming blanket and fluid warming device with careful temperature monitoring so as to avoid the risks of inadvertent hyperthermia.

As the duration of surgery may exceed 6 hours, meticulous attention should be paid to patient positioning.

- For most craniofacial procedures a supine 'head-up' tilt position is adopted.
- Prone positioning of the patient is used for posterior vault expansion, anterior–posterior shortening procedures and total calvarial remodelling.
- In all cases, pressure points should be adequately padded in order to avoid cutaneous or peripheral nerve injury.
- The eyes should be well lubricated and adequately protected. This may be difficult in patients with marked exorbitism in whom suturing of the palpebral fissures is often required.
- It is also important to ensure that the abdomen is free when in the prone position to facilitate unrestricted diaphragmatic movement with ventilation and to avoid venous congestion.
- Cerebral venous congestion may be reduced further by adopting a 'head-up' position.

Management of blood loss

Extensive blood loss and major transfusion is often unavoidable and remains the greatest risk to infants and children undergoing major craniofacial surgery. Haemorrhage may arise from the extensive scalp incision, bone edges or less commonly from sinus and extradural venous tears. While the intra-operative blood loss may easily exceed a child's estimated blood volume, accurate assessment of this loss is frequently difficult. This is due to blood loss onto the surgical drapes and gowns as well as dilution by irrigation fluid used for the surgical power tools.

Intravascular volume replacement and transfusion requirements must therefore be guided by careful monitoring of the following:

- Vital signs: heart rate, blood pressure, arterial waveform, capillary refill time, core–peripheral temperature gradient, central venous pressure (CVP) and urine output;
- Acid–base status;
- Haemoglobin concentration and haematocrit;
- Coagulation parameters and platelet count.

The goals of fluid management are to maintain a normal circulating volume, an appropriate haemoglobin concentration, normal electrolyte balance and normoglycaemia. Of paramount importance is the avoidance of hypovolaemia and maintenance of adequate organ perfusion. This is achieved by meticulously matching transfusion volumes to blood loss using a combination of a balanced salt solution, colloid solution and packed red cells as required. As the fluid dynamics may change very rapidly, a proactive approach should be adopted with blood being transfused early. It is the author's practice to use a colloid solution after approximately 20–$30 \, \text{ml kg}^{-1}$ of crystalloid have been administered and thereafter a combination of blood and colloid to maintain an acceptable haemoglobin concentration ($7 \, \text{g dl}^{-1}$ is considered adequate in a haemodynamically stable child). As large volumes of fluid are being transfused relatively quickly it is important that all fluids are warmed before infusion. Transfusion practice may also depend to some extent on the experience of the anaesthetist. Note that while anaesthetists tend to underestimate blood loss, the risks of over-transfusion still remain, particularly in infants and young children.

Reducing allogeneic blood transfusion

Although donor blood is extensively tested and monitored, it is not without risk from viruses, reactions or the incorrect blood being transfused. Furthermore, the complications associated with the massive transfusion of allogeneic blood, including metabolic acidosis, hyperkalaemia, hypocalcaemia and coagulopathy, may cause significant morbidity. Strategies should therefore be employed to reduce or even avoid the use of allogeneic blood.

Pre-operative measures

- Iron supplements should be used in patients with iron deficiency anaemia.
- Recombinant erythropoietin therapy. Although pre-operative elevation of haemoglobin with erythropoietin has been shown to reduce transfusion requirements in children undergoing craniofacial surgery, an unfavourable cost–benefit ratio limits its usefulness.
- Pre-operative autologous blood donation is not used routinely in children in the United Kingdom.

Intra-operative measures

- Patient positioning ('head-up tilt');
- Scalp infiltration with an adrenaline-containing tumescent solution;
- Meticulous surgical technique;
- Induced hypotension may be beneficial in the older child undergoing midfacial advancement. There are a number of agents that may be used to achieve moderate intra-operative hypotension, a commonly used combination being remifentanil and clonidine. The use of induced hypotension in infants and young children undergoing craniosynostosis repair is controversial and is not practised at the author's institution.
- Acute normovolaemic haemodilution is limited by the child's relatively small circulating blood volume and so has limited value.
- Antifibrinolytic agents such as tranexamic acid may be employed but are not routinely used at the author's institution.
- Intra-operative cell salvage. This can be a safe and effective means of reducing intraoperative allogeneic blood use. The newer blood salvage machines have relatively fast processing times and low processing volumes and provide a continuous supply of washed red cells in proportion to the rate at which the patient is bleeding. Despite this, cell salvage alone is unable to cope with the rapid and massive volume replacement requirements of infants undergoing craniofacial surgery. The overall efficacy of red cell recovery by cell salvage is dependent on the ability to recover the blood lost in a usable form. This comprises suction

losses as well as blood loss to surgical swabs, the latter of which can account for between 30 and 50% of the total blood lost. Washing the blood-soaked swabs in a normal saline/heparin solution has been found to favourably increase the amount of recoverable blood.

Post-operative measures

- Lowering the transfusion threshold in otherwise healthy children (currently $7.0 \, g \, dl^{-1}$ at the author's institution);
- Iron supplements. Oral iron therapy should be given to children with low haemoglobin;
- Post-operative cell salvage involves the collection of blood from surgical drains followed by re-infusion, with or without a wash cycle. Although there have been concerns about the safety of transfusing unwashed red cells, post-operative cell salvage is commonly used in orthopaedic surgery. Despite the potential benefits, post-operative cell salvage is not used for craniofacial surgery in the United Kingdom.

Management of dilutional coagulopathy

Dilutional coagulopathy occurs commonly in patients undergoing craniofacial surgery. It is the author's practice to administer fresh frozen plasma ($10–15 \, ml \, kg^{-1}$) intra-operatively once the patient has lost approximately one estimated circulating blood volume. Thereafter the need for further fresh frozen plasma is based on clinical evaluation, the magnitude of drain losses and serial measurement of the coagulation profile. As fresh frozen plasma is deficient in fibrinogen and factor VIII, cryoprecipitate ($5–10 \, ml \, kg^{-1}$) may be required if blood loss persists in the presence of a low fibrinogen level ($<0.8 \, g \, l^{-1}$).

Platelets are rarely required in patients undergoing major surgery although they may be necessary following the massive blood loss associated with complex major surgery. While platelets ($10 \, ml \, kg^{-1}$) are generally given in response to a demonstrable thrombocytopenia ($<50 \times 10^9 \, l^{-1}$), they may be given empirically once a patient has lost more than twice their estimated circulating blood volume.

Intra-operative complications

Intra-operative complications are fortunately uncommon but may include the following:

- Accidental extubation, endobronchial intubation or severing of the pilot tube.
- Acute bradycardia secondary to the oculocardiac reflex. This may occur in response to orbital manipulation and responds in the majority of cases to immediate cessation of the stimulus. Occasionally a vagolytic such as glycopyrrolate or atropine may be required.
- Venous air embolism (VAE). As patients are in a 'head-up' position they are at increased risk for VAE. At the author's institution capnography is used to monitor for clinically significant VAE.
- Sudden major blood loss resulting in hypotension. This responds to fluid resuscitation in the majority of cases although a vasopressor may occasionally be required.
- Significant metabolic acidosis. Children undergoing craniofacial surgery may develop a varying degree of intra-operative metabolic acidosis as measured by the base deficit. This occurs despite the patient being haemodynamically stable and clinically well perfused and is most likely due to the infusion of acidic fluids resulting in hyperchloraemic acidosis.

Post-operative care

The majority of children can be extubated at the end of surgery. Following a period of stabilisation on the recovery ward, further post-operative care is provided on the neurosurgical high-dependency unit where invasive monitoring is continued. Admission of a patient to the intensive care unit for mechanical ventilation is uncommon at the author's institution but may occasionally be required in the event of an unexpected or significant intra-operative complication.

Bilateral nasopharyngeal airways are routinely used in children at risk of post-operative upper airway obstruction following complex major surgery. They may remain *in situ* for up to 5 days or until such time as the oedema has settled.

Frost sutures (between the lower eyelid and eyebrow) may also be used in this group of patients to protect the cornea. In order to reduce the potential for continuing facial oedema within the initial 24–48 hour post-operative period, patients are nursed in a 'head-up' position.

Fluid management

As significant fluid losses may continue into the initial post-operative period, meticulous attention should be paid to post-operative fluid management (see Figure 25.4). Haemodynamic parameters, drain losses and coagulation profile should be monitored carefully. A falling haematocrit in association with minimal drain losses should alert one to the possibility of an intracranial haemorrhage. This constitutes an emergency for which an immediate neurosurgical opinion should be sought.

Pain management

It is important that adequate pain control is achieved prior to transfer of a patient to the neurosurgical high-dependency unit. This may involve carefully titrating further doses of intravenous morphine in the recovery ward. Thereafter satisfactory analgesia is achieved in most patients with a combination of regular intravenous paracetamol ($15\,\mathrm{mg\,kg^{-1}}$ 6 hourly), oral morphine ($200\,\mathrm{mcg\,kg^{-1}}$ 4 hourly) on an 'as required basis' and a NSAID such as diclofenac ($1\,\mathrm{mg\,kg^{-1}}$ PO 8 hourly) or ibuprofen ($5\,\mathrm{mg\,kg^{-1}}$ PO 6 hourly) once the clotting profile has normalised.

Post-operative nausea and vomiting is common following craniofacial surgery and an antiemetic such as ondansetron should be administered regularly. Intravenous morphine delivered via a patient- or nurse-controlled analgesia device can also be used but may be associated with an increased incidence of nausea and vomiting and delayed mobilisation of some patients.

Specific craniofacial procedures
Fronto-orbital remodelling

Metopic synostosis produces a characteristic triangular deformity of the frontal bone with lateral forehead deficiency (trigonocephaly). Coronal synostosis may be unilateral or bilateral. Unicoronal synostosis results in flattening of the ipsilateral forehead with bossing of the contralateral side (frontal plagiocephaly). Bicoronal synostosis, which may be syndromic or an isolated abnormality, produces a more spherically shaped head with a wide and flattened forehead (brachycephaly).

Surgical reconstruction for both metopic and coronal synostosis involves fronto-orbital remodelling which entails a bifrontal craniotomy, release of the

Post-operative fluid replacement in children after craniofacial surgery

Figure 25.4 Post-operative fluid replacement in children after craniofacial surgery.

Objectives
- Maintain normal circulating blood volume by continuous assessment and reassessment of fluid balance and replacement with appropriate fluids
- Maintain haemoglobin at an appropriate level
- Maintain normal electrolyte balance and normoglycaemia

Fluid replacement
- Give **maintenance** fluids
- Replace on-going **blood losses** (drain losses, haematoma) with gelofusin and/or packed red cells (see below)

  A falling haemoglobin (Hb) in association with minimal drain losses may indicate an intracranial haematoma which is a neurosurgical emergency. Please ensure that the craniofacial fellow is called immediately

---

MAINTENANCE FLUID
- 2.5% dextrose /0.45% saline
- **Give 50% of full maintenance in recovery and 2/3 once on the ward**

MODERATE BLOOD LOSS (≥ 10 ml kg^{-1} h^{-1})
- Measure losses at **half hourly** intervals and replace at the appropriate **hourly** rate (i.e. if blood loss in first half hour is 25 ml h^{-1}, replace at a rate of 50 ml h^{-1}). Monitor fluid balance hourly in order to avoid over or under transfusion
- Measure Hb after transfusion of each 20 ml kg^{-1} blood
- **Replace with blood or colloid in order to maintain Hb >7 g dl^{-1}**
  (4 ml kg^{-1} packed cells raises Hb by approximately 1 g dl^{-1}. Minimise donor exposure when blood is used by making full use of a unit of blood – transfuse to a Hb of ~ 12 g dl^{-1} and avoid opening a new unit unless necessary)

MAJOR BLOOD LOSS (>10 ml kg^{-1} h^{-1})
If there is major blood loss post-operatively an urgent medical review should be sought. Blood losses should be replaced to maintain normal circulating blood volume and Hb.

- **If Hb 10-12 g dl^{-1}** give blood:colloid 1:1
  i.e. if blood loss 100 ml, give 50 ml blood, 50 ml colloid
- **If Hb >12 g dl^{-1}** give blood:colloid approx 1:2
  i.e. if blood loss 100 ml, give 30 ml blood, 70 ml colloid
- **If Hb <10 g dl^{-1}** give blood: colloid approx 2:1
  i.e. if blood loss 100 ml, give 70 ml blood, 30 ml colloid

Coagulation profile should be checked after each 80 ml kg^{-1} Infusion (i.e. after infusion of estimated blood volume [EBV]) and repeated serially)
- FFP (10 ml kg^{-1}) usually required after rapid transfusion of 1 x EBV
- Platelets (5 ml kg^{-1}) usually required after transfusion of 2 x EBV

NB. The coagulation results should be taken in the context of the clinical status of the patient and should **not** be treated in isolation

---

HYPOVOLAEMIA IS THE MOST COMMON PROBLEM AFTER CRANIOFACIAL SURGERY

Signs	▪ Tachycardia ▪ Delayed capillary refill (>2 seconds) ▪ Cool, mottled peripheries ▪ Hypotension – this is a late sign
Immediate treatment	**Give an immediate bolus of gelofusin (10 ml kg^{-1})** **Reassess and repeat as necessary**

DdB/BB April 2009

affected suture and simultaneous supraorbital and frontal reconstruction. The ideal timing of surgery varies; proponents for early reconstruction (before 12 months of age) claim that greater bony pliability results in a better result while those who prefer to delay surgery until 15 to 18 months of age do so in order to reduce the chance of recurrence.

Anaesthetic implications
- Patient position: supine 'head-up' tilt;
- Surgical approach: coronal incision ('Alice band');
- Surgical duration: 3–4 hours;
- Preformed south-facing RAE orotracheal tube;
- Lacrilube ointment only to eyes (no tape);
- Two peripheral venous cannulae;

- Femoral central venous line recommended;
- Arterial line essential;
- Monitor oropharyngeal/rectal temperature;
- Intra-operative cell salvage may be useful.

Anterior–posterior shortening with barrel staving osteotomies and total calvarial remodelling

Sagittal craniosynostosis is the commonest form of synostosis and results in a skull shape that is typically long and narrow (scaphocephaly). The timing of reconstructive surgery is important in terms of both the nature and extent of the surgical procedure performed. If surgery is performed within 6 months of birth when the cranial bones are still very compliant, an anterior–posterior shortening procedure with barrel staving osteotomies is performed. This relatively short procedure involves a combination of wide sagittal craniectomy with plication of the parietal bones after they have been divided vertically (barrel staving osteotomies) thus allowing lateral expansion of the skull and contraction of the anterior–posterior dimension.

Correction of sagittal synostosis in the older child (≥18 months) involves rearrangement of the calvarium or total calvarial remodelling. This is a more extensive procedure involving reconstruction of at least the anterior two-thirds if not all of the calvarium.

Anaesthetic implications

- Patient position: modified prone position with neck extension;
- Surgical approach: coronal incision;
- Surgical duration: anterior–posterior shortening 2–3 hours, total calvarial remodelling 3–4 hours;
- Reinforced oral tracheal tube with full neurosurgical strapping;
- Two peripheral venous cannulae;
- Femoral central venous line recommended for total calvarial remodelling;
- Arterial line essential;
- Monitor nasopharyngeal temperature;
- Intra-operative cell salvage may be useful for total calvarial remodelling.

Posterior calvarial vault expansion

Unilateral lambdoid synostosis is the least common form of craniosynostosis and produces an asymmetric flattening of the occiput (posterior plagiocephaly). Reconstructive surgery involves the removal and reshaping of a large part of the posterior skull and is commonly performed at 6 months of age or younger.

Anaesthetic implications

The anaesthetic implications and surgical aftercare for posterior vault expansion are as for anterior–posterior shortening.

Spring-assisted surgery (spring cranioplasty)

Dynamic distraction with steel springs is increasingly being used in the management of scaphocephaly and posterior plagiocephaly. Spring-assisted scaphocephaly correction has a number of advantages over traditional surgery including: shorter operating time (~45 min), smaller scar with minimal dural dissection, minimal blood loss with blood transfusion rarely being required, rapid recovery and a shorter hospital stay. Surgery is usually performed between 4 and 6 months of age as the development of frontal bossing in late infancy precludes the use of this technique. Spring-assisted posterior vault expansion is also associated with a shorter operating time (~1.5 h) and hospital stay and reduced blood loss compared with traditional surgery. However, blood transfusion may still be required in this group of patients. A disadvantage of spring-assisted surgery is the requirement for further surgery, albeit relatively minor, to remove the springs.

Anaesthetic implications

The anaesthetic implications and surgical aftercare for spring-assisted surgery are as for traditional surgery apart from the fact that patients undergoing scaphocephaly correction do not usually require invasive monitoring (still recommended for posterior vault expansion) as is the case for spring removal.

Monobloc frontofacial advancement with distraction osteogenesis (RED frame)

Children with Apert, Crouzon and Pfeiffer syndromes often have functional problems including raised intracranial pressure, severe exorbitism with or without subluxation of the globe, upper airway obstruction with severe obstructive sleep apnoea and feeding problems. Monobloc frontofacial advancement allows correction of all these problems in a single procedure.

The operation combines transcranial frontal advance and extracranial Le Fort III midfacial advance with the frontal bones and maxilla being brought forward in one piece either immediately at surgery or more slowly by distraction using a rigid external distractor (RED frame). The RED frame (Figure 25.3) comprises a halo device which is attached to the mobilised facial skeleton through a combination of cranial pins, rods and wires. Distraction at a rate of ~1.5 mm per day is achieved post-operatively by progressively shortening the wires. Once the midface has advanced the required distance and following a consolidation period of 6 weeks the distractor is removed under general anaesthesia.

Since monobloc frontofacial advancement may be associated with high morbidity especially in young infants and children, timing of surgery is crucial. Ideally the procedure should be delayed until skeletal maturity has been achieved at around 12 years of age. However, it may be considered in infants less than 1 year of age if the severity of the functional problems is such that surgery can no longer be delayed.

Anaesthetic implications

- Patient position: supine 'head-up' tilt;
- Surgical approach: combined intra-oral and transcranial (coronal) incisions;
- Surgical duration: 6–8 hours;
- Reinforced oral tracheal tube secured with a circum-mandibular wire (a nasotracheal tube sutured to the septum may also be used). In patients with a tracheostomy, a reinforced tracheal tube is placed via the tracheostome and sutured to the anterior chest wall;
- A throat pack not only protects the airway from blood and bony fragments but also assists in securing the tracheal tube;
- Lacrilube ointment followed by temporary tarsorrhaphies are used to protect the eyes intra-operatively. These are replaced with Frost sutures for 48 h post-operatively;
- At least two large peripheral venous cannulae;
- Femoral central venous line recommended especially in the younger child;
- Arterial line essential;
- Urinary catheter;
- Intra-operative cell salvage routinely used;
- A rapid infusor may be useful in older patients;

- Particular care should be taken to ensure that all pressure points are padded;
- Antiembolism compression stockings (TEDS) for older teenagers;
- Bilateral nasopharyngeal airways and a nasogastric tube are inserted at the end of surgery;
- While some centres electively ventilate patients for a few days post-operatively, it is common practice at the author's institution to extubate all patients at the end of surgery provided that they are haemodynamically stable and have no respiratory compromise;
- As the external distractor is a bulky device it may impede access to the airway making reintubation very difficult. If there are any post-operative airway concerns the halo may be placed with the suspension frame left until later.

Removal of rigid external distractor (RED frame)

In the older child, removal of a rigid external distractor is relatively simple, involving disconnection of the halo device followed by removal of the cranial pins. In infants, however, insertion of titanium mesh sheets to prevent penetration of the skull by the cranial pins necessitates removal of the distractor and sheets via a coronal incision. As the presence of a RED frame may make airway management difficult it is important to ensure that the necessary tools and expertise required to remove the frame are readily available before induction of anaesthesia. In cooperative children the suspension frame may be removed prior to induction of anaesthesia. If this is not feasible, the facemask may have to be inverted and then changed for a laryngeal mask airway once the patient is adequately anaesthetised as the frame's wires and bars makes conventional placement of a facemask impossible. Laryngoscopy and intubation may also be difficult if not impossible, and for procedures other than removal of the frame where intubation is deemed necessary, it is advisable that the surgeon removes the wires and bars.

Frontofacial bipartition (midline fasciotomy)

A facial bipartition occurs naturally as part of a midline facial cleft. A midline split can also be created surgically as an extension of a monobloc frontofacial advancement in the treatment of orbital hypertelorism (horizontal dystopia) and Apert syndrome. Following mobilisation of the maxilla and orbits, removal of a midline segment of bone and extension of the central osteotomy down to the incisors allows rotation of the two hemifacial segments together thereby narrowing the interorbital distance and expanding the maxilla. It also corrects any downgoing slant to the eyes which is a feature of Apert syndrome.

Anaesthetic implications

The anaesthetic implications and surgical aftercare for facial bipartition are as for monobloc frontofacial advancement.

Orbital box osteotomy

Orbital box osteotomy is used in the treatment of hypertelorism and vertical orbital dystopia particularly when lateral movement of a single orbit is required. It involves making a 360° osteotomy around one or both orbits, thereby allowing them to be moved medially either upwards or downwards. As the osteotomy runs between the orbital floor and the roots of the permanent dentition, this procedure should only be performed once puberty has been reached.

Anaesthetic implications

The anaesthetic implications and surgical aftercare for orbital box osteotomy are as for monobloc fronto-facial advancement.

Key points

- The successful peri-operative management of infants and children undergoing craniofacial surgery depends on careful evaluation of the patient, an understanding of the proposed surgical procedure and anticipation and prompt treatment of the many potential problems that may arise.
- Children who have undergone previous corrective surgery may be difficult to intubate.
- Blood loss and major transfusion remain the greatest risk to infants and children undergoing major craniofacial surgery. Blood loss, which may be dramatic or insidious, and dilutional coagulopathy, should be managed proactively.
- Intra-operative cell salvage is useful in reducing the use of allogeneic blood particularly in prolonged major or complex major surgical cases.
- The majority of patients can be extubated at the end of surgery and post-operative care continued on the neurosurgical HDU with continued invasive monitoring.

Further reading

Jones B, Dunaway D, Hayward R. Surgery. In: Hayward R, Jones B, Dunaway D, Evans R, eds. *The Clinical Management Of Craniosynostosis*. Cambridge University Press. 2004;374–401.

Levine M. Craniofacial malformations: Anesthetic considerations and post-operative management. In: Bissonnette B, Dalens D, eds. *Pediatric Anaesthesia Principles and Practice*. McGraw-Hill. 2002.

Mallory S, Bingham R. Anaesthesia for craniosynostosis surgery. In: Hayward R, Jones B, Dunaway D, Evans R, eds. *The Clinical Management of Craniosynostosis*. Cambridge University Press. 2004;355–73.

Chapter

26

Anaesthesia for neurosurgery in children

Su Mallory

Introduction

This chapter focuses on the particular challenges faced by the paediatric neuroanaesthetist. In addition to delivering an appropriate anaesthetic for the underlying condition and procedure, the anaesthetist must also consider the specific needs of the child and family. Flexibility and an intimate understanding of neurophysiology are key. Normal development and brain physiology will be reviewed, addressing how disease processes and anaesthesia may affect them. Essential peri-operative anaesthetic considerations are discussed, as well as some specific neurosurgical procedures and their problems.

Anatomy and physiology

In the neonate the calvarium is composed of ossified plates covering the dura, and these are separated by fibrous sutures and two fontanelles. The posterior fontanelle closes during the second or third month while the anterior fontanelle usually closes between 10 and 18 months. Both fontanelles fully ossify in the second decade. These fontanelles and non-fused sutures can separate up to early adolescence, providing some protection from a chronic increase in intracranial pressure. However, absorption of acute changes is prevented by the dura mater. The fontanelles also facilitate clinical assessment of intracranial pressure in infancy.

Intracranial pressure

Intracranial pressure (ICP) in neonates and infants is normally in the range 0–6 mmHg. It increases until adulthood, when values of 7–17 mmHg are normal. Brain tissue, blood and cerebrospinal fluid (CSF) are contained within the cranium in the proportions 80%,

10% and 10% respectively. Consequently, intracranial pressure may be increased by cerebral oedema, or rises in cerebral blood or CSF volumes. As the skull is essentially a closed box ICP rises rapidly once compensatory mechanisms have been exhausted. Clinical signs of increased ICP include vomiting, irritability, drowsiness, bulging fontanelles, 'sun-setting eyes' (downward gaze) and increased head circumference. If ICP continues rising, Cushing's response of systolic hypertension, bradycardia and respiratory irregularity occurs which are signs of imminent coning, coma and death. ICP can be affected by surgery and anaesthesia, and a clear understanding of the many factors involved is essential knowledge for those undertaking neuroanaesthesia.

Cerebral blood flow and perfusion pressure

Much of neuroanaesthesia is directed towards controlling ICP, when appropriate and feasible. Central to this is the ability to manipulate cerebral blood flow (CBF) which is usually intimately related to cerebral blood volume (CBV) and in turn to ICP. CBF varies with age (see Table 26.1), and is affected by a number of additional factors, some of which can be directly manipulated by the anaesthetist in order to reduce ICP when this is indicated by the clinical situation.

Cerebral blood supply is usually coupled to demand, which is dependent on cerebral metabolic rate. There is normally autoregulation with cerebral vasoconstriction or vasodilation to meet the metabolic demand of the cerebral tissue. These metabolic demands may be increased in conditions such as sepsis or seizures. Here blood flow may increase leading to a rise in cerebral blood volume and consequently ICP. In conditions of decreased metabolic activity such as hypothermia, the reverse is true and

Core Topics in Paediatric Anaesthesia, ed. Ian James and Isabeau Walker. Published by Cambridge University Press. © 2013 Cambridge University Press.

Table 26.1 Cerebral blood flow: normal range at different ages

Age	Cerebral blood flow (ml min^{-1} 100 g^{-1})
Neonate	40–42
6 months to 3 years	90
3–12 years	100
Adult	50

blood flow decreases. Cerebral metabolic rate is higher in children than in adults, as is the demand for both glucose (child 6.8 mg min^{-1} 100 g^{-1}, adult 5.5 mg min^{-1} 100 g^{-1}) and oxygen (infant 5.8 ml min^{-1} 100 g^{-1}, adult 3.5 ml min^{-1} 100 g^{-1}). In the presence of oxygen, the main source of energy for cerebral metabolism is glucose. There are limited stores of glucose and glycogen in cerebral tissue, so normal cerebral blood flow is essential to maintain glucose and oxygen levels. The increased metabolic rate in infants and children increases the impact of any interruption in cerebral blood supply.

Cerebral perfusion is controlled by autoregulatory mechanisms within the normal range of MAP. If excessive hypo- or hypertension, hypoxia, hypercapnia or cerebral ischaemia occurs, these mechanisms fail and cerebral perfusion becomes dependent on systolic blood pressure. Where there is anaemia or haemodilution, leading to decreased blood viscosity, then viscosity autoregulation also plays a role. Lower viscosity increases oxygen delivery and vasoconstriction occurs. Here CBV decreases although CBF is constant.

Cerebral perfusion pressure (CPP) is calculated according to the formula:

$$CPP = MAP - (ICP + CVP)$$

where MAP is mean arterial pressure, ICP is intracranial pressure and CVP is central venous pressure.

Volatile anaesthetic agents inhibit autoregulation via dose-dependent cerebral vasodilation. In children, the lower level of autoregulation is presumed to be related to the lower mean arterial blood pressure. Sick neonates have impaired autoregulation, and CBF in this group is dependent on systolic pressure. Fluctuations in blood pressure may explain the occurrence of intraventricular haemorrhage in this patient group.

The effects of carbon dioxide on CBF appear to be the same as in adults, but a linear relationship exists between PaCO$_2$ and CBF in the sick neonate. Hyperventilation has been demonstrated to restore autoregulation in the neonate. Cerebral steal may occur in some circumstances; hypercapnia results in vasodilation of normal vessels and diversion of blood away from abnormal vessels, for example in tumours or ischaemic areas. Inverse steal may occur in the presence of hypocapnia; normal vessels become constricted and there is preferential flow to the abnormal vasculature, which is less able to regulate flow.

Control of PaCO$_2$ is an essential tool for the reduction of CBF and therefore ICP. In raised ICP, the interventions that can help to reduce it are mild hyperventilation, moderate hypothermia, cessation of seizure activity, treatment of sepsis and haemodilution. Hypoxia, vasodilators and high concentrations of volatile agent as well as pathological changes (tumour, abscess, trauma) will also adversely affect autoregulation, potentially increasing CBF and consequently ICP.

Cerebrospinal fluid

Cerebrospinal fluid (CSF) provides a degree of support and protection against trauma, as well as a constant internal environment for the brain. CSF is mainly produced by the choroid plexus. It flows from the lateral ventricles through the foramen of Monro into the third ventricle, then through the cerebral aqueduct of Sylvius to the fourth ventricle and out via the foramina of Luschka and the foramen of Magendie to the subarachnoid space where it is absorbed by the arachnoid villi. CSF production can be reduced by furosemide or acetazolamide in an effort to control ICP. The contribution of these interventions to ICP regulation is, however, very small and manipulations of CBF and CBV have far greater impact. CSF production is relatively constant in children and adults, but there is a lower storage capacity for CSF in children, so disturbed CSF reabsorption has a far greater effect.

Principles of anaesthesia for the neurosurgical patient

Pre-operative management

Assessment should include neurological status. It is essential to note signs of raised ICP, altered conscious level and any focal findings. Vomiting due to raised ICP may cause dehydration and electrolyte imbalance. Brain stem lesions can be associated with bulbar palsies that may result in aspiration and pulmonary consolidation. Some groups of children are likely to have multisystem disease, such as ex-premature infants (chronic lung disease), those with cerebral abscesses (e.g. cyanotic heart disease) and those with major spinal defects (renal disease).

Pre-operative investigations should include a full blood count for all patients, and electrolytes in those with a history of vomiting or a ventricular drain. Neurosurgery in children can be associated with large blood loss if sinuses or dilated veins from raised ICP are disrupted. Blood must be cross-matched for children undergoing craniotomy. A clotting screen may also be required as anticonvulsant treatment can cause coagulopathy.

Sedative premedication is avoided in children with significantly raised ICP, as further elevation of ICP due to hypercapnia may be catastrophic. Pooling of oral secretions in the prone or the sitting position may result in reduced adhesion of tracheal tube fixation tape. Atropine or glycopyrrolate can reduce these secretions and may also enhance cardiovascular stability.

Induction of anaesthesia

General anaesthesia remains the norm for craniotomy in children, although awake craniotomy has been reported in the older child. Induction of anaesthesia may be inhalational or intravenous. The anaesthetist needs to be mindful of the ICP. A calm patient and family who have had the options and induction process explained are the ideal. They should be aware that the chosen technique might have to be adapted to avoid upset should cannulation prove awkward.

- Sevoflurane has become the volatile agent of choice for gaseous induction in children. It causes cerebral vasodilation, but this may have less effect on the intracranial pressure than an intravenous induction accompanied by crying or breath-holding.
- If intravenous induction is preferred and feasible, then propofol is commonly used.
- A non-depolarising muscle relaxant is used, such as atracurium or vecuronium.
- Suxamethonium may be used if a rapid sequence induction is indicated, although there is the theoretical risk of raising ICP.

Surges in arterial pressure at laryngoscopy should be avoided using fentanyl or remifentanil at intubation, and the airway should be secured with an armoured tracheal tube of appropriate size to avoid undue leak and hypoventilation. Satisfactory bilateral lung ventilation should be assessed with the head in a neutral position and then once more in its position for surgery, as neck flexion will cause the tracheal tube to move towards the carina. Cerebral venous obstruction should be avoided by careful patient positioning, 'head-up' tilt, and taping rather than tying the tracheal tube. The tape must be moisture-proof as surgical prep solutions or blood can jeopardise its security.

Intra-operative monitoring

Routine monitoring includes ECG, non-invasive blood pressure, pulse oximetry, capnography, temperature probes (both central and peripheral), and a peripheral nerve stimulator. All major cases require direct arterial pressure measurement. As well as monitoring appropriate ventilation, capnography alerts the anaesthetist to the occurrence of venous air embolism (VAE). If central venous pressure monitoring is required for assessment of intra-operative fluid balance, the most appropriate route is via the femoral vein. This avoids potential obstruction of cerebral venous drainage. Additionally, two peripheral cannulae are required in case rapid fluid resuscitation becomes necessary. Urinary catheters are not used routinely but may be indicated in patients at risk of diabetes insipidus, those undergoing prolonged surgery or where large blood loss is anticipated.

The large surface area to volume ratio of paediatric neurosurgical patients may make temperature control difficult. It is essential to monitor body temperature, aiming to maintain a temperature of 36–36.5 °C.

- Patient warming devices and fluid or blood warmers should be available.
- If the patient's temperature rises, all warming devices should be switched off, and this is usually sufficient to reduce temperature.
- Lowering the temperature may have a cerebral protective effect, therefore allowing surgery to be completed if cerebral perfusion is compromised.
- Moderate hypothermia of 34–36 °C post-ischaemia can also have neuro-protective benefits without additional risk of cardiac arrhythmias and metabolic changes.
- Post-ischaemic neurological function and cerebral histopathology appear to be detrimentally affected

by 1–2 °C increases in temperature, and hyperthermia should therefore be avoided.

- Post-operative hyperpyrexia, which is more likely after craniopharyngioma resection and hypothalamic, pontine and mid-brain manipulations, should be treated aggressively, especially if the temperature exceeds 40.5 °C.

Anaesthetic agents

Balanced anaesthesia should be maintained, with 0.5–1.0 MAC of isoflurane or sevoflurane in air/oxygen or nitrous oxide/oxygen. Nitrous oxide should be avoided when ICP is critically raised or there is a risk of venous air embolism. The ideal agent for neuroanaesthesia should maintain cerebrovascular autoregulation, allow the continued coupling between CBF and metabolism, avoid an increase in CBV or ICP, have no impact on the EEG and have both neuroprotective and anticonvulsant potential.

Volatile agents at low dose cause cerebral vessels to constrict by suppressing metabolism. Isoflurane has cerebrovascular stability at 0.5–1.0 MAC and used to be the gold-standard volatile agent for neuroanaesthesia. Sevoflurane has been demonstrated to have a better profile and is the least vasoactive volatile agent, with less vasodilation for the same depth of anaesthesia, and little or no effect on autoregulation, CBV and ICP below 1 MAC. Its fast elimination also allows neurological status to be assessed more reliably in the immediate post-operative period. With increasing concentrations of either isoflurane or sevoflurane, vasodilatory effects predominate, and while ICP may only increase marginally, the effects on CPP are clinically significant owing to a decrease in MAP.

Propofol does not impair autoregulation; it decreases CBF and ICP and has a lesser effect on electrophysiological monitoring. This has resulted in total intravenous anaesthesia (TIVA) techniques being widely adopted in adult neurosurgical practice, but there remain concerns about TIVA in children for long procedures.

Ventilation

Mild to moderate hyperventilation (PaCO$_2$ approx. 3.8–4.2 kPa) will reduce cerebral blood volume via vasoconstriction. Cerebral ischaemia has been described if PaCO$_2$ is allowed to fall below 3.5 kPa, although the paediatric population with their healthy blood vessels appear to be less prone to focal ischaemia.

Positive end-expiratory pressure (PEEP) increases intra-thoracic pressures and if possible should be avoided in neurosurgical patients. Hyperoxia with a PaO$_2$ greater than 20 kPa may be beneficial. This will increase tissue oxygenation in areas of poor flow following cerebral oedema and can be achieved in patients with healthy lungs with a FiO$_2$ of 0.35. Prolonged hyperoxia should be avoided in neonates and ex-premature infants.

Analgesia

Intra-operative analgesia can be provided with fentanyl, which does not increase CBF or ICP, unlike alfentanil and sufentanil. Unless the procedure is prolonged or post-operative ventilation is planned, the maximum dose should not exceed 7–10 mcg kg^{-1}. Remifentanil is widely used in adult practice and appears to be a reasonable alternative to fentanyl in children, as its short duration of action means it can be titrated to surgical stimulus. Titration of adequate post-operative analgesia following remifentanil infusion is necessary. On completion of surgery, muscle relaxation is reversed as necessary with neostigmine and atropine or glycopyrrolate. Glycopyrrolate has the theoretical advantages of less tachycardia and fewer central effects than atropine. Children should be extubated when breathing well with a normal end-tidal carbon dioxide. Excessive coughing should be avoided by deep extubation if possible.

Fluid replacement and cardiovascular parameters

In the normal brain, osmotic forces produce fluid fluxes. A fall in osmotic pressure of 5–10 mOsmol kg^{-1} may result in cerebral oedema. Intra-operatively, a balanced fluid such as Hartmann's solution may be used as maintenance, although where large volumes of fluid are required this mildly hypo-osmolar solution is not ideal and normal saline may be preferable. Hyperglycaemia is associated with adverse outcome in head injuries, and blood sugar should be monitored regularly in the peri-operative period. Glucose-containing infusions are reserved for use only if specifically required.

It is difficult to measure blood loss accurately in neurosurgery, and the relatively large head size of children results in proportionately larger blood loss compared with adults. Appropriate replacement can be achieved by assessing all cardiovascular parameters, in particular heart rate and arterial pressure. Exchange transfusions are not unusual in small children and are well tolerated provided clotting, blood gases and potassium levels are checked regularly. Rapid and large transfusion of blood carries a number of risks in the infant and is discussed in Chapter 14.

The optimal surgical field is associated with a relatively slow heart rate, and this is usually achieved with deep anaesthesia and normovolaemia. Induced hypotension should be used with great caution. If it is required, good oxygenation, normovolaemia and direct arterial pressure monitoring are mandatory. A β-blocker, with or without an α-blocker, such as propranolol or labetalol, may achieve a suitable blood pressure. Other vasodilator agents such as sodium nitroprusside have also been used, but will compromise cerebral autoregulation. Acute rises in ICP can usually be managed with moderate hyperventilation and mannitol. Dexamethasone may be used to decrease cerebral oedema but should be used with caution in the presence of infection such as cerebral abscess.

Post-operative management

The majority of patients do not require post-operative ventilation, but the decision to ventilate may be made pre-operatively where specific indications exist, or intra-operatively. This may be necessary if surgery has been unexpectedly prolonged, the patient has been cardiovascularly unstable or if there is a neurological surgical indication.

Patients undergoing craniotomy require high-dependency care post-operatively. Direct arterial pressure monitoring should be instituted for 24 hours, and cardiorespiratory function, fluid balance and neurological status should be monitored. Analgesia for these patients includes regular intravenous paracetamol and an opioid, with the addition of diclofenac if no contraindication exists. Codeine phosphate has been the traditional opioid of choice as it provides analgesia without altering conscious level or pupil size. Oral morphine is increasingly used. Patient or nurse-controlled intravenous morphine analgesia is useful, particularly for patients who have had posterior fossa craniotomy or spinal surgery. Control of post-operative nausea and vomiting is with ondansetron.

Specific considerations

Acute head injury

The force required to produce a skull fracture in a child is large, so an associated brain injury is more likely than in an adult. Rapid increase in ICP from cerebral oedema and subdural haematoma may necessitate urgent surgical intervention. Secondary injury, scalp lacerations resulting in large blood loss, facial injuries causing airway compromise and additional thoracic, abdominal or limb injuries need to be considered.

Brain tumours

These may be vascular lesions and may be suitable for pre-operative embolisation of large feeding vessels in order to reduce operative blood loss. However, surgery is still not without significant risk of morbidity and mortality. The majority of brain tumours in children occur in the posterior fossa. Surgery performed with the child in the sitting position provides excellent surgical access, improved cerebral venous drainage, decreased blood loss, lowering of ICP and improved post-operative recovery including preservation of cranial nerve function. This position provides an anaesthetic challenge as there is increased risk of VAE, and it can be associated with cardiovascular instability, pneumocephalus, and quadriplegia due to spinal cord infarction. Hypotension is unusual in the paediatric population provided the patient is adequately fluid loaded.

Posterior fossa syndrome is a unique post-operative complication of this procedure. It consists of a number of components including ataxia, nerve palsies, hemiparesis, irritability and cortical blindness. It is often associated with symptoms of cerebellar mutism resulting in the loss of speech and occasionally loss of ability to eat or drink. Recovery over time is variable and has been reported to take anything from days to years. The cause remains debated but focal decrease in cerebral blood flow is considered most probable.

Venous air embolus

VAE is uncommon in children owing to a lower negative intracranial venous pressure compared with adults, and morbidity is rare. PEEP is not routinely employed during ventilation as it increases cardiovascular instability, increases the risk of paradoxical air embolus and appears to confer no benefit. A patent foramen ovale is associated with increased risk from paradoxical VAE. Nitrous oxide should not be used in cases where there is a risk of VAE.

Diagnosis of VAE can be made using a number of methods including oesophageal stethoscope, pre-cordial Doppler or trans-oesophageal echocardio-graphy. Most units in Britain monitor for VAE using capnography; the alarm limits are set close to the end-tidal carbon dioxide level (ETCO$_2$), so that the anaesthetist is immediately alerted if the ETCO$_2$ falls. Significant emboli are those which cause a fall in blood pressure of more than 10%, or changes in heart rate and in particular arrhythmias. If VAE is suspected, immediate management should be to flood the surgical site with fluid to seal the veins, provide 100% oxygen, administer jugular venous compression and resuscitate with fluid to raise the venous pressure and limit the embolus size. Head-down tilt or even CPR may become necessary, and the anaesthetist should know how to release the child from the sitting position should this uncommon event occur.

Craniopharyngioma

Craniopharyngioma is a slow-growing cystic supra-sellar tumour arising from remnants of the cranio-pharyngeal duct. It has benign histology, but insidious growth may produce significant mass effects, including progressive neurological and endo-crine deterioration as the tumour expands into the hypothalamus, optic nerves and pituitary stalk. These children are often either small owing to growth failure or obese as a result of hypothalamic dysfunction. The major problems in the peri-operative period are likely to be related to blood loss or to diabetes insipidus (DI), the latter due to failure of ADH secretion from the posterior pituitary. The anaesthetist must take guidance from the endocrine team as these patients may be on steroids, and synthetic vasopressin (DDAVP) will be required in the peri-operative period to control DI. Involvement of the endocrin-ology team is essential. Central venous pressure monitoring, arterial access and an indwelling catheter are essential, as measuring peri-operative urine spe-cific gravity and plasma osmolality will be needed to assess DI. There is also an increased incidence of seizures and hyperpyrexia requiring treatment after craniopharyngioma surgery.

Epilepsy surgery

There are two major types of surgery for intractable epilepsy:

- Excision of a specific seizure focus (e.g. temporal lobe resection);
- Interruption of neural transmission (e.g. corpus callosotomy).

Implantation of a vagal nerve stimulator is a more recent treatment. Developmental delay and behav-ioural issues as well as co-existing disease make anaes-thesia for epilepsy patients a challenge. Anaesthetic agents display pro- and anticonvulsant properties at differing doses. Less than 1 MAC isoflurane minim-ises the effects on the EEG and facilitates mapping of the lesion. Anticonvulsant treatments may produce a number of side effects including sedation, altered drug metabolism (both enhanced and inhibited), platelet abnormalities, liver dysfunction, metabo-lic acidosis and increased risk of idiosyncratic drug reactions. An increased tolerance to neuromuscular blockade and opioid analgesia is of particular importance. Awake craniotomy techniques have been used in older children to minimise iatrogenic injury during epilepsy surgery.

Neural tube defects

Uncovered neural tube defects, such as encephalocoele or myelomeningocoele in newborn infants, should be repaired as an emergency. Early surgery may be indicated for large lesions, or where there is a risk of rupture and meningitis. In many other instances surgery can be deferred until all investigations, including imaging, have been completed.

Traditionally intubation has been in the left lateral position, but the supine position can be used if the lesion is protected adequately from pressure. A Montreal mattress (Figure 26.1) with the head and body supported and the defect in the central space of the mattress is often ideal. Surgery is usually per-formed in the prone position, and care is needed to avoid inferior vena cava compression, which causes engorgement of the paraspinal veins. Haemangiomas in the surrounding tissues may increase surgical blood loss. Intra-operative opioids are avoided or minimised unless post-operative ventilation is planned. Wound infiltration with 0.25% bupivacaine and paracetamol suppositories usually provides effective analgesia.

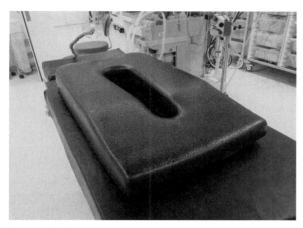

Figure 26.1 Montreal mattress.

Hydrocephalus

Hydrocephalus can arise as a result of many processes, either acquired (e.g. intra-uterine infection, meningitis, tumour, haemorrhage) or congenital (e.g. Arnold Chiari malformation, myelomeningocoele). Consequently these patients may present as neonates for surgery. Ventriculo-peritoneal (VP) shunt insertion is the usual treatment for this condition. In the premature infant, co-existing inguinal hernias may have to be repaired to prevent CSF accumulating in the hernial sacs. The peritoneal route is avoided if there is intra-abdominal pathology that may require surgical intervention in the future. Ventriculo-atrial shunts are rarely employed because of the potential complications of bacterial endocarditis. Alternatively, a ventriculo-pleural shunt may be used, but this is usually reserved for cyst or subdural fluid drainage.

Many infants requiring a VP shunt will have required neonatal intensive care and will be less than 44 weeks gestation at surgery. These babies present all the problems associated with surgery in the ex-premature neonate (see Chapter 9). Exposure of skin surfaces and the surgical field preparation make temperature control difficult. Although blood loss is minimal, there is a potential risk of air embolism with catheter insertion, and excessive drainage of CSF can result in cardiac instability.

Spinal and cranio-cervical surgery
Congenital abnormalities

Those in the lumbar region include dermal sinus tracts and thickened filum terminale. They present with minimal clinical features but a dermal pit or hair tuft may be apparent. Dermal sinus tracts predispose to meningitis and may present with progressive paraplegia. Tethered filum terminale may present with leg weakness or bowel and bladder symptoms. These abnormalities are usually avascular and intra-operative transfusion is rare. Spinal monitoring may be used, and an anaesthetic technique that permits intra-operative neurophysiological studies is required, for instance low doses of agents known to reduce evoked potential responses, such as isoflurane. The patient is positioned prone with all the potential problems that this may present.

Spinal tumours

Extramedullary spinal tumours tend to arise from abnormal embryogenesis or as metastases from a different site. Intramedullary tumours, most commonly astrocytomas or ependymomas, are a greater surgical challenge as they involve the spinal cord itself.

Spinal tumours are often extremely vascular and despite optimal positioning and induced hypotension, they may require large transfusions. Surgical manipulations of the spinal cord may be associated with arrhythmias and hypotension. Inadequate anaesthesia may contribute to this picture.

Instability of the craniocervical spine

This may be acquired or congenital. Many congenital cases may be associated with inherited disorders, e.g. Down syndrome, Morquio disease and pseudo-achondroplasia. Atlanto-axial subluxation (Figure 26.2) may be posterior but is much more commonly anterior.

Subluxation creates a kyphosis over C2. The spinal cord, tethered by the dentate ligament, is compressed primarily by the dens. Flexion is more hazardous than extension, with sudden flexion causing cord contusion.

Instability of the craniocervical spine in patients presenting for corrective surgery presents a number of significant problems. The main problem initially is inducing anaesthesia and intubation prior to fixation of the neck in a halo jacket or surgery. Intubation is usually achieved by standard techniques, but the neck must be held in line by an assistant, who prevents flexion or extension. In adult practice, sedated fibre-optic intubation (FOI) or use of an intubating laryngeal mask airway (LMA) are the first choices for

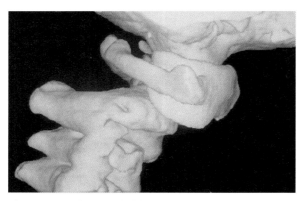

Figure 26.2 Atlanto-axial subluxation.

securing the airway; in paediatric practice, however, asleep FOI is the method of choice where difficulty is anticipated. Cricoid pressure is contraindicated.

Depending on the lesion, the surgical approach will either be postero-lateral or trans-oral. With the latter approach the child remains intubated post-operatively until all oral swelling has settled, usually within 24–48 hours. Once the child is in the halo jacket it is essential to appreciate that the previous laryngoscopic view is altered by the fixation position and may no longer be straightforward. The standard laryngoscope handle normally clashes with either the lateral rods or the top of the jacket, and therefore a polio handle is advantageous. The option of FOI should always be available when anaesthetising a child in a halo jacket, although many procedures can be performed safely with an LMA. The LMA not only provides an airway but may also facilitate intubation where indicated.

Stereotactic surgical techniques

Stereotactic surgery allows precise mapping and access to small deep-seated lesions of the brain, with decreased neurological morbidity. In the past, the application of the stereotactic head-frame in children required general anaesthesia and involved moving the anaesthetised patient between CT scanner and operating theatre. These devices have now been superseded by frameless stereotaxy, for which general anaesthesia is still required, but movement of the anaesthetised patient between different areas is not. External markers on the patient's scalp act as reference points for a pair of cameras above the operating field, which feed back the position of the tip of a chosen surgical tool to a 3D computer-generated

image. Stereotactic procedures can be time-consuming. There is minimal surgical stimulation, but hypotension is unusual.

Neuroendoscopic techniques

Neuroendoscopy is a helpful technique in the treatment of a number of disorders including hydrocephalus, cyst puncture and periventricular tumour biopsy. Indications and applications continue to expand. The procedure requires minimal anaesthesia once the burr hole has been made. The patient's age and clinical state usually dictate anaesthetic technique with such a minimally invasive technique. Improved video facilities now allow the anaesthetist as well as the surgeon to have a view of the surgery as it proceeds, and this has improved communication. Patient positioning can be varied and access limited. In selected or prolonged cases, invasive monitoring may be indicated.

Third ventriculostomy

Third ventriculostomy is an alternative to the VP shunt. It involves fenestration of the floor of the third ventricle, allowing it to communicate with the basal cisterns, and so facilitating reabsorption of CSF. It is relatively contraindicated in individuals with abnormal ventricular anatomy, ventricular haemorrhage or with a history of meningitis. Endoscopic ventriculostomy eliminates the risk of shunt-related complications and therefore decreases the necessity for the repeated operations that follow insertion of a VP shunt.

Complications of third ventriculostomy include haemorrhage, particularly injury to the basilar or perforating arteries (which have resulted in intra-operative deaths) and transient or permanent sequelae from midbrain manipulation (variable cardiovascular instability, bradycardia and asystole). Increases in ICP due to pre-existing disease, irrigation fluid or bleeding are also possible, and rather than the classic Cushing's reflex, hypertension and tachycardia may offer the most reliable clue to the development of significantly raised ICP.

Post-operatively, altered mental state, cranial nerve palsies, vomiting and aspiration, syndrome of inappropriate antidiuretic hormone (SIADH) and ventriculitis may all complicate recovery. Electrolyte imbalance post-operatively has been attributed to a number of factors including irrigation fluid,

Table 26.2 Considerations for paediatric neurosurgery

Procedure	Pre-operative considerations	Intra-operative considerations	Post-operative considerations
Acute head injury	Secondary damage Airway compromise Blood loss Limb/organ injury	Fluid management Blood loss ICP	May require HDU/ICU
Sitting craniotomy	Oral secretions and stability of ETT	VAE Cardiovascular instability Pneumocephalus	HDU Cord infarction Posterior fossa syndrome
Craniopharyngioma	Increased BMI Endocrine review DDAVP	Risk of DI Central monitoring/urinary catheter	Risk of DI Endocrine follow-up
Epilepsy surgery	Developmental delay/behavioural issues Co-existing disease Medication effects (coagulopathy)	Idiosyncratic drug reactions Altered drug metabolism Intra-operative monitoring (EEG effects)	Increased risk of seizures Increased risk of hyperpyrexia
Neural tube defects	Timing of procedure Neonates/ex-premature infants Intubation position	Prone position Blood loss Temperature control	May require ICU
Hydrocephalus	Co-existing conditions Prematurity	Temperature control VAE Cardiac instability with CSF drainage	May require ICU
Spinal surgery	Instability of C-spine FOI may be required Halo/jacket *in situ* Associated syndromes	Agents allowing for neurophysiological studies Prone position Arrhythmias/hypotension Blood loss	Halo/jacket *in situ* +/– altered laryngoscopic view May require ICU
Transphenoidal surgery	Endocrine review	Cardiovascular instability Blood loss +/– central monitoring	Airway management (pharyngeal blood/nasal packs) Acute haematoma
EC–IC bypass	Premedication Associated disease process Anti-platelet therapy +/– Pre-operative fluids	Maintain normocapnia/normotension/normothermia	Maintain normocapnia/normotension/normothermia Adequate analgesia

disturbance of the hypothalamic nuclei and hormonal imbalance.

Endoscopic transphenoidal surgery

Endoscopic transphenoidal surgery can be used for removal of a variety of lesions, including pituitary tumours and craniopharyngiomas. Surgical access to the pituitary gland is achieved without brain retraction, and the associated morbidity and mortality are decreased.

- Pre-operative assessment is as for other pituitary tumours. It is useful to insert central access at induction as these patients may require repeated blood tests to monitor endocrine function post-operatively.
- Intra-operatively, cardiovascular instability may be encountered on application of nasal

epinephrine, and the potential for haemorrhage is also present.

- On emergence from anaesthesia, the airway may be difficult to manage and jeopardised in obligate nasal breathers by pharyngeal blood, gastric blood and nasal packs. Acute haematoma may present with sudden blindness, ophthalmoplegia, hypotension and decreased conscious level.

Re-vascularisation surgery/ extracranial–intracranial bypass

The paediatric patient group presenting for this procedure are those with Moyamoya disease, a progressive chronic occlusive cerebrovascular disease. It usually presents in childhood with symptoms from stenosis of the arteries of the circle of Willis and the internal carotid arteries. These children may have had transient ischaemic attacks or strokes, indicating significantly compromised cerebral blood flow. Medical treatment consists of antiplatelet therapy with aspirin in most cases.

The anaesthetist's aim is to avoid possible ischaemia and its sequelae. Pre-operative fluids may be advisable to maintain hydration and blood pressure prior to surgery. Crying and stress need to be minimised and premedication is advisable.

Normocapnia should be maintained intraoperatively as hyperventilation may reduce cerebral blood flow and precipitate an ischaemic event; carbon dioxide retention may cause 'steal' from compromised vessels by areas of healthy vasculature. Normocapnia is also of continued importance in the post-operative period with adequate analgesia to decrease hyperventilation and crying.

Normothermia, normovolaemia and normotension are also essential during recovery. Careful control of these parameters peri-operatively may avoid hyperperfusion injury. Hyperperfusion of previously hypoperfused regions of the brain where autoregulation is no longer functioning can be detrimental. Hyperperfusion injury may result in nausea, vomiting, seizures, haemorrhage and permanent neurological deficit.

Conclusion

Paediatric neuroanaesthesia is a complex balance. It requires knowledge of neuroanatomy, neuropathology and pharmacology as well as an insight into what may or may not be practical in the infant or child. Some of the points to consider are summarised in Table 26.2. With suitable planning and preparation, the peri-operative and intra-operative course can be managed to optimise the outcome for the patient and their family.

Key points

- Paediatric neuroanaesthesia is sometimes a compromise between theory and practicality.
- Knowledge of neurophysiology and the ability to manipulate it is key.
- Pre-operative assessment must pay particular attention to the symptoms and signs of raised ICP.
- Extreme vigilance is required in certain environments where VAE is a risk.
- Provision for appropriate post-operative facilities is essential.

Further reading

Baykan N, Isbir O, Gercek A *et al.* Ten years of experience with pediatric neuroendoscopic third ventriculostomy. *J Neurosurg Anesthesiol* 2005;**17**(1):33–7.

Engelhard K, Werner C. Inhalational or intravenous anaesthetics for craniotomies? Pro inhalational. *Curr Opin Anaesthesiol* 2006; **19**(5):504–8.

Harrison EA, Mackersie A, McEwan A *et al.* The sitting position for neurosurgery in children: a review of 16 years experience. *Br J Anaes* 2002;**88**(1):12–17.

Szabo EZ, Luginbuehl I, Bissonnette B. Impact of anaesthetic agents on cerebrovascular physiology in children. *Paed Anaes* 2009;**19**(2):108–18.

Chapter

27

Anaesthesia for ophthalmic surgery in children

Ian James

Introduction

Ophthalmic surgery is undertaken across the entire paediatric age range, from the newborn with a congenital cataract to the teenager with a lens dislocation. The most common procedures are listed in Table 27.1. Unlike adults, children undergoing eye surgery will nearly always require general anaesthesia. Many of these children are ASA class 1 and will be managed as routine day-cases. In others the eye problem may be associated with a congenital or metabolic abnormality, and anaesthesia may not be so straightforward.

Pre-operative assessment

It is important to establish potential anaesthetic difficulties in those patients whose eye problem is part of a syndrome. This may be limited to developmental delay but may on occasion pose significant airway difficulty.

Most congenital cataracts are idiopathic, and some are hereditary. Occasionally they occur after intra-uterine infection with rubella, cytomegalovirus or toxoplasmosis with attendant associated anomalies. Congenital cataracts can also be associated with a chromosomal abnormality such as Down syndrome or the Pierre Robin anomalad. Neonatal cataracts are also a feature of Hallerman–Strieff syndrome which, although very rare, is associated with a particularly difficult airway. Squints and glaucoma may be seen in other syndromes in which there may be major airway and intubation difficulties, such as the craniosynostoses or the mucopolysaccharidoses (see Table 27.2). Glaucoma and early retinal detachments are seen in Stickler syndrome, an inherited disorder of collagen which has airway problems similar to Pierre Robin, with micrognathia and a cleft palate.

Table 27.1 General anaesthesia may be required for the following procedures

Procedure	
Examination of the eye	General examination Measurement of intraocular pressure Retinoblastoma follow-up
Extraocular procedures *On the lids and orbit*	Steroid injection of haemangioma Excision of meibomian cysts Excision of orbital dermoids/tumours Ptosis surgery Tarsorrhaphy
On the nasolacrimal system	Syringing and probing of ducts Insertion of Crawford tubes Dacryocystorhinostomy (DCR)
On the eye	Squint surgery Episcleral dermoid excision Enucleation/evisceration Laser surgery/cryotherapy
Intraocular procedures	To reduce intraocular pressure – goniotomy – trabeculectomy Lensectomy ± artificial lens insertion Vitreoretinal surgery Corneal grafting Intra-vitreal injection

Other disorders that are associated with eye lesions requiring surgery include homocystinuria, Marfan syndrome and the phakomatoses.

Homocystinuria is a metabolic disorder in which hypoglycaemia and thromboembolic episodes occur

Table 27.2 Syndromes with eye disorders and airway difficulties

Syndrome associated with airway disorder	Ophthalmic condition
Mucopolysaccharidoses	Corneal clouding, glaucoma
Craniosynostoses –Crouzon, Apert, Pfeiffer	Squints, proptosis, glaucoma
Craniofacial syndromes –Goldenhar, Treacher Collins, Smith Lemli Opitz, Pierre Robin	Nasolacrimal duct obstruction, lid colobomas, squints Congenital cataract
Hallerman–Strieff	Neonatal cataracts
Stickler's	Retinal detachment

readily. Patients may have dislocated lenses that will require extraction. It is advisable to start an intravenous glucose infusion pre-operatively to ensure adequate hydration and blood glucose in these children. Patients may be on low-dose aspirin or other antithrombotic medication which should be continued in the peri-operative period to minimise the risk of thromboembolic episodes.

Dislocated lenses also occur in patients with Marfan syndrome, a disorder due to deficiency of the structural protein fibrillin. Cardiac abnormalities such as mitral regurgitation, mitral valve prolapse and aortic root dilation are common in children, although most have no cardiovascular symptoms; many patients will be on β-blockers. Hypertension should be avoided. There is a small risk of spontaneous pneumothorax in these patients, and particular care must be taken with patient positioning because of their hyperextensible joints.

The congenital phakomatoses are neuro-oculo-cutaneous disorders and may have ocular lesions that require surgery. This group includes Sturge–Weber syndrome, neurofibromatosis and tuberous sclerosis, disorders that are associated with seizures and other intracranial lesions, cardiac lesions, and in von Hippel–Lindau disease with phaeochromocytoma. These patients will require careful pre-operative assessment and management.

General principles of anaesthesia

Most children undergoing eye surgery are otherwise healthy, day-case patients, but some will have very poor vision. Particular care is necessary in approaching and handling those children who may not be able to see or be fully aware of what is happening. Many children, particularly those with glaucoma or cataracts, may need to undergo repeated anaesthetics over a number of years. They too will need sympathetic handling as they can become increasingly uncooperative.

Premedication and induction are a matter of personal and patient preference. Spontaneous ventilation via a facemask will suffice for simple eye examinations, although it is more convenient to use a laryngeal mask airway (LMA) to allow the ophthalmologist unrestricted access to the eyes. Spontaneous ventilation with an LMA is also satisfactory for the shorter procedures such as laser surgery, and for most of the extraocular cases such as excision of an orbital dermoid. Many orbital dermoids are superficial and are simple to excise. Some, however, can be very deep, and may require extensive surgery behind the globe. It is important to discuss the exact nature of these with the surgeon, as the anticipated length of surgery may influence airway management. There may also be the potential for bleeding.

The surgeon will require a 'quiet' eye for intraocular procedures, which is best achieved using paralysis and controlled ventilation. Because of the inaccessibility of the airway when the face is covered with sterile drapes, a secure airway is absolutely essential. The lower incidence of coughing at the end of the procedure associated with an LMA offers some advantage over a tracheal tube. It should be borne in mind, however, that the surgeon's and their assistants' hands are perilously close to the airway, particularly in small infants, and can dislodge a poorly secured LMA. If there is any doubt about the security or position of an LMA a tracheal tube should be used. A preformed RAE tracheal tube is generally used but the fixed length of the endotracheal portion of these tubes is often too long in infants, and can result in endobronchial intubation. It is possible to insert some form of padding under the curve of the tube at the mouth to prevent this. It is my practice to use a reinforced, flexible tracheal tube in infants under 6 months to ensure proper tube position.

A dilated pupil is necessary for many surgical procedures. The mydriatic agents most commonly used peri-operatively are the parasympatholytic drug cyclopentolate 0.5% or 1%, or the sympathomimetic drug phenylephrine 2.5%. These are normally administered pre-operatively, but occasionally adequate pupillary dilation is not achieved. Further drops can be applied once the child is asleep which are usually well tolerated, although hypertension and pulmonary oedema have been reported owing to systemic absorption of these agents. On occasion the surgeon will inject subconjunctival mydricaine, a mixture of adrenaline, atropine and procaine, to improve pupillary dilation. It is prudent to avoid a high concentration of volatile agent in this scenario and to avoid hypercapnia to minimise the risk of dysrhythmias should there be systemic absorption of the midricaine.

Most surgical procedures involving the eye and orbit are well managed with intravenous paracetamol, topical anaesthetic agents and post-operative analgesia with oral paracetamol and a non-steroidal analgesic such as ibuprofen. Evisceration of the eye, cryotherapy and vitreoretinal surgery are usually associated with more severe peri-operative pain, and fentanyl $1-2 \, mcg \, kg^{-1}$ should be administered intraoperatively.

Protective eye goggles need to be worn during laser surgery on the eyes. It is important to be aware that there are several different types of laser, each requiring different goggles.

Specific procedures
Examination of the eyes

General anaesthesia for examination of the eyes is necessary in very young children and some older children who are too uncooperative to allow an adequate examination when awake. This can be carried out satisfactorily using a facemask although an LMA is preferable when the examination is likely to be lengthy, or where it is necessary to use the operating microscope. As many of these children require regular examinations and repeated anaesthetics, it is essential that induction is managed in as sympathetic a manner as possible.

Measurement of intraocular pressure

Special consideration is required if intraocular pressure (IOP) is to be measured, as most anaesthetic agents reduce IOP. It is always a concern that IOP will be lowered to such an extent by injudicious anaesthesia that a high IOP may be masked, potentially compromising treatment and vision. Some anaesthetists therefore use ketamine, which does not reduce IOP. When it is not possible to obtain venous

access, a dose of $5-10 \, mg \, kg^{-1}$ ketamine intramuscularly will result in a child who is quiet and still enough to permit a thorough eye examination within a few minutes. It is essential to ensure the airway is well maintained. Ketamine may lead to a slight increase in IOP, although there are conflicting reports about this, but it is probably safer to have a falsely high IOP than a falsely low one that might result in IOP treatment being delayed.

Many paediatric anaesthetists are reluctant to use intramuscular ketamine, and an alternative technique is to undertake an inhalation induction using sevoflurane. The ophthalmologist should be close by during induction and ready to measure the IOP as soon as the child stops moving, and while the eyes are still central. It is important to try to limit the sevoflurane to minimise the fall in IOP. Care must be taken to ensure that the facemask does not encroach upon the eye as this may elevate IOP.

Both techniques are acceptable. As these children are likely to have repeated measurements to assess efficacy of treatment perhaps the more important issue is to ensure that the same technique is used when comparing IOP measurements over a period of time. IOP measurements should be taken before laryngoscopy or LMA insertion, even though the latter does not appear to raise IOP.

Nasolacrimal duct obstruction

Children with blocked nasolacrimal ducts usually present within the first year of life. Initial treatment involves probing of the punctum of the duct in the eyelid with a small blunt needle and irrigation with $1-2 \, ml$ of saline, sometimes with some dye such as fluorescein in it. This is a short procedure and can be safely managed with an LMA. It is helpful to place a fine suction catheter in the nasal cavity to aspirate the irrigation fluid. Where a simple probing has failed, a Crawford tube or other fine silicone catheter is passed through the duct into the nose and secured in place for a few weeks. This may be preceded by a dacryocystogram (DCG) in which about $1 \, ml$ of radio-opaque dye is injected into the duct and the course of the duct confirmed radiographically. Rarely, the surgeon will manipulate or 'fracture' the inferior turbinate to relieve any obstruction at the lower end of the duct. A very small amount of saline or blood may appear in the nose or nasopharynx, which should be suctioned before removal of the LMA.

When the duct is completely blocked, usually by bony obstruction, a dacryocystorhinostomy (DCR) will be undertaken. This involves surgical exposure of the lacrimal sac below the medial canthus and the creation of a new opening from it through the bony upper lateral aspect of the nose into the nasal cavity. This can result in modest amounts of blood trickling into the nasopharynx, so airway protection with a tracheal tube and throat pack is necessary. Opioid analgesia, for example fentanyl, should be administered. A mild head-up tilt and a modest degree of hypotension should be induced to minimise bleeding. Topical vasoconstrictor to the nasal mucosa may be beneficial. The pharynx should be suctioned fully before removal of the throat pack and tracheal tube.

Minimally invasive endoscopic DCR is now being performed, in conjunction with ENT surgeons, and can include the use of an endoscopic laser; a similar anaesthetic technique will be necessary.

Squint repair

Repair of squint is the most common ophthalmic surgical procedure in children. It is usually performed on a day-case basis, but there is a high incidence of post-operative vomiting (POV) which occasionally results in unplanned overnight admission. Squint surgery is also associated with the oculocardiac reflex (OCR), a bradycardic response to extraocular muscle traction which can be profound. It has been postulated that POV and the OCR might be associated. There is reportedly an increased incidence of malignant hyperpyrexia (MH) in patients with a squint. Although this is very rare a high index of suspicion should be maintained for this. Suxamethonium should be avoided, and temperature monitoring should be utilised (Box 27.1).

Box 27.1 Squint surgery

Commonest paediatric ophthalmological surgical procedure
- Watch out for oculocardiac reflex
- High incidence of PONV – give antiemetics
- Opiates increase the risk of PONV
- Topical anaesthesia, intravenous paracetamol and NSAID usually satisfactory
- MH risk – but very rare

If a spontaneous ventilation technique is employed during squint surgery, sevoflurane is more suitable than halothane as it is associated with less OCR. Hypercapnia has been shown to double the incidence of significant bradycardia, and some surgeons prefer a completely immobile eye, so controlled ventilation may be more suitable. Atracurium is associated with a greater incidence of OCR than pancuronium but the shorter duration of action of atracurium makes this a more appropriate relaxant. Rocuronium appears to attenuate the OCR.

Squint surgery is one of the most painful ophthalmic procedures, but intra-operative opioids undoubtedly increase the incidence of POV. Peribulbar block is effective in producing good analgesia, as well as reducing the incidence of OCR. Most paediatric anaesthetists remain cautious about using this technique in children, however, because of the risks of retrobulbar haemorrhage and globe perforation, and it is not recommended.

Post-operative pain relief can be enhanced significantly if the surgeon administers a sub-Tenon block at the end of the procedure. Tenon's capsule is the fascial layer that extends from the limbus, fusing posteriorly to the optic nerve, separating the globe from orbital fat. Sensation of the eye is provided by ciliary nerves that cross the episcleral space after emerging from the globe. Strabismus surgery on the extraocular muscles is carried out within this space, so instilling local anaesthetic here can be very effective. Alternatively, satisfactory analgesia following squint surgery can be obtained using either diclofenac 0.1% or oxybuprocaine 0.4% eye drops alone. If these are administered selectively to the operative site by the surgeon prior to suturing the conjunctiva, the problems associated with an anaesthetic cornea can be minimised.

Adequate post-operative analgesia can usually be achieved satisfactorily using topical anaesthesia, paracetamol and a non-steroidal analgesic such as diclofenac or ibuprofen. Where analgesia is inadequate, as it may be for the more painful myopexy repair or repeat surgery, ketorolac has been shown to be effective. On occasion it may be necessary to administer stronger analgesia such as an opioid.

In some older, cooperative children, the surgeon may place an adjustable suture as part of the technique. Fine adjustments to the repair can be made, using topical anaesthesia, when the patient is awake. In some patients with strabismus a minute quantity of botulinum toxin, a paralytic, is injected directly into one or more extraocular muscles. This is often done using electromyographic (EMG) control so muscle paralysis should be avoided.

The oculocardiac reflex

OCR is common during squint surgery, occurring in approximately 60% of cases. It is evoked by traction on the extrinsic eye muscles or pressure on the globe, causing a sinus bradycardia. The bradycardia reverts almost immediately the stimulus is removed and it is unusual to see a more serious rhythm disturbance. However, very occasionally sinus arrest or major dysrhythmias may occur. It is generally believed that OCR occurs most commonly when the medial rectus muscle is manipulated, but traction on any of the extraocular muscles can evoke the reflex. Children with a positive OCR appear to be more likely to develop POV than those with no obvious reflex, leading to suggestions that preventing the OCR may reduce the incidence of POV. Blocking the afferent limb of the reflex using a peribulbar block is one way of achieving this, but this carries a risk of perforating the globe and is not undertaken in children. Administering atropine 10 mcg kg^{-1} at induction and accepting the resultant modest tachycardia is effective and preferable. The administration of atropine is especially helpful if propofol, which has a bradycardic effect, is used for induction or maintenance of anaesthesia (Box 27.2).

Vomiting following strabismus surgery

Nausea alone is a difficult entity to quantify in children, who generally have a higher incidence of post-operative vomiting than adults. POV is a well-recognised complication following strabismus surgery, particularly in children over the age of 2 years,

with experience indicating that more than half of children undergoing strabismus surgery will be sick if no preventative measures are taken. Vomiting may not start until several hours after surgery, and parents should be warned about this at the pre-operative assessment.

The precise mechanism for the increased incidence of vomiting following squint surgery remains unknown but may well be part of an oculo-emetic reflex, involving the ophthalmic division of the trigeminal nerve and the vomiting centre in the medulla. Blocking the afferent nerves by way of a retrobulbar or peribulbar block reduces the incidence. Local anatomical reasons probably play a part as different surgical techniques affect the incidence of vomiting. In particular, the Faden myopexy technique of squint repair has a significantly higher incidence of POV than the simpler muscle recession/resection technique.

Many different strategies have been suggested to reduce the incidence of vomiting following squint surgery, with varying success. These include the use of anticholinergic agents, dimenhydrinate, dexamethasone, clonidine, antiemetics such as metoclopramide, droperidol or ondansetron, or utilising the putative antiemetic properties of propofol either for induction or as part of a TIVA technique. These publications have been comprehensively reviewed (see Further reading).

Unfortunately it is not possible to compare the studies relating to strabismus surgery and POV satisfactorily because they involve very different underlying anaesthetic techniques, and have often not taken into account different surgical techniques. It is clear, however, that the introduction of the 5HT$_3$ (serotonin) antagonists has led to a significant reduction in the incidence of POV, and they should be administered intra-operatively. Ondansetron alone is very effective, although combination therapy is better, for example using ondansetron 100 mcg kg^{-1} with dexamethasone 150 mcg kg^{-1}. It is possible to reduce the incidence of vomiting to less than 10% using a multimodal approach adopting several of these methods.

Enucleation/evisceration

Removal of the whole eye, enucleation, may be necessary because of retinoblastoma or when there is an unsightly blind eye. The surgical technique involves

---

Box 27.2 Oculocardiac reflex

Common during squint surgery, particularly with traction on medial rectus muscle

Also occurs in enucleation, vitreoretinal surgery, pressure on globe, and surgery on maxilla

Results in bradycardia, rarely sinus arrest

Reverts when muscle traction released

Associated with increased PONV

Best prevented with IV atropine at induction

---

dissection of each of the extraocular muscles off the globe, so the oculocardiac reflex may readily be evoked. Anaesthetic management should be as for strabismus surgery.

In evisceration the contents of the globe are removed rather than the whole eye, leaving the sclera behind. There are no specific anaesthetic problems but the procedure can be very painful and appropriate analgesia, including an intra-operative opioid such as fentanyl, should be administered.

Intraocular surgery

Intraocular surgery in children may be for the management of glaucoma, or for cataract extraction with or without an intraocular lens implant. Lens implants are being inserted now even in infants. Congenital cataracts will frequently need surgery in the first weeks of life to prevent permanent loss of vision. Neonates are at risk of post-operative apnoea, and arrangements should be made for appropriate post-operative monitoring. The principal surgical drainage procedures to treat glaucoma include goniotomy, trabeculotomy and trabeculectomy.

Intraocular pressure (IOP)

- Normal IOP is between 10 and 22 mmHg.
- IOP depends on the balance between the production of aqueous humour, mainly from the ciliary body in the posterior chamber, and its drainage via a trabecular meshwork to the canal of Schlemm in the anterior chamber.
- Most paediatric glaucoma is a result of an intrinsic disorder of aqueous outflow, and medical therapy is of limited value.
- Venous drainage from the eye is valveless and any rise in venous pressure, for example with coughing or straining, leads to an immediate rise in IOP by altering the volume of the choroid, and by impeding aqueous drainage via the canal of Schlemm.
- Generally, arterial pressure has little effect on IOP.

It is essential that the eye is motionless during intraocular procedures. Sudden rises in IOP should be avoided to prevent the extrusion of intraocular contents through the incisions. Neuromuscular paralysis and controlled ventilation provide optimum operating conditions; ideally, neuromuscular blockade should be monitored using a peripheral nerve stimulator. A modest dose of fentanyl is beneficial.

It is good practice to try to prevent an increase in IOP at the end of the procedure caused for example by coughing on the tracheal tube at extubation. This is less critical than it used to be with the advent of very fine suture material allowing complete closure of the ocular wounds. Anaesthesia can be maintained until neuromuscular blockade has been reversed, the patient is breathing spontaneously and extubation has been performed. A small dose of propofol ($0.5\,mg\,kg^{-1}$) given immediately prior to extubation is useful in obtaining a smooth extubation. Topical anaesthesia to the airway can be helpful in older children, although this should be avoided in infants as the simplest way to avoid the elevated IOP associated with crying in the immediate post-operative period is to offer them an early feed.

An LMA can be used for intraocular surgery, even in small children, and has the advantage of smoother extubation with less coughing and reduced likelihood of acute IOP elevation than with a conventional tracheal tube. However, if an LMA is used, it is imperative to ensure that it is perfectly positioned and well secured before proceeding with surgery. If there is any doubt, a tracheal tube should be used.

Most intraocular surgery is not particularly painful, although a small dose of fentanyl is usually administered. The combination of paracetamol and diclofenac is usually satisfactory for post-operative pain relief. The exception is corneal grafting, which benefits from stronger analgesic provision.

Corneal grafting (penetrating keratoplasty)

Anaesthesia for corneal grafting is similar to that outlined above for intraocular surgery, but is a longer procedure. It is particularly important to maintain a motionless eye and prevent sudden rises in IOP as a large defect is created over the cornea. Acetazolamide, which reduces aqueous production, or mannitol may be administered intravenously during these procedures to lower the IOP, and it may be beneficial to induce modest hypotension. Intra-operative opioids are warranted. The surgeon may suture a ring around the cornea to support the eye during the procedure. Isoflurane appears to produce a quieter eye than sevoflurane.

Vitreoretinal surgery

Repair of retinal detachment generally takes place in very specialised centres. This involves the creation of a chorioretinal scar using cryotherapy and the placement of a scleral buckle towards the back of the eye to obtain apposition of the retinal pigment epithelium and the neuroretina. An intraocular gas bubble containing sulfur hexafluoride (SF6) or per-fluoropropane (C3F8) may be injected into the eye to tamponade the detached surfaces together while adhesions develop. Nitrous oxide must not be administered when these gases are used, as it will rapidly diffuse into the gas bubble and alter its size. The intraocular gases may remain in the eye for several weeks, and diffusion of nitrous oxide from a subsequent anaesthetic during this period into an existing intraocular gas bubble can result in rapid expansion of the bubble and an acute rise in pressure within the globe. This can cause irreversible ischaemic damage to the retina and optic nerve, so patients and their carers must be given very clear instructions about passing this information on to other anaesthetists, should they require further surgery during this time.

Opioid analgesia should be administered peri-operatively, as vitreoretinal surgery is painful. In adults a sub-Tenon block has been shown to be very effective in providing analgesia and is likely to be equally effective in children.

Emergency eye surgery

Penetrating eye injury is often a true emergency and may require removal of any foreign bodies and early wound closure to salvage vision. This has been a contentious issue for anaesthesia. The possibility of a full stomach would conventionally dictate a rapid induction–intubation sequence using suxamethonium. However, it has been traditionally taught that any acute rise in IOP, such as that caused by suxamethonium, may cause extrusion of ocular contents through even very small wounds, leading to total loss of vision in that eye.

There are in fact no well-documented reports describing vitreous extrusion following the use of suxamethonium, and in those difficult situations where the eye is at risk and regurgitation is a concern, there is no good reason to avoid suxamethonium as part of a conventional rapid sequence induction, particularly if there are any concerns about the airway.

In small children who are at risk of a 'full stomach', most experts advocate a modified rapid sequence induction in which atracurium or rocuronium are utilised, and gentle ventilation continued until intubation to avoid hypoxaemia. Premature attempts at intubation should be avoided as this may provoke coughing which significantly raises intraocular pressure. A nerve stimulator may be helpful in indicating when full relaxation has occurred.

Retinopathy of prematurity (ROP)

Severe ROP still occurs despite meticulous neonatal care, and can lead to total blindness. Infants at risk of severe ROP are:

- Those ≤31 weeks gestational age; and/or
- Those with birthweight ≤1500 g.

ROP is characterised by abnormal blood vessel growth in the retina and is classified in five stages, ranging from mild (stage 1) to severe (stage 5). Infants who develop severe ROP (stage 3 or more) are at significant risk of retinal detachment and blindness. The outcome of the disease process can be improved by cryotherapy or laser therapy, which ablates the peripheral retina and removes the stimulus to new growth. This needs to be done early in the disease, so early identification is essential. Eye examinations in at-risk infants should take place between 6 and 7 weeks postnatal age and continued 2-weekly until the risk has passed.

In some centres the examination and treatment may take place within the neonatal unit. Frequently, however, these premature infants are transferred to theatre for their treatment. The usual precautions for managing preterm infants should be adopted (see Chapter 9), particularly in relation to temperature control. Cryotherapy is a painful procedure and warrants administration of opioid analgesia such as fentanyl. This has implications for the post-operative care of these babies who will be at increased risk of apnoeic episodes following anaesthesia. Appropriate facilities for post-operative monitoring and ventilation must be arranged for these babies. Many of these infants will have other systemic disorders consequent upon their extreme prematurity, such as bronchopulmonary dysplasia, which may influence both the conduct of anaesthesia and the need for post-operative support, and they will need careful assessment.

271

Key points

- Bradycardia is readily produced by traction on extraocular muscles or pressure on the globe – the oculocardiac reflex.
- Squint surgery is associated with a high incidence of post-operative vomiting.
- Avoid nitrous oxide in vitreoretinal surgery.
- Suxamethonium is not contraindicated in non-fasted patients with a penetrating eye injury.

Further reading

Olutoye O, Watcha MF. Management of post-operative vomiting in pediatric patients. *Int Anesthesiol Clin* 2003;**41**(4):99–117.

Vachon CA, Warner DO, Bacon DR. Succinylcholine and the open globe: tracing the teaching. *Anesthesiology* 2003;**99**(1):220–3.

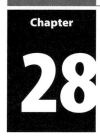

Anaesthesia for plastic surgery in children

Michael W. Frost

Introduction

Plastic surgeons treat a range of congenital and acquired conditions in children from birth to adolescence, and paediatric work makes a significant contribution to the plastic surgery caseload. Procedures are classified as 'reconstruction' or 'cosmetic', but this distinction is often blurred in children as many abnormalities are unsightly and impair physical function as well.

Common procedures such as correction of anomalies of the ears, hands and feet will be described in this chapter. Repair of cleft lip and palate is covered in Chapter 23. Urological surgeons undertake hypospadias repair in some centres and this topic is covered in Chapter 34.

A number of skin conditions are amenable to treatment with targeted laser surgery. Modern lasers have allowed many lesions to be treated in childhood, with less scarring, better cosmetic outcomes and reduced need for treatment in later life. Anaesthetists need to understand the principles of lasers, the attendant risks and the precautions required for safe use.

Pre-operative assessment

The majority of children undergoing plastic surgical procedures are ASA 1 and ASA 2, and require minimal investigation prior to surgery. Most children can be managed on a day-case basis. A routine plastic surgery list may include infants and adolescents, and key anaesthetic requirements are adaptability and close attention to detail. A friendly and supportive environment is vital as many children will attend for repeated visits and bad experiences will lead to future problems. Time and effort spent building rapport with the parent and child will pay dividends.

General principles

Distraction techniques in the anaesthetic room are helpful and premedication is rarely required. Induction technique depends on individual anaesthetist's preference, taking the age of the patient into consideration. Success with venous access in small infants is related to skin temperature and it helps if the child is kept warm prior to arrival in the anaesthetic room. Pain on injection may be reduced by using 0.5% propofol or by adding 1 ml of 1% lidocaine per 100 mg propofol. A strong light source for transillumination or ultrasound may be used to find hidden veins after inhalational induction.

The laryngeal mask airway (LMA) may be used in most plastic surgical procedures. Care should be taken to avoid displacement in infants, during surgery involving the face, or during bilateral bat ear correction. A reinforced LMA may be more stable, but there should be a low threshold to using a tracheal tube in these patients. Care should be taken to protect vulnerable areas such as the eyes, and in the application of tourniquets.

Surgical procedures on the limbs are usually performed under tourniquet to provide a clear surgical field and reduce blood loss. Relative hypotension may be helpful in some procedures; blood pressure of no more than 20% below baseline appears to be safe in healthy older children. It is safer to aim for normotension in infants, as adverse cardiovascular events are more common in this age group (bradycardia, myocardial depression from deep volatile anaesthesia). A combination of remifentanil and sevoflurane provides good control of blood pressure. Great care must be taken to flush infusion lines at the end of surgery to avoid inadvertent boluses of drugs such as remifentanil.

Core Topics in Paediatric Anaesthesia, ed. Ian James and Isabeau Walker. Published by Cambridge University Press. © 2013 Cambridge University Press.

Pain management

Effective pain control is essential for plastic surgery. Apart from humanitarian concerns, inadequate analgesia during surgery leads to labile blood pressure, poor operating conditions and increased risk of rebound bleeding after surgery. Wound infection is more common if there is a post-operative haematoma. It is important to have a good understanding of the surgery as surgical stimulation can vary enormously during a plastic surgical procedure.

Multimodal analgesia is especially relevant to paediatric plastic surgery. General anaesthesia should be combined with regional anaesthesia, local block or field infiltration where possible. It is helpful to inject local anaesthetic prior to incision, as this reduces hypnotic and analgesic requirements, and improves recovery. If the surgeon is planning a complex procedure, local infiltration may have to be delayed until the end of the procedure to prevent interference with mapping of incisions or finding the right 'plane' in the surgical field. It is also important to anticipate analgesic requirements when the block wears off.

Remifentanil is ideal intra-operatively, as it blocks virtually all surgical stimulation, provides excellent cardiovascular stability, reduces hypnotic dosage and is simple to use in children of all ages. We commonly use a remifentanil infusion in our unit for procedures expected to take an hour or more. An initial bolus of $1 \, \text{mcg} \, \text{kg}^{-1}$ IV is followed by an infusion, normally at $0.1–0.2 \, \text{mcg} \, \text{kg}^{-1} \, \text{min}^{-1}$. Morphine $50–100 \, \text{mcg} \, \text{kg}^{-1}$ IV should be given to provide analgesia post-operatively, particularly where remifentanil is used, and is best given early in the operation. Intravenous paracetamol provides a useful contribution to post-operative analgesia. Post-operatively, a combination of ibuprofen and paracetamol should be prescribed regularly, with morphine $200 \, \text{mcg} \, \text{kg}^{-1}$ PO ($80 \, \text{mcg} \, \text{kg}^{-1}$ in infants) hourly as required.

Congenital limb deformities and hand surgery

There is an enormous variety of congenital limb deformities, with most corrective surgery in the upper limb undertaken by plastic surgeons, particularly hand surgery. The aims of surgery are primarily to improve function and secondly to improve appearance. Manual dexterity develops at an early age, so surgery is often undertaken within the first 2 years,

which allows for improved function. There are over 100 recognised syndromes with associated hand abnormalities, but this still only represents a small fraction of congenital hand abnormalities. A classification of upper limb abnormalities proposed by Swanson has been adopted internationally (see Table 28.1):

- Failure of formation
- Failure of differentiation
- Duplication
- Overgrowth
- Undergrowth
- Constriction band syndromes
- Generalised skeletal abnormalities

Correction of many congenital limb deformities involves some form of skin cover, either as a full thickness graft from an area such as the groin or as a split skin graft from the thigh or medial arch of the sole of the foot. This needs to be discussed with the surgeon in advance to allow appropriate preparation and to anticipate analgesia requirements both during and after skin grafting. The child may become cold during long operations if multiple sites are exposed. Standard warming measures should be used.

Most hand and foot surgery is carried out using a tourniquet to minimise blood loss and to provide a bloodless surgical field. Poor application will make dissection of tissue planes and identification of individual nerves very difficult, so it is vital to check that the tourniquet is the correct size, is functional and has been properly positioned with appropriate padding, before draping.

- Tourniquets may be used for 2 hours, but long tourniquet times are associated with increased post-operative oedema.
- In infants, the tourniquet becomes less effective after 2 hours owing to excellent collateral blood supply via bones, which cannot be occluded.
- Blood loss should be anticipated when the tourniquet is released if there has been extensive dissection.
- It is good practice to release the tourniquet briefly and re-inflate, to allow the surgeon to identify the major bleeding points.
- After the tourniquet is deflated it is best to remove it fully to prevent venous congestion.

Regional blockade is ideal for limb surgery, and has the added advantage of sympathetic block and

Table 28.1 International classification of upper limb congenital abnormalities

	Example	Notes
Type I – Failure of formation	Hypoplasia of thumb	Failure of formation may be in: • Transverse axis (any level from shoulder to thumb) • Longitudinal axis (pre-axial (radial), central or post-axial (ulnar)
Type II – Failure of differentiation of parts	• Soft tissue – syndactyly, camptodactyly, trigger finger • Skeletal – clinodactyly • Vascular/neurological	• Two or more digits fused together • Complex syndactyly as part of a syndrome (e.g. Apert)
Type III – Duplication	• Polydactyly	• Extra digits • May occur as part of syndrome • Pre-axial (thumb) • Central (ring, middle and index) • Post-axial (little finger) most common • 2 in every 1000 live births
Type IV – Overgrowth	• Macrodactyly	Localised gigantism
Type V – Undergrowth	• Radial hypoplasia • Brachydactyly • Brachysyndactyly	e.g. Radial club hand, thumb hypoplasia • Shortness of fingers and toes • Short and fused digits
Type VI –Constriction band syndromes	• Amniotic band syndrome	• Entrapment of fetal parts (usually a limb or digits) in fibrous amniotic bands while *in utero*
Type VII – Generalised anomalies	• Atypical cleft hands	

After Swanson AB, Swanson GD, Tada K. A classification for congenital limb malformation. *J Hand Surg Am* 1983;**8**:693–702.

vasodilation. This is useful for procedures involving microscopic anastomosis of vessels, such as toe-to-hand digit transfers. Axillary brachial plexus block can be performed using a single injection placed under ultrasound guidance (see Chapter 16).

Digit relocation and transplantation

With a hypoplastic or missing thumb but normal fingers, the usual treatment is pollicisation of the index finger, which involves shortening and rotation of the index finger on its neurovascular supply to occupy the position of the thumb. With congenitally short (brachydactyly) or absent digits, microsurgical techniques now allow reconstruction of digits by using one or more toes.

The principal aims of reconstruction are focused on improvement in function. Surgery has the greatest impact when the missing digit is a thumb or where there are several digits missing. The second toe is the most common digit transplanted, as it is relatively long, has a reliable blood supply and has the ability

to grow. Removing the second toe does not appear to have a great impact on the function or appearance of the foot. The big toe is rarely used to reconstruct digits, but a partial flap called a 'wrap around flap' may be created from the pulp and nail of the big toe, with the donor site being covered with a skin graft.

Digit transfer operations take 2–3 hours. Careful planning is required to make sure all equipment is available and the child is appropriately positioned for microsurgical access. A vacuum bean mattress can be very helpful to reduce the risk of pressure-related injury. Antibiotics should be given 5 minutes prior to inflation of the tourniquet to allow for good tissue penetration. A peripheral block at the donor site and an axillary plexus block are ideal.

Syndactyly and polydactyly

Syndactyly (fusion of digits) and polydactyly (accessory digits) are the two most common congenital abnormalities of the hand. Syndactyly tends to affect the ring and little finger but can affect all

(a)

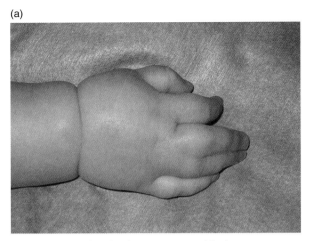

(b)

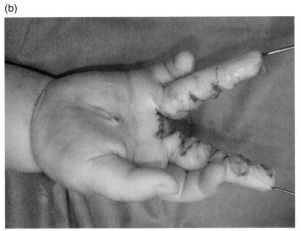

Figure 28.1 Syndactyly release in a 1-year-old infant.

fingers. It may vary in severity from a single slightly displaced web to a full fusion up to the tips of the nails affecting many digits with bony abnormalities included. With increasing complexity of syndactyly there is the additional risk of complex neurovascular arrangements especially when associated with osseous abnormalities.

Peripheral nerve blockade at the wrist is effective, safe and relatively easy to perform for many congenital hand operations, including syndactyly release. The ulnar nerve can easily be blocked by inserting 2 ml of plain local anaesthetic under the flexor carpi ulnaris muscle just proximal to the pisiform bone. The median nerve is located between the tendons of flexor carpi radialis and palmaris longus, which can be identified by gentle flexion of the wrist. A 27G needle gently inserted between these tendons at the wrist with 2 ml of plain local anaesthetic inserted into the bursa will allow blockade of the median nerve. The radial nerve block is essentially a field block with the injection site just lateral and distal to the radial styloid over the anatomical snuffbox and then extended laterally using about 3 ml. The radial nerve block at the wrist is useful for trigger thumb surgery.

Ear surgery

Correction of prominent ears

This condition is associated with loss of the antehelical fold of cartilage. Surgery aims to correct this to allow the pinna to lie parallel to the head.

Pinnaplasty is usually delayed until the age of 4–5 years when the ear cartilage is more rigid. This operation has traditionally been associated with a higher than normal risk of post-operative nausea and vomiting. The use of propofol infusion combined with local anaesthetic infiltration and minimal opioid helps to reduce this risk. Careful attention has to be given to bandaging post-operatively to reduce the risk of haematoma, at the same time avoiding excessive pressure on the cartilage of the pinna, which may also increase PONV. A flexible LMA is often used so that the head can be turned easily during the procedure. It is important to ensure the head is not rotated more than 65° from the midline to avoid neck injury, including atlanto-axial dislocation.

Ear reconstruction

Approximately 1 in 6000 infants are born with microtia. This can be corrected by a two-stage reconstruction using costal cartilage. A tracheal tube should be used for the first stage as it takes several hours, involves rib harvest, and has the potential for pneumothorax. A continuous infusion of levobupivacaine provides good quality post-operative analgesia after the first stage, using a fine catheter in the costal wound for 24 hours. As with bat ear repair, attention must be paid to the bandaging of the ears to minimise the risks of ischaemia of the grafts. Mini vacuum-suction drains are usually inserted to avoid haematoma. The second stage is a shorter procedure but incorporates a skin graft, usually from the thigh.

Accessory auricles

Accessory auricles are abnormal segments of ear tissue commonly in the pre-auricular region but sometimes on the cheek and neck. They may contain cartilaginous remnants and require adequate exposure and removal. Surgery is generally performed when the infant is 3 to 6 months old.

Dermoid cysts

These commonly occur at the outer border of the eyebrow (external angular dermoid cyst). In this location they are generally superficial and are removed via a small incision adjacent to the eyebrow. Dermoid cysts also occur in the midline of the nose. The problem here is that there may be a sinus with an epithelial lined track extending deeply into the nasal septum and possibly to the base of the skull. Always consider the possibility for the need for deep exploratory surgery and choose a secure airway technique.

Tongue tie

Tongue tie release to free up mobility of the tongue is a short procedure commonly performed in infants. A flexible LMA may be used, with carefully positioned throat pack and local infiltration of the area.

Poland's syndrome

Poland's syndrome comprises congenital breast hypoplasia associated with unilateral absence of pectoralis major muscle and an ipsilateral hand deformity. The aim is to achieve a natural shaped breast and chest wall symmetry. Surgery using tissue expanders and implants is normally carried out in late adolescence.

Gynaecomastia

Gynaecomastia is excessive breast formation in boys and usually occurs as a result of oestrogen and testosterone imbalance at puberty. Surgery is undertaken either by liposuction or direct excision via the areolar margin of the breast tissue. Surgical excision is associated with increased post-operative bleeding and haematoma. It is important that the blood pressure is normal prior to closure of the wound so that good haemostasis can be obtained, especially if local anaesthetic with adrenaline has been used. The adrenaline in the infiltration solution will wear off after 2 hours, which may increase the risk of bleeding and haematoma formation.

Laser surgery

Lasers are used to treat a range of congenital and acquired skin conditions, most of which respond well to treatment. The use of lasers presents a variety of challenges in children. Vascular and pigmented lesions such as port wine stains change in their pigmentation as the child gets older, making the lesion more resistant to laser intervention. Lesions are now treated at an earlier age so that fewer treatment sessions are required, with fewer complications as a result.

Principles of laser surgery

Chromophores are pigmented targets that selectively absorb certain wavelengths of light. Laser light is intense monochromatic light, the wavelength of which is determined by the medium (gas, liquid or solid) through which the light passes. Laser irradiation can be used to selectively target chromophores (water, haemoglobin or melanin) in the skin by selecting an appropriate wavelength along with an appropriate pulse and energy setting. The net result is intense localised production of heat in the chromophore resulting in vaporisation in the target tissue. To target specific tissues precisely, it is necessary to take into account the thermal relaxation time of the chromophore. This is defined as the time necessary for the target chromophore to cool to half its peak temperature after irradiation. The pulse time of the laser must be equal to or less than this to prevent damage to surrounding tissues and allow time for appropriate cooling and dissipation of energy.

Early laser technology used continuous-wave mode for treating vascular skin lesions and was associated with a high degree of scarring because of uncontrolled heating effects. This led to the development of pulsed dye lasers (PDL), with wavelengths of 585 nm or 595 nm, which have become the mainstay for treatment of vascular lesions in terms of efficacy and low risk of adverse scarring. The PDL emits a laser beam with wavelength close to one of the maximum absorption peaks of oxyhaemoglobin. Transient bruising lasting several days is common after use of PDL lasers. Recent advances include dynamic surface cooling, which increases the efficacy of the laser (e.g. Candela laser) and very short pulse duration, which improves the clinical result and helps minimise adverse effects.

Laser surgery and anaesthesia

The choice of laser and laser settings need to be adjusted to take account of the smaller vessels in children and the unpredictable nature of scarring. The laser is applied in multiple 'dots' to cover the birthmark to produce a controlled burn, and wound aftercare is a vital part of the treatment process. Aloe vera is commonly used for cooling the skin. If the treatment results in an open wound, a topical antiseptic such as mupirocin ointment is usually applied.

Each shot of the laser feels like being flicked with an elastic band, so many children will require general anaesthesia. The aim is to keep the patient immobile, warm and well-perfused so the surgeon can clearly visualise the vessels at the site of surgery. The airway can generally be managed with an LMA, and it is helpful to avoid tapes to secure the LMA if lasering around the mouth. Analgesia such as fentanyl, paracetamol and ibuprofen should be given, and cool facepacks help to reduce discomfort. A stat dose of dexamethasone reduces facial swelling after treatment. Some children will be able to undergo laser treatment with just a topical anaesthetic cream applied an hour before surgery. Whichever method is undertaken, efforts should be made to ensure the experience for the child is pleasant, as four to six treatments may be required at 6-monthly intervals. Children should avoid sun exposure before, during and after laser treatment as it may decrease the efficacy of the procedure or contribute to post-operative pigmentation changes.

Laser safety

Universal safety precautions are mandatory:

- Wet swabs should be used to protect the child's eyes, and staff should wear protective goggles appropriate to the specific laser used.
- The theatre doors should be locked or alarmed and notices displayed to indicate laser treatment in progress.
- The CO_2 laser is particularly associated with fires, and stringent fire precautions must be taken.
- Risks include burning holes in drapes, or ignition of flammable substances such as Tincture of Benzoin. It is sensible to reduce the inspired

oxygen as low as possible when lasering in the region of the airway. A fire extinguisher must be immediately to hand and wet swabs used to cover potential ignition points.

- Scavenging systems need to be in place and facemasks should be worn when lasers are used to remove viral warts, as an aerosol of vaporised tissue is produced with the potential risk of viral DNA being inhaled.
- There is a potential for electrical injury or an accident from tripping over cables when several lasers are used in the same theatre, and extra vigilance is required.
- Forgetting to change goggles when switching lasers is another potential problem.

Lesions amenable to treatment by laser surgery

Vascular birthmarks are relatively common in infants and can be separated into two distinct categories:

- Vascular tumours otherwise known as haemangiomas;
- Vascular malformations such as port wine stains.

It is important to identify the type of lesion correctly as they have quite different natural histories and treatments. Most infantile haemangiomas are uncomplicated and do not require any intervention as they will naturally involute with time. Some haemangiomas undergo rapid proliferation and may threaten vital structures or have the potential to cause major disfigurement. Lasers can be used to target symptomatic superficial haemangiomas, with specific indications being bleeding, rapid proliferation and ulceration.

The most commonly used laser for this is the PDL (585 nm or 595 nm) targeting oxygenated haemoglobin. For more deeply embedded haemangiomas the 755 nm alexandrite or the 1064 nm Nd:YAG laser may be used for higher penetration (see Figure 28.2). A course of treatments over several weeks is often necessary, and residual telangiectasias may require further treatment again with the PDL laser. Laser therapy for such lesions will invariably involve general anaesthesia for this age group of patients.

Vascular malformations such as port wine stains are less common than infantile haemangiomas and do not undergo rapid growth followed by involution. They tend to grow with the child and become

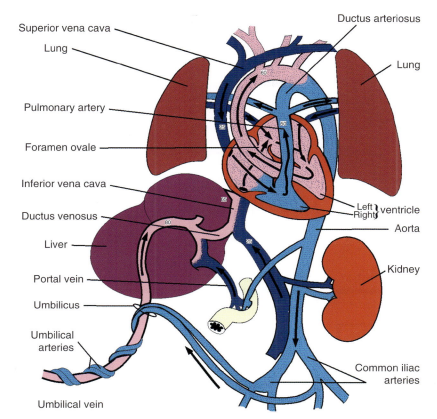

Superior vena cava

Lung

Pulmonary artery

Foramen ovale

Inferior vena cava

Ductus venosus

Liver

Portal vein

Umbilicus

Umbilical arteries

Umbilical vein

Ductus arteriosus

Lung

Left ventricle
Right

Aorta

Kidney

Common iliac arteries

Figure 1.1 The fetal circulation. The numbers indicate oxygen saturation. From Murphy PJ. The fetal circulation. *Contin Educ Anaesth Crit Care Pain* 2005;5(4):107–112, with permission.

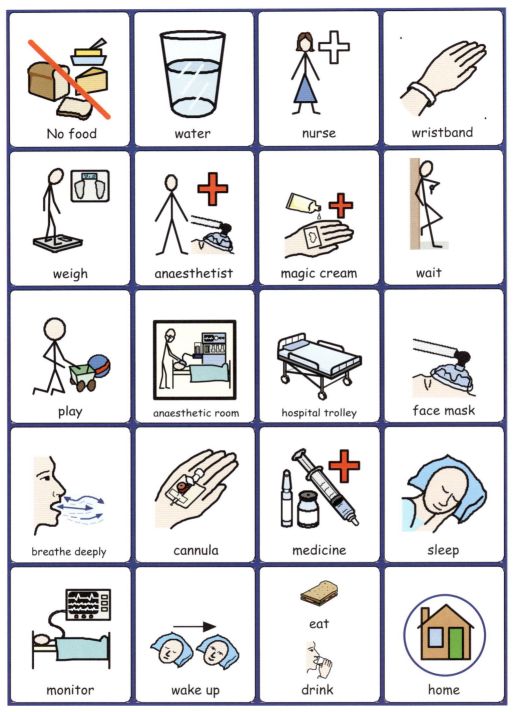

Figure 3.1 An example of a symbol system, used to create a time-line of a hospital visit. Used with permission from Widgit Symbols © Widgit Software. 2002–2011 www.widgit.com

Figure 11.1 Surgical Safety Checklist.

Surgical Safety Checklist: aide memoire GOSH

NHS

Theatre team brief at start of the session:

- Who is on the team today?
- What are we doing?
- Do we have the equipment?
- Are there any staffing issues?

- Any outside issues?
- Any time issues?
- Is the list order correct?

Sign-in: immediately prior to induction, led by the anaesthetist

- Consent form checked
- Surgical site marking checked
- Ward checks completed
- Allergies checked
- Metal check (MRI)

- Anaesthesia drugs and equipment checks completed
- Check blood available in fridge (if applicable)
- Airway/aspiration risk assessed – assistance and equipment available (if necessary)

- Remember stop before you block

Time-out: immediately prior to incision, led by the circulating nurse

- **Surgeon, anaesthetist and scrub nurse/ODP: confirm consent and site. Refer to the relevant imaging (if applicable)**
- Discuss the procedure briefly:
  - Anaesthetist: introduce case, confirm allergies, ASA score; any concerns?
  - Surgeon: review case; any critical or unusual steps?
  - Scrub nurse/ODP: confirm sterile equipment available, any other concerns?

- If relevant – perfusionist: bypass plans, any other concerns?
- Confirm antibiotic prophylaxis has been given (if necessary)
- Confirm appropriate warming measures in place
- Confirm thromboembolic prophylaxis undertaken (if necessary)
- Are there any new team members?

Sign-out: at completion of surgery, led by the circulating nurse

- Confirm swab, needle and instrument counts are correct
- Confirm procedure to be written in Theatre book
- Confirm specimen has been labelled (if appropriate)

- Any equipment issues to address/incident form to complete?
- Surgeon/Anaesthetist/Nurse: review the post-operative plans

Checklist Group 2011

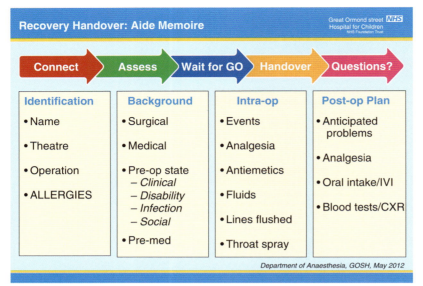

Figure 11.4 Recovery handover aide-memoire.

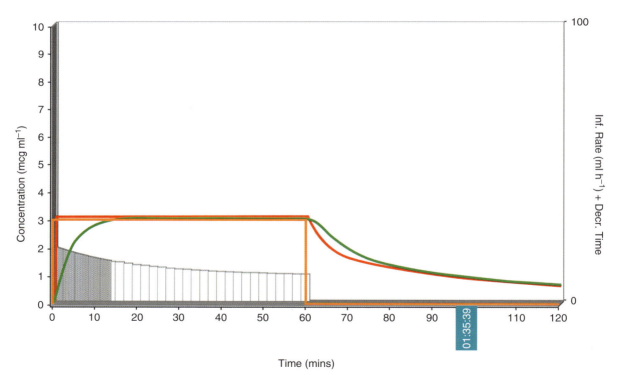

Figure 15.2 Blood targeted infusion of propofol in a child using the Paedfusor PK model. This diagram represents a 60 minute infusion of propofol where the blood target concentration (orange line) has been set at 3 mcg ml^{-1} and then the infusion is switched off (blood target 0). The red line represents the predicted blood concentration while the green line represents the effect-site concentration, which correlates with depth of sedation or anaesthesia. The effect-site concentration lags behind the blood concentration, and it takes around 10 minutes to reach an effect-site concentration equal to the target. The context-sensitive half-time is represented by the time it takes for the blood concentration to drop from 3 mcg ml^{-1} to 1.5 mcg ml^{-1}, which is in this case after 60 minutes of infusion approximately 20 minutes. Inf, infusion.

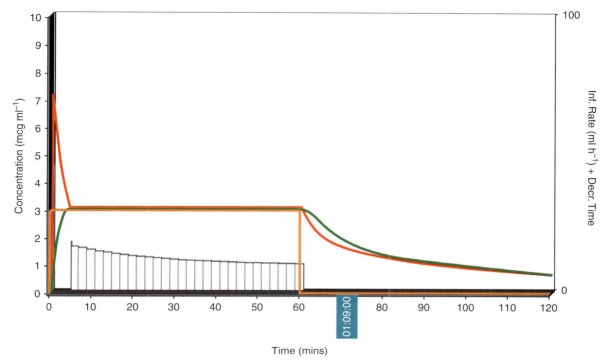

Figure 15.3 Effect-site targeted infusion of propofol in a child using the Paedfusor PK model. This diagram represents a 60 minute infusion of propofol where the effect-site target concentration (orange line) has been set at 3 mcg ml^{-1} and then the infusion is switched off (blood target 0). As in Figure 15.2, the red line represents the predicted blood concentration while the green line represents the effect-site concentration, which correlates with depth of sedation or anaesthesia. Although the effect-site concentration still lags behind the blood concentration, it takes only around 3 minutes to reach an effect-site concentration equal to the target. This is because a larger bolus is given to increase the blood concentration quickly to a higher peak which drives the propofol along a concentration gradient into the effect-site much more quickly. Thus induction of anaesthesia will be quicker but at the expense of potential adverse effects related to the higher peak blood concentration such as hypotension and bradycardia.

(a)

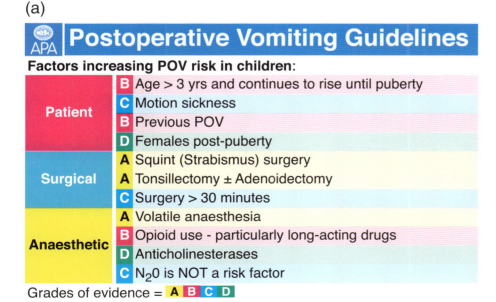

Figure 19.1 a and b, Copies of the POV 'credit card' provided to members of the Association of Paediatric Anaesthetists of Great Britain and Ireland, summarising factors increasing POV risk in children and recommendations for prevention and treatment of POV in children.

(b)

Recommendations for the prevention of POV in children:

Increased Risk	**A**	IV ondansetron 0.15 mg.kg⁻¹ at induction (max. 4mg)
	B	Give intraoperative IV fluids No mandatory oral fluids post-operatively
High Risk (including Squint Surgery & Adeno-tonsillectomy)	**A**	IV ondansetron 0.05 mg.kg⁻¹ and IV dexamethasone 0.15 mg.kg⁻¹
	D	Consider IV anaesthesia and alternatives to opioids

Recommendations for the treatment of established POV in children:

B	IV ondansetron 0.15 mg.kg⁻¹ if not administered in previous 6 hrs
D	If already given ondansetron give: IV dexamethasone 0.15 mg.kg⁻¹ injected slowly

POV Guidelines Group: AS Carr (Chair), L Brennan, S Courtman, D Baines, H Holtby, PA Lönnquist, N Morton, J Pope, S Jacobson

Full POV Guidelines (2010) at www.apagbi.org.uk

Figure 19.1(b) *(cont.)*

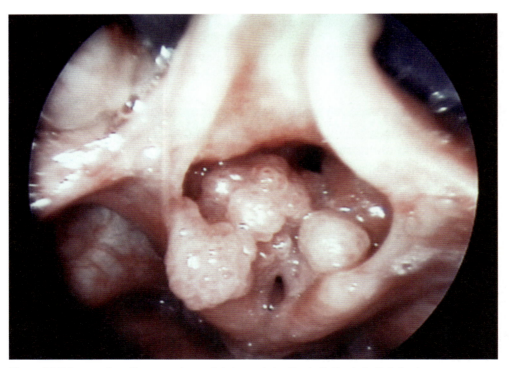

Figure 21.2 Laryngeal papillomas causing partial airway obstruction (with thanks to Dr S. Bew).

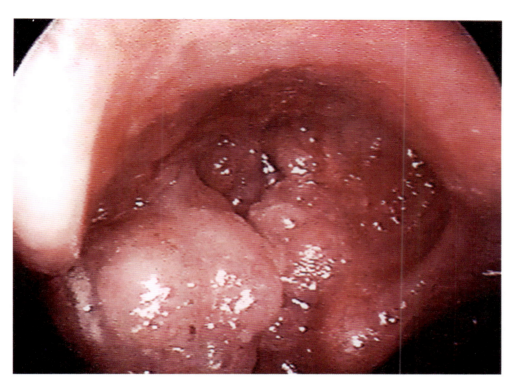

Figure 21.3 Laryngeal papillomas causing severe airway obstruction (with thanks to Dr S. Bew).

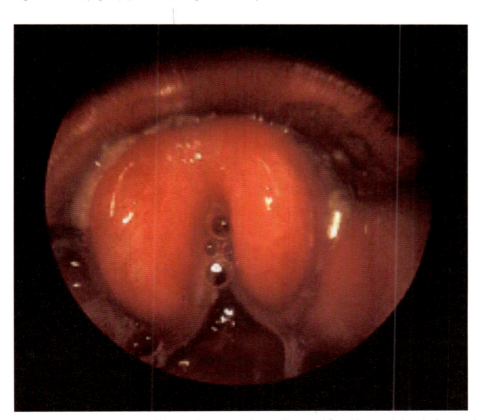

Figure 21.4 Endoscopic view of the epiglottis in epiglottitis. (Reprinted from Hammer J. Acquired upper airway obstruction. *Paed Resp Rev* 2004;**5**:29, with permission from Elsevier.)

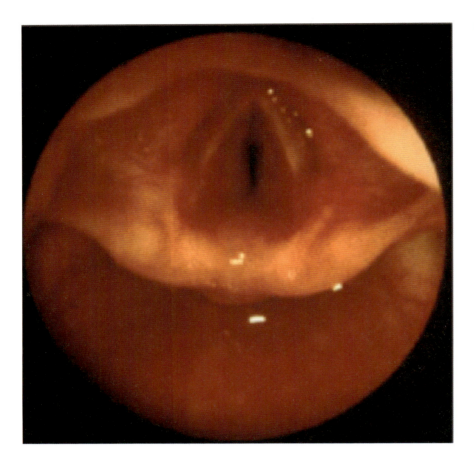

Figure 21.5(a) Endoscopic view of the larynx in croup (a).

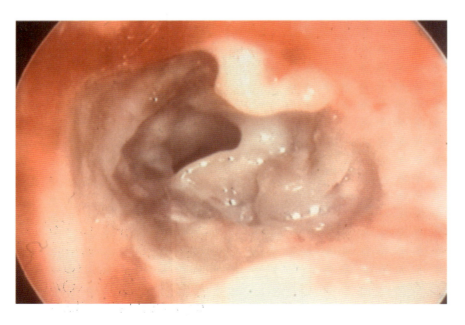

Figure 21.6 Endoscopic view of the trachea in bacterial tracheitis.

The soft palate

Resting position of soft palate

Position of soft palate during speech (arrows indicate flow of air)

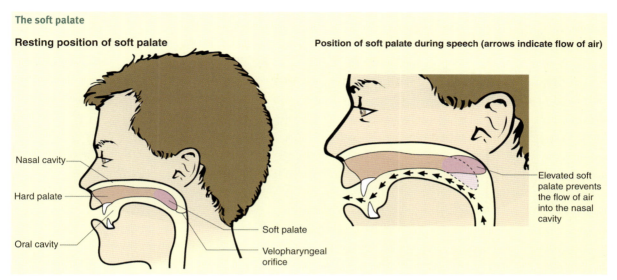

Nasal cavity

Hard palate

Oral cavity

Soft palate

Velopharyngeal orifice

Elevated soft palate prevents the flow of air into the nasal cavity

Figure 23.2 The position of the soft palate at rest and during speech. (Reprinted from Mosahebi A. Kangesu L. Cleft lip and palate. *Surgery (Oxford)* 2006;**24**:34–37, with permission from Elsevier.)

Palate repair

Before

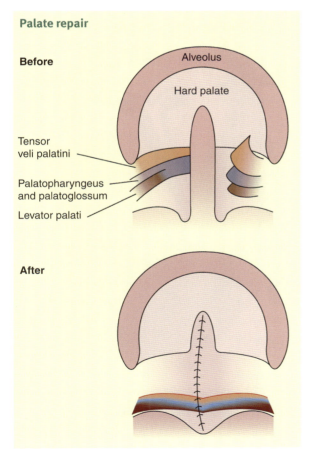

Alveolus

Hard palate

Tensor veli palatini

Palatopharyngeus and palatoglossus

Levator palati

After

Figure 23.3 Primary cleft palate repair – muscles of soft palate are realigned transversely. (Reprinted from Mosahebi A. Kangesu L. Cleft lip and palate. *Surgery (Oxford)* 2006;**24**:34–37, with permission from Elsevier.)

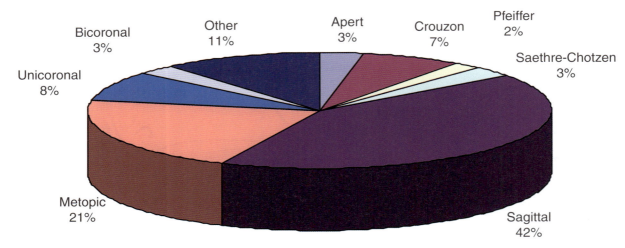

Figure 25.1 Distribution by diagnosis amongst 122 children undergoing cranial vault surgery (GOSH 2008–2009).

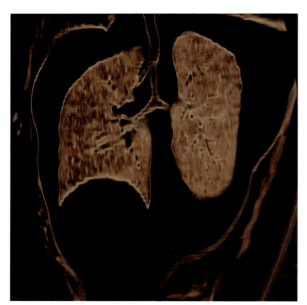

Figure 30.3 Scan showing aberrant tracheal bronchus.

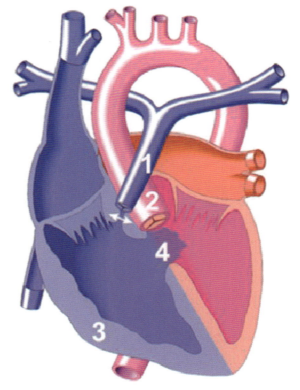

Figure 31.2 Tetralogy of Fallot. Narrowed pulmonary valve and artery (1) with narrowed right ventricular infundibulum (arrows), with aorta (2) over-riding a ventricular septal defect (4), and hypertophied right ventricle (3). From the PedHeart Resource (www.HeartPassport.com). Courtesy of Scientific Software Solutions, Inc.

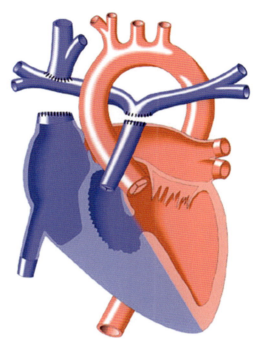

Figure 31.3 Bidirectional Glenn shunt (BDG) in tricuspid atresia, showing anastomosis of the superior vena cava to the right pulmonary artery. From the PedHeart Resource (www.HeartPassport. com). Courtesy of Scientific Software Solutions, Inc.

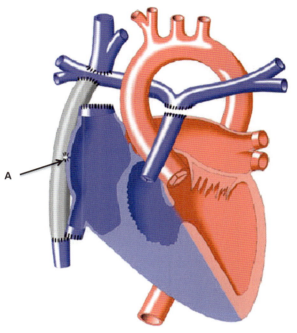

Figure 31.4 Total cavopulmonary connection (TCPC) in tricuspid atresia. Both the superior and inferior vena cavae are connected to the right pulmonary artery. There is a fenestration (A) between the IVC to PA conduit and the atrium. From the PedHeart Resource (www. HeartPassport.com). Courtesy of Scientific Software Solutions, Inc.

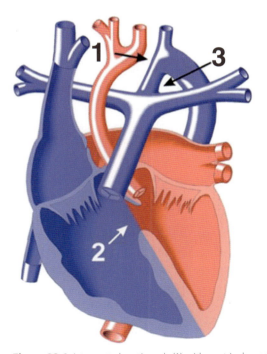

Figure 33.1 Interrupted aortic arch (1) with ventricular septal defect (2). A patent ductus arteriosus (3) provides distal aortic blood flow. From the PedHeart Resource (www.HeartPassport.com). Courtesy of Scientific Software Solutions, Inc.

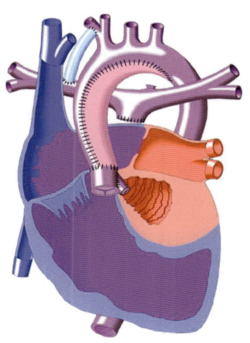

Figure 33.2 Norwood first stage repair of HLHS. The main pulmonary artery has been used to create a neo-aorta. A modified Blalock–Taussig shunt provides pulmonary blood flow. From the PedHeart Resource (www.HeartPassport.com). Courtesy of Scientific Software Solutions, Inc.

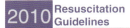
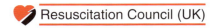
Paediatric Basic Life Support
(Healthcare professionals with a duty to respond)

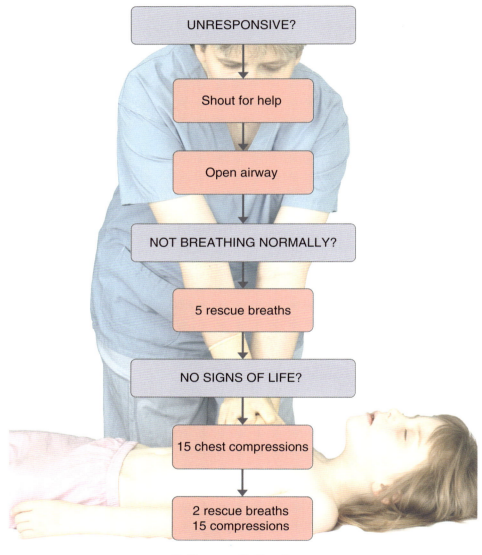

UNRESPONSIVE?

Shout for help

Open airway

NOT BREATHING NORMALLY?

5 rescue breaths

NO SIGNS OF LIFE?

15 chest compressions

2 rescue breaths
15 compressions

Call resuscitation team

October 2010

5th Floor, Tavistock House North, Tavistock Square, London WC1H 9HR
Telephone (020) 7388-4678 . Fax (020) 7383-0773 . Email enquiries@resus.org.uk
www.resus.org.uk . Registered Charity No. 286360

Figure 38.1 Paediatric basic life support.

Paediatric choking treatment algorithm

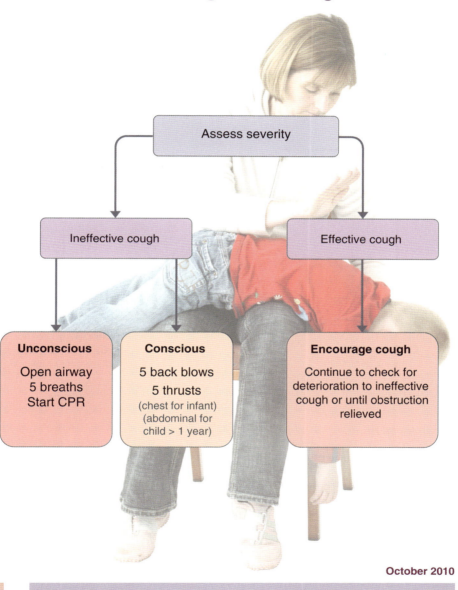

Assess severity

Ineffective cough

Effective cough

Unconscious

Open airway
5 breaths
Start CPR

Conscious

5 back blows
5 thrusts
(chest for infant)
(abdominal for
child > 1 year)

Encourage cough

Continue to check for
deterioration to ineffective
cough or until obstruction
relieved

October 2010

5th Floor, Tavistock House North, Tavistock Square, London WC1H 9HR
Telephone (020) 7388-4678 • Fax (020) 7383-0773 • Email enquiries@resus.org.uk
www.resus.org.uk • Registered Charity No. 286360

Figure 38.2 Paediatric choking treatment algorithm.

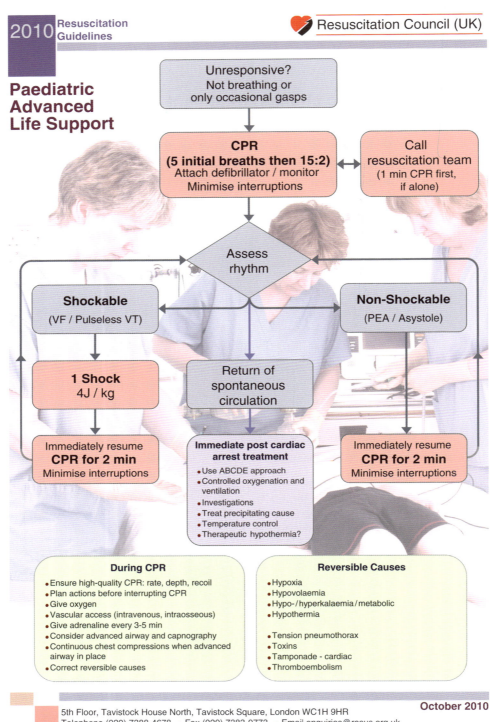

Paediatric Advanced Life Support

Unresponsive?
Not breathing or
only occasional gasps

CPR
(5 initial breaths then 15:2)
Attach defibrillator / monitor
Minimise interruptions

Call resuscitation team
(1 min CPR first,
if alone)

Assess rhythm

Shockable
(VF / Pulseless VT)

Non-Shockable
(PEA / Asystole)

1 Shock
4J / kg

Return of spontaneous circulation

Immediately resume
CPR for 2 min
Minimise interruptions

Immediate post cardiac arrest treatment
- Use ABCDE approach
- Controlled oxygenation and ventilation
- Investigations
- Treat precipitating cause
- Temperature control
- Therapeutic hypothermia?

Immediately resume
CPR for 2 min
Minimise interruptions

During CPR
- Ensure high-quality CPR: rate, depth, recoil
- Plan actions before interrupting CPR
- Give oxygen
- Vascular access (intravenous, intraosseous)
- Give adrenaline every 3-5 min
- Consider advanced airway and capnography
- Continuous chest compressions when advanced airway in place
- Correct reversible causes

Reversible Causes
- Hypoxia
- Hypovolaemia
- Hypo-/hyperkalaemia/metabolic
- Hypothermia

- Tension pneumothorax
- Toxins
- Tamponade - cardiac
- Thromboembolism

October 2010

5th Floor, Tavistock House North, Tavistock Square, London WC1H 9HR
Telephone (020) 7388-4678 • Fax (020) 7383-0773 • Email enquiries@resus.org.uk
www.resus.org.uk • Registered Charity No. 286360

Figure 38.3 Paediatric advanced life support.

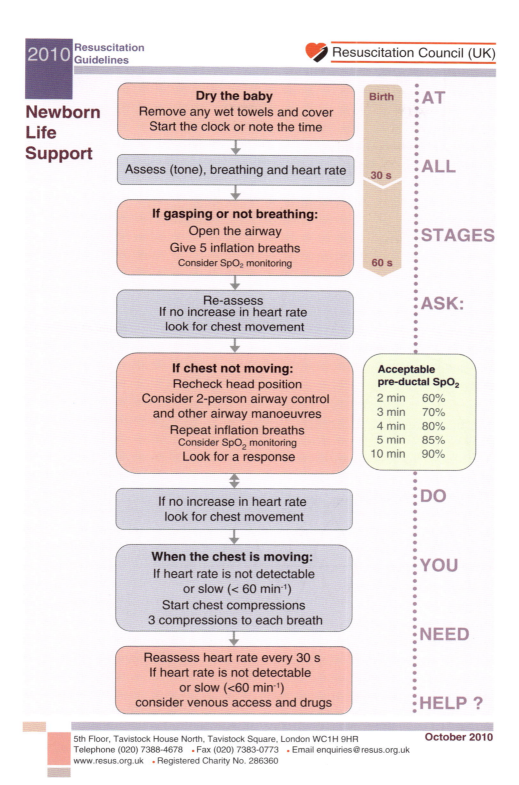

2010 Resuscitation Guidelines

Resuscitation Council (UK)

Newborn Life Support

Dry the baby Remove any wet towels and cover Start the clock or note the time	Birth
Assess (tone), breathing and heart rate	30 s
If gasping or not breathing: Open the airway Give 5 inflation breaths Consider SpO_2 monitoring	60 s

AT

ALL

STAGES

ASK:

Re-assess
If no increase in heart rate
look for chest movement

If chest not moving:
Recheck head position
Consider 2-person airway control
and other airway manoeuvres
Repeat inflation breaths
Consider SpO_2 monitoring
Look for a response

Acceptable pre-ductal SpO_2

2 min	60%
3 min	70%
4 min	80%
5 min	85%
10 min	90%

If no increase in heart rate
look for chest movement

DO

When the chest is moving:
If heart rate is not detectable
or slow (< 60 min^{-1})
Start chest compressions
3 compressions to each breath

YOU

Reassess heart rate every 30 s
If heart rate is not detectable
or slow (<60 min^{-1})
consider venous access and drugs

NEED

HELP ?

5th Floor, Tavistock House North, Tavistock Square, London WC1H 9HR
Telephone (020) 7388-4678 • Fax (020) 7383-0773 • Email enquiries@resus.org.uk
www.resus.org.uk • Registered Charity No. 286360

October 2010

Figure 38.4 Newborn life support.

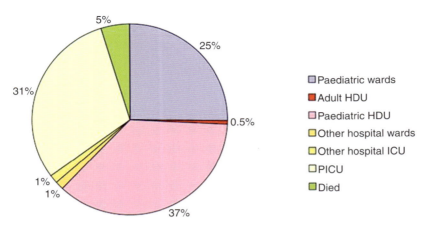

Figure 41.1 Discharge destinations for paediatric admissions to general intensive care units (aggregated data for southwest region 2006–7).

5%

25%

31%

☐ Paediatric wards
■ Adult HDU
☐ Paediatric HDU
☐ Other hospital wards
☐ Other hospital ICU
☐ PICU
■ Died

0.5%

1%
1%

37%

Total = 217 ICU admissions

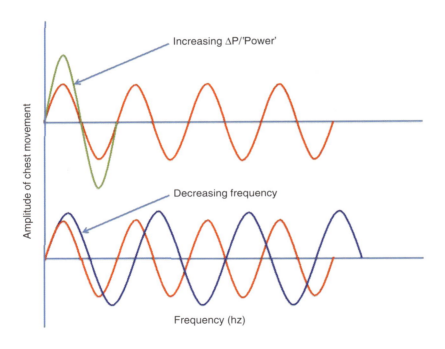

Figure 41.6 Effect of 'power' and frequency on amplitude of oscillation.

Increasing ∆P/'Power'

Amplitude of chest movement

Decreasing frequency

Frequency (hz)

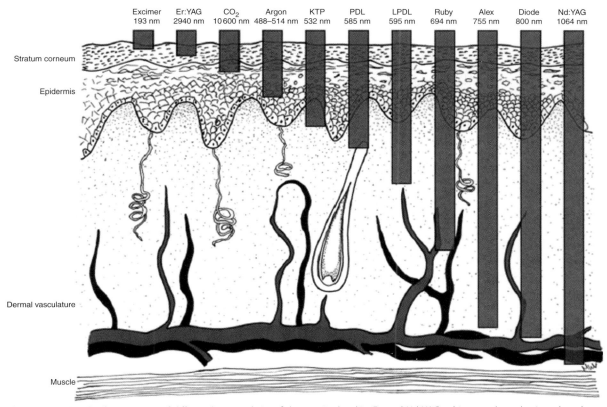

Figure 28.2 Depth of penetration of different lasers and site of damage in the skin. Er- and Nd-YAG, erbium- and neodymium-doped yttrium aluminium garnet; KTP potassium titanyl phosphate; PDL, pulsed dye laser; LPDL, long-pulse dye laser; Alex, Alexandrite laser. Adapted from Figure 1.13 of JS Dover, KA Arndt, RG. Geronemus, *Illustrated Cutaneous and Aesthetic Laser Surgery*, 2nd edition McGraw-Hill. 1999.

prominent during puberty. A number of unusual conditions may be associated with port wine stain:

- Glaucoma (port wine stain around the eye);
- Sturge–Weber syndrome (malformation affects superficial vessels of the brain, associated with developmental delay, hemiplegia and seizures);
- Klippel–Trenaunay syndrome (vascular malformation affecting arm or leg, associated with hypertrophy and venous and lymphatic malformations);
- Proteus syndrome (associated with hemihypertrophy, lymphangioma, lipoma and macrocephaly).

The underlying pathology is associated with an increased number of ectactic vessels in the papillary and reticular dermis. They can also be treated by targeting oxygenated haemoglobin in the vascular compartment with the PDL laser. This is effective in reducing the visual impact of lesions by around 80%.

However, the response to treatment is hugely variable and will depend on the depth of the lesion, with deeper structures being more difficult to treat. Timing of treatment is controversial, but earlier intervention during childhood is generally felt to be helpful, to reduce psychological impact and reduce the need for intervention at a later stage. When planning a course of laser treatment it is helpful to undertake a test patch to show the parents the effect and demonstrate the post-operative bruising associated with the procedure.

Childhood pigmented lesions are amenable to treatment with Q-switched lasers which have a very short pulse duration but very high peak power. They produce largely non-thermal mechanical damage with shock waves, vaporisation of tissue and destruction of melanin pigment. Ruby (694 nm) and Alexandrite (755 nm) laser light are well absorbed by melanin but not haemoglobin. They are effective in the treatment of epidermal lesions such as sebaceous naevus and naevus of Ota and can be used in non-pulsed mode for the removal of hair. If the density of pigment is relatively low, laser surgery is often combined with local anaesthesia infiltration, but if used for depilatory action then application of ice is usually adequate for pain relief.

Key points

- Multimodal analgesia techniques are key to success in paediatric plastic surgery.
- Use local anaesthesia field infiltration, local blocks or regional blockade where possible.
- Administer long-acting opioids early.
- Good communication between the anaesthetist and surgeon is vital.
- Safety is paramount when undertaking anaesthesia for laser surgery.

Further reading

Cantatore JL, Kriegel DA. Laser surgery: An approach to the paediatric patient. *J Am Acad Dermatol* 2004;**50**:165–83.

Fenlon SM. Anaesthesia for plastic surgery in children. *Curr Anaes Crit Care* 2002; **13**:87–91.

Pittaway A. Pediatric dermatological procedures performed outside the operating room. *Curr Opin Anaesthesiol* 2012;**25**:498–500.

Chapter

29

Anaesthesia for orthopaedics, including scoliosis surgery, in children

Steven Scuplak

Introduction

Anaesthetic requirements for children undergoing orthopaedic surgery can be very varied, ranging from simple to complex. Complexity is introduced by the invasiveness of the procedure, or by the association of an underlying medical condition. Anatomical, physiological or biochemical abnormalities can make even minor surgery hazardous, but when combined with highly invasive procedures, such as spinal surgery, the situation can easily become very high risk. This chapter will discuss the general principles of elective orthopaedic anaesthesia, the common procedures and underlying medical conditions, and outline the principles of anaesthesia for scoliosis surgery. Anaesthesia for hand surgery is discussed in Chapter 28.

Orthopaedic anaesthesia

Orthopaedic procedures can be broadly classified into elective or emergency cases. Emergency surgery is most commonly associated with trauma (see Chapter 39), although infection and compartment syndrome after elective procedures may require urgent intervention.

Pre-operative preparation for elective surgery

Orthopaedic patients often require repeat surgery and prolonged hospital admissions. Negative experiences must be minimised and individualised strategies adopted to minimise distress.

The patient history should seek to identify conditions that have an orthopaedic association as this will influence the focus of examination and further investigations. Examples include:

- Cerebral palsy (gait correction surgery, hip surgery, scoliosis)
- Muscular dystrophy (scoliosis surgery)
- Osteogenesis imperfecta (fractures, scoliosis)
- Arthrogryposis (joint contractures, scoliosis)
- Craniofacial syndromes e.g. Apert syndrome (hand surgery)
- Neurofibromatosis (pseudoarthrosis of the tibia)
- VATER/VACTERL association (scoliosis surgery, hand surgery)

Special note should be taken if the child suffers from muscle spasm and requires antispasmodics, as post-operative muscle spasm may be severe if the limb is immobilised post-operatively. Post-operative spasm should be anticipated and aggressively managed. Many children will be receiving medication such as anticonvulsants that need to be continued throughout the peri-operative period.

Pre-operative blood tests should be guided by the history and examination. Tourniquets are used routinely for peripheral orthopaedic surgery so blood transfusion is rarely required. Children undergoing major procedures such as hip surgery require at minimum a group and antibody screen. Treatment of pre-existing anaemia will minimise the risk of transfusion. Correction of nutritional deficiencies is straightforward, but occasionally erythropoietin is indicated in chronic disease.

Ionising radiation is commonly used during orthopaedic surgery, so the possibility of pregnancy must be excluded in any girl after the menarche. Deep vein thrombosis (DVT) is uncommon in children, but prophylaxis should be considered in high-risk groups and should be discussed with the surgeon. Risk factors include:

Core Topics in Paediatric Anaesthesia, ed. Ian James and Isabeau Walker. Published by Cambridge University Press. © 2013 Cambridge University Press.

- Teenage years
- Obesity
- Oral contraceptive pill
- Prolonged immobility
- Lower limb fractures, pelvic, hip or spinal surgery
- Previous DVT
- Conditions associated with a thrombotic tendency (antiphospholipid syndrome, factor V Leiden, protein C, S or antithrombin III deficiency)

Anaesthesia techniques

Orthopaedic surgery offers ample opportunity for wrong site surgery. There needs to be a special focus on pre-induction checks during the sign-in phase of anaesthesia, particularly the consent for surgery, the nature and site of surgery and the surgical site marking, which is confirmed during the time-out prior to incision.

The method of induction will depend on patient preference and underlying medical concerns.

Gaseous induction

Medical factors favouring gaseous induction include management of a difficult airway and difficult venous access.

In certain circumstances gaseous induction is contraindicated. This can be absolute, as for malignant hyperthermia susceptibility (MHS), or relative where there is insufficient clinical evidence to guarantee safety, as in the case of the muscular dystrophies (see below). MHS is a specific autosomal dominant inherited disorder, and there are only a few rare diseases linked to MHS. These are:

- Core myopathies (particularly central core disease)
- King–Denborough syndrome
- Brody disease

Children with these conditions should all receive a non-triggering anaesthetic. No other diseases have a proven association with MHS.

Muscle relaxants

Neuromuscular abnormalities are common in patients presenting for orthopaedic surgery, many of which are difficult to categorise. The possibility of an adverse reaction to suxamethonium leading to hyperkalaemia and cardiac arrest is ever present, and suxamethonium can never be considered to be safe in these patients. If neuromuscular blockade is required then a judicious dose of a non-depolarising agent should be used (taking into account the severity of the neuromuscular condition).

Continued neuromuscular blockade after intubation is contraindicated when motor nerve function needs to be monitored. Percutaneously applied wires and struts may cause nerve damage during limb lengthening surgery and application of an external frame. This risk is minimised if it is possible to detect a motor response if nerve irritation occurs. Neuromuscular blockade must be discontinued if motor pathways need to be monitored during spinal surgery.

Maintenance of anaesthesia

Maintenance of anaesthesia should provide safe operating conditions, good analgesia, rapid recovery and minimal complications, such as post-operative nausea and vomiting. Maintenance of anaesthesia is usually by inhalational agent, although total intravenous anaesthesia (TIVA) may be needed if inhalational agents are contraindicated.

Antibiotics

Antimicrobial prophylaxis is indicated if metalwork is to be implanted, and local policy should dictate the agents of choice. These should be administered as soon as possible after induction, so that tissue concentrations can be maximised – this is most important when a tourniquet is used.

Analgesia

The principles of best practice are to maximise the use of local anaesthetic blocks, minimise the use of opioids and avoid deep planes of anaesthesia in vulnerable patients. Multimodal analgesia is central to pain management, with regular paracetamol and non-steroidal anti-inflammatory drugs (NSAIDs) indicated for most cases. This combined with local anaesthetic infiltration is adequate for simple procedures. Immobilisation of the operative site, either by plaster cast or fixator, tends to limit the degree of post-operative pain. The exception is in knee surgery when a passive motion machine may be used.

NSAIDs

Animal and human studies suggest that fracture healing and ossification is reduced by NSAIDs, probably owing to their effects on cyclo-oxygenase-2 and mesenchymal cell differentiation, but this is controversial and not all studies are consistent. If bone healing is a major concern, NSAIDs should probably be limited to the first 48 hours post-operatively.

Regional techniques

The following regional techniques are performed routinely, provided there are no contraindications:

- *Axillary nerve block*: upper limb surgery.
- *Single shot caudal* and *lumbar epidural blocks*: lower limb surgery; combinations of local anaesthetic and clonidine are commonly used for single shot caudal analgesia.
- *Continuous epidural blockade*: limited use in the post-operative period because of the need to monitor for nerve injury and compartment syndrome. Consider elective top-up of the block at the end of surgery before removing the catheter.
- *Peripheral nerve blocks*: require specific expertise and are less reliable. Ultrasound guidance improves success, so with increasing availability of equipment and experience, these techniques will become more common.

Elective bladder catheterisation should be considered if an epidural is used, also after prolonged surgery, large intra-operative fluid loads and in the presence of lower-limb plaster casts. Catheterisation will prevent acute post-operative urinary retention but also simplify patient care and prevent soiling of plaster casts.

Opioid analgesia

Opioid analgesia is used as part of balanced anaesthesia during surgery and to supplement local anaesthetic blocks. Post-operatively, opioids are often required as neural blocks regress. As a general rule, oral opioids are adequate for soft tissue surgery, but IV opioids should be used for bone-disrupting surgery, ideally by means of a nurse-controlled or patient-controlled device.

Parenteral opioids are rarely needed after the first 24 hours, although they are useful for dressing changes and the manipulation of external fixators.

Enteral fluid and feeding can usually be started immediately post-operatively, especially if opioids have been avoided. Oral morphine can then be used to manage breakthrough pain.

Tourniquets

Pneumatic tourniquets are placed in approximately 50% of procedures and inflation pressures should be determined by systolic blood pressure. Lower-limb inflation pressures should be set at approximately 150 mmHg above systolic and upper-limb 100 mmHg above. Adequate padding under the tourniquet is essential and must be protected from any ingress of irritant fluids. Inflation times should be limited to 75 minutes and simultaneous bilateral inflation avoided. Inflation times above 90 minutes lead to a progressive rise in core temperature.

Specific orthopaedic conditions
Congenital dislocation of the hip

Congenital dislocation of the hip occurs in approximately 4 in 1000 live births, with females more affected than males, and if undetected can lead to permanent dislocation, dysplasia and eventual osteoarthritis. Treatment should begin in the neonatal period. Treatment is aimed at reducing the dislocation and optimising the position of the femoral head in the acetabulum, thus promoting healthy growth. This can be achieved non-invasively by traction or closed reduction with application of a hip frog plaster (hip spica). Invasive procedures are needed in difficult cases; this may involve adductor tendon releases (to improve mobility and relocation of the femoral head), open reduction of the joint, femoral rotational osteotomy to improve femoral head engagement and acetabular procedures to improve the coverage of the femoral head.

Anaesthetic management

Major hip surgery may result in significant blood loss, and blood should be grouped and antibody status determined as a minimum. Often the exact nature of the surgical intervention is unknown until after further examination under anaesthesia and an arthrogram has been performed. The insertion of a regional block can be delayed until the indication is clear. Single-shot caudal or lumbar epidural are beneficial for all invasive procedures, although opioids are often required to cover skin incisions over the iliac crest by the end of extensive procedures. Nurse- or patient-controlled opioid analgesia will be required post-operatively. Post-operative immobilisation is often achieved using a hip spica – this limits the use of a lumbar epidural catheter, as there is minimal access to the lumbar spine. Post-operatively the legs should be raised to reduce swelling and a post-operative haemo-globin level checked. Capillary refill and distal pulses should be regularly examined to detect circulatory compromise.

Hip spica

This extensive hip plaster cast forms the cornerstone of treatment to maintain hip position in smaller children. To apply it, the patient must be suspended on a casting table. Control of the airway may be difficult, and even as a sole procedure, intubation should be considered. Moving the patient onto the spica table is stimulating, and may reveal a lighter plane of anaes-thesia than expected, particularly if the surgical site is covered by a regional block; take care to maintain an appropriate depth of anaesthesia. Application of a hip spica can take 40 minutes – it can be challenging to keep the child warm. Double nappies are used to avoid soiling of the cast and should be in place before the child wakes up. Urinary catheterisation simplifies immediate post-operative care after extensive surgery.

Congenital talipes equinovarus

Congenital talipes equinovarus (CTEV), or clubfoot, is a common congenital deformity occurring in approximately 1 in 1000 live births. Most cases are idiopathic but can be associated with neuromuscular abnormalities. Early treatment is by soft tissue manipulation and serial casting. Percutaneous Achil-les tendon lengthening or soft tissue release may be required to aid correction and in later stages osteo-tomy maybe needed. Rarely the correction is achieved by application of an external frame and gradual correction.

Anaesthetic management

Occasionally the patient will need to be positioned prone. A caudal epidural block should be standard practice and if an osteotomy is performed then par-enteral opioids will be required post-operatively. Any procedure involving the stretching of muscles com-bined with post-operative casting will be associated

with post-operative muscle spasm. Severe intermit-tent cramping pain may become apparent as the caudal recedes, and is not responsive to opioids. Spasm responds to oral diazepam, and this should be prescribed pre-operatively rather than pursuing increasing doses of opioids.

Cerebral palsy

Cerebral palsy results from central nervous damage caused either antenatally or in the immediate peri-natal period. It is characterised by motor dysfunction, which can be classified into spastic (most common), dyskinetic, ataxic or mixed. The clinical picture is highly variable, and normal intellect can be masked by difficulties in communication. During the pre-operative visit it is essential to enquire about levels of comprehension and not to make assumptions that will alienate the child.

The area of the brain affected will dictate any associated problems. Epilepsy occurs in about 40% and intellectual or cognitive problems are common. Swallowing and feeding problems are frequent and can result in malnutrition and recurrent chest infec-tion. These patients are at risk of developing chronic respiratory insufficiency. Gastro-oesophageal reflux is common and many have anti-reflux procedures, often with a gastrostomy. Enthusiastic feeding can rapidly develop into obesity with little appreciation of the underlying lack of muscle mass. Difficult venous access is common. Scoliosis is common, and this can further impact on respiratory function. Many children have had ventriculo-peritoneal shunts inserted for the treatment of hydrocephalus, and damage to these systems must be avoided. Latex allergy occurs with greater frequency in this group of patients.

Orthopaedic surgery is aimed at improving func-tion, mobility and reducing pain. The simplest pro-cedure is injection of botulinum toxin into the spastic muscles combined with post-operative physiotherapy and splinting. Hip surgery can be performed to reduce painful dislocation or enhance function by rotational femoral osteotomy to achieve realignment of the limb. Fixed flexion deformities require extensive soft tissue releases and casting to maintain the correction.

Anaesthetic management

Gastro-oesophageal reflux and respiratory impair-ment is common, so in all but minor procedures the child should be intubated and ventilation controlled.

In the absence of a gastrostomy the placement of a nasogastric tube simplifies the post-operative administration of anticonvulsant therapy. Difficult venous access increases the need for central access; care must be taken to avoid damage to ventriculo-peritoneal drainage systems. Temperature regulation is often disordered and in severe cases the basal metabolic rate so low that severe hypothermia may occur rapidly.

Pain assessment is difficult in the post-operative period owing to general irritability and poor communication. Muscle spasm must be aggressively managed, and the early use of oral diazepam is encouraged. Opioids must be used when indicated, although atypical responses are common. The simplest and safest method of administration of opioids is to titrate intravenously post-operatively and accept that high-dependency support will be required. The balance between the safe provision of analgesia and respiratory compromise is narrow, and post-operative respiratory infections are common and can be life threatening.

Muscular dystrophy

The dystrophinopathies include Duchenne muscular dystrophy, and the less common Becker muscular dystrophies. Muscle weakness is progressive leading to respiratory failure and cardiomyopathy that can progress to circulatory failure. Recent advances that have extended survival and reduced morbidity include non-invasive ventilatory support, steroids and a variety of cardiovascular drugs. Scoliosis is common and the decision to proceed to surgery must be balanced against the high risks.

The use of inhalational agents and suxamethonium in the muscular dystrophies has been associated very rarely with rhabdomyolysis, hyperkalaemia and cardiac arrest. The metabolic derangement is distinct from MH and can first appear on emergence from anaesthesia with the onset of spontaneous movement. Exposure to inhalational agents in the muscular dystrophies should be avoided and a TIVA technique employed. Blood loss during surgery is increased because the contraction of arteriolar smooth muscle is impaired. Poor cardiac function and respiratory reserve require expert management.

Osteogenesis imperfecta

Osteogenesis imperfecta (OI) is a group of rare inherited connective tissue disorder that results in increased bone fragility. Surgery is usually indicated for the treatment of fractures and scoliosis. Airway management, positioning and blood pressure measurement can result in fractures. Suxamethonium should be avoided because of unpredictable effects of fasciculations, but OI is not associated with malignant hyperpyrexia. Bleeding is increased from exposed abnormal bone matrix and can be severe and difficult to control.

Arthrogryposis

Arthrogryposis describes the condition of congenital non-progressive symmetrical joint contractures arising from a variety of causes of fetal immobility. Neurogenic causes are present in the vast majority and often associated with a reduction in muscle mass. The involvement of the temporomandibular joint may limit mouth opening and if combined with micrognathia may make intubation difficult. Vascular access can be extremely difficult owing to the abnormal and featureless appearance of the limbs. There is a common association with congenital heart disease. Surgery is often needed to improve posture and joint mobility and for scoliosis.

Scoliosis surgery

Scoliosis is an abnormal lateral curvature of the spine and can be classified into congenital, idiopathic (infantile, juvenile, adolescent) and acquired. Congenital scoliosis is commonly associated with other abnormalities and often progresses rapidly at an early age. The major causes of acquired scoliosis are neuromuscular diseases, particularly cerebral palsy and the muscular dystrophies. Surgical treatment is indicated when the degree of curvature or its rate of acceleration puts other organs at risk or when pain intervenes. The commonest procedures requiring anaesthesia are posterior spinal surgery, anterior spinal surgery and application of plaster jackets.

The largest group requiring surgery comprises teenagers with idiopathic scoliosis. These patients are fit and healthy, and pre-assessment should concentrate on imparting information and the detection of anaemia. At the other end of the spectrum are patients with progressive end-stage neuromuscular disease, where multidisciplinary discussions are required to focus on consideration of the benefits and the risks of surgery.

All patients requiring scoliosis surgery should be pre-assessed, and multidisciplinary involvement is mandatory. Pre-assessment allows for the detection and optimal management of any underlying disease and secondary morbidity. Risks of anaesthesia need to be openly discussed and can sometimes limit the surgical options. Post-operative care needs to be planned and the likelihood of elective post-operative ventilation evaluated.

Pre-operative assessment

Respiratory function is probably the most crucial area to concentrate on. For many children the formal assessment of respiratory function is difficult because of a lack of cooperation. Frequent chest infections, poor cough or symptoms suggestive of sleep apnoea warrant further investigation that may include blood gas analysis, respiratory function tests and most usefully, sleep study analysis. Sleep studies monitor continuous SpO_2 and transcutaneous CO_2 and provide useful information as to the need for post-operative respiratory support. This information can also be used to monitor the progression of neuromuscular disease and guide pre-operative intervention and the possibility of non-invasive respiratory support. The increased use of home ventilation, either by non-invasive mask support, or by tracheostomy and more formal ventilation, has increased the number of patients being offered surgery despite the presence of advanced respiratory disease.

Cardiomyopathy may be a feature of the muscle pathology leading to scoliosis, or a structural cardiac anomaly may be part of an associated syndrome. Severe chest wall deformity rarely leads to primary cardiac insufficiency. Severe pulmonary disease can lead to elevated pulmonary vascular resistance and right ventricular dysfunction. Cardiac surgery itself may predispose to scoliosis by disrupting chest wall growth secondary to damage to the ribs and sternum. The severity of cardiac disease can be masked in wheelchair-bound patients by lack of activity, and surgery can produce unique stresses that may result in acute decompensation. A routine pre-operative ECG should be performed, and further investigation with echocardiography is frequently indicated. Children with progressive neuromuscular disease require an up-to-date echo before surgery.

Nutrition needs to be optimised pre-operatively and any feeding difficulties resolved. Supplementary enteral feeding may need to be started. Anaemia should be investigated and fully treated before embarking upon major surgery.

Epilepsy is common and therapy should be continued over the peri-operative period with a management plan for breakthrough seizure activity.

Spinal cord injury and monitoring

Spinal cord damage is a prime concern during scoliosis surgery. Damage can be caused by direct mechanical trauma or more commonly secondary to vascular insufficiency. Mechanical trauma can be from instrumentation or from compression during spinal manipulation. Vascular insufficiency may result from vascular spasm or disruption to the arterial supply of the cord during spinal manipulation. These injuries will be intensified by hypotension and major blood loss.

Spinal cord function can be monitored using sensory evoked potentials or motor evoked potentials and occasionally by performing a 'wake up' test. Sensory potentials relate to posterior cord function and motor potentials relate to anterior cord function. The posterior third of the cord has a vascular supply derived from two spinal arteries while the anterior two-thirds part has only a single supply. This has led to the increased use of motor monitoring, as ischaemia is more likely to develop in the larger anterior single vessel territory. Ideally both modalities are monitored and recorded continuously by specially trained staff, with any significant changes brought to the attention of the anaesthetist and surgeon immediately. Relevant changes are apt to occur:

- During spinal instrumentation, for example pedicle screw insertion;
- During times of spinal manipulation, such as rod insertion and curve correction;
- During periods of cardiovascular instability.

The potentials are measured between surface or subcutaneous electrodes placed on all limbs, scalp and cervical area, with the occasional use of an epidural catheter placed intra-operatively. The production of motor potentials requires high-energy transcranial stimulation and may lead to inadvertent masseter contraction; a bite block to protect the lips, tongue and tracheal tube from damage is essential.

The anaesthetic technique has to be modified to optimise the recordings. Sensory potentials are maximised with low levels of inhalational agents; motor monitoring requires the total avoidance of inhalational agents and no continued neuromuscular blockade. Improved neuromuscular monitoring has reduced the need for 'wake up' testing to minimal levels. A wake up test requires the withdrawal of anaesthesia and ideally the conscious movement of the toes. Fortunately with opioid-based techniques these events are not usually remembered.

Posterior spinal surgery

Posterior spinal surgery is increasingly performed alone to correct scoliosis. This change has occurred because of the technological advancements in the equipment used to correct the spinal deformity and increased ability to monitor cord function during major manipulations. Spinal fixation is usually achieved by attaching a pair of suitably curved rods to the bony spine. In the past this was achieved with a combination of pedicle screws in the lumbar region and laminar hooks or wires in the thoracic and cervical spine. Increasingly, pedicle screws are used throughout the spine and provide a more robust attachment. This enables the bony spine to be manipulated to a greater degree and assume a closer to normal correction.

Anaesthetic management

The technique for induction of anaesthesia can be as preferred but the needs of intra-operative spinal monitoring will dictate further management. Total intravenous anaesthesia (TIVA) is required for successful motor monitoring and neuromuscular blockade can only be used to aid intubation. High-dose intra-operative opioids provide optimal conditions, and propofol/remifentanil-based TIVA is a common choice.

Analgesia

Pain relief intra-operatively is best provided by high dose opioids, usually fentanyl or a continuous infusion of remifentanil. On recovery it is desirable that spontaneous lower limb movements occur as soon as possible so that neurological integrity can be established. In paediatric patients, the use of propofol-based TIVA as a target-controlled infusion (TCI) over a prolonged period of time can result in delayed post-operative recovery due to the accumulation of propofol. It is advisable to decrease the infusions or terminate them early and possibly change to inhalational-based anaesthesia while closing the wound. Post-operatively, pain control requires large doses of opioid, ideally administered by IV infusion initially and continued as an NCA. Extensive surgery makes PCA impractical initially. Post-operatively the patients usually have to lie supine for 12 hours to tamponade the wound and reduce bleeding. Paracetamol should be given regularly and NSAIDs are useful if excessive bleeding has not occurred; their use should be limited to the first 48 hours post-operatively to reduce the incidence of failed fusions.

The two major concerns for anaesthesia for posterior spinal surgery are the anticipated blood losses and surgery in the prone position.

Blood loss

Blood losses can be life-threatening if the fusion involves the whole spine down to pelvis. Blood loss is increased by increased tissue disruption, length of surgery, and the appearance of coagulopathy. In extreme cases haemostasis is only achieved by judicious premature surgical closure of the wound. Blood should be immediately available for all but limited posterior procedures.

Venous access is dictated by anticipated blood loss. Two large-bore peripheral cannulae are desirable, one used for fluid administration and the other for TIVA and as a backup. A system for rapid infusion should be available, preferably with integrated warming. Central venous access is indicated when large losses are expected, peripheral access is limited, when coexisting disease adds complexity, or by the need for extended post-operative venous access. Intra-operative arterial access is desirable in all but the most limited cases.

Intra-arterial blood pressure monitoring is essential as blood pressure can change rapidly owing to fluid loses and occasionally as a result of spinal cord disruption, and is a constant guide to spinal perfusion pressures. Intra-operatively the blood pressure should be controlled to reduce blood losses. Profound hypotension may compromise cord perfusion, and if spinal monitoring detects deterioration then this needs to be aggressively reversed. Urinary catheterisation is standard to assess fluid balance and will be required in the post-operative period. Antimicrobial therapy is essential as the amount of metalwork is extensive and the consequences of infection are devastating.

Blood loss during surgery is reduced by controlled hypotension and avoiding hypertension, and by administration of the antifibrinolytic tranexamic acid ($10 \, mg \, kg^{-1}$ IV). Blood salvage should be routine, using an automated cell saver for suction blood, and the blood from swabs can be rinsed out in physiological saline. In many cases blood transfusion can be avoided, provided post-operative anaemia is acceptable. Massive blood transfusion leads to coagulopathy, which should be anticipated and treated aggressively to prevent escalation. Cord injury can occur during periods of hypotension and cord monitoring should be used to assess adequacy of resuscitation. Bleeding occurs from the traumatic detachment of muscle from the spine and from bone. For definitive spinal fixation to occur, the periostium of the bony elements must be removed and the interarticular joints need to be disrupted. This, combined with bleeding from the pedicle marrow, provides a vast area over which bleeding can occur.

Prone positioning

Airway control in the prone position needs to be secure. Reinforced flexible tracheal tubes are ideal and placement of a bite guard reduces possible damage to lips, tongue and tracheal tube. A nasogastric tube is necessary to decompress the stomach and is usually retained into the post-operative period; a nasopharyngeal temperature probe is placed to assess core temperature.

Positioning the patient prone requires time, coordination with the theatre team and familiarity with the equipment available to support the body. Vascular access must be secure, the abdomen must remain unrestricted, the head must be well supported in a neutral position without pressure on the orbits or nose, and all peripheral pressure points must be padded. The arms must drape comfortably, without undue compression or extension that may lead to brachial plexus or peripheral nerve injury. The simplest way to assess posture is to replicate it on oneself to judge the degree of comfort and then modify as appropriate. Responsibility for positioning should be clear – the anaesthetist should control positioning of the upper body as a logical minimum. A fenestrated warm air body warmer enhances the ability to maintain normothermia. Clear drapes improve the ability to assess the patient.

Post-operative care

All patients should be managed in a HDU environment post-operatively as a minimum requirement. Elective admission to PICU will depend on patient factors and the extent of surgery. The presence of neuromuscular disease, respiratory disease or severe coexisting disease will necessitate a period of elective ventilation so that stability can be established prior to extubation. Wheelchair-bound patients with neuromuscular disease often undergo more extensive surgery, as the spinal fusion may extend to the pelvis. Normothermia, correction of coagulopathy and optimisation of fluid balance and pain control are essential prior to extubation. Occasional unplanned PICU admission may be necessary if massive blood loss has occurred. Patients undergoing extensive combined anterior–posterior spinal surgery should electively be admitted to PICU for post-operative ventilation, even if there are no underlying medical concerns.

Growth rod insertion

Spinal fixation prior to the cessation of normal growth will arrest further growth. Growth rods provide dynamic stabilisation and correction of scoliosis in younger patients and permit further growth over time. The two rods are attached posteriorly with limited attachment to spine. They overlap and can be distracted over years to decrease the degree of abnormality and adapt to the growing spine. These remain in place until definitive posterior fixation is feasible. Blood loss is not a major issue since there is only limited exposure of the spine, but spinal cord monitoring is necessary so will influence the conduct of anaesthesia. The surgery for further distractions involves even less exposure, but again spinal monitoring will dictate anaesthetic technique.

Anterior spinal surgery

Anterior spinal surgery is usually performed to release the spine and enhance mobility. It is usually followed immediately or at intervals by posterior fusion. The problems of anterior surgery are related to those of thoracotomy and therefore one-lung ventilation and post-operative pain relief. Surgery often involves a thoraco-abdominal incision in the lateral position with disruption to the diaphragm. This type of surgery is inappropriate in patients with severe coexisting disease and significant respiratory impairment.

The conduct of anaesthesia is again influenced by techniques used to monitor cord function. A standard tracheal tube is adequate as exposure of the spine is by lung retraction and ventilation/perfusion mismatch rarely results in significant changes in oxygenation. Of greater concern is retraction resulting in compression of major blood vessels or mediastinal shift. For this reason invasive arterial monitoring is essential. Blood loss is usually well controlled and transfusion is very rarely indicated. Central venous access is only required if peripheral access is difficult or if there is complicating coexisting disease.

Optimal pain relief in the post-operative period is essential to prevent lung collapse and infection. Coughing is inhibited by wound pain and irritation from the chest drain. Intra-operative infiltration of the intercostal nerves can be performed by the surgeon, and epidurals can also be used. A multimodal approach to analgesia is best with regular paracetamol, NSAIDs and morphine NCA that can be augmented with ketamine. Post-operative ventilation is rarely required as patient selection implies that respiratory reserve is adequate, but patients should be nursed in an HDU environment.

Wound debridement for wound infection

Wound infection is a devastating and life-threatening complication of scoliosis surgery, owing to the amount of implanted material and underlying poor medical condition of many patients. Antimicrobial agents are routinely continued post-operatively until the wound becomes dry. Patients presenting for exploratory surgery with wound infection must be managed aggressively. Superficial infections may be connected to deep extensive lesions producing widespread tissue necrosis. Debridement can result in massive blood loss and this must be anticipated. Long-term venous access is required to provide access for antimicrobial agents and often to supplement nutrition.

Plaster jacket application

The use of plaster jackets offers a non-surgical management of scoliosis in young patients where significant growth is yet to occur. The child must be intubated and the tracheal tube securely fixed, as the application requires significant movement and precarious positioning. The fixed thoracoabdominal jacket will impede ventilation and an aperture must be cut as soon as possible to allow abdominal movement.

Key points

- Children presenting for elective orthopaedic surgery may have associated medical conditions, and a careful history should be taken, particularly to identify associated neuromuscular disorders.
- Multimodal analgesia should be used, although NSAIDs should be limited to 48 hours if there is a concern about bone healing.
- Procedures involving muscle stretch and casting may be associated with post-operative muscle spasm.
- All children undergoing scoliosis surgery should be assessed pre-operatively in a multidisciplinary clinic. The major concerns peri-operatively are bleeding and spinal cord function.
- TIVA is the anaesthesia technique of choice if spinal cord monitoring is used.

Chapter 30

Anaesthesia for thoracic surgery in children

Simon R. Haynes

Introduction

Anaesthesia for thoracic surgery in children poses different problems to those encountered in adult thoracic anaesthetic practice. It is a low volume specialty largely confined to specialist paediatric hospitals. Anaesthesia may be required for a heterogeneous range of conditions, will frequently be of an urgent or emergency nature and can very often be challenging. This chapter will cover the management of congenital and acquired lung abnormalities, intrathoracic masses, intrapleural collections and pectus surgery. Patient positioning, surgical retraction of the lung and the underlying disease processes involved all contribute to the demands placed on the paediatric thoracic anaesthetist. Thoracotomy for cardiac surgery, for example for coarctation repair, is covered in Chapter 31 and thoracotomy for oesophageal anomalies is covered in Chapter 20.

Congenital abnormalities of the lung
Congenital lobar emphysema

This condition is due to bronchial cartilaginous dysplasia that generates a ball-valve effect to allow pathological emphysematous accumulation of air within the affected lobe, and is associated with poor deflation of that lobe. Usually a single lobe is affected, most commonly the left upper. There is a spectrum of disease which usually presents in the neonatal period. Presentation may be that of a coincidental X-ray finding; alternatively, a neonate may present *in extremis*, with hypoxia, hypercapnia and mediastinal shift caused by hyperinflated lung tissue (Figure 30.1). When a child is presenting acutely, urgent lobectomy is indicated.

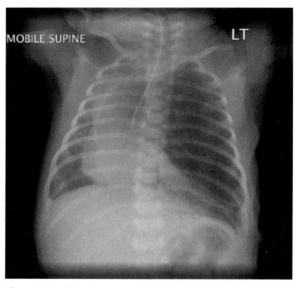

Figure 30.1 Chest X-ray showing congenital lobar emphysema.

Congenital cystic abnormalities of the lung

There are three main types of cystic congenital abnormalities

- Congenital cystic adenomatous malformations (CCAM)
- Pulmonary sequestration
- Bronchogenic cysts

In common with congenital lobar emphysema, there is a spectrum of disease. Symptoms can be caused by mass effect, or by secondary infection.

Congenital cystic adenomatous malformation

CCAM results from localised arrest of maturation of fetal lung. A disorganised mass of air and/or blood

Core Topics in Paediatric Anaesthesia, ed. Ian James and Isabeau Walker. Published by Cambridge University Press. © 2013 Cambridge University Press.

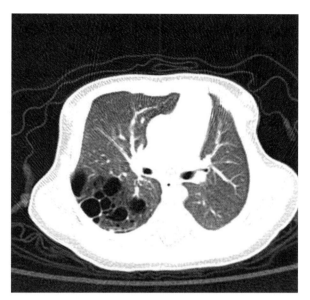

Figure 30.2 CT scan showing congenital cystic adenomatous malformations in the lung.

filled cysts is present which does not usually communicate with normal lung (see Figure 30.2). An antenatal diagnosis is often made, but the immediate course of action depends on the clinical condition of the child once born. Resection of the abnormal area may be required urgently to relieve compression – this is not usually as marked as with congenital lobar emphysema. The affected area may be removed electively later in childhood to prevent infection and to remove the abnormal tissue, which has potential to undergo malignant change.

Pulmonary sequestration

This is a separate bronchopulmonary mass or cyst which is disconnected from the bronchial tree and has a separate blood supply arising from the aorta. It forms when a supernumerary lung bud arises from the primitive foregut. Other congenital abnormalities are present in 65% of cases. Appropriate pre-operative investigation is required to identify the blood supply.

Bronchogenic cysts

These are solitary, unilocular and often mucus filled. They are often an incidental radiographic finding, but may become infected.

Acquired pathology
Thoracic tumours in children

Primary lung malignancies are rare in children. Extensive intrathoracic tumours such as neuroblastoma may require de-bulking or resection through a thoracotomy. Such tumours are not usually intrapulmonary. Thoracotomy may be required for metastatectomy.

Anterior mediastinal mass

Anterior mediastinal masses are a common presenting feature of haematological malignancy such as lymphoma, or occasionally due to primary malignancy. Histological diagnosis of a mediastinal mass is essential to direct therapy. Mediastinal masses can compress trachea, bronchi or great vessels. Respiratory symptoms are frequently the presenting feature and may be rapidly progressive. Occasionally a child with a mediastinal mass presents *in extremis* with airway obstruction. The presence of stridor or respiratory difficulty at rest forewarns of difficulty, particularly the child who has to sit forward to obtain a position of comfort. CT scan images obtained pre-operatively are particularly helpful to identify compression of major structures. Pre-operative steroids may relieve symptoms to some extent in haematological malignancy, but may make the mass shrink quickly and provoke tumour lysis syndrome.

Although most children requiring anaesthesia for biopsy of a mediastinal mass tolerate the procedure without major incident, catastrophic airway and cardiovascular compromise can occur. Alterations in chest wall muscle tone, for example following administration of a muscle relaxant, or minor postural changes can provoke total airway obstruction or occlude venous return. Such a complication must be anticipated following induction of anaesthesia. Splinting the obstruction with a rigid bronchoscope and turning the patient prone may retrieve the situation. If this does not relieve the obstruction, the only solution may be the emergency provision of cardiopulmonary bypass. For this reason, all surgery for mediastinal masses should be performed by paediatric cardiac surgeons in a cardiac surgical unit.

Pleural collections

Pleural drainage became incorporated into surgical practice in 1917 to treat empyema associated with the influenza pandemic. Pleural drainage removes air, blood or other fluid from the pleural space, allowing lung re-expansion and eliminating mediastinal shift. Negative intrapleural pressure during spontaneous respiration cannot be achieved if gas or fluid intervenes between the two pleural layers.

Empyema

Empyema is associated with bacterial pneumonia, usually pneumococcal. It results in inflammatory debris forming a thick, inelastic covering of the lung, restricting expansion, often accompanied by a purulent pleural effusion. Areas of lung may be necrotic, with the potential for the development of a bronchopleural fistula.

Surgical decortication is the standard treatment for established empyema. The thick inflammatory debris encapsulating the lung is excised. Extensive decortication can be performed through a small thoracotomy incision. Children with this condition are frequently systemically unwell with fever and bacteraemia, and may have been ill for several days before presenting for surgery. Oxygenation is often marginal at presentation. Pre-operative attention to ensure that hydration is adequate is important, with appropriate fluid resuscitation where necessary. Some children will be bacteraemic and haemodynamically compromised. Blood should be cross-matched; many of these children have become anaemic during the illness, and blood loss from the inflamed lung surface is occasionally significant. Severely ill children may require a period of optimisation in intensive care before proceeding to surgery, and may require post-operative ventilation. Most previously well children improve markedly after decortication.

Lung abscess

This may be associated with primary bacterial infection but may also be precipitated by foreign body inhalation. It may require lung resection. Destruction of lung tissue and erosion into a bronchus with bronchopleural fistula formation may have occurred. Although single lung ventilation (SLV) may not assist with the surgical field, its use may prevent soiling of the non-operative lung, and may be necessary at intubation in the presence of a bronchopleural fistula.

Bronchiectasis

Chronic infection damages the muscular and elastic components of affected bronchi. It is a feature of cystic fibrosis. In children it is often associated with underlying immune compromise or immune suppression and is a common long-term complication of children receiving organ transplants in early life. Surgical resection of localised disease is indicated to prevent infection of normal lung tissue. Provision of SLV is strongly indicated during resection to prevent soiling and infection of the healthy lung.

Chest wall deformity

Pectus excavatum is more common than pectus carinatum. Unless extremely severe, the indication for correction is cosmetic, and children undergoing this surgery should be old enough to understand and to consent to surgery themselves. The Ravitch procedure involves a major incision across the chest, detachment of costal cartilages from the sternum and surgical re-modelling of the sternum. The more recently introduced and popular Nuss procedure for pectus excavatum is less invasive and requires a small incision on each side of the chest. A curved steel bar is inserted under endoscopic guidance under the sternum and then rotated 180° to raise the sternum. Safe insertion of the Nuss bar requires thoracoscopy with CO_2 insufflation to create space anterior to the mediastinum for its insertion. Whichever procedure is used the major issue is the control of post-operative pain, and epidural analgesia should be employed.

Anaesthesia for thoracic surgery: specific considerations

Hypoxic pulmonary vasoconstriction (HPV)

HPV is the mechanism by which the body limits blood flow through unventilated or hypoxic areas of lung. If HPV is inhibited, then the flow of deoxygenated blood increases through non-ventilated areas of lung. Much has been written about the inhibitory effects of inhalational anaesthetic agents on HPV, but in practice, it is not a problem unless high concentrations of inspired agent are used.

Lateral decubitus position

Most thoracic surgical procedures require the patient to be in the lateral decubitus position, operative side uppermost. Increased ventilation/perfusion (V/Q) mismatch may result in hypoxaemia:

- Surgical retraction of the upper (operative) lung or single lung ventilation causes collapse of the operative lung.
- The dependent lung may be compressed by the mediastinum and abdominal organs.
- HPV may be impaired by inhalational anaesthetic agents.

The effect of the lateral decubitus position on V/Q mismatch may be more marked in infants compared with older children and adults. In adults and older children with unilateral lung disease, oxygenation is usually better when the patient is in the lateral decubitus position with the healthy lung 'down'. The hydrostatic pressure difference between upper and lower lungs diverts blood flow away from the upper lung to the healthy lower lung. This pressure gradient is less in infants, making this phenomenon less important. Also, infants have a compliant thoracic wall, which supports the lower lung less effectively; during tidal ventilation airway closure is more likely to occur because functional residual capacity (FRC) approaches closing volume. Consequently, in infants with unilateral lung disease oxygenation is improved with the healthy lung 'up', although this is clearly not practical during surgery.

The effect on oxygenation is noticeable during surgery in the lateral decubitus position in infants and young children. A predictable sequence of events occurs:

- FRC increases when moved from supine to the lateral position;
- On opening the pleural space, FRC decreases to 25% below baseline, falling further to 50% of baseline during lung retraction (if single lung ventilation is not used);
- FRC then returns to the baseline on completion of surgery.

Oxygenation follows a similar sequence, and provided it is within defined boundaries, modest hypoxaemia is acceptable, and surgery can usually proceed without too much concern.

Lung retraction

Surgical access to the operative lung can be facilitated by ventilating only the dependent lung, allowing the operative lung to collapse. In adults and older children, one-lung ventilation is achieved relatively easily. In smaller children this is harder to achieve, so the surgeon will need to retract the lung on the operative side for adequate exposure. This necessitates effective dialogue between surgeon and anaesthetist, particularly as there may also be some mediastinal distortion.

When lung is retracted, there is decreased lung compliance. This may be accompanied by hypoxaemia; typically the haemoglobin saturation (SpO_2) will decrease to 85–90%. If there is no further perturbation in the surgical field, SpO_2 will gradually increase as hypoxic pulmonary vasoconstriction lessens the volume of blood passing through the collapsed lung. Lung retraction should be gentle, to avoid both lung contusion and mediastinal compression, which occludes venous return to the heart which in turn causes haemodynamic compromise. Positive end expiratory pressure (PEEP) should be used during a thoracotomy. This maintains lung volume in the 'down' lung, both aiding oxygenation and supporting the mediastinum (which then maintains its position in the chest cavity).

Single lung ventilation (SLV)

'Isolating' the two lungs is standard practice when anaesthetising for thoracic surgery in adults. The non-operative lung alone is ventilated, allowing the operative lung to deflate. This improves surgical access, shortens operating times and minimises lung trauma caused by surgical retraction. Contamination of the non-operative lung and trachea by blood or pus draining from the operative lung may be minimised.

In adults, SLV is readily achieved using a double lumen tube; one lumen lies in a mainstem bronchus, the other in the trachea, the inflatable cuff around the bronchial lumen allowing lung isolation. Double-lumen tubes are not available in small sizes, so SLV in children requires alternative strategies. The smaller the child, the harder it is to achieve, so greater justification for its use is required. Strategies for SLV in children include use of a single lumen tracheal tube, bronchial blockers, a Univent tube or a conventional double lumen tube. These are discussed below.

Single lumen tube

This is the simplest method in a small child and can usually be achieved in babies from around 3 kg upwards, although the smaller the patient the more difficulty is encountered. The mainstem bronchus on the non-operative side is intubated with a conventional tube that is 0.5 mm in diameter smaller than normal. It is a fallacy that in children younger than 3 years a tube advanced beyond the carina has an equal chance of entering either bronchus. The right bronchial angle is invariably smaller, and in the absence of abnormal anatomy, a tube usually enters the right main bronchus. To intubate the left bronchus, the tube is rotated through 180° after traversing the glottis, the child's right shoulder is raised and the child's head is turned towards the right. The tracheal tube is then advanced until breath sounds are no longer audible on the right. If a tube is advanced without these manoeuvres it will usually enter the right main bronchus.

Tube placement may be assisted by direct airway visualisation with a fibre-optic bronchoscope passed through the tube, advancing the tube over the bronchoscope into position. In small babies this is not simple; the bronchoscope is easily dislodged as the tracheal tube is advanced. If right bronchial intubation cannot be achieved easily, and a fibre-optic bronchoscope is not available to guide placement, a mirror image technique of that used for left-sided intubation helps.

Tolerances in small children for correct tube position are as little as 2–3 mm, and positioning the tube to ensure that the upper lobe is ventilated can be awkward. The upper lobe bronchus on either side may originate very close to the carina, and its orifice may be occluded by the tube tip or cuff. Failure to ventilate the upper lobe is suggested by persistently low oxygen saturation and is confirmed by failure to hear breath sounds at the lung apex. This is a particular problem on the right side because of the shorter distance between the carina and the origin of the upper lobe bronchus. Difficulty may also occur when selectively intubating the right main bronchus, as the upper lobe bronchus can arise at the carina, or directly from the trachea (Figure 30.3). The right upper lobe bronchus arises from the trachea in pigs, and so-called 'pig bronchus' is a normal variant in up to 2% of humans.

Chest auscultation to check tube position is important after positioning for surgery is completed. Moving a child, especially a small infant, frequently disrupts what seemed to be perfect one-lung ventilation. The commonest problem is failure to provide an adequate seal of the tube in the bronchus, especially with an uncuffed tube. A tube with a low pressure cuff

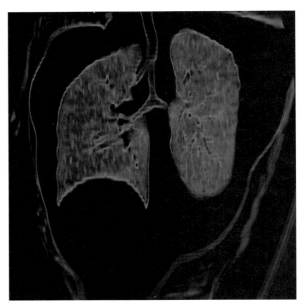

Figure 30.3 Scan showing aberrant tracheal bronchus. See plate section for colour version.

in the main bronchus helps lung isolation, but placing the cuff without occluding the upper lobe bronchus can be problematic. Suction cannot be performed on the operated lung with this technique.

Balloon-tipped bronchial blockers

The trachea is conventionally intubated, and the bronchus on the operative side is occluded by a balloon-tipped device with a central lumen through which the lung deflates allowing only the non-operative side to be ventilated. An end hole balloon wedge catheter, a Fogarty embolectomy catheter, and more recently, wire-guided endobronchial blockers (WEB) have all been used. The balloon may dislodge from the bronchus into the trachea, causing complete airway obstruction.

The smallest commercially available WEB is the 5 Fr Arndt device (Cook Critical Care, Bloomington, IN, USA). With the balloon deflated this has a maximum outer diameter of 1.7 mm. Placement is guided by fibre-optic bronchoscopy, both the WEB and the bronchoscope being passed through a tracheal tube. This balloon length is 1.0 cm, corresponding to the average length of the right main stem bronchus in a 2 year old. If a 2.2 mm bronchoscope is used, the smallest tracheal tube the device can be placed through has a 4.5 mm internal diameter. It has been formally evaluated in children undergoing surgery for anterior correction of scoliosis, with good effect in children as small as 9.7 kg. In practice, this technique cannot be used during the first year of life, the usual age when surgery for congenital lung anomalies is performed. In older children it generally allows more reliable lung separation than that provided by selective endobronchial intubation.

Univent tube (Fuji Systems Corporation Tokyo)

This is a conventional tracheal tube with a second lumen through which a bronchus blocker is advanced. Because the second lumen is an integral part of the tube, displacement of the blocker is unlikely unless the tube itself is dislodged. The Univent tube is bulky; a tube with an internal diameter of 3.5 mm has the same external diameter as a 5.0 mm internal diameter Portex 'ivory' uncuffed tube. Like the Arndt blocker it is unsuitable for use in chidren under the age of approximately 2 years. The balloon is low volume and high pressure.

Double lumen tubes (DLT)

These are two tubes of unequal length moulded together. There are right and left sided tubes; the shorter tube opens in the trachea and the longer in the bronchus. There are tracheal and bronchial cuffs. Inflating the bronchial cuff allows diversion of ventilation to either lung, according to whether the bronchial or tracheal lumen is ventilated. The cuff protects each lung from contamination by infected debris or blood from the contralateral side. Insertion is straightforward; the DLT is advanced through the larynx, then rotated through 90° to the appropriate side and the bronchial component is advanced into the appropriate bronchus. A DLT allows suction of the operative side, and can augment oxygenation when CPAP is applied to the operative lung. Although bulky and rigid, there are few reports of airway trauma associated with its use.

DLTs are of limited use in children, being too big to be used before adolescence. An extra-small 'Robertshaw' tube has an external diameter at the tracheal cuff of 10 mm – the same as most conventional tracheal tubes with an internal diameter of 7.0 mm. The smallest Mallinckrodt 'Bronchocath' is a left-sided 28 Fr with an external diameter of 9.3 mm and an internal diameter of 3.1 mm. The smallest right-sided version (35 Fr) has an external diameter of 11.7 mm, and internal of 4.8 mm.

Indications for SLV

Single lung ventilation is difficult to achieve in children and so should be justified in its use.

- Strong indication for SLV:
  - Major gas trapping in one lung or pleural space, e.g. bronchopleural fistula, congenital lobar emphysema
  - Lobectomy for bronchiectasis or similar need to prevent airway soiling by blood or infective material
  - Minimally invasive thoracic surgery
- Moderate indication for SLV:
  - Lobectomy or pneumonectomy for cystic malformations or tumour
  - Anterior spinal surgery
  - Oesophageal or aortic surgery
- Contraindication to SLV:
  - Unacceptable hypoxia after institution of SLV
  - Technical inability to isolate one lung safely

Bronchoscopy

The anaesthetist undertaking paediatric thoracic work should be able to use both rigid and flexible bronchoscopes to assist with accurate tracheal tube or bronchus blocker placement, as well as to allow tracheobronchial toilet. The author routinely performs bronchoscopy prior to tracheal intubation in all children undergoing pulmonary surgery. This assists lung isolation, allows identification of anatomical variants such as a tracheal bronchus (Figure 30.3) and obtains airway secretions for microbiological testing.

Bronchoscopy may also be used to investigate stridor, or recurrent pulmonary infection, and to evaluate tracheal injury. Tracheomalacia, bronchomalacia, subglottic stenosis, or extrinsic airway compression are examples of diagnoses reached at bronchoscopy.

The smallest flexible fibre-optic instruments with a suction channel have a diameter of 2.8 mm, and without suction, 2.2 mm. A fibre-optic instrument can be introduced either through a laryngeal mask airway in a spontaneously breathing patient, or transnasally. Nasal introduction gives more information; laryngeal and pharyngeal pathology is visualised and a dynamic examination of the upper airway can be performed.

Techniques for rigid bronchoscopy in adults cannot simply be transposed to small children.

A Sander's injector may cause barotrauma in children with normal lungs and cannot be recommended for paediatric practice. When lungs are poorly compliant or there is airway obstruction, air is poorly entrained. In children, ventilation through a rigid bronchoscope is performed by attaching a Mapleson F breathing system to the side arm of a Storz bronchoscope (see Figure 21.1), occluding the main channel by a diaphragm, window, or the operator's thumb. If there is airway obstruction, for example caused by an impacted foreign body, air trapping in the lungs can be problematic and expiration must be unimpeded and of adequate duration. A rigid telescope inserted through a small bronchoscope also causes expiratory embarrassment. A 1.9 mm telescope inside a 3.0 mm internal diameter bronchoscope, or a 2.8 mm telescope in a 3.5 mm bronchoscope are the smallest acceptable combinations.

Maintenance of anaesthesia during rigid bronchoscopy can be with inhalational agents, but this is unpopular with nursing and surgical staff because of difficulty scavenging gas. Intravenous anaesthesia may be used as an alternative.

Video assisted thoracoscopic surgery (VATS)

As in other surgical specialties, minimally invasive surgery has developed in thoracic surgery, and has its advocates particularly for empyema drainage. Satisfactory surgical exposure requires distancing of the lung from the chest wall. In older children this can be achieved reliably by use of SLV. Alternatively this can be achieved by intra-pleural insufflation of carbon dioxide as used for intra-abdominal minimally invasive surgery. Care by the operator is required to avoid compromising venous return by creating excessive intrapleural pressure.

Pleural drains

There are three important components to a pleural drain:

- A tube. This should be large enough. Small drains are adequate for gas, larger drains may be required for fluid, blood or pus.
- A one-way valve is required (usually an underwater seal). This allows expulsion of air during spontaneous expiration or positive pressure inspiration, and prevents re-entry of air through the drain during spontaneous inspiration.
- A collecting chamber. This may be single or the unit may have several drains in series to prevent increased resistance to drainage as fluid levels increase.

Suction applied to the collecting chamber increases the pressure gradient between pleural space and collecting chamber. Bilateral pleural drains should not be connected to the same suction source lest differential resistance to drainage results in mediastinal shift. Pleural drains should not be clamped or inadvertently occluded, especially in patients receiving positive pressure ventilation – failure to drain pleural air can quickly cause a tension pneumothorax. A drain connected to a suction unit with the suction turned off has the same effect as clamping the drain. Stopping suction on a pleural drain requires disconnection from the suction unit.

Principles of anaesthesia for thoracic surgery

The importance of pre-operative assessment and communication with the surgical and operating theatre staff cannot be overstated, and the adoption of the WHO Safe Surgery Guidelines to ensure the correct side is operated on is mandatory. If lung separation is planned, topical local anaesthetic to the larynx and trachea is indicated since repeated manipulation may be required to position a tracheal tube correctly. Nitrous oxide is contraindicated in thoracic anaesthesia as it may diffuse into and expand any gas-filled cavity.

Vascular access

Thoracic surgery may involve the mobilisation of large blood vessels, or operating on inflamed, friable tissue. Intra-operative bleeding can be brisk during tumour surgery, and significant plasma losses from either raw tissue surfaces or consequent to lymphatic disruption can occur during the post-operative period. Adequate intravenous access is essential for fluid replacement, and cross-matched blood should be available. Central venous pressure monitoring can be misleading in the lateral decubitus position, but central venous cannulation is indicated if haemodynamic instability is anticipated or if there is inadequate peripheral venous access. Invasive arterial pressure monitoring is helpful because of the potential for intraoperative haemodynamic instability and for blood gas analysis.

Ventilation strategies

Open thoracotomy precludes spontaneous ventilation, as there is an inability to generate negative intrapleural pressure, and mediastinal shift prevents lung expansion. Occasionally, spontaneous ventilation is preferred until lung isolation is achieved to prevent a tension pneumothorax, or to prevent gas trapping. In practice this is rarely immediately life-threatening, and muscle relaxation and positive pressure ventilation are usually safe.

In severe congenital lobar emphysema, novel ventilatory modes may be needed to allow some exhalation. Trial and error may identify the best means of ventilating the child until the chest wall has been opened, or alternatively, spontaneous ventilation may be maintained. When the author has managed severely affected cases in the newborn period, a very slow respiratory rate without PEEP, and tolerance of fairly extreme hypercapnia resulted in adequate oxygenation until the chest wall was opened. Haemodynamic compromise caused by mediastinal shift resolves instantly the pleural space is opened and the hyperinflated lobe delivered through the chest wall. SLV may be impossible to achieve safely in cases presenting acutely because of hypoxia and distorted tracheobronchial anatomy. In asymptomatic cases, SLV prevents or, at worst, reduces, gas trapping in the emphysematous lobe caused by the instigation of positive pressure ventilation.

During surgery, ventilation is tailored to the individual patient, and may require unusual settings. Modified ventilatory strategies to optimise exhalation may be required. The whole surgical team should be aware of the need for either urgent pleural drainage or thoracotomy. A modern ventilator offering spirometry is useful; manual ventilation may be necessary in small infants. Permissive hypercapnia may be prudent. A sudden change in compliance may reflect either surgical manipulation or tube displacement, and dialogue between surgeon and anaesthetist is essential. End-tidal capnography may underestimate $PaCO_2$ particularly if SLV is used.

Post-operative management and analgesia

Children undergoing intrathoracic surgery require admission to a high-dependency unit post-operatively as complications are frequent, and adequate provision must be made for pain management, chest physiotherapy and non-invasive CPAP. Full ventilatory support is sometimes necessary, and paediatric intensive care facilities must be available.

Thoracic surgery is very painful. Pain after thoracotomy has been described as one of the most intense possible. Intra- and post-operative analgesia for thoracotomy requires a combination of regional anaesthetic technique with systemic analgesia, both opioid and non-steroidal. The choice of technique is influenced by the age of the child, the underlying pathological process and the preference of the anaesthetist.

Regional anaesthesia

Intercostal nerve blocks (several nerves require blockade for a thoracotomy incision) will provide satisfactory intra-operative analgesia, but only a brief effect in the post-operative period. A catheter placed in the sub-pleural space by the surgeon at the end of the procedure allows local anaesthetic to be administered that will reach the paravertebral space. This usually provides good analgesia confined to the operative side. Epidural analgesia is provided either by a catheter inserted at the level of the operation, or in smaller children it may be threaded up the epidural space after caudal insertion. Epidural analgesia requires careful post-operative supervision. Intrapleural instillation of local anaesthetic agents has been described, but the author has not found this technique to be particularly effective. It must be remembered that local anaesthetic drug absorption from all these routes is significant, and care must be taken to avoid accumulation and toxicity, especially in infants.

Systemic analgesia

Opioid infusion, preferably with patient-controlled or nurse-controlled superimposed boluses, is essential for the first 48 hours after thoracotomy. This is in addition to a regional technique unless the regional technique offers perfect analgesia. Regular paracetamol and non-steroidal anti-inflammatory drugs should also be prescribed. Good analgesia allows early mobilisation, and helps to prevent problems with sputum retention.

297

Key points

- Surgical access to the operative lung can be facilitated by ventilating only the dependent lung, allowing the operative lung to collapse. In small children this is hard to achieve as double-lumen tubes are only available for children over the age of 8–10 years.
- Anaesthetising a child with an anterior mediastinal mass can precipitate total airway collapse. It may be necessary to insert a rigid bronchoscope to maintain an airway.

- In the infant with congenital lobar emphysema, positive pressure ventilation can lead to acute hyperinflation of the affected lobe with severe respiratory and haemodynamic compromise. It may be necessary to try various ventilatory strategies to identify the best means of ventilating the child until the chest wall has been opened.
- Thoracic surgery can be very painful. Regional and local analgesia should be employed wherever possible, supplemented by patient- or nurse-controlled morphine infusion and regular paracetamol and NSAIDs.

Further reading

Chernick V, Boat TF, Wilmott RW, Bush A. *Kendig's Disorders of the Respiratory Tract in Children*, 7th edition. Saunders Elsevier. 2006.

Hammer G. Single-lung ventilation in infants and children. *Paed Anaes* 2004;14;98–102.

Haynes SR, Bonner S. Anaesthesia for thoracic surgery in children. *Paed Anaes* 2000;10:237–51.

Zur KB, Litman RS. Pediatric airway foreign body retrieval: surgical and anesthetic perspectives. *Paed Anaes* 2009;19 (Suppl 1): 109–17.

Chapter

31

Anaesthesia for cardiac surgery in children

Ian James and Sally Wilmshurst

Introduction

Most children presenting for paediatric cardiac surgery have a congenital cardiac disorder, the incidence of which is around 1 in 150 births. The commonest are listed in Table 31.1. Without surgical intervention, around 50% of children with congenital heart disease (CHD) would die during childhood. Acquired diseases such as rheumatic fever, endocarditis or Kawasaki disease are rare although there is an increasing need for anaesthesia in cardiomyopathy for placement of a mechanical support device or cardiac transplantation.

About 3600 cardiac surgical procedures are carried out annually on children in the UK, 20% of which are undertaken in neonates. Traditionally, these procedures are classified as 'open' where cardiopulmonary bypass (CPB) is required, or 'closed'. The latter includes procedures such as the creation of a systemic to pulmonary artery shunt, ligation of a patent ductus arteriosus (PDA) or simple coarctation repair, and these procedures are frequently performed via thoracotomy. Cardiopulmonary bypass is also used occasionally for non-cardiac surgery, such as complex tracheal repairs or to facilitate removal of tumours adjacent to the heart or major vessels. Technological developments that have allowed miniaturisation of the cardiopulmonary bypass circuit mean it is now feasible to undertake complex repairs on infants under 2 kg. Surgery may be either corrective, such as ventricular septal defect (VSD) repair, or palliative as in the establishment of a single ventricle circulation.

Staged surgery is necessary for many complex lesions, so many children will return for further surgery. Survival to adulthood is increasing such that there is an increasing need for expertise in the field of 'grown up congenital heart' disease (GUCH). This chapter will cover the principles of anaesthesia for cardiac surgery in children.

Overview of surgery for congenital heart defects

Congenital heart disease is often classified as cyanotic or non-cyanotic, but this is not particularly useful in terms of planning anaesthetic management. The haemodynamic consequences of a lesion and its effect on ventricular function are of more relevance. A simplistic classification is shown in Table 31.2. It should be recognised that there is a wide spectrum of abnormality in many of the lesions such that there can be substantial differences in the physiological and haemodynamic consequences within a single lesion. In many lesions early survival is dependent upon preservation of blood flow through the ductus arteriosus, and the administration of prostaglandin infusion may be necessary to maintain ductal patency.

Table 31.1 Congenital cardiac lesions and their frequency

Lesion	Frequency
Ventricular septal defect	17%
Tetralogy of Fallot	12%
Transposition of the great arteries	11%
Coarctation of the aorta	11%
Atrial septal defect	10%
Hypoplastic left heart syndrome	5%
Atrioventricular septal defect	3%
Pulmonary atresia	1%

Core Topics in Paediatric Anaesthesia, ed. Ian James and Isabeau Walker. Published by Cambridge University Press. © 2013 Cambridge University Press.

Children with inadequate pulmonary blood flow such as tricuspid or pulmonary atresia, often referred to as having a right to left shunt, will generally be cyanosed at birth. Many will require early surgical intervention to augment pulmonary blood flow. The high PVR in the newborn means that this needs to be supplied from the systemic circulation, usually a modified Blalock–Taussig shunt (BTS) using a Gore-Tex™ tube from the inominate or subclavian artery to the pulmonary artery (see Figure 31.1). This is usually performed without CPB via a thoracotomy or sternotomy, although CPB will be needed if adequate oxygenation cannot be maintained during the procedure. Occasionally a central shunt directly from the aorta will be necessary. Pulmonary stenosis may be amenable to dilation by interventional cardiac catheterisation or surgical dilation; if not a shunt will be required. There is a very wide spectrum of severity of lesion in tetralogy of Fallot (ToF), some of whom will need a BTS in infancy.

Children with excessive pulmonary blood flow, usually referred to as having a left to right shunt, suffer from cardiac failure. This can often be managed medically with diuretics until they are suitable for full surgical correction. Untreated excessive pulmonary artery (PA) flow will lead to irreversible pulmonary vascular disease, so if the failure cannot be controlled medically and early surgical repair is not feasible, then PA banding may be necessary. This is most easily undertaken through a sternotomy, without CPB, and involves placing a band around the main PA to restrict pulmonary blood flow. This is usually adjusted to reduce PA pressure distal to the band to about half or less of systemic pressure. Oxygen saturation will generally fall to around 85%. The band is removed when definitive surgery is undertaken.

Table 31.2 Classification of cardiac surgical disorders

Category	Specific condition
Inadequate pulmonary blood flow (right to left shunts)	Tricuspid atresia Pulmonary atresia Pulmonary stenosis Tetralogy of Fallot
Excessive pulmonary blood flow (left to right shunts)	Patent ductus arteriosus Atrial septal defect Ventricular septal defect Atrioventricular septal defect Aortopulmonary window
Abnormal connections (complex shunts)	Transposition of the great arteries Hypoplastic left heart syndrome Truncus arteriosus Total anomalous pulmonary venous connection
Left ventricular outflow tract obstruction	Aortic coarctation Interrupted aortic arch Aortic stenosis Hypertrophic obstructive cardiomyopathy

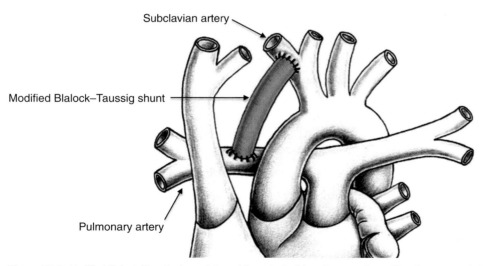

Subclavian artery

Modified Blalock–Taussig shunt

Pulmonary artery

Figure 31.1 Modified Blalock–Taussig shunt. Adapted from the PedHeart Resource (www.HeartPassport.com). Courtesy of Scientific Software Solutions, Inc.

Children with complex abnormal connections have a variable combination of cyanosis and heart failure and usually require surgery involving CPB in the neonatal period.

Children with transposition of the great arteries (TGA) and hypoplastic left heart syndrome (HLHS) will generally need prostaglandin infusion to maintain ductal patency while waiting for surgery. In HLHS and truncus arteriosus it is necessary to ensure that pulmonary blood flow does not increase, with a corresponding fall in systemic blood flow, as pulmonary vascular resistance falls in the first few days of life.

Infants may have total anomalous pulmonary venous drainage (TAPVD) in which all the pulmonary veins drain to the right atrium. In supracardiac TAPVD this may be via an abnormal bridging vein in the thorax, and if there is no obstruction to venous return it may not be detected immediately. In infracardiac TAPVD the pulmonary veins may drain into the IVC, usually via the hepatic veins. This invariably causes significant pulmonary venous obstruction and requires urgent surgery immediately after birth. The engorged pulmonary veins and profound hypoxaemia lead to it occasionally being misdiagnosed initially as meconium aspiration. TAPVD may pose difficulties with pulmonary hypertension post-operatively.

Obstructive lesions of the left ventricle frequently result in left ventricular hypertrophy and a consequent increased myocardial oxygen demand. Patients are at risk of acute myocardial ischaemia if oxygen demand is increased by tachycardia or if coronary perfusion pressure falls during anaesthesia. Patients with Williams syndrome and supra-aortic stenosis are particularly challenging and have a high risk of sudden death in the peri-operative period. Some obstructive lesions of the left side of the heart such as critical aortic stenosis and interrupted aortic arch will require surgery in the newborn period. Simple coarctation of the aortic arch is generally repaired via thoracotomy in both infants and older children.

Pre-operative assessment

Successful anaesthesia for CHD surgery requires a meticulous, anticipative approach that starts in the pre-operative period. Key features of pre-operative assessment include:

- Understanding the anatomy, physiology and haemodynamics of the presenting disorder;

- Understanding the proposed surgical procedure, and the consequences of any previous surgery;
- Determining the clinical condition of the child, particularly cardiac function.

Most patients presenting for elective cardiac surgery will have undergone some form of joint cardiology and cardiac surgical review in which the lesion and proposed treatment will be detailed. This will generally include details of previous surgery, current clinical status and medication, and a recent echocardiogram. On occasion additional information may be available from cardiac catheterisation and other imaging such as cardiac MRI or CT. Chest X-ray (CXR) may be instructive in demonstrating features such as dextrocardia or the classic boot-shaped heart commonly seen in ToF, and over- or under-perfusion of the lungs. A new CXR should be obtained if there is a history of worsening heart failure or signs of respiratory infection.

The following are of particular importance to the anaesthetist:

- *Is the patient 'duct-dependent'?* Some newborns with inadequate pulmonary blood flow, such as pulmonary atresia, will be dependent on prostaglandin infusion to keep the ductus arteriosus open and allow blood flow to the pulmonary circulation from the aorta. For some other newborns, such as those with HLHS or severe coarctation, keeping the duct open is equally important but in this situation it is to allow blood flow from the PA to the aorta. For infants dependent upon on a patent duct or a systemic-to-pulmonary artery shunt, it is important that flow through the shunt is 'balanced', that is that systemic and pulmonary artery blood flow is roughly equal. This 'balance' is determined by systemic vascular resistance (SVR) and pulmonary vascular resistance (PVR), and it is important to minimise changes to this balance during induction of anaesthesia. Injudicious use of anaesthetic agents may drop SVR, increasing systemic perfusion at the expense of pulmonary blood flow, and may precipitate profound hypoxaemia, bradycardia and cardiac arrest. Conversely, over-ventilation or the administration of high inspired oxygen concentration should be avoided in patients dependent upon their duct or shunt for systemic perfusion, as this will drop pulmonary vascular resistance and increase pulmonary blood flow at the expense of diminished systemic blood flow. Similar considerations will apply in truncus arteriosus where the pulmonary arteries originate from a common aortic trunk. PVR must be kept high to maintain adequate flow to the systemic circulation. For many of these patients oxygen saturations around 80% represent an appropriate 'balance'.

- *Degree of cyanosis.* Children with cyanotic CHD presenting for surgery may be profoundly desaturated, with polycythaemia and coagulopathy. It is essential to understand the underlying lesion in hypoxaemic patients. For some patients, as noted above, it is important to resist the temptation to deliver high inspired oxygen concentration to correct hypoxaemia, as this may lead to profoundly low systemic blood flow and acidosis.

- *Is myocardial function impaired?* In some lesions, such as obstructive lesions of the left side of the heart, anomalous origin of the left coronary artery from the pulmonary artery (ALCAPA) or dilated cardiomyopathy, there can be severely impaired left ventricular function. It is important to avoid tachycardia and other causes of increased myocardial oxygen consumption, or a fall in coronary perfusion. Some of these patients may already be dependent on inotropic support. Echocardiography is crucial in determining the degree of left ventricular dysfunction pre-operatively. The ejection fraction (EF) is a useful estimation of ventricular function, and in healthy hearts is 50–70%. An EF of less than 30% is indicative of poor function.

- *Is there significant pulmonary hypertension?* If so, any hypoxaemia or hypercapnia during induction and intubation will be poorly tolerated. If the right ventricle is significantly hypertrophied and distorting the left ventricle, systemic hypotension may compromise coronary artery perfusion and lead rapidly to acute biventricular failure. Pulmonary hypertension is the major cause of anaesthesia-related mortality in children.

- *Is there an atrial septal defect?* If present, it is important to be meticulous in ensuring that no air bubbles enter the venous system, as they can lead to paradoxical cerebral air emboli. All infusion lines must be checked meticulously.

- *Previous surgery.* Has there been a previous sternotomy? If so, there may be fibrous adhesion of the heart to the back of the sternum with the risk of inadvertent injury and significant bleeding during re-sternotomy. This can be a particular problem if there is an artificial conduit sitting on the front of the heart. It is customary during repeat sternotomy to leave one of the groins available to the surgeon for cannulation for elective or emergency femoral or iliac bypass. This has implications for placement of monitoring lines.

- *Is there an existing shunt?* Arterial pressure monitoring can be inaccurate if placed in the same arm as a BTS.

- *Is there a pacemaker or implantable cardioverter defibrillator (ICD) in place?* It is important to understand the underlying rhythm disturbance. It may be necessary to re-programme a pacemaker to fixed pacing or disable the ICD before cautery can be used safely.

- *Intercurrent illness.* CHD with high pulmonary blood flow can lead to increased susceptibility to chest infections. Undergoing CPB with an acute respiratory tract infection may result in significant post-operative morbidity and increased ICU stay. It can be difficult to differentiate acute upper respiratory tract infection from heart failure in some symptomatic children. The decision to proceed with surgery needs to be considered on an individual basis; delay of elective surgery is usually indicated in the presence of fever or an elevated white cell count, but a mild cough or runny nose is generally not a reason to cancel surgery.

- *Syndromes.* Although most children with CHD are otherwise healthy, the disorder may be associated with a congenital syndrome, such as Trisomy 21 or CHARGE. Infants with a conotruncal anomaly, such as interrupted aortic arch, truncus arteriosus or ToF, should be presumed to have DiGeorge syndrome (22q11 deletion) until proven otherwise. This is associated with parathyroid and thymic dysfunction. Hypocalcaemia may be problematic, and irradiated blood should be used to avoid graft versus host disease (GVHD).

- *Medications.* Some children will be dependent on prostaglandin infusion or inotropic support, and it is important these are not interrupted. Others may be on anti-failure medication such as diuretics or captopril. Some children with ToF who suffer from severe hypercyanotic 'tet' spells may be on propranolol. Some children will be on some form of anticoagulant therapy such as warfarin or antiplatelet drugs. Platelet transfusion may be necessary after surgery. It is important not to stop anticoagulation for too long in patients wholly dependent upon a shunt, nor to allow them to become dehydrated. Some patients may be on heparin, which is usually stopped 2 hours before surgery.

- *Laboratory investigations.* Long-standing cyanosis can result in polycythaemia and a coagulopathy. Thrombocytopenia and clotting factor deficiency may be present. Furthermore, these patients may be taking aspirin or other anticoagulant medications up to the day of surgery. Children taking diuretics or in severe cardiac failure may have metabolic derangements such as hypokalaemia.
- *Fasting time* is of particular importance in small children dependent on a small shunt. Their hyperviscosity due to polycythaemia leaves them prone to shunt thrombosis if prolonged starvation leads to dehydration. Clear fluids should be given until 2 hours prior to surgery, and IV fluids should be started if there is uncertainty about theatre time.

An important aspect of the pre-operative visit is to discuss the proposed procedure to the parents and where appropriate the child, including type of induction and post-operative analgesia and intensive care. Premedication and topical analgesia is prescribed as necessary.

Induction

Haemodynamic stability is the goal in the anaesthetic room. Essential monitoring – ECG, audible pulse oximetry and blood pressure – should be started prior to induction of anaesthesia. In some children this may be poorly accepted but should be applied at the earliest opportunity. Ideally intravenous access should be obtained prior to induction, but this is not always achievable. Where this is the case and in those patients expressing a preference for inhalational induction, intravenous access should be established as soon as feasible.

Sevoflurane is widely used for inhalational induction and is generally very safe. Uptake of anaesthetic agents from the lungs is slowed in the presence of a large right to left shunt although this is rarely of practical significance. Importantly, any relative overdose of agent will be equally slow to reverse.

For most patients there is no definite advantage of one intravenous induction agent over another. All anaesthetic agents have haemodynamic effects and should be used with caution. Propofol is suitable if ventricular function is good but should be avoided where a fall in SVR or diastolic pressure is to be avoided.

When ventricular function is impaired, intravenous induction can be very challenging.

- *Ketamine* is a direct myocardial depressant, but it usually maintains or increases blood pressure, heart rate and cardiac output via sympathomimetic stimulation. It is a commonly used agent particularly when it is important to avoid a fall in SVR. However, in patients who may be surviving on maximal sympathomimetic drive, such as those with end-stage cardiomyopathy, ketamine's unopposed direct myocardial depressant action may lead to a profound fall in cardiac output.
- *Fentanyl*, which is perceived to be a cardio-stable agent, may also have detrimental cardiac effects in patients whose cardiac output is maintained by a sympathomimetic drive. It very effectively suppresses the stress response, which can lead to a fall in blood pressure. It also reduces heart rate, an important component in maintaining cardiac output in some children.
- *Etomidate* has negligible effect on myocardial contractility or blood pressure and is probably the best agent for patients with very limited myocardial reserve, despite concerns about short-term adrenal suppression and pain on injection.

For patients with very poor myocardial function and low cardiac output, such as those presenting for heart transplantation, it is important to remember:

- Circulation times may be slow, so drug effect may be delayed;
- There is preferential blood supply to key organs such as the brain so smaller induction doses are needed.

The following is the authors' preferred means of induction in such patients: a small dose of fentanyl, 0.5–1.0 mcg kg^{-1}, is followed by slow increments of midazolam 50 mcg kg^{-1} over 10–15 minutes until the patient is having difficulty keeping their eyes open. At this point, etomidate 0.2 mg kg^{-1} is administered together with the muscle relaxant. Blood pressure should be measured at short intervals throughout induction.

Pancuronium is the most commonly used muscle relaxant because of its long duration of action. Its modest increase in heart rate is beneficial in opposing the reduced heart rate commonly seen with fentanyl, but it should be avoided where a tachycardia may be detrimental.

Oral intubation is generally used in older children and in those in whom early extubation is planned. Nasal intubation is preferred in infants and in those in whom prolonged intensive care is anticipated, and may also be preferable when transoesophageal echocardiography (TOE) is used, as the tube is less likely to be dislodged during probe manipulation.

Maintenance of anaesthesia

Anaesthesia for CPB surgery is usually maintained using a combination of moderate to high dose opioid, typically fentanyl in the dose range 15 to 30 mcg kg^{-1}, combined with a volatile agent such as isoflurane in air or an air/oxygen mix. Nitrous oxide is useful during inhalational induction but should be avoided for maintenance of anaesthesia. Isoflurane and sevoflurane both cause only a modest fall in SVR and blood pressure at 1–1.5 MAC and are widely used. Volatile agents can produce a profound fall in blood pressure and cardiac output in infants less than 6 months, and it is preferable to limit their dose and to use a higher dose of fentanyl in these patients. There is increasing interest in the use of continuous infusions of propofol and/or remifentanil for maintenance, but there are limited studies to date.

Neuraxial blockade, in the form of spinal or epidural anaesthesia, has attractive theoretical benefits in attenuating the stress response associated with cardiac surgery. It is used in some centres, but anxiety about epidural haematoma has prevented widespread adoption.

Antibiotic prophylaxis is essential in cardiac surgery. The choice of antibiotics will generally depend upon local protocols and they should be administered in the 60-minute period prior to skin incision.

Monitoring

ECG, pulse oximetry, capnography and invasive arterial and central venous pressure monitoring are required for all cardiac cases. End-tidal CO_2 is inaccurate in patients with cyanotic CHD and can be 2 kPa lower than arterial CO_2 but can provide a useful trend of ventilation. Non-invasive blood pressure monitoring should be used while arterial access is being achieved. A urinary catheter should be placed in all patients undergoing CPB.

Invasive arterial and central venous lines must be secure and reliable and should be placed under full aseptic conditions. For CPB cases it is customary to insert a multi-lumen central venous line in addition to a good peripheral line. In most cases this will be via the internal jugular or femoral vein. Thrombosis of central veins is an unfortunate complication of central venous cannulation in small infants. In neonates with univentricular physiology where cavopulmonary connections will be necessary later, such as those with HLHS, it is preferable to avoid the internal jugular veins if possible as SVC thrombosis will compromise subsequent successful repair. In newborn infants the umbilical vein may be usable.

Where central venous access is technically difficult the external jugular vein can be used for pressure monitoring and to provide access for administration of drugs. Rarely, it may be necessary to start surgery with peripheral access only; a direct transthoracic right atrial line can be placed by the surgeon once the chest is open.

Arterial access is usually via the radial, femoral or occasionally the axillary artery. The smaller peripheral arteries are occasionally used but may become shut down and display an inaccurately low pressure as the patient is cooled. It is best to avoid the ipsilateral upper limb if a BTS is present or planned, as it is likely to under-read the true pressure. It is important to place the arterial line in the right arm during non-CPB coarctation repair as the surgeon will clamp the aortic arch proximal to the origin of the left subclavian artery during repair. During re-sternotomy one groin is usually left free for the surgeon should there be a need to use the femoral or iliac vessels for CPB.

Core (usually nasopharyngeal) and peripheral temperature monitors should be placed in all cases. Core temperature is essential for the conduct of CPB, and is also important in ensuring there is mild hypothermia prior to clamping the aorta during coarctation repair.

Transoesophageal echocardiography (TOE) offers great advantages peri-operatively enabling confirmation of the diagnosis, detection of a small patent foramen ovale (PFO) not seen on transthoracic echo, detection of air within the heart after cardiotomy, and assessment of surgical repair and ventricular function. There are now probes suitable for children as small as 4 kg. TOE may be undertaken by a cardiologist or an anaesthetist. It is important to ensure that the TOE operator is not also solely responsible for the anaesthesia.

Near infrared spectroscopy (NIRS) provides a measure of cerebral and somatic oximetry as a function of regional blood flow. Cerebral NIRS can be useful in monitoring changes in cerebral perfusion related to CPB and to malposition of the CPB cannulae. In some centres, especially in North America, its use is routine.

The pre-bypass period

For sternotomy the patient is placed in the supine position with the arms by the sides and a small roll under the shoulders to bring the sternum forward. All lines, monitors and the catheter should be secured and accessible. Passive cooling is allowed prior to bypass. A warming mattress and forced air warmer are used for rewarming and temperature maintenance following CPB.

Sternotomy is known to be very stimulating, and adequate opioid and/or volatile anaesthetic is required to blunt a hypertensive response. Following sternotomy anaesthesia requirements are reduced. During 'first time' sternotomy, ventilation is discontinued momentarily to prevent lung injury from the saw. Chest compliance often increases following sternotomy and ventilatory parameters should be monitored.

Haemodynamic instability can occur during mediastinal dissection due to manipulation of the great vessels, impaired venous return, arrhythmias, bleeding or labile pulmonary vascular resistance. Extreme vigilance is required if there is a shunt or duct-dependent circulation, as distortion may interfere with pulmonary or systemic perfusion, and it may be necessary to ask the surgeon to pause to allow recovery.

Prior to CPB a dose of heparin is administered (400 IU kg^{-1}) to prevent clotting of the extracorporeal circuit. Heparin should always be administered into a secure line. The adequacy of heparinisation is checked after 2–3 minutes, usually by the activated clotting time (ACT) which should be above 400 seconds.

Cardiopulmonary bypass

CPB requires the drainage of the systemic venous return from the patient and, following oxygenation, return via a cannula placed in the ascending aorta. The aortic cannula is placed first, and its correct placement is vital. NIRS may be of value in demonstrating a fall in cerebral oxygenation on the rare occasion that the cannula tip is misplaced.

Unlike the majority of adult cardiac cases where a single venous cannula is placed in the right atrium, paediatric CPB usually requires that venous cannulae are placed separately in the SVC and IVC. Very occasionally, there may be an additional major source of venous drainage to the heart, such as a left-sided SVC which may also need to be cannulated. Venous return to the bypass circuit is passive and requires appropriately sized cannulae to ensure complete emptying of the heart. CVP should fall to near zero. An advantage of measuring CVP in the internal jugular vein is that obstruction to cerebral venous return by the SVC cannula will be apparent. NIRS may also detect a fall in cerebral blood flow.

Once the cannulae are satisfactorily secured, the surgeon instructs the perfusionist to start bypass. Often this may start with just one venous cannula in place. Lung ventilation is continued until both cannulae are in place and the patient is on 'full flow', and can then be discontinued.

It is usual to give a supplementary bolus of fentanyl immediately prior to CPB, as the blood level will fall substantially owing to haemodilution and adsorption to the CPB circuit. Isoflurane is administered into the CPB sweep gas by the perfusionist to maintain anaesthesia during CPB. Hypothermia reduces the MAC of volatile agents and reduces the metabolism of drugs so these measures are usually sufficient in maintaining adequate anaesthesia. In children in whom CPB is conducted at only mild hypothermia a hypnotic agent such as midazolam or a propofol infusion may be administered to minimise the risk of awareness.

Management of bypass varies and is usually the responsibility of the surgeon and the perfusionist, although in some centres the anaesthetist is also involved. Blood flow on CPB is non-pulsatile with flow rates generally around 3 l min^{-1} m^{-2}. An in-line venous oxygen saturation monitor will generally indicate whether flow and tissue perfusion are adequate.

Mean blood pressure on CPB is generally maintained at around 35–60 mmHg. The pressure often falls markedly on institution of CPB, owing to haemodilution and vasodilation, but usually rises after a few minutes. If there is a PDA or a BTS this will need to be ligated to prevent flow into the lungs. Other sources of arterial run-off and low pressure, such as aorto-pulmonary collaterals, can be more difficult to manage. If blood pressure remains low then it may be necessary to administer a vasoconstrictor such as phenylephrine. NIRS may be useful in monitoring adequacy of cerebral perfusion on CPB. Haematocrit is normally maintained at around 20–25% on CPB; raising this may also improve blood pressure and cerebral oxygenation.

Most surgery is performed with cooling between 30 and 34 °C to reduce systemic and cerebral metabolic demands, although there is an increasing trend to undertake surgery in many cases at near normal temperature. For longer, more complex procedures the temperature may be reduced to 25–30 °C. Some surgery requires hypothermia to 18 °C to allow total cessation of bypass. This is known as deep hypothermic circulatory arrest (DHCA) and is discussed below.

For most paediatric cardiac procedures it is necessary to stop the heart, which involves administering a cardioplegic solution into the aortic root. The aorta is cross-clamped to ensure the potassium-containing solution goes to the coronaries. Traditionally this solution was cooled to around 4 °C to assist myocardial preservation but, increasingly, warm blood cardioplegia solutions are being used. Cardioplegia, which is important for myocardial preservation, is usually repeated every 20 minutes or so. Very occasionally, if the procedure is likely to be very short, the heart is fibrillated to prevent ejection and the risk of air embolism while repair is undertaken.

Deep hypothermic circulatory arrest (DHCA)

If surgery is required on the aortic arch or the head and neck vessels, and in some other complex repairs, the patient is cooled to 15–18 °C and the circulation stopped to allow the aortic cannula to be removed. At least 20 minutes of cooling should occur before the circulation is stopped. Ice packs should be applied to the head to aid brain cooling. It is difficult to quantify the long-term impact of this technique on

neurodevelopmental outcome, but DHCA times of greater than 40 minutes are associated with an increased risk of cerebral injury. Because of the risks of cerebral injury, some centres use selective cerebral perfusion during DHCA. After the circulation is restarted an adequate period of reperfusion and rewarming is required after DHCA before stopping CPB.

Discontinuing bypass

Once the surgical repair is completed the patient is rewarmed to 36 °C in preparation for coming off CPB. Electrolytes, particularly potassium and calcium, are corrected by the perfusionist, and a varying degree of ultrafiltration to raise the haematocrit above 30% may have been possible. Blood glucose frequently rises during CPB but rarely high enough to warrant administration of insulin.

Tracheal suction should be used to remove airway secretions prior to restarting and confirming adequacy of ventilation. Unless there is a physiological contraindication, ventilation is initially with high inspired oxygen together with low dose volatile agent. Although rewarming increases drug metabolism and cerebral blood flow, the concentration of anaesthetic agents increases after separation from CPB because of sequestration in under-perfused organs. Therefore extra doses of fentanyl are not usually required. The volatile agent can be increased and inspired oxygen reduced depending upon the haemodynamic and ventilatory parameters after successfully discontinuing CPB.

CPB causes a variable amount of myocardial dysfunction, so it is common to start an inotropic infusion prior to coming off. Choice of inotrope varies according to local practices and preferences, and may need to be adjusted post-CPB to address any particular haemodynamic issues. Rhythm disturbances need to be addressed and it may be necessary to pace the heart to ensure an adequate heart rate. TOE is very useful in demonstrating ventricular function and ensuring that air has been evacuated from the ventricles.

If cardiac output or blood pressure is unsatisfactory it may be necessary to go back on CPB to allow the myocardium more time to recover, to resolve rhythm disturbances, to increase inotropic support, or to review the surgical repair. On occasion, acute rhythm disturbance and ventricular dysfunction is due to air bubbles in the coronary arteries. This is associated with acute ECG changes and will usually resolve over a short period. Increasing the blood pressure, for example with an inotropic agent, to improve coronary perfusion is usually beneficial.

Modified ultrafiltration

After successful separation from CPB some patients will undergo modified ultrafiltration (MUF). This reduces total body water and raises haematocrit and mean arterial pressure whilst removing various inflammatory cytokines. As MUF returns warm, haemoconcentrated, oxygenated blood into the right side of the heart it lowers pulmonary vascular resistance, which can be useful in attenuating pulmonary hypertension.

Protamine administration and management of coagulopathy

Once the patient is stable and further bypass runs are unlikely, protamine is administered to reverse the heparin. It is important to ensure the perfusionist has discontinued the CPB pump suckers before administering protamine to avoid clotting the circuit. In vitro, 1.3 mg protamine reverses 1 mg (100 IU) of heparin so 1 to 1.5 times the dose of heparin is commonly given. Protamine can cause haemodynamic instability and should be administered slowly, although reactions are rare in children.

The adequacy of reversal is usually assessed by measuring ACT.

Coagulopathy can persist following protamine reversal particularly in neonates, cyanotic patients or those on anticoagulants. Infusions of platelets, cryoprecipitate and fresh frozen plasma may be required and thromboelastography (TEG) may be useful in guiding management. In life-threatening haemorrhage, recombinant factor VII may be necessary.

In complex patients and those with repeat sternotomies in whom bleeding is anticipated, antifibrinolytic therapy can be used from the start of the case to limit bleeding. The use of aprotinin in children is controversial owing to increased complications following its use in adult patients but still used in some centres successfully. Tranexamic acid is an alternative, but the correct dosing strategy and its efficacy have yet to be proven in children.

For most patients we would aim to ensure that Hb is above $10\,g\,dl^{-1}$ in the post-operative period. For those patients with palliated repairs who continue to have oxygen saturations in the 80s, Hb should be maintained above $12\,g\,dl^{-1}$.

Further management

Following satisfactory haemostasis, epicardial pacemaker leads are attached, chest drains are inserted and the chest is closed. Most cardiac surgery patients are managed post-operatively on the intensive care unit. Termination of volatile agent for transfer causes lightening of anaesthesia, and adequate sedation and analgesia should be ensured. A propofol infusion can be useful for transfer. A clear and comprehensive handover to the intensive care team is essential.

In some infants, particularly neonates who have undergone long and complex surgery, sternal closure leads to a mechanical tamponade of the heart with impaired function. In these infants the sternum may be left open and the wound protected with a silicon membrane. The chest is closed after 2–3 days when cardiac function has improved.

Pacemakers in cardiac surgery

Rhythm disturbances may occur after paediatric cardiac surgery and epicardial pacemaker wires are routinely placed. Heart block may occur after repairs involving the ventricular septum, and atrial dysrhythmias may occur because of suture lines in the atrium. For some lesions, such as univentricular repairs and heterotaxy, dysrhythmias are poorly tolerated. As some patients will require pacemaker support post-bypass, it is important to understand pacemaker codes and which settings to use.

The pacemaker code is a series of letters describing the type of pacing. The first letter represents the chamber being paced, the second the chamber being sensed and the third the response to sensing. The chambers are atria (A), ventricle (V), both/dual (D) or none (O). Pacing is inhibited (I), triggered (T) or both (D) on sensing; if pacing carries on regardless of sensing it is none (O). Permanent pacemakers that are more sophisticated often have a fourth and fifth letter in the code, but the three-letter code is generally employed.

In the presence of complete heart block, dual chamber pacing is required and DDD mode is selected. If second degree block or slow sinus rhythm requires treating then the atria are paced using AAI or AOO.

Fast-track surgery

Pressure on healthcare resources has led to renewed interest in the early extubation, occasionally in theatre, and short-stay intensive care management of certain cardiac conditions such as simple ASD or VSD. The spectrum of suitable conditions is growing, but should fulfil minimal criteria of adequate haemostasis, normothermia, minimal inotropic support and minimal ventilatory requirements.

For patients in whom early extubation is planned, adequate multimodal analgesia should be started in the operating theatre. This will include intravenous paracetamol, local analgesic infiltration to the sternal wound and the commencement of an intravenous morphine infusion (PCA or NCA).

The historical use of high-dose opioid anaesthesia hinders early extubation and fast-tracking. Moderate doses of fentanyl, $15–20 \, \text{mcg kg}^{-1}$, and shorter acting muscle relaxants with reversal are more appropriate.

Some specific conditions

Blalock–Taussig shunt

A modified BTS is a GoreTex tube from the subclavian artery to the pulmonary artery (see Figure 31.1). It may be undertaken via thoracotomy or via sternotomy. Where possible the arterial line should not be placed in the ipsilateral arm. Heparin, $100 \, \text{IU kg}^{-1}$, is usually given once the subclavian end of the shunt has been completed. It is important to maintain an adequate blood pressure to ensure blood flow through the shunt, and on occasion inotropic support may be necessary. Oxygen saturations of 70–80% should be expected following completion of the shunt. If there is excessive flow through the shunt there can be diminished systemic flow with signs of low cardiac output, together with high oxygen saturations. On occasion, if there is very high run-off from the systemic circulation into the shunt, there can be a very low diastolic pressure leading to severe myocardial ischaemia. This can occur post-operatively as PVR falls during the first week of life, and may necessitate shunt revision.

Tetralogy of Fallot

In this condition there is right ventricular outflow tract obstruction (RVOTO), a VSD, an aorta that 'over-rides' the VSD and right ventricular hypertrophy (see Figure 31.2). There is a wide spectrum of severity. At one end is the patient with virtually no more than a VSD – the 'pink tetralogy'. At the other end is the very cyanosed patient with total right ventricular outflow tract obstruction due to pulmonary atresia and right-to-left shunting across the VSD. On occasion the main and possibly the branch pulmonary arteries are hypoplastic; these patients can be very difficult to manage. Another variant has an absent pulmonary valve, which results in a hugely dilated pulmonary artery that can cause significant airway compression, in particular of the left main bronchus.

The classic ToF has a variable degree of RVOTO due to a combination of thick infundibular muscle bundles and a narrowed pulmonary valve annulus, so the degree of cyanosis is variable. Some children have intermittent hypercyanotic spells known as 'tet' spells, in which spasm of the right ventricular infundibulum occurs increasing right-to-left shunting through the VSD. The muscular infundibulum is sensitive to the effects of catecholamines, so spells can be brought on by stress and can be ameliorated using beta-blockers.

Hypercyanotic spells can be triggered by crying, a fall in SVR at induction of anaesthesia and surgical manipulation. An audible pulse oximeter signal can warn of a developing spell when the anaesthetist is placing monitoring lines. The management of a spell includes administering 100% oxygen, giving a fluid bolus, a dose of opioid such as fentanyl, and physical measures to increase SVR such as pushing the patient's knees up to the chest. If these measures are unsuccessful a vasoconstrictor such as noradrenaline or phenylephrine $1–5 \, \text{mcg kg}^{-1}$ should be administered. Some experts advocate beta-blockade with propranolol $50–100 \, \text{mcg kg}^{-1}$ if the heart rate is high. Esmolol $500 \, \text{mcg kg}^{-1}$ over 1 minute followed by an infusion at $50–200 \, \text{mcg kg}^{-1} \, \text{min}^{-1}$ is an alternative.

Tetralogy of Fallot is repaired using a patch to close the VSD and excising hypertrophied muscle bundles from the right ventricular outflow tract. It may be necessary to enlarge the outflow tract or the valve annulus with a patch. Widening the pulmonary valve with a transannular patch will produce

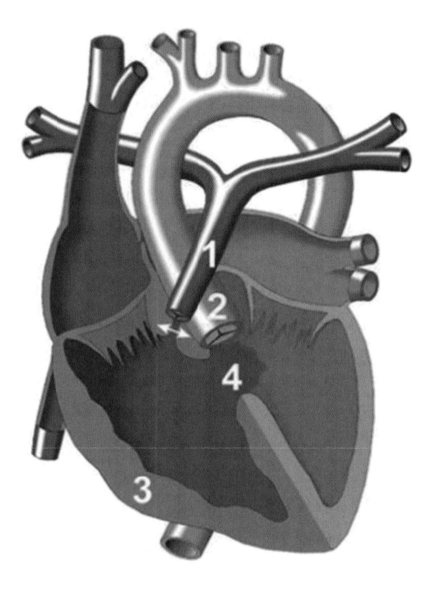

Figure 31.2 Tetralogy of Fallot. Narrowed pulmonary valve and artery (1) with narrowed right ventricular infundibulum (arrows), with aorta (2) over-riding a ventricular septal defect (4), and hypertophied right ventricle (3). From the PedHeart Resource (www. HeartPassport.com). Courtesy of Scientific Software Solutions, Inc. See plate section for colour version.

pulmonary regurgitation. Together with a poorly compliant, hypertrophied right ventricle, this can make post-bypass management challenging. Adequate cardiac output requires a high filling pressure rather than increased inotropic support. Surgery carries a risk of heart block post-operatively as the conduction tissue passes close to the borders of the VSD. Occasionally a sinister dysrhythmia known as junctional ectopic tachycardia (JET) occurs which may lead to very poor output. This is treated with cooling and amiodarone infusion, and by minimising inotropic support.

Transposition of the great arteries (TGA)

In TGA the aorta arises from the right ventricle and the PA from the left. A VSD may also be present. The condition is incompatible with life unless there is a source of mixing such as an ASD, VSD or PDA, otherwise oxygenated pulmonary venous blood cannot reach the systemic circulation. Patients are usually managed on a prostaglandin infusion preoperatively and a balloon atrial septostomy is performed if there is inadequate mixing.

The arterial switch operation (ASO) involves disconnecting the great arteries and attaching them to the correct ventricle. The coronary arteries will need to be transposed. Unsatisfactory coronary artery re-anastomosis leading to myocardial ischaemia and poor cardiac output is a major cause of post-operative problems. Following bypass, the left ventricle can be very non-compliant, and fluid boluses should be administered very cautiously to avoid left atrial enlargement and coronary distortion. Milrinone and adrenaline are useful in combination following the ASO.

The origin of the coronary arteries sits very close to the PA following repair. Elevation in PA pressure can occlude the coronaries, compromising left ventricular function, so measures to minimise pulmonary vascular resistance are important. A direct left atrial pressure line is usually sited to monitor left ventricle function and to guide fluid and inotrope administration. The sternum is frequently left open to prevent further deterioration in left ventricular compliance due to myocardial swelling.

Single ventricle circulation

Historically, children with defects where the right ventricle was inadequate, for example tricuspid atresia, would be managed with a systemic to pulmonary artery shunt but would die in late childhood or early adulthood. In the 1960s Fontan described an operation where pulmonary blood flow was achieved by directly connecting the right atrium to the pulmonary arteries. Although this 'single ventricle' solution was a major advance, complications such as atrial dysrhythmias were significant, and long-term survival was poor. The Fontan procedure has undergone a number of modifications and now involves the staged connection of the SVC and the IVC directly to the pulmonary artery with much improved long-term, good quality survival. The total cavopulmonary connection (TCPC), as it is now termed, can be used whichever ventricle is underdeveloped, the 'usable' ventricle becoming the systemic ventricle.

Creating a single ventricle circulation usually involves three stages. During the neonatal period PVR is high and a BTS is performed. As PVR falls, venous pressure becomes adequate to supply pulmonary blood flow.

The second stage, a Glenn (cavopulmonary) shunt involving the anastomosis of the SVC to the

right PA, is created at around 4 to 6 months of age and the BTS taken down (see Figure 31.3). The original Glenn shunt involved end-to-end anastomosis of the SVC to the right PA. Current practice is for an end-to-side anastomosis so blood perfuses both lungs, the bidirectional Glenn (BDG). Oxygen saturation will usually be in the 80s after a BDG. It is important to recognise that pressure measured in the internal jugular vein reflects pulmonary perfusion pressure. This 'venous pressure' has to be maintained higher than normal, often 12–15 mmHg, to ensure an adequate driving pressure of blood across the lungs. Patients benefit from a low intrathoracic pressure and being in a slightly head-up position.

The third stage, TCPC completion, in which the IVC is anastomosed to the PA, is undertaken usually between the age of 1 and 5 years. This will only be successful if PVR is reasonably low. Ideally the transpulmonary gradient after the TCPC, the difference between systemic venous pressure and atrial pressure, should be less than 10 mmHg.

If PVR is high there will need to be high systemic venous pressure to drive blood across the lungs, with poor filling of the systemic atrium and low cardiac output. Transpulmonary gradient will be high, and there may also be poor oxygenation, pleural effusions, ascites and renal dysfunction. In this situation the surgeon may 'fenestrate' the TCPC by creating a small hole between the GoreTex tube and the systemic atrium, allowing systemic venous blood to shunt through this fenestration to the systemic atrium (see Figure 31.4). This can improve preload and cardiac output, but this will be at the expense of lower oxygen saturation. Intrathoracic pressure should be kept low, and these patients benefit from early transition to spontaneous ventilation and extubation. Dysrhythmias are poorly tolerated and pacing may be necessary.

Hypoplastic left heart syndrome

In HLHS there is an inadequately developed left ventricle and aortic arch; distal aortic blood flow is initially dependent upon ductal flow from the pulmonary artery. The Norwood operation for HLHS makes use of the right ventricle as the systemic ventricle and creates a neo-aorta utilising the main pulmonary artery. The right and left PAs are disconnected from the main PA, and are supplied by

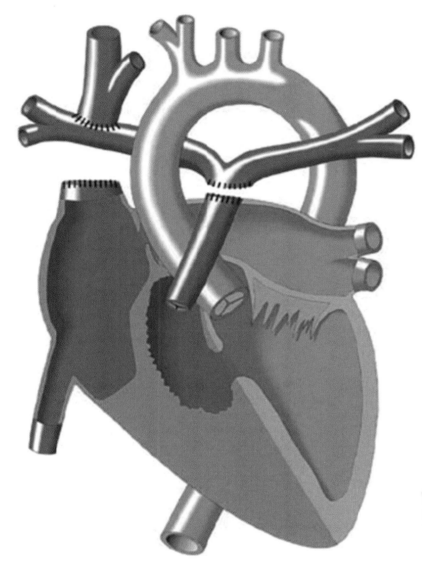

Figure 31.3 Bidirectional Glenn shunt (BDG) in tricuspid atresia, showing anastomosis of the superior vena cava to the right pulmonary artery. From the PedHeart Resource (www.HeartPassport.com). Courtesy of Scientific Software Solutions, Inc. See plate section for colour version.

either a BTS or, in the Sano modification, a shunt from the ventricle.

As both the pulmonary and systemic circulation are supplied from the same ventricle, it is important to balance SVR and PVR to maintain adequate pulmonary and systemic perfusion (see Table 31.3). This usually necessitates low inspired oxygen and a moderately raised $PaCO_2$ to keep PVR up. When appropriately balanced, oxygen saturation will be around 75–80%. These patients can be very challenging peri-operatively as they can rapidly develop very poor systemic output if PVR is allowed to fall. Progression via a Glenn to a TCPC is as above.

Coarctation repair

Coarctation may present in the neonatal period or later in childhood. Neonatal coarctation often presents with severe shock when the duct closes at around 4 days of age, and can be mistaken for sepsis. Immediate management is to re-open the duct if possible with prostaglandin to allow

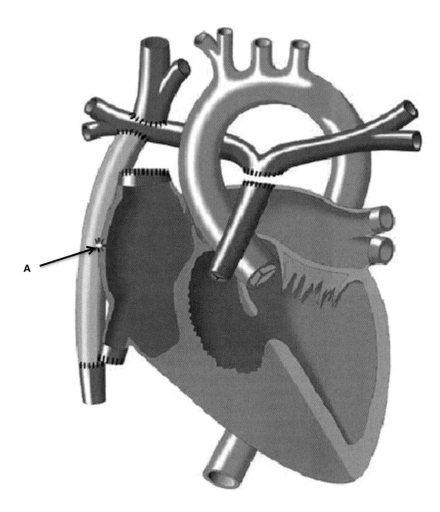

Figure 31.4 Total cavopulmonary connection (TCPC) in tricuspid atresia. Both the superior and inferior vena cavae are connected to the right pulmonary artery. There is a fenestration (A) between the IVC to PA conduit and the atrium. From the PedHeart Resource (www. HeartPassport.com). Courtesy of Scientific Software Solutions, Inc. See plate section for colour version.

perfusion of the distal aorta from the pulmonary artery. There may be severe left ventricular dysfunction and ventilatory and inotropic support may be required. Surgery to repair the coarctation is undertaken when cardiovascular and metabolic stability has been restored. Volatile agents are poorly tolerated in these neonatal patients, and high-dose fentanyl is the safest technique.

Surgery is usually via a left thoracotomy, although occasionally in neonates it can be easier to undertake it via a sternotomy. During the repair the surgeon will clamp the aorta, usually for a period of around 15–20 minutes, which places spinal cord perfusion at risk. Moderate central cooling should be achieved before the clamp is applied. In older patients blood pressure (measured in the right arm) may rise significantly during this period, and it may be necessary to increase

the volatile agent or start a vasodilator. It is important to stop these a few minutes before the aortic clamp is removed to avoid a catastrophic fall in blood pressure, and to have volume replacement ready. Dialogue with the surgeon is essential.

Ligation of patent ductus arteriosus

This is generally undertaken in the newborn period via left thoracotomy. In very low birth weight premature infants it is often easiest to carry this out in the NICU to avoid the hazards of transfer to the operating theatre. With the anxieties surrounding anaesthetic neurotoxicity in these infants, our preferred technique is to use high-dose fentanyl alone. Non-invasive blood pressure monitoring is generally acceptable in these infants, and central venous

Table 31.3 Manipulating PVR and SVR

Direction of change of vascular resistance	Intervention
PVR ↑	Hypercapnia Hypoxia Acidosis PEEP High airway pressure Atelectasis
PVR ↓	Hypocapnia Alkalosis High FiO_2 Low haematocrit Nitric oxide Prostacyclin (epoprostenol) Milrinone Low airway pressure
SVR ↑	Vasoconstrictors Hypothermia Raising haematocrit
SVR ↓	Vasodilators Anaesthetic agents Low haematocrit Warming

access is unnecessary provided that there is a secure good intravenous line. One of the major potential complications of the procedure is inadvertent ligation of the descending aorta, as the duct is often larger than the aorta. If there is no lower-limb arterial line in place it is essential to place a pulse oximeter on the foot so that persistence of aortic pulsation can be confirmed.

Key points

- Successful anaesthesia for CHD surgery requires a meticulous, anticipative approach that starts in the pre-operative period.
- Many infants with CHD have a 'balanced circulation' in which changes in pulmonary or systemic resistance with anaesthesia can lead to severe adverse haemodynamic disturbances.
- Patients with unrepaired tetralogy of Fallot with severe right ventricular outflow tract obstruction can develop life-threatening profound hypoxia during induction if systemic resistance falls, and may need vasoconstrictor support.
- Children who are very cyanosed and polycythaemic will often have abnormal coagulation.

Further reading

Andropoulos DB, Stayer SA, Russell IA, Mossad EB, eds. *Anesthesia for Congenital Heart Disease*, 2nd edition. Wiley-Blackwell. 2010.

Chapter

32

Anaesthesia for cardiac catheterisation and other investigative procedures in children

Ian James and Sally Wilmshurst

Introduction

Cardiac catheterisation generally describes those procedures in which the heart and major vessels are imaged under X-ray control using catheters and other devices inserted through distal vessels. It is both a diagnostic tool and an interventional modality, and an outline of the most common procedures undertaken is shown in Table 32.1.

As a diagnostic tool catheterisation has been popular since the 1940s, but with the increasing sophistication of echocardiography and technological advances in other non-invasive modalities, such as cardiac CT and MRI, there has been a substantial reduction in the need for cardiac catheterisation for the diagnosis of congenital heart disease (CHD). There has, however, been a significant increase in the use of interventional techniques, in some instances obviating the need for surgical procedures. About 2500 children undergo interventional procedures in the UK annually, about 10% of whom are neonates. PDA occlusion and ASD closure are the most frequently performed.

Most cases are elective and many patients are relatively well, albeit with an underlying cardiac disorder. However, a significant number of procedures are undertaken in haemodynamically compromised patients, some of whom may be in a precarious clinical condition. Examples of these patients include those with critical valve stenosis, patients with end-stage cardiac disease undergoing assessment for heart transplantation, patients with severe pulmonary hypertension, and patients with cardiomyopathy requiring an implantable cardioverter defibrillator (ICD). In such patients anaesthesia can be more challenging than for patients undergoing major cardiac surgery. Cardiac catheterisation may also be necessary

Table 32.1 Cardiac catheter laboratory procedures

	Procedure
Diagnostic	Diagnostic catheter/ angiography Coronary angiography Endomyocardial biopsy Pulmonary vascular resistance study Transoesophageal echocardiography
Interventional	Septal defect closure Vessel occlusion Valvoplasty Angioplasty Stent placement Balloon atrial septostomy Percutaneous valve placement
Electrophysiological studies (EPS)	Conduction system mapping Ablation of arrhythmogenic focus Pacemaker insertion Reveal® insertion Placement of implantable cardioverter defibrillator (ICD) Cardioversion
Miscellaneous	Drainage of pericardial effusion

in unstable patients from the critical care unit who are failing to progress following cardiac surgery. In all cases it is essential that the anaesthetist understands the haemodynamic and physiological consequences of the underlying lesion and undertakes a thorough assessment of such patients pre-operatively. The key principles outlined in Chapter 31 for the pre-operative assessment of children undergoing cardiac surgery are equally applicable for patients undergoing cardiac investigative and interventional procedures.

Risk

Recent data indicate that the risk of cardiac arrest during paediatric cardiac catheterisation is around 0.5%, with a mortality of 0.08%; these figures are some 20 times higher than for routine paediatric anaesthesia. The risks are even higher for patients with pulmonary hypertension who represent the highest anaesthesia-related mortality cohort in paediatrics. An added complication is that the cardiac catheter suite is frequently an isolated site, remote from the main complex of theatres and ready assistance. Good communication and teamwork is thus an essential component of safe anaesthesia for these procedures. It is important to identify those cases in which it is prudent to ensure additional expertise is present.

Diagnostic cardiac catheterisation

Diagnostic catheterisation involves the collection of haemodynamic data that cannot fully be obtained from echocardiography. Measurement of arterial, mixed venous, pulmonary venous and pulmonary arterial oxygen saturations allows determination of cardiac output (Qs), pulmonary blood flow (Qp) and the pulmonary to systemic shunt ratio, commonly referred to as Qp:Qs (Box 32.1). Measurement of oxygen consumption is cumbersome, requiring a mass spectrometer and the collection of all expired gases. Standard assumed values are often used. In older children thermodilution is an alternative method of determining cardiac output, although this is inaccurate in the presence of a cardiac shunt.

Direct pressure measurements in the heart chambers and blood vessels can be used with blood flow values to provide systemic and pulmonary vascular resistance. Many of the measurements are indexed to body surface area (BSA). Indexed pulmonary vascular resistance (PVR) is referred to in Wood Units and should be under 3. Pressure measurements also provide important information about cardiac function and obstructions to flow across valves and vessels, and are more accurate than those derived using echocardiography.

Box 32.1 Haemodynamic calculations

Flow: (based on the Fick Equation):

$$\text{Cardiac output (Qs)} = \frac{VO_2}{C_{ao}O_2 - C_{mv}O_2}$$

$$\text{Pulmonary flow (Qp)} = \frac{VO_2}{C_{pv}O_2 - C_{pa}O_2}$$

Oxygen content $(C_xO_2) = (S_xO_2 \times Hb \ (g \ dl^{-1}) \times 1.34 \times 10 \ ml \ l^{-1}) + (PaO_2 \ mmHg \times 0.003)$

VO_2 = oxygen consumption; ao = aorta; mv = mixed venous; pa = pulmonary artery; pv = pulmonary vein

Shunt fraction:

Because of the technical difficulties of measuring oxygen content for shunt calculation, in practice it is often calculated using saturation measurements from a number of different sites by the following equation:

$$\text{Pulmonary to systemic (Qp:Qs)} : = \frac{S_{ao}O_2 - S_{mv}O_2}{S_{pv}O_2 - S_{pa}O_2}$$

Mixed venous saturation $(S_{mv}O_2)$ can be approximated from:

$$\frac{3(SaSVC) + (SaIVC)}{4}$$

Resistance:

$$\text{Systemic (SVR)} = \frac{AoP - RAP}{Qs}$$

$$\text{Pulmonary (PVR)} = \frac{PAP - LAP}{Qp}$$

RAP = right atrial pressure; LAP = left atrial pressure

Additional diagnostic information is obtained using angiography, which involves the injection of contrast medium to outline the heart structures, great vessels, venous connections and any abnormal vessels such as collaterals. This can be crucial in establishing the exact anatomical nature of some complex cardiac anomalies. Coronary angiography may be undertaken when echocardiography is unable to answer concerns about coronary anatomy or perfusion. Coronary artery disease is an unfortunate complication of heart transplantation, and coronary angiography is part of the routine annual follow-up of these patients. Intravascular ultrasound (IVUS), in which a very fine ultrasound catheter is passed down the coronary artery, is more sensitive at identifying early plaque formation and is increasingly used in children over the age of about 10 years.

Contrast medium is iodine-based and of varying osmolality. Hyperosmolar solutions are avoided in children as they are associated with flushing, hypotension, bradycardia and renal impairment. Adequate hydration is essential in children undergoing angiography, particularly those with pre-existing renal dysfunction, because of the small risk of contrast-induced nephropathy. Anaphylactic reactions to contrast can occur but are rare.

Interventional cardiac catheterisation

Interventional procedures involve the passage of a variety of devices into the heart or major vessels. These may be:

- Balloons, which are dilated with contrast or a gas, usually carbon dioxide, to distend valves or vessels;
- Stents, which are expanded by a balloon and left in place to widen a vessel;
- Devices that can be deployed to close holes;
- Coils that can be positioned to obstruct vessels;
- More recently it has become possible to implant artificial valves via a percutaneous route.

There is greater potential for haemodynamic instability in these patients than those undergoing diagnostic procedures, and the anaesthetist needs to remain particularly vigilant.

Access

The right side of the heart and pulmonary arteries are usually accessed via the femoral vein. The internal jugular vein is preferred for endomyocardial biopsy as it provides easier access to the right ventricle, and may be necessary in other cases if the femoral or iliac vessels are blocked. Internal jugular vein access will also be required if it is necessary to measure pressure in a Glenn shunt, in which the SVC is connected to the pulmonary artery.

The left side of the heart and major arterial vessels are usually accessed from the femoral artery, or via a septal defect or puncture. The cardiologist may insert a femoral arterial monitoring line even when left heart catheterisation is not planned. An alternative, indirect method of assessing left atrial pressure is the pulmonary capillary wedge pressure, obtained by wedging a balloon-tipped catheter into a small pulmonary artery, and measuring the pressure distal to the balloon. This can be useful when measuring pulmonary vascular resistance.

Catheters are inserted through a sheath placed using the Seldinger technique. Relatively large sheaths are sometimes required to pass devices through, and insertion of the sheath is usually the most stimulating time for the patient. Heparin is often given when arterial or left atrial catheters are inserted to prevent thrombosis. At the end of the procedure it is important that satisfactory haemostasis at the puncture site is achieved before anaesthesia is terminated as it can be very difficult to control bleeding in a restless, wakening child.

Anaesthesia

Cardiac catheterisation is seldom painful, apart from the initial placement of cannulae in the vessels. In a few older children some diagnostic procedures can be undertaken under local anaesthesia, supplemented if necessary with light sedation. However, most procedures in children can be prolonged and general anaesthesia is necessary.

In most cases the main requirement from the anaesthetist is for a still patient with stable haemodynamics throughout the procedure, preferably with parameters as near to normal as possible. Inappropriate anaesthesia and ventilation can adversely affect the haemodynamic data being collected, so the anaesthetist must have a thorough knowledge of these potential changes as well as of the procedures being performed. For example, oxygen saturation data for accurate blood flow measurement are best achieved with inspired oxygen as near to 21% as can be tolerated. Normocapnia is particularly important when pulmonary vascular resistance is being assessed. Hypovolaemia and hypotension may lead to inaccurate determination of flows and shunts. Good communication with the cardiologist is essential before and during these procedures.

Induction

Where possible, full monitoring should be applied prior to induction. Inhalational or intravenous induction is suitable for cardiac catheterisation and will usually depend on the child's age and preferences. Sevoflurane is an ideal agent for inhalational induction. For intravenous induction propofol is usually suitable unless a fall in SVR is to be avoided, in which case ketamine may be preferred. As most procedures are conducted through femoral vessels it is generally preferable to avoid the lower-limb veins for venous access.

Airway management

An LMA may be appropriate for many straightforward diagnostic cases in older infants and children. For small infants, patients who are clinically unstable, and those undergoing interventional procedures a tracheal tube should be employed. Intubation is also recommended for patients in whom internal jugular venous access is required. If the cardiologist needs to collect all expired respiratory gases to measure oxygen consumption a cuffed tracheal tube should be used. A cuffed tube will also be advantageous when it is necessary to ensure steady carbon dioxide tension during pulmonary vascular resistance studies.

Controlled ventilation is indicated in most cases, as it allows careful control of the blood gases for haemodynamic data collection, and facilitates the short periods of apnoea that are occasionally necessary for accurate pressure measurement and high quality angiographic pictures.

Maintenance

Nitrous oxide should be avoided during cardiac catheterisation. Isoflurane is usually well tolerated and is generally the volatile agent of choice. Desflurane appears to be more dysrhythmogenic than isoflurane. The concentration of volatile agent can usually be reduced once the catheters have been inserted.

A small dose of fentanyl ($1–2\,mcg\,kg^{-1}$) may be given prior to passing a transoesophageal echo (TOE) probe, if this is being used, to blunt the pressor response it induces. Opioid analgesics are otherwise seldom required. Many procedures are undertaken as day-cases, so a plan for post-discharge analgesia should be made. Local anaesthetic infiltration to the puncture site is usually adequate for post-catheter pain relief along with paracetamol, administered either intravenously during the procedure or orally afterwards. There is a significant incidence of nausea and vomiting following cardiac catheterisation despite avoidance of opioids, so an antiemetic should be given.

Monitoring

Full monitoring should be used for all catheterisation procedures. Multilead ECG is generally part of the routine cardiac electrophysiological data displayed, so a separate anaesthetic ECG is not usually required after induction. If a lower-limb digit is used for the pulse oximeter, the contralateral limb to that used for catheter access should be chosen. Capnography can be significantly affected by cyanotic heart disease, owing to venous admixture and impaired pulmonary blood flow, and may underestimate $PaCO_2$ by $2\,kPa$. In general, the greater the degree of cyanosis the greater the end-tidal to arterial pCO_2 disparity. Invasive blood pressure monitoring is seldom required in diagnostic catheterisation, but may be indicated in unstable children and patients with severe pulmonary hypertension.

Intravenous fluids are required for all but the shortest procedures, especially if contrast is being used.

Positioning

For most procedures where biplane X-ray imaging is used, the patient is positioned supine with the arms above the head. Care must be taken that the brachial plexus is not stretched. Exposure is less than during surgical procedures but temperature monitoring and the facilities for active warming should be available. Because procedures can take many hours, pressure areas must be protected.

Interventional procedures

- *Septal defect device closure*: Closure of an atrial septal defect, with an umbrella-like device, is the most commonly performed interventional procedure. Patients are generally well, and the procedure is straightforward. TOE is necessary to ensure correct placement. This procedure is only suitable where there is a rim of septal tissue for the device to anchor upon. Very occasionally the device can dislodge and may impinge on an atrioventricular valve, necessitating urgent open-heart surgery to retrieve it. More rarely, transcatheter closure of a VSD can be undertaken, but this is technically more challenging and is associated with more complications, particularly heart block and valve damage.

- *Vessel occlusion*: This is most commonly performed for patent ductus arteriosus, although it is occasionally used for aorto-pulmonary collaterals or veno-venous connections. These patients are usually relatively well, although on occasion there can be a degree of high output failure. Again, there is always the risk of the occlusion device embolising necessitating retrieval.

- *Valvotomy*: This may be carried out in the early newborn period for critical pulmonary valve stenosis or for critical aortic valve stenosis. Both these groups of patients can be seriously ill and will require prostaglandin infusion to maintain a patent ductus arteriosus. In both procedures a balloon is dilated across the valve for several seconds, resulting in a short period of no output.

- *Critical aortic stenosis*: This has a significant procedural mortality as there is often a hypertrophied ischaemic left ventricle, and inflation of the balloon tends to obstruct coronary perfusion. Volatile agents are poorly tolerated, and it is our practice to use high-dose fentanyl and oxygen. Hypovolaemia is also poorly tolerated, and inotropic support may be necessary. Resuscitation drugs should be close at hand. Not infrequently, dilation damages the valve and causes acute aortic regurgitation, which may need urgent surgical repair. These patients will nearly always need pre- and post-operative intensive care support.

- *Critical pulmonary stenosis*: There will be profound cyanosis, and acidosis is common. There is usually a poorly functioning right ventricle which may be further compromised during occlusion of the pulmonary valve. Pulmonary regurgitation may be produced, though this is better tolerated than aortic insufficiency. Post-procedural inotropic support may be necessary.

- *Balloon dilation* of the aortic and pulmonary valves may be necessary in older children, and the greater the obstruction the greater the likelihood of ventricular hypertrophy and dysfunction.

- *Angioplasty and stent placement*: Re-coarctation of the aorta, pulmonary artery stenosis or narrowing of the superior vena cava is often amenable to balloon angioplasty. It may be necessary to place an endovascular stent to maintain adequate vessel patency although this necessitates a larger catheter, with a higher risk of vascular damage. Acute complications include rupture of the vessel being dilated, which may require urgent surgery. Most centres will ensure that surgical cover is provided. Although rare, there is the possibility of displacement and embolisation of the stent.

- *Balloon atrial septostomy (BAS)*: In some cardiac lesions, such as transposition of the great arteries (TGA), it is essential that there is adequate mixing of systemic and pulmonary venous blood in the period prior to surgery. Where this is inadequate, it will be necessary to create a communication at atrial level. This is usually performed by passing a balloon-tipped catheter across from the right to left atrium through the foramen ovale, inflating it and then withdrawing it sharply back into the right atrium, tearing the septum in the process. It may be necessary to repeat this a few times to achieve an adequate hole. These neonatal patients are usually extremely desaturated and may be acidotic, but rapidly improve once the septostomy has been made. It is usual to undertake these cases in the catheter suite with full radiological imaging, but on occasion the procedure is performed in the intensive care unit under echocardiographic guidance.

- *Percutaneous valve placement*: The development of a pulmonary valve, fashioned from a titanium stent and bovine jugular vein, that can be inserted percutaneously has revolutionised the management of right ventricular outflow tract obstruction which would otherwise require major open-heart surgery. As with other procedures, there is a risk of device migration, and damage to intracardiac structures and vessels. There is also the risk of coronary artery distortion from the device.

Hazards/complications

Although most diagnostic procedures are uncomplicated, for some children the nature of the cardiac lesion being investigated is such that induction of anaesthesia may be hazardous. For example, a fall in SVR or blood pressure in children in whom coronary perfusion is borderline can lead to significant haemodynamic compromise and cardiac arrest. Particular care should be taken with infants with severe pulmonary hypertension and cardiomyopathy. In addition to the risks of device embolisation already mentioned there are a number of potential complications associated with cardiac catheterisation in general that mean vigilance is essential. These include:

- *Dysrhythmias:* these can be precipitated by catheters within the heart or at the coronary ostia. Withdrawal of the catheter usually resolves the problem. Very occasionally antiarrhythmics or cardioversion may be necessary.

- *Coronary ischaemia:* ECG changes may be seen during coronary angiography. If these do not resolve following withdrawal of the catheter, glyceryl trinitrate (GTN) can be administered by the cardiologist directly into the aortic root. GTN is occasionally administered just before the catheter is introduced into the coronary to prevent vessel spasm and it is important to correct any hypovolaemia or hypotension before this as the blood pressure is likely to fall.

- *Hypotension:* This can be caused by impaired ventricular function exacerbated by volatile anaesthetic agents, by hypovolaemia, or by rhythm disturbances.

- *Impaired cardiac output:* Balloon dilation of aortic or pulmonary valve stenosis will totally obstruct flow from the ventricle. This is for a few seconds only and is usually well tolerated. On occasion it can lead to profound decompensation and cardiac arrest.

- *Hypoxaemia:* Passing catheters into vessels that are the only or the main source of pulmonary blood flow can lead to profound desaturation.

- *Perforation of cardiac chambers or major vessels:* Although rare, it is important to consider the possibility of perforation of a cardiac chamber resulting in tamponade, or of a major vessel, if there is an otherwise unexplained fall in blood pressure or signs of reduced cardiac output during or after the procedure. An echo should be obtained urgently to assess this. Retroperitoneal haematoma from a perforation in the abdominal or iliac vessels should also be considered,

particularly if there has been difficulty advancing a catheter from the femoral vessels.

- *Vascular injury:* Thrombosis of the artery used for catheterisation is a known complication, and a small dose of heparin is often administered at the time of catheterisation. Regular assessment of the limb pulses and temperature is an important part of routine post-operative management, and there should be a protocol in place for the management of a limb with signs of arterial insufficiency.

- *Haematoma:* this may occur at the site of vascular access at the end of the procedure or several hours later, particularly if heparin has been given during the procedure.

Electrophysiological studies

Children present for electrophysiological studies (EPS) to identify the source of an arrhythmia and to ablate an abnormal focus or pathway. Most of these patients have normal ventricular function, and many suffer from paroxysmal supraventricular tachycardias. Most commonly these are re-entry or accessory pathway tachycardias such as sinoatrial node re-entrant tachycardia (SARNT), AV nodal re-entrant tachycardia (AVRNT) or Wolff–Parkinson–White syndrome, an atrioventricular re-entry tachycardia (AVRT).

The procedure involves the insertion of catheters with multiple electrodes along their length in the right atrium, across the tricuspid valve, in the right ventricle and in the coronary sinus to stimulate and map the electrical pathways in the heart. Access can be from the femoral or from the subclavian vein. Once the abnormal pathway has been identified it is ablated by radiofrequency energy delivered by another catheter. The size of the 'burn' necessary to fully ablate the focus varies and the procedure can be prolonged. Where the abnormal focus lies close to the AV node radiofrequency carries a high risk of heart block; a newer technique involving cryoablation with a supercooled catheter appears to be safer.

Anaesthesia is generally straightforward as these children are usually otherwise well. Many arrhythmias are provoked by stress, and it is important that deep anaesthesia is avoided as it may then prove difficult to identify the focus. Isoflurane at 1–1.5 MAC is appropriate, supplemented with a small dose of fentanyl. Adenosine may be given to help identify an aberrant pathway, and isoprenaline may sometimes be given to provoke the dysrhythmia. The use of dexamethasone as an antiemetic should be avoided in these patients as its anti-inflammatory effect may ameliorate the 'burn' and compromise the ablation. Adenosine may induce bronchospasm, and should be avoided in children with asthma. The procedures can be prolonged; appropriate methods to monitor and maintain temperature should be used.

Implantation of pacemakers and other devices

Some permanent pacemakers are implanted in the catheter laboratory, usually in the left subclavicular region, with transvenous pacing leads inserted into the subclavian vein. Where the nature of an intermittent dysrhythmia cannot be identified a Reveal® device, a small subcutaneous ECG recorder, may be implanted in the same area. Anaesthesia is generally straightforward and should include intravenous and topical analgesia, together with prophylactic antibiotics.

Implantable cardioverter defibrillator (ICD)

A number of disorders are associated with sudden death in childhood due to an arrhythmia which may be prevented by an ICD. These include:

- Hypertrophic obstructive cardiomyopathy (HOCM)
- Dilated cardiomyopathy (DCM)
- Arrhythmogenic right ventricular dysplasia
- Long QT syndrome
- Brugada syndrome

Many of these patients will have experienced a life-threatening arrhythmia or have a family history of sudden cardiac death. The procedure requires the placement of ventricular pacing leads via the subclavian vein and device insertion in the subclavicular or axillary area. The device is designed to detect ventricular tachycardia or fibrillation and deliver a defibrillation shock. It will also pace where necessary. Once inserted it is necessary to test that it is working satisfactorily by inducing ventricular fibrillation. Full resuscitation drugs should be on hand, and external defibrillation pads should be placed lest the device does not work properly. Inducing a period of ventricular fibrillation can lead to severe cardiac decompensation in some of these patients, such as those with severe cardiomyopathy, and invasive arterial pressure monitoring and central venous access should be used.

Induction of anaesthesia can be challenging in patients with impaired ventricular function. For those with DCM it is important that blood pressure and coronary perfusion do not fall during induction. A combination of fentanyl $1-2 \, \mathrm{mcg \, kg^{-1}}$ and etomidate $0.2-0.3 \, \mathrm{mg \, kg^{-1}}$ works well. Sevoflurane is used where intravenous induction is not appropriate. For patients with HOCM it is important not to increase myocardial activity or heart rate, and to maintain filling pressures.

Pericardial effusion drainage

Insertion of a pericardial needle or drain to relieve a pericardial effusion is usually performed under echocardiographic guidance. General anaesthesia can be challenging as these patients may have severely compromised cardiac function. Ketamine is the induction agent of choice. Profound hypotension can occur when the effusion is drained as the heart becomes acutely underfilled, and it is important that the effusion is drained slowly. Adequate venous access for rapid volume administration is essential. The situation is not helped by the need for the patient to be semi-erect to facilitate the effusion gravitating to the base of the heart. In adolescents it is safer to undertake this under local anaesthesia.

Cardiac MRI and CT

Cardiac MRI and magnetic resonance angiography (MRA) is increasingly used in the diagnosis and assessment of CHD, and is particularly useful in demonstrating three-dimensional anatomical relationships and in quantifying flows. It has the advantage that there is no radiation, although there is the disadvantage of the need for MRI-compatible equipment and a general anaesthetic as the scans are long. There is generally a need for short periods of apnoea, so controlled ventilation and tracheal intubation is required.

These investigations are often undertaken to plan further surgical procedures in patients reliant upon a systemic to pulmonary shunt and who may be polycythaemic. It is vitally important to avoid dehydration, and clear oral fluids should be maintained until 2 hours before the procedure. Where this is not possible, intravenous fluids should be administered before anaesthesia.

Key points

- Some children undergoing procedures in the cardiac catheter laboratory can present greater challenges than those undergoing cardiac surgery.
- Children with pulmonary hypertension undergoing cardiac catheterisation pose the highest risks for cardiac arrest and mortality under anaesthesia.

- Dexamethasone should not be administered as an antiemetic to children undergoing arrhythmia ablation procedures as it can reduce the effect of the 'burn'.

Further reading

Andropoulos DB, Stayer SA, Russell IA, Mossad EB, eds. *Anesthesia for Congenital Heart Disease*, 2nd edition. Wiley-Blackwell. 2010.

Anaesthesia for children with heart disease undergoing non-cardiac surgery

Anthony Moriarty, Alet Jacobs and Ian James

Introduction

The likelihood of an anaesthetist encountering a child with heart disease requiring non-cardiac surgery is increasing, in large part owing to the improved outcomes from infant cardiac surgery and to the innovative techniques that have led to survival from previously untreatable lesions.

Approximately 1 in 150 children have congenital heart disease (CHD), and about a quarter of these will have an additional non-cardiac defect. This may be part of a well-described association. For example, children with Down syndrome may have duodenal atresia and an atrioventricular septal defect, while tracheo-oesophageal fistula, anal atresia and tetralogy of Fallot may be seen in children with VACTERL association (Vertebral, Anorectal, Cardiac, Tracheo-Esophageal, Renal, Limb anomalies). Some children with heart disease will present for coincidental surgery, such as appendicitis or adenotonsillectomy. Anaesthesia may also be required for children with acquired or late onset heart disease, such as those with cardiomyopathy or pulmonary hypertension. Scoliosis is a common feature of the muscular dystrophies in which severe cardiomyopathy may be present, while children with pulmonary hypertension may require the placement of long-term venous access. The improving long-term survival of patients after heart transplantation presents another group of patients who may require anaesthesia for incidental surgery.

This is an extraordinarily heterogeneous group of patients, and it is not possible to describe an anaesthetic technique that is suitable for all patients. This chapter will outline the key principles that are important in anaesthetising patients with heart disease, and provide an overview of some of the lesions that are likely to be encountered.

Risk

The peri-operative and 30-day mortality of children with heart disease undergoing anaesthesia and surgery is significantly increased compared with the normal population. Data indicate that more of these children die during non-cardiac procedures than during cardiac surgery, although this may reflect the greater number of non-cardiac procedures. Most are aged less than 2 years. Children at highest risk include those with:

- Pulmonary hypertension
- Heart failure, particularly those with cardiomyopathy
- Left ventricular outflow tract obstruction, particularly aortic stenosis
- Single ventricle circulation
- Cyanosis
- Multiple co-morbidity
- Emergency procedures

General principles of anaesthesia for children with heart disease

When presented with a child with heart disease requiring non-cardiac surgery, it is important to understand the cardiac lesion, and the alterations in blood flow or myocardial performance that may be present. It is usually then possible to anticipate the effects that manipulation of the circulation and ventilation will have on cardiac output or oxygen saturation. A simple classification of cardiac disorders is shown in Table 33.1. For children with uncorrected CHD the physiological derangements and effects of anaesthesia will be essentially the same as for those undergoing cardiac surgery, and these are discussed

Core Topics in Paediatric Anaesthesia, ed. Ian James and Isabeau Walker. Published by Cambridge University Press. © 2013 Cambridge University Press.

Table 33.1 Classification of cardiac disorders

Type of disorder	Specific condition
Inadequate pulmonary blood flow (right to left shunts)	Tricuspid atresia Pulmonary atresia Pulmonary stenosis Tetralogy of Fallot
Excessive pulmonary blood flow (left to right shunts)	Patent ductus arteriosus Atrial septal defect Ventricular septal defect Atrioventricular septal defect Aortopulmonary window
Abnormal connections (complex shunts)	Transposition of the great arteries Hypoplastic left heart syndrome Truncus arteriosus Total anomalous pulmonary venous connection
Left ventricular outflow tract obstruction	Aortic coarctation Interrupted aortic arch Aortic stenosis Hypertrophic obstructive cardiomyopathy

in the opening section of Chapter 31. It is not just the effect of anaesthetic drugs that is important; posture, dehydration, sudden blood loss and changes in intra-cavity pressures (as in laparascopic or thoracoscopic surgery) may all have detrimental effects.

Most corrective congenital cardiac surgery is undertaken in the first year of life. After this time children with continuing manifestations of CHD are most likely to have residual problems, such as valvar stenosis or regurgitation, or impaired ventricular function. In general, a ventricle that has been subjected to pressure overload, as in outflow obstruction, will become hypertrophied, often with poor diastolic function. Systolic function may be well-preserved initially but the ventricle will be prone to myocardial ischaemia. It is important to maintain coronary perfusion pressure in these patients. A ventricle subjected to volume overload, as in a large intracardiac shunt or aortic or pulmonary valve incompetence, will become dilated. In this scenario there will be primarily systolic ventricular dysfunction.

In some CHD one of the ventricles is hypoplastic and unable to contribute to an effective, two-ventricle

circulation. In tricuspid or pulmonary atresia it is the right ventricle while in hypoplastic left heart syndrome (HLHS) it is the left ventricle that is ineffective. For such patients with a 'univentricular heart' a series of staged surgical procedures is undertaken to establish a single-ventricle circulation in which the effective ventricle drives the systemic circulation, while the pulmonary circulation relies on passive flow. Patients may be encountered who are in one of the stages of the establishment of a single-ventricle circulation. For those who rarely encounter these patients it can be challenging to understand the haemodynamics of the staged or palliative procedures, and this is discussed later.

Common to many cardiac disorders, both unrepaired and palliated, is the important concept of maintaining a balanced circulation.

The balanced circulation

Ideally, output from the right and left side of the heart should be equal. This is often referred to as Qp:Qs of 1:1 (Qp is pulmonary blood flow, Qs is systemic blood flow). In some CHD lesions such as ventricular septal defect (VSD) or patent ductus arteriosus (PDA), there may be significant blood flow from the left to the right side of the heart – a left-to-right shunt – causing excessive pulmonary and ventricular overload, resulting in the typical features of cardiac failure and pulmonary congestion. A Qp:Qs of 2:1 or more is usually associated with significant failure. Factors that reduce pulmonary vascular resistance (PVR) or increase systemic vascular resistance (SVR) may exacerbate this shunt, worsening the failure. It is important to recognise when anaesthetising such patients that high inspired oxygen and hyperventilation reduce PVR.

Conversely in a patient with right-to-left shunt in whom Qp is impaired, such as unrepaired tetralogy of Fallot (ToF), reducing the SVR will increase the right-to-left shunting and may lead to profound hypoxaemia. This is particularly relevant during induction of anaesthesia in these patients.

The duct-dependent circulation

The concept of the balanced circulation is particularly important in patients with a duct-dependent circulation. In some newborn infants with complex CHD, maintaining blood flow through the ductus arteriosus from pulmonary artery to aorta, or vice versa, is

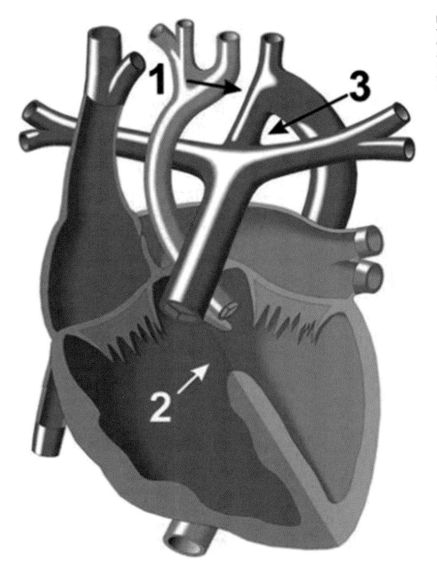

Figure 33.1 Interrupted aortic arch (1) with ventricular septal defect (2). A patent ductus arteriosus (3) provides distal aortic blood flow. From the PedHeart Resource (www.HeartPassport.com). Courtesy of Scientific Software Solutions, Inc. See plate section for colour version.

necessary to maintain adequate systemic or pulmonary perfusion. These include newborns with:

- HLHS
- Interrupted aortic arch (IAA)
- Transposition of the great arteries (TGA)

Prostaglandin infusion will usually be necessary to keep the duct open until surgery can be undertaken. In these children, maintaining adequate pulmonary and systemic blood flow is achieved by manipulating the resistances of the two circulations. Where ductal patency is required to provide systemic perfusion, as in HLHS or IAA (see Figure 33.1), this involves attempting to keep PVR high and SVR low. These patients should be maintained in room air, with a modest hypercapnia and respiratory acidosis. A well-balanced circulation will result in an arterial oxygen saturation of around 75–85%. High-inspired oxygen and hyperventilation must be avoided as these will drop PVR leading to increased pulmonary blood flow at the expense of systemic blood flow. This can lead to profoundly low systemic tissue perfusion, metabolic acidosis and, if unchecked, cardiac arrest. Oxygen saturations in the 90s would suggest that pulmonary blood flow is excessive and needs to be reduced. Rarely, this necessitates

Table 33.2 Congenital syndromes and associated cardiac lesions

Anomaly	Common cardiac lesion	Associated problems
Trisomy 21	Ventricular septal defect Atrioventricular septal defect	Prone to pulmonary hypertension Neck instability
DiGeorge (22q11 deletion)	Arch anomalies Tetralogy of Fallot	Absent thymus and parathyroid, so immune deficiency and hypocalcaemia Need irradiated blood
Velocardiofacial	Ventricular septal defect	Cleft palate
VACTERL anomaly	Tetralogy of Fallot Ventricular septal defect	Tracheo-oesophageal fistula
CHARGE	Ventricular septal defect	Choanal atresia
Goldenhar	Ventricular septal defect	Intubation difficulty
Duchenne's muscular dystrophy	Cardiomyopathy	Respiratory muscle weakness

intubating the infant to ensure modest hypoventilation and a respiratory acidosis.

Pre-operative assessment

In addition to routine pre-assessment it is necessary to establish the current status of the cardiac lesion. For most children with successfully repaired CHD it is unlikely that there will be any impact upon the anaesthesia and surgery. For those children with residual defects, unrepaired defects or palliated defects, the history and examination should focus on establishing the exact diagnosis, and stage of repair.

Although carers may be able to provide some details it is important to review the most recent cardiological summary to establish:

- Diagnosis and previous interventions
- Residual lesions, such as valvar stenosis or incompetence
- The presence of a PDA, or surgical shunt
- The degree of cyanosis
- Whether there have been any hypercyanotic spells
- Ventricular function
- If there have been rhythm disturbances or syncopal attacks
- Whether there is a pacemaker
- Current medications, including anticoagulation
- Current clinical status including intercurrent infections

An assessment must be made of any associated congenital syndrome as these may have anaesthesia-related factors. Some of the more common are shown in Table 33.2.

Echocardiogram

A recent echocardiogram will be necessary to determine ventricular function. Cardiologists identify different cardiac chambers by their echo appearance, and use standard terminology to describe findings using a system termed 'sequential segmental analysis'. The echo report will include a description of the following:

- Atrial position and systemic and pulmonary venous drainage
- Atrioventricular (AV) connections and the ventriculo-arterial (VA) connections
- Abnormal shunts and direction of flow
- Ventricular dimensions and function
- Coronary anatomy

Common terms include:

- 'Atrial situs' – the sidedness of the atrial chambers.
  - *Situs solitus* – normal arrangement of atria and the abdominal organs
  - *Situs inversus* – mirror image atria and abdominal organs
  - *Situs ambiguus* – no clear lateralisation of the thoracic and abdominal organs
  - *Left atrial isomerism* – two morphologically left atria
  - *Right atrial isomerism* – two morphologically right atria

- Atrioventricular connections
  - *Concordant AV connection* – usual connection of the atria to the ventricles
  - *Discordant AV connection* – left atrium is connected to right ventricle, right atrium is connected to left ventricle
  - *Absent left- or right-sided AV connection* – mitral or tricuspid atresia
  - *Double inlet left or right ventricle* – two-ventricle heart but there is >50% override of right or left atrial connection to the left or right ventricle respectively owing to malalignment of atrial and ventricular septa
- Ventriculo-arterial connections
  - *Concordant VA connection* – usual connection of the ventricles to the aorta and pulmonary trunk
  - *Discordant VA connections* – left ventricle connected to pulmonary trunk, right ventricle connected to aorta, as in transposition of the great arteries.
  - *Single outlet VA connection* – aortic or pulmonary atresia
  - *Double outlet right ventricle* – two-ventricle heart, but there is >50% override of the aorta from the right ventricle
- Cardiac position
  - *Levocardia* – normal position of cardiac mass
  - *Dextrocardia* – right-sided cardiac mass
- Connections between atria or ventricles and direction of flow (e.g. ASD, VSD). *Restrictive* means small; *non-restrictive* means large
- Description of valves and valve sizes in comparison to normal values using the *z* score (describes standard deviation from the mean)
- Measurement of velocity of gradients between chambers using Doppler flow, which may be converted to pressure using the formula:

$$P = 4\,v^2$$

where P = pressure (mmHg) and v = velocity (m s^{-1}).

A small amount of tricuspid regurgitation (TR) is usual, and the velocity of the regurgitant jet can be used to estimate the pressure difference between the right atrium and right ventricle. This is useful in pulmonary hypertension to estimate the pressure in the right ventricle, hence the pulmonary artery pressure. A TR jet of >4 m s^{-1} indicates severe pulmonary hypertension.

Examination

This should determine whether there are signs of cardiac failure, which include:

- Failure to thrive
- Feeding difficulties
- Tachypnoea
- Sweaty episodes
- Tachycardia
- Enlarged liver
- Recurrent chest infections

Children in significant failure will be receiving diuretics, and occasionally an ACE-inhibitor. These should not be stopped prior to surgery. If cardiac failure is poorly controlled it may be necessary to increase anti-failure medication before undertaking surgery. This should be done in conjunction with the cardiology service.

Intercurrent respiratory tract infection

Chest infection in the child with heart disease should be considered a contraindication to routine surgery, as the risks of haemodynamically destabilising hypoxaemia or changes in PVR during the peri-operative period are increased.

Many children with excessive pulmonary blood flow, as in left to right shunts, are susceptible to recurrent chest infections. It is not always clear whether abnormal chest signs are due to failure or to chest infection, and it can sometimes be difficult to decide whether to proceed in such patients. A raised temperature or rise in infective blood markers should be considered contraindications to non-urgent surgery.

Cyanosis

Many children with CHD may be functioning well at home with oxygen saturations in the 70–80s. Most of these will be dependent upon a Blalock–Taussig (BTS) or Glenn shunt (see below). There will usually be a compensatory polycythaemia and a coagulopathy. Many patients will be on antiplatelet drugs or warfarin. The haematocrit should not be allowed to fall too low in these patients, and blood transfusion should be started early if there is significant blood loss. We would aim to keep the Hb greater than

$11-12\,\mathrm{g\,dl}^{-1}$. The aim during anaesthesia is to maintain the oxygen saturation that the child is used to. Indeed, in children with a fixed intracardiac shunt it will not be possible to achieve 'normal' oxygen saturations, although oxygen saturations may rise slightly with higher inspired oxygen and a fall in PVR. End-tidal CO_2 is inaccurate in cyanosed patients, often reading 2 kPa less than arterial CO_2, but may provide a useful trend of ventilatory adequacy.

Laboratory investigations

Those that are of most use are:

- Haematocrit, which may be high if the patient is very cyanosed;
- Clotting studies, if the patient is taking anticoagulants or is very cyanosed;
- Urea and electrolytes, if the patient is receiving diuretics;
- Liver function tests, if there are signs of cardiac failure;
- Infective markers, if there are signs of respiratory tract infection.

Antibiotic prophylaxis for infective endocarditis

Guidance has changed recently, and the routine administration of antibiotics is no longer recommended for patients with heart lesions, even for those children undergoing dental procedures. Antibiotic prophylaxis is now recommended only for susceptible patients (see Table 33.3) undergoing gastrointestinal or genito-urinary procedures at a site with suspected infection. The organisms most likely to cause endocarditis are *Staphylococcus aureus*, streptococci and enterococci. Local protocols will dictate the choice of antibiotics to cover these organisms.

Anaesthesia technique

Once the underlying condition has been elucidated, a careful anaesthetic regimen can be devised. Often, the usual anaesthetic technique for the particular procedure will be used provided due consideration is given to those lesions in which it is important not to disturb a balanced circulation. Most anaesthetic drugs will reduce systemic vascular resistance, myocardial contractility, heart rate and rhythm, all of which can lead to haemodynamic

Table 33.3 Infective endocarditis prophylaxis

Patients with the following conditions are at risk for infective endocarditis:
- Acquired valve disease with stenosis or regurgitation
- Valve replacement
- Previous infective endocarditis
- Hypertrophic cardiomyopathy
- Structural congenital heart disease

  o including surgically corrected or palliated structural conditions

Patients with the following are not at risk:
- Isolated atrial septal defect
- Fully repaired ventricular septal defect
- Fully repaired patent ductus arteriosus
- Endothelialised closure devices

instability. No single induction agent is ideal for all children with CHD and effects are dose-dependent. Prolonged spontaneous ventilation with high-dose volatile agent is potentially hazardous for many children with CHD; a balanced technique with controlled ventilation and the administration of an opioid to reduce the dose of volatile agent is usually more appropriate. The use of regional analgesia should be considered carefully in patients taking anticoagulants.

Propofol

Both bolus administration and infusion of propofol can cause significant decreases in SVR and myocardial contractility. It is widely used in children with CHD but is best avoided in patients with impaired myocardial function, pulmonary hypertension and those in whom a fall in SVR will increase a right to left shunt.

Ketamine

Ketamine is a useful agent for patients who have poor cardiac reserve as heart rate, blood pressure, cardiac output and SVR are maintained by sympathetic stimulation. This effect is lost in the catecholamine-depleted patient such as a child with severe cardiomyopathy, in whom ketamine must be titrated carefully to minimise its underlying negative inotropic effect. Ketamine can be used in children with severe pulmonary hypertension.

Volatile agents

Volatile agents are associated with a dose-dependent decrease in SVR (and probably PVR) and myocardial contractility, and have variable effects on heart rate and rhythm. The newer volatile agents sevoflurane, isoflurane and desflurane have less effect on SVR than halothane and are all routinely used to maintain anaesthesia as part of a balanced anaesthetic technique, although high concentrations should be avoided. Sevoflurane is widely used as an induction agent.

Opioids

Fentanyl, remifentanil and sufentanil have minimal effects on either systemic or pulmonary vascular resistance. They can attenuate the pulmonary hypertensive response to noxious stimuli and are useful for patients at risk of pulmonary hypertensive crisis. Opioids very effectively block the stress response, so they should be used with great caution in children in severe cardiac failure whose cardiac output is maintained by sympathetic stimulation.

Benzodiazepines

Midazolam has minimal effects on CO, HR or vascular resistances and can be used in small doses in combination with other induction agents to reduce the total dose of induction agent required. It is also useful for its anxiolytic and amnesic effects.

Some specific cardiac conditions
Left-to-right shunt (ASD, VSD, AVSD, PDA)

These patients may be in significant cardiac failure, and may have disordered electrolytes owing to diuretic therapy. They may need higher inspired oxygen concentrations and increased ventilator pressures owing to interstitial oedema and poor pulmonary compliance, but care must be taken not to cause a significant fall in PVR as this may increase the shunt.

Some patients in severe failure from a large VSD or AVSD in whom early corrective surgery is not possible may undergo pulmonary artery banding to reduce pulmonary blood flow. Oxygen saturation in these patients may be 80–90%. As there is a physical restriction to pulmonary blood flow there is usually little detrimental effect from a fall in PVR.

Children with a long-standing left-to-right shunt are at risk of pulmonary hypertension.

Tetralogy of Fallot

This is the most common cyanotic cardiac defect and is often associated with non-cardiac defects. In the classic ToF (Figure 31.2) there is:

- A VSD;
- An over-riding aorta (the aorta sits over the VSD and receives blood from both ventricles);
- Right ventricular outflow tract obstruction (RVOTO), usually a narrowed pulmonary valve annulus and thickened RV muscle bundles in the infundibulum below this;
- Right ventricular hypertrophy.

Patients will usually be cyanosed because of a right-to-left shunt of blood from right ventricle to aorta.

However, there is a wide spectrum of severity in this lesion. The RVOTO can be trivial so that the patient has little more than a VSD (the 'pink Fallot'), or can be very extensive with severe narrowing extending from the mid-cavity of the right ventricle through a very stenotic pulmonary valve to small main and branch pulmonary arteries. These patients may be very cyanosed. Where there are very thickened muscle bundles in the RVOTO, patients may have a history of hypercyanotic 'spells', probably due to infundibular muscle spasm. Some of these patients will have been started on propranolol to try to reduce the dynamic element of this muscular obstruction. These patients are prone to profound desaturation if SVR is reduced during induction of anaesthesia, as right ventricular output will preferentially enter the aorta. Pulse oximetry and ECG should be in place prior to induction, and it is essential that there is a clear action plan should desaturation occur. This will generally involve attempting to increase SVR and reduce PVR by:

- Increased oxygen administration;
- Giving a fluid bolus, 10–$20\,\mathrm{ml\,kg^{-1}}$;
- Physical measures to increase SVR, such as:
  - compressing the thighs of an infant
  - bringing the knees up to the chest;
- Administering a vasoconstrictor, such as noradrenaline or phenylephrine (0.5–$2\,\mathrm{mcg\,kg^{-1}}$).

Some authorities advocate a bolus of propranolol (10–$50\,\mathrm{mcg\,kg^{-1}}$) although our experience is that a vasoconstrictor is more effective during a spell.

Many infants with ToF who have frequent hyper-cyanotic spells and in whom early corrective cardiac surgery is not feasible will have a BTS. These patients are unlikely to spell during anaesthesia.

Repaired ToF

Some infants with repaired ToF will have a degree of pulmonary valve incompetence, while others may continue to have some right ventricular outflow tract obstruction and poor right ventricular compliance. These patients will generally need higher than normal central venous pressures to maintain cardiac output, and they do not tolerate hypovolaemia well.

Left ventricular outflow tract obstruction

LVOTO includes aortic stenosis at subvalvar, valvar and supravalvar levels, narrowing of the aortic arch and coarctation. These patients can be deceptively difficult, particularly those with aortic valvar stenosis which can be difficult to treat completely; many patients have residual stenosis after repair. The additional work that the left ventricle has to do leads to left ventricular hypertrophy, with increased myocardial oxygen demand, the degree of which depends on the gradient across the valve and how long the stenosis has been present. It is important to avoid a further increase in left ventricular afterload or tachycardia, so good peri-operative analgesia is important. Equally importantly, a fall in SVR will decrease coronary artery perfusion leading to myocardial ischaemia in the hypertrophied myocardium. High-dose volatile agents should be avoided. Patients with a gradient across the aortic valve greater than about 40 mmHg are at high risk of cardiac arrest during anaesthesia, and should only be managed in specialist centres. Cardiological input and an echocardiogram to assess the degree of obstruction and ventricular performance are essential prerequisites to anaesthesia.

Blalock–Taussig shunt

Some newborns with severe cyanosis due to inadequate pulmonary blood flow, such as those with pulmonary or tricuspid atresia or severe ToF, need an augmented blood supply to the lungs in early infancy. The high PVR in the newborn means that this needs to be supplied from the systemic circulation. This is most commonly a modified Blalock–Taussig shunt (mBTS) using a GoreTex™ tube from the subclavian artery to the pulmonary artery, but

on occasion may be a central shunt from the aorta (see Figure 31.1). It is important to maintain an adequate blood pressure to ensure blood flow through the shunt, and on occasion inotropic support may be necessary. These patients are acutely sensitive to hypovolaemia or hypotension, which can result in reduced pulmonary blood flow and profound hypoxaemia.

As with the duct-dependent circulation, high inspired oxygen or hyperventilation during anaesthesia may lower PVR, causing excessive blood flow through the shunt to the lungs at the expense of reduced systemic flow, causing low cardiac output.

These patients will usually be taking some form of anticoagulation, commonly aspirin, to prevent the shunt blocking and this should not be stopped before surgery. For major surgery it may be necessary to administer platelets. Patients commonly have oxygen saturations in the 70–80% range, and may be polycythaemic. Prolonged pre-operative starvation should be avoided as dehydration may cause shunt thrombosis. Sudden profound cyanosis during the perioperative period should be attributed to shunt occlusion until proven otherwise.

Glenn shunt

Many infants with a mBTS will proceed to full surgical repair of their CHD when they are bigger. For those in whom corrective surgery is not possible, PVR will usually have fallen sufficiently after the first few months of life to allow systemic venous augmentation of the pulmonary circulation. This is achieved with a Glenn (cavo-pulmonary) shunt, involving anastomosis of the SVC to the right pulmonary artery (Figure 31.3). As blood will perfuse both lungs this is often referred to as a bidirectional Glenn (BDG). The mBTS is taken down at this time.

These patients remain cyanosed with oxygen saturations generally in the 80s. It is important to recognise that pressure measured in the internal jugular vein reflects pulmonary perfusion pressure. This 'venous pressure' has to be maintained higher than normal, often 12–15 mmHg, to ensure an adequate driving pressure of blood across the lungs. Patients do not tolerate hypovolaemia, and increases in intrathoracic pressure may impede pulmonary blood flow. Patients benefit from being in a slightly head-up position and the Trendelenburg position is best avoided.

Total cavo-pulmonary connection (TCPC, Fontan circulation)

This is the final stage of the creation of the single ventricle circulation. In addition to the BDG, the IVC is connected to the pulmonary artery using an intra-cardiac or extracardiac GoreTex tube (Figure 31.4). The single ventricle thus supplies systemic blood flow, while the entire pulmonary blood flow is essentially passive, and dependent on systemic venous pressure and low PVR. These patients do not tolerate hypovolaemia or dysrhythmias. Oxygen saturations should be in the mid-90s after successful TCPC.

Anything that elevates PVR will impede pulmonary blood flow and, by reducing systemic atrial and ventricular filling, may lead to low cardiac output. Spontaneous ventilation is generally better for short, simple procedures. Positive pressure ventilation can reduce pulmonary blood flow but can be used for major surgery provided airway pressure is kept low and hypovolaemia is avoided. Surgical procedures that increase intrathoracic or intra-abdominal pressure, such as laparascopic procedures, may be poorly tolerated so invasive pressure monitoring should be used. There should be a clear understanding between anaesthetist and surgeon that it may be necessary to convert to an open procedure.

The poorly functioning Fontan

In the patient with a poorly functioning Fontan circulation, for example due to high PVR and/or a failing ventricle, it will be necessary to maintain a very high systemic venous pressure to obtain pulmonary perfusion and oxygenation and to fill the systemic ventricle to maintain adequate cardiac output. This high venous pressure can lead to persistent pleural effusions, ascites, renal dysfunction and protein-losing enteropathy. There may be low cardiac output in addition to the high venous pressure. In the borderline patient the surgeon may have 'fenestrated' the TCPC, i.e. created a small hole between the GoreTex tube and the systemic atrium (see Figure 31.4). In the event of high systemic venous pressure, blood will shunt through this fenestration to the systemic atrium. This can improve preload and cardiac output, but as this is desaturated blood, it will be at the expense of lower oxygen saturations. It is essential in patients with a fenestration to be meticulous about avoiding

air in intravenous infusions and when giving drugs to prevent paradoxical air embolism.

These patients can be very challenging, as they usually have poor ventricular function, low cardiac output, acidosis and hypoxaemia. Induction of anaesthesia and the institution of positive pressure ventilation can lead to rapid deterioration and arrest. They should only be managed in specialist centres.

Hypoplastic left heart syndrome

The improved results from the Norwood procedure mean that many more children with HLHS are surviving into childhood, and may need anaesthesia for non-cardiac surgery. For example, neonates may present with necrotising enterocolitis after their first stage repair.

In HLHS there is in essence a small, ineffective left ventricle, usually with a very small aorta. At birth these infants are dependent on a PDA to provide systemic perfusion via the pulmonary artery. The Norwood procedure, undertaken in the first few days after birth, utilises the right ventricle as the systemic ventricle; the main pulmonary artery is used to augment the aorta, creating a neo-aorta. The pulmonary arteries are disconnected from the main pulmonary artery, and are perfused by a mBTS (see Figure 33.2), or in the Sano modification by a conduit from the ventricle.

After this first stage operation, the patients remain in a very delicate 'balanced shunt' situation, as both systemic and pulmonary blood flow are supplied by the single right ventricle. Balancing the resistances of the systemic and pulmonary circulations is crucial to maintain adequate systemic and pulmonary blood flow. As with the duct-dependent circulation, high inspired oxygen and hyperventilation must be avoided as these will increase pulmonary perfusion and reduce systemic output. Oxygen saturations are best maintained around 70–80%. Maintaining patency of the mBTS is also crucial, and these patients will be anticoagulated, usually with anti-platelet drugs such as aspirin. Dehydration is very poorly tolerated, and intravenous fluids should be administered if minimal starvation time cannot be ensured. There is a high risk of sudden death in these patients.

The second stage of management of HLHS is the establishment of a BDG at around the age of 4 months. TCPC is the third stage, usually undertaken

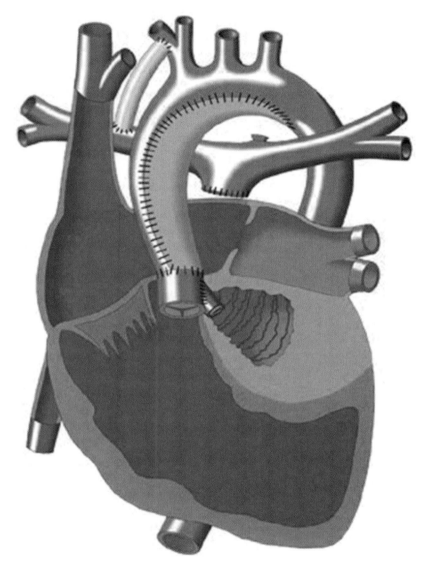

Figure 33.2 Norwood first stage repair of HLHS. The main pulmonary artery has been used to create a neo-aorta. A modified Blalock–Taussig shunt provides pulmonary blood flow. From the PedHeart Resource (www.HeartPassport. com). Courtesy of Scientific Software Solutions, Inc. See plate section for colour version.

at 1–3 years. It is important to be aware that after completing the TCPC, the HLHS patient is left with a morphological right ventricle as the systemic ventricle, and this is prone to medium-term failure. In contrast, children with a single ventricle circulation due to a right-sided lesion have a morphological left ventricle and may cope well into adulthood.

Pulmonary hypertension

Pulmonary hypertension (PH) is usually defined as a mean pulmonary artery pressure at rest of 25 mmHg or more. Over 50% are idiopathic. PH may be secondary to congenital heart disease, chronic lung disease and rarer causes such as sickle cell disease or thromboembolic disease. The risk of peri-operative cardiac arrest and mortality is substantially increased in these patients but it is difficult to put a sensible figure on this, as there is a wide spectrum of severity of PH. Patients at highest risk are those in whom pulmonary artery pressure is equal to or greater than systemic pressure, and those in whom there is a dilated right ventricle compressing the left side. For these patients the risk of peri-operative cardiac arrest may be 5% or more. Children with PH should be transferred to specialist centres for both elective and emergency surgery.

The key principle of anaesthesia for these children is to avoid a rise in PVR which may precipitate acute right ventricular failure. Hypoxia, acidosis, increased $PaCO_2$ or increased sympathetic activity secondary to inadequate level of anaesthesia must all be scrupulously avoided. Meticulous attention to the airway and ventilation is as important during emergence and recovery as during induction. A fall in SVR or hypovolaemia following induction must also be avoided as these may lead to impaired coronary perfusion, myocardial ischaemia and biventricular failure. Inhaled nitric oxide should be available for these patients.

Cardiomyopathy

Cardiomyopathy (CM) is rare, but presents a severe challenge for the anaesthetist. It is not always symptomatic, and is a major cause of sudden, unexpected death in children. Wherever possible these patients should be managed in a specialist centre. There are several forms:

- Dilated (DCM), approx. 60%
- Hypertrophic (HOCM), approx. 25%
- Ventricular non-compaction, 9%
- Restrictive (RCM), 2%
- Arrhythmogenic right ventricular (ARVC), approx. 4%

DCM: there is decreased systolic and diastolic ventricular function and ventricular dilation which can lead to mitral regurgitation. Cardiac output may be very poor, and inotropic support, commonly milrinone, may be necessary pre-operatively. Coronary perfusion depends on maintaining adequate filling and diastolic pressure, but it is important not to increase SVR or heart rate as the myocardium may not tolerate an increased workload. All anaesthetics decrease myocardial contractility; etomidate may be the safest induction agent. Ketamine is an alternative, but is dependent upon sympathomimetic stimulation to maintain cardiac output. As the myocardium may be catecholamine depleted in DCM (and in other causes of heart failure), there may be a fall in output with this agent.

HOCM: there is usually severe ventricular muscle thickening causing dynamic LVOTO. Increased myocardial contractility and tachycardia should be avoided,

so adequate anaesthesia and analgesia are important. There is diastolic dysfunction and impaired left ventricular filling. It is important to maintain preload and afterload. A fall in SVR must be avoided as it can rapidly lead to myocardial ischaemia; it may be necessary to administer a small bolus of phenylephrine, $0.5-1 \text{ mcg kg}^{-1}$. Propofol should be avoided.

RCM: this is rare. Cardiac output is very dependent upon maintaining heart rate and adequate filling. Pulmonary hypertension is often present.

Life-threatening dysrhythmias are a risk in all forms of CM and appropriate precautions should be in place.

Hereditary arrhythmogenic syndromes

These comprise a heterogeneous group of myocardial ion channel disorders, sometimes referred to as cardiac channelopathies, and are also a cause of sudden, unexpected death in children. They predispose patients to life-threatening peri-operative arrhythmias and include:

- Long QT syndrome (LQTS)
- Brugada syndrome
- Congenital sick sinus syndrome (SSS)
- Arrhythmogenic right ventricular cardiomyopathy (ARVC)
- Catecholaminergic polymorphic ventricular tachycardia (CPVT)

LQTS: LQTS is a generic term describing a group of disorders in which there is a prolonged QT interval, which predisposes to polymorphic ventricular tachycardia and cardiac arrest. There are a number of different genotypes, associated with different ion channel dysfunction and management; LQTS can also be an acquired problem.

The QT interval is measured from the start of the QRS complex to the completion of the T wave, measured in leads II, V5 and V6. It varies with heart rate so is often expressed as corrected QT:

$$QTc\,(\text{msec}) = \frac{QT\,(\text{msec})}{\sqrt{RR}(\text{sec})}$$

where RR is the interval (in seconds) between two R waves on the ECG. Normal QTc is ≤ 420 msec.

Several commonly used peri-operative drugs can prolong the QTc and should be avoided, such as ondansetron, droperidol, ketamine, suxamethonium and most adrenergic agents. Inhalational agents may prolong the QTc but there is conflicting advice about their safety. Pre-operative correction of electrolytes, good analgesia, maintenance of normal haemodynamic and ventilatory parameters and normothermia are mainstays of management. Peri-operative infusion of magnesium sulfate 30 mg kg^{-1} is advocated.

Peri-operative management of patients with channelopathies can be challenging and is described in detail in the review article by Staikou *et al.* in Further reading.

Management of the patient with a heart transplant

Survival following heart transplantation has improved markedly in the past decade, with a median survival now of 15 years.

Most heart-transplanted patients are followed up regularly and are likely to be well, but it should be noted that there is a significant incidence of early coronary disease. Most patients will be receiving a statin. In patients presenting for coincidental surgery who exhibit signs of myocardial dysfunction, such as reduced exercise tolerance, the possibility of coronary disease or acute rejection should be considered and cardiological advice sought.

The prime issue of importance to anaesthetists is that these patients have a denervated heart, commonly with a basal heart rate of around 90–100. Atropine will have no effect on heart rate. The lack of sympathetic innervation results in a blunted and delayed haemodynamic response to pain or stress, and the absence of heart rate changes cannot be used to gauge depth of anaesthesia or hypovolaemia. Patients readily become hypotensive and it is wise to administer intravenous fluids early. Patients take an array of immunosuppressive drugs, and strict aseptic techniques are essential. Renal dysfunction is a feature of many of these drugs, such as tacrolimus, and should be assessed pre-operatively. Some patients may be receiving steroid therapy.

The neonate with a cardiac lesion requiring surgery

It is not uncommon to be faced with a neonate who needs urgent general surgery but who also has a cardiac lesion. This may be for an intestinal atresia, tracheo-oesophageal fistula or necrotising enterocolitis, for example. These infants need urgent referral to a specialist centre.

Management, including determining the priority of the various interventions, will depend upon the nature of the lesions. Relatively simple cardiac defects such as ventricular or atrioventricular septal defects are not usually an impediment to urgent anaesthesia, provided cardiac failure is managed appropriately. A child with a complex cardiac anomaly such as TGA may be stable while receiving prostaglandin, so an urgent general procedure can take precedence. Conversely, a severely cyanosed infant with tricuspid atresia or ToF may need an urgent systemic-to-pulmonary artery shunt before any other surgery can take place. Comprehensive echocardiographic investigation, expert cardiological input and multi-disciplinary discussion is essential.

It is important to remember that the neonatal myocardium has reduced contractility and a reduced ability to relax, so they tolerate poorly an increase in afterload and a decrease in preload. Maintaining a normal serum calcium is very important in these patients. The ventricles are very interdependent so failure of one ventricle quickly leads to failure of both. The poor response to volume loading means they are very dependent on heart rate. Parasympathetic innervation of the heart is better developed in neonates than sympathetic innervation, so vagal responses and bradycardia can occur with ease. Atropine should be available at all times.

Heterotaxy syndromes

Heterotaxy refers to an abnormal right–left arrangement of the thoracoabdominal organs. Complex cardiovascular malformations are frequently present, and there may be defects of other organs, such as intestinal malrotation, biliary atresia, splenic, skeletal and urinary tract abnormalities. Paired organs, such as the lungs and kidneys, are often mirror images of each other.

In *right atrial isomerism,* the left atrium is a mirror image of the right, the left lung will have three lobes like the right, there may be asplenia (absent spleen), and the liver may be on the left side. Because of the asplenia patients require long-term antibiotic prophylaxis, particularly against pneumococcus.

In *left atrial isomerism,* the right atrium is a mirror image of the left. There may be an absent or abnormally sited sino-atrial node, so rhythm disturbances and heart block are common. The child may have multiple spleens (polysplenia).

Key points

- There is an increased peri-operative mortality in children with heart disease undergoing anaesthesia for non-cardiac procedures.
- Children with heart disease that is causing minimal restriction of activity can often be managed in non-specialist centres, but there are some that are particularly high risk and should always be referred to a specialist centre. These include children with:
  - Pulmonary hypertension
  - Left ventricular outflow tract obstruction
  - Single ventricle circulation
  - Cardiomyopathy.
- Avoiding changes in the balance of systemic and pulmonary vascular resistance is crucial in many children with congenital heart lesions.

Further reading

Andropoulos DB, Stayer SA, Russell IA, Mossad EB, eds. *Anesthesia for Congenital Heart Disease*, 2nd edition. Wiley-Blackwell. 2010.

Ing RJ, Ames WA, Chambers NA. Paediatric cardiomyopathy and anaesthesia. *Br J Anaes* 2012;**108**:4–12.

Staikou C, Chandrogiannis K, Mani A. Peri-operative management of hereditary arrhythmogenic syndromes. *Br J Anaes* 2012;**108**(5):730–44.

Chapter

34

Anaesthesia for urological surgery in children

Angus McEwan

Introduction

Urological surgery accounts for a large part of the paediatric anaesthetist's workload. Procedures range from minor interventions such as cystoscopy and circumcision through to major surgery such as nephrectomy and bladder reconstruction. Children presenting for urological procedures are generally well, but some may have impaired renal function or associated medical conditions such as congenital adrenal hyperplasia (CAH). This chapter will describe anaesthetic management of minor and major urological surgery.

Minor procedures

Common minor procedures include:

- Cystoscopy
- Resection of posterior urethral valves
- Circumcision
- Insertion of suprapubic catheter
- Hypospadias repair
- Orchidopexy

In general these children are well, with the exception of neonates presenting for resection of posterior urethral valves where severe urethral obstruction *in utero* may lead to renal impairment. All children require routine pre-operative evaluation including urine culture if there is a possibility of urinary tract infection. Children presenting for repeat surgery may be particularly anxious, and may require support from a play specialist and/or sedative premedication. Topical local anaesthetic cream is routine for those having intravenous induction.

Cystoscopy

Indications for cystoscopy vary from investigation of minor renal tract abnormalities to follow-up after major reconstructive or tumour surgery.

Airway management for these cases is usually with spontaneous respiration with a laryngeal mask airway (LMA) or facemask, except in the neonatal period when intubation and ventilation is more appropriate (see below). Cystoscopy can be surprisingly stimulating. This may result in hyperventilation, tachycardia or laryngospasm unless adequate analgesia and depth of anaesthesia is provided. Without adequate analgesia the child may be very uncomfortable in the immediate post-operative period. Intravenous opioid, either fentanyl $1–2 \, \text{mcg kg}^{-1}$ or morphine $50–100 \, \text{mcg kg}^{-1}$, is useful both to improve intra-operative conditions and to provide good post-operative pain relief, but should be given several minutes before the start of the procedure to provide adequate analgesia before surgery commences. Alternatively, caudal analgesia may be indicated, particularly if the child is to have a urinary catheter after surgery. Antibiotics such as an aminoglycoside (gentamicin, amikacin), cephalosporin or co-amoxiclav should be given according to local antibiotic protocols, as instrumentation of the renal tract in the presence of urinary infection is an important cause of post-operative sepsis.

Post-operative analgesia should be provided with paracetamol $15 \, \text{mg kg}^{-1}$ PO 6 hourly, ibuprofen $5 \, \text{mg kg}^{-1}$ PO 6 hourly and morphine $200 \, \text{mcg kg}^{-1}$ PO if required.

Resection of posterior urethral valves

Posterior urethral valves (PUVs) are associated with an abnormal fold of tissue in the male urethra that

Core Topics in Paediatric Anaesthesia, ed. Ian James and Isabeau Walker. Published by Cambridge University Press. © 2013 Cambridge University Press.

leads to obstruction of urine flow. The severity of the obstruction varies widely. In the most severe cases, obstructive uropathy leads to renal impairment *in utero* with oligohydramnios and pulmonary hypoplasia. This presents with respiratory distress and renal failure in the neonatal period, which may not be compatible with life. More commonly, bilateral hydronephrosis is diagnosed using antenatal ultrasound, but renal function is not severely impaired. Delayed presentation may be with sepsis due to urinary infection, incontinence or renal impairment due to chronic obstruction. These boys typically have a high-pressure small capacity bladder with vesicoureteric reflux and may occasionally require bladder augmentation in later life to preserve renal function. The effects of PUVs on the renal tract are life-long; one-third of boys progress to end-stage renal failure, and 10–15% of children undergoing renal transplantation have a diagnosis of PUVs.

Cystoscopy is diagnostic and allows transurethral resection of PUVs. This is the mainstay of surgical treatment, ideally performed in the few days of life, with follow-up cystoscopy 1–2 months later. Preoperative assessment of renal function is important. Creatinine and electrolytes will reflect the mother's renal function in the first 24 hours; serial assessments should be performed over several days to assess the true renal function of the neonate. Children require long-term monitoring of renal function, the results of which should be known prior to subsequent interventions.

In infants <5 kg undergoing resection of PUVs, tracheal intubation with intermittent positive pressure ventilation (IPPV) is generally utilised. Larger infants can be managed with an LMA and spontaneous ventilation. The patient is positioned in a modified lithotomy position at the far end of the operating table; long ventilator tubing may be required. This position can make warming awkward, but this is important as the patients are often small. Resection of PUV is a painful procedure, and caudal block provides excellent analgesia. The addition of clonidine 1 mcg kg^{-1} to the caudal solution improves the quality and duration of the analgesia, but should be avoided in neonates owing to concerns about sedation and respiratory depression. Alternatively, intravenous opioids can be used. Prophylactic antibiotics should be given.

Post-operative pain relief is provided with oral paracetamol. Careful post-operative fluid management is required if large volumes of urine are produced after relief of the obstruction.

Circumcision

Medical indications for circumcision include phimosis, paraphimosis, balanitis and recurrent urinary infection, and boys who require intermittent catheterisation to prevent urinary infection. Circumcision may be performed on neonates, infants or older children, usually as a day-case procedure.

Spontaneous ventilation with LMA or facemask is appropriate. However, in small infants tracheal intubation with IPPV may be preferable. Analgesia is provided with a caudal block, penile block or penile ring block.

Post-operative analgesia is provided with simple analgesics: paracetamol, NSAIDs if renal function is normal, with the addition of oral morphine if required. Parents should be encouraged to give regular analgesia at home post-operatively.

Hypospadias repair

Hypospadias occurs in 1:250 boys. It most commonly occurs in isolation without other congenital anomalies, and renal function is not impaired. Hypospadias refers to malposition of the urethral meatus. Instead of opening at the tip of the penis the external urethral opening is proximal to the urethral tip on the ventral surface of the penis. Hypospadias varies from very mild to very severe when the urethral opening is in the scrotum. Between 15 and 50% of patients have an associated curvature of the penis known as chordee. A number of different operations have been described to repair the defect. Repair may be undertaken as a single-stage or two-stage procedure, using preputial mucosa to form a graft for the reconstructed urethra in the two-stage operation. Occasionally additional tissue is required in order to repair larger defects. Graft tissue may be taken from the buccal mucosa or from behind the ear (posterior auricular graft).

Anaesthesia is usually with LMA and spontaneous ventilation. If buccal mucosa is required for a urethral graft, intubation is usually employed with controlled ventilation. Nasal intubation is most convenient for the surgeon, but oral intubation with a RAE tube positioned to one side of the mouth is also acceptable. A throat pack is advisable as there may be some bleeding into the mouth. Local anaesthetic with adrenaline is injected before a posterior auricular graft is taken to reduce bleeding and to provide post-operative analgesia. A caudal block provides excellent analgesia for hypospadias surgery, and the addition of clonidine extends its duration. Prophylactic antibiotics should be given.

Post-operative analgesia should be provided with paracetamol, NSAIDs and oral morphine. Children who have a urinary catheter post-operatively may suffer from painful 'bladder spasm' due to irritation of the trigone muscle. Oral oxybutynin 1.25–2.5 mg PO 8–12 hourly may be helpful in this situation and should be continued whilst the catheter is *in situ*. Minor hypospadias can be managed on a day-stay basis. Most children undergoing more complex procedures can be discharged from hospital the day after surgery, but may need to return the following week for dressing change under anaesthesia.

Orchidopexy

Orchidopexy is performed for cryptorchidism, or undescended testes, which is the most common genital abnormality in boys. Normal descent of the testes into the scrotum occurs at 28–40 weeks gestation; maldescent is seen in 30% of premature infants, 3% of term babies and 1% of boys aged 6 months to 1 year. Spontaneous descent is uncommon after 1 year of age. Occasionally a short course of hormonal treatment with human chorionic gonadotropin (hCG) is used to facilitate descent of the testis into the scrotum. Corrective surgery is usually performed in children aged 6 months to 2 years. The testis may be felt in the superficial inguinal pouch or inguinal canal in 80% of cases, or it may be non-palpable if the testis is in the abdominal cavity. Occasionally the testis is absent, probably owing to perinatal torsion. There is an increased incidence of testicular cancer in patients with undescended testis (mainly involving intra-abdominal testis). Orchidopexy is performed to facilitate self-examination, to improve fertility, to reduce the risk of trauma or torsion, to treat an associated hernia (seen in 90% of cases) and for psychological reasons.

The aim of the operation is to secure the testis in the scrotum. For testes that are palpable in the inguinal canal and can be brought down without tension, an open procedure involving an inguinal incision and small scrotal incisions may be performed. If the testis is not palpable, a diagnostic laparoscopy is performed. This may identify blind-ending spermatic vessels due to an earlier torsion, with or without a nubbin of testicular tissue remaining. Abnormal or atrophic testicular tissue is removed via the laparoscope to reduce the risk of later malignancy. Many surgeons perform contralateral fixation if earlier torsion is suspected. Alternatively, the testis may be intra-abdominal, or cord structures may be seen entering the inguinal ring, in which case the surgeon will explore and proceed to orchidopexy if the testis is normal.

Orchidopexy for intra-abdominal testis is performed as a single-stage procedure if the cord structures can be brought down into the scrotum without tension, or the Fowler Stephens operation may be performed. This involves division of the testicular vessels, so that the blood supply to the testis is via the vas deferens. Second-stage laparoscopic fixation is performed 6–9 months later, after the collateral blood supply to the testis from the vas deferens is fully developed.

Simple orchidopexy is performed with spontaneous ventilation using an LMA. In unilateral surgery in infants an ileo-inguinal local anaesthetic block may be used. This does not block the pain from the small scrotal incision but in practice this does not appear to be a problem. For bilateral orchidopexy or orchidopexy in older boys, a caudal block is more appropriate.

For laparoscopic techniques, tracheal intubation and controlled ventilation is required. Caudal analgesia may be used. Post-operative analgesia is provided by paracetamol and NSAIDs with the addition of oral morphine if required. Orchidopexy is usually performed as a day case in young children under 2 years; older boys may have more severe post-operative pain and nausea and vomiting, and may benefit from overnight stay.

Major urological procedures

Common procedures include:

- Pyeloplasty
- Nephrectomy
- Ureteric reimplantation
- Resection of nephroblastoma (Wilms' nephrectomy)

Less common procedures include:

- Surgery for repair of bladder exstrophy

- Bladder augmentation and formation of Mitrofanoff
- Renal transplantation

Pyeloplasty

Pyeloplasty is performed to relieve hydronephrosis due to pelviureteric junction (PUJ) obstruction. The abnormality is usually unilateral. Renal function on the affected side may be compromised, but the contralateral kidney is often not affected and overall function is usually adequate. Until recently the majority of these procedures were performed open. Many are now performed laparoscopically via the retroperitoneal space, which allows better access to the PUJ obstruction, although the procedure is technically more difficult.

Nephrectomy

A nephrectomy or heminephrectomy is performed either for severe hydronephrosis or to remove a small non-functioning kidney or the part of the kidney that is non-functioning. An increasing number of these operations are also being performed laparoscopically.

Anaesthesia for pyeloplasty and nephrectomy involves tracheal intubation with controlled ventilation. Bleeding is seldom a problem with pyeloplasty or nephrectomy, but is more common with heminephrectomy.

A suggested protocol for ordering blood is:

- Pyeloplasty: No crossmatch
- Nephrectomy: Group and save
- Heminephrectomy: Crossmatch required

There are a number of different options with respect to intra-operative and post-operative analgesia for open procedures. Some advocate an opioid technique using morphine or fentanyl intra-operatively. This is combined with local anaesthetic infiltration and simple analgesics followed by nurse-controlled analgesia (NCA) or patient-controlled analgesia (PCA) with morphine post-operatively, or, for infants in whom a small non-functioning kidney is removed, oral morphine. Others advocate the use of an epidural technique with either a single-shot epidural followed by either NCA or PCA with morphine, or a continuous epidural. Either of these techniques is effective. Invasive monitoring is not required.

If the procedure is undertaken laparoscopically, field blocks or local infiltration in combination with intra-operative opioids can be used. Post-operatively the child requires simple analgesics in combination with morphine NCA or PCA.

Ureteric reimplantation

Vesicoureteric reflux occurs when urine passes retrogradely from the bladder to the ureter. Reflux may be due to an anatomical abnormality, for instance an abnormality of the distal ureteral orifice where it enters the bladder, or due to distal obstruction, for instance because of PUVs. Reflux may be asymptomatic, or it may lead to recurrent urinary infections, pyelonephritis and renal scarring, which in turn may lead to hypertension or renal failure.

Medical treatment includes prophylactic antibiotics to prevent urinary infections, and prompt treatment of proven infections to reduce renal scarring. Ureteric reimplantation is performed in children who have frequent breakthrough infections, in those with severe reflux leading to renal scarring, or in older girls with milder reflux that persists on long-term follow-up. Reimplantation as an isolated procedure involves a lower abdominal transverse incision with the patient supine; in children with PUVs major reconstruction may be required (see below).

Anaesthesia is with tracheal intubation and controlled ventilation. Bleeding is seldom a problem although blood should be grouped and saved. Prophylactic antibiotics are given. Invasive monitoring is not required. Intra-operative and post-operative analgesia is ideally provided with a continuous lumbar epidural. Alternatively, intra-operative opioids followed by local infiltration, morphine PCA or NCA, and paracetamol can be used. If renal function is compromised, NSAIDs should be avoided.

Wilms' tumour (nephroblastoma)

Wilms' tumour is the most common primary malignant renal tumour in children, and accounts for more than 50% of abdominal tumours and 6–7% of all childhood malignancies. Long-term survival of >90% is expected with current treatment regimens, although intensive chemotherapy and radiotherapy for high-risk patients may be associated with significant long-term side effects such as cardiotoxicity, scoliosis, infertility and secondary malignancy.

Nephroblastoma usually presents as a palpable mass in children around 3–5 years of age, but 5–10% may present with bilateral disease or multifocal disease in a single kidney. Wilms' tumour is familial in 1–2% of patients. Children are usually relatively asymptomatic and often present late with fevers, weight loss and a large mass. They may present with abdominal pain or haematuria if the tumour bleeds or extends into the renal pelvis or ureter. Extension of tumour into the inferior vena cava (IVC) is seen in 4% of cases and may be associated with cardiac failure, hepatomegaly, ascites or varicocoele. Metastatic spread is to the lungs and bone marrow. Paraneoplastic syndromes may result in hypertension, hypercalcaemia or acquired von Willebrand's disease. Hypertension is usually due to renal ischaemia mediated via the renin–angiotensin system. Catecholamine levels are usually normal as are levels of homovanillic acid (HVA) and vanillylmandelic acid (VMA). Wilms' tumour may be associated with a number of congenital syndromes including:

- Aniridia (congenital absence of the iris, 1% of patients)
- Danys Drash syndrome (hypospadias, undescended testes and Wilms' tumour)
- Beckwith–Wiedemann syndrome with hemihypertrophy (10% of patients)
- Neurofibromatosis

Initial staging requires ultrasound, CT and MRI scans, tumour biopsy and bone marrow aspirate to determine tumour histology and spread. Treatment consists of 6–12 weeks of chemotherapy to reduce the size and vascularity of the tumour, followed by radical nephrectomy, followed by further chemotherapy +/− radiotherapy to treat residual disease. Partial nephrectomy may be considered in children with bilateral disease or where the tumour is limited to one pole of the kidney. If there is residual disease in the IVC after chemotherapy, tumour excision on cardiopulmonary bypass may be required as a joint procedure between the urologists and cardiothoracic surgeons.

Surgery is undertaken in between courses of chemotherapy, and careful pre-operative review of full blood count and clotting is required. Antihypertensive drugs should also be reviewed and continued pre-operatively. If chemotherapy has been given a Hickman line will usually be in place. This can be used for induction of anaesthesia and monitoring of the central venous pressure (CVP). It is important that a sterile technique is used to access the line and that the line is aspirated and flushed carefully to remove residual anaesthetic drugs at the end of surgery.

Wilms' nephrectomy is major surgery. It involves a large transverse abdominal incision, which may be associated with considerable post-operative pain. There is potential for haemodynamic instability due to compression or kinking of the IVC during surgical manipulation, or major haemorrhage associated with the tumour resection (particularly heminephrectomy) or bleeding from major vessels. Three adult units of blood should be cross-matched, clotting abnormalities should be corrected pre-operatively, and blood pressure controlled carefully intra-operatively.

Anaesthesia will require tracheal intubation and IPPV. Very large tumours may cause atelectasis, reduced respiratory reserve or delayed gastric emptying. Invasive monitoring is required, and if no Hickman line is present an internal jugular line should be placed (avoid the femoral route). Secure IV access in the upper limbs is required as it may be necessary to clamp the IVC. A urinary catheter is inserted. Temperature should be monitored, and a warming blanket and a fluid warmer should be used. Epidural analgesia (high lumbar or low thoracic) provides excellent intra- and post-operative analgesia. The bowel is exposed during surgery, and third space and evaporative fluid losses may be considerable, and reduced by the use of a bowel bag. Fluid balance and tissue perfusion should be monitored carefully during surgery (routine monitoring of blood gases), but post-operative ventilation is seldom required.

Bladder exstrophy and epispadias

This rare congenital abnormality affects between 1 in 20 000 and 1 in 50 000 live births. It affects boys three times more commonly than girls. This is the most common abnormality in a spectrum of rare conditions from isolated epispadias to complete exstrophy of the cloaca exposing bladder and rectum. Cryptorchidism is usual in boys.

Exstrophy arises from failure of fusion of midline structures. In cloacal exstrophy there is an associated omphalocoele and there may also be involvement of the spinal structures. Sacral agenesis is common, as is tethering of the spinal cord. Epidural anaesthesia should be avoided in cloacal exstrophy. This does not appear to be the case in simple bladder exstrophy, but it may be advisable to exclude spinal abnormalities by a spinal ultrasound if there is a sacral pit or other obvious abnormality.

Diagnosis is often made in the antenatal period by ultrasound scan; the rarity of this condition means that it is best dealt with in a small number of specialist centres, and the baby should be transferred as soon as possible after birth.

In simple bladder exstrophy the bladder is laid open on the anterior abdominal wall. There is complete epispadias and the pubic bones are widely splayed, which makes surgical closure difficult. If closure is delayed more than 48 hours the condition of the bladder deteriorates; it becomes progressively more hyperaemic and oedematous, and the risk of infection increases. Delayed closure also increases the risk of renal damage because of obstruction to urine flow in the ureters and also increases the risk of bladder carcinoma in later years.

Pre-operatively the defect should be covered with a thin plastic film to prevent fluid and heat loss and to reduce the risk of infection. Renal function should be checked and one adult unit of blood should be cross-matched.

The surgical approach to bladder exstrophy is evolving and varies from centre to centre. The aim of surgery is to close the bladder, oppose the pelvic bones, repair the epispadias and produce continence with a bladder of adequate volume. The surgical debate centres largely on the timing and extent of surgery. Some surgeons advocate radical surgery in the neonatal period with closure of the bladder, pelvic osteotomies and repair of epispadias. This takes 3–4 hours and involves major blood and fluid losses. Others advocate a more limited approach with simple bladder closure in the neonatal period, with a more radical surgery involving epispadias repair and bladder neck reconstruction at 6 months or a year. Simple bladder closure is relatively quick (approx. 2 h) and is not associated with large blood or fluid losses. Antibiotic cover is required for surgery. At the conclusion of surgery a plaster of Paris hip spica may be applied to oppose the pelvic bones. The bladder and ureters are drained with multiple catheters which should be clearly marked, and which must not be displaced. In cloacal exstrophy, neurosurgical repair takes precedence if myelomeningocoele is present. A colostomy is required to separate gastrointestinal and genito-urinary tracts, and bladder repair is performed as in classical exstrophy.

All the considerations of neonatal anaesthesia apply. Tracheal intubation and controlled ventilation are required. Good IV access is required, preferably in the upper limbs. Femoral access is avoided because of proximity to the surgical field. An internal jugular line may be necessary if adequate peripheral access is not possible. Temperature is monitored, and warming of patient and of fluids is required. Bleeding is not usually extensive but blood transfusion is likely to be needed and blood should be available.

The intra-operative and post-operative analgesia plan depends on the surgical strategy. In simple bladder closure some surgeons prefer babies to be ventilated post-operatively to reduce the incidence of wound dehiscence. If the baby is to be ventilated post-operatively the anaesthetic technique can be based on a high-dose opioid. If the baby is to be extubated at the end of surgery, intra-operative and post-operative analgesia is ideally provided by epidural analgesia. Epidural analgesia should be avoided in cloacal exstrophy because of the high incidence of spinal abnormalities, as described above.

Radical surgery includes bladder closure, epispadias repair and pelvic osteotomies. Large blood losses are common and an arterial line is required. Post-operative ventilation is usually required.

These children often require surgery later in life, mainly bladder augmentation and bladder neck reconstruction to attempt to achieve urinary continence. Children with cloacal exstrophy may have a later pull-through procedure, although it is difficult to achieve faecal continence.

Augmentation cystoplasty and Mitrofanoff

The aim of augmentation cystoplasty is to increase bladder capacity, reduce urinary infection, achieve urinary continence and reduce pressure in the upper renal tracts to preserve renal function. It is indicated in children with neuropathic bladder who do not respond to simple interventions such as intermittent catheterisation or cystoscopic injections of Botox, many children with bladder exstrophy, and occasionally in children with posterior urethral valves. A 'continent' stoma is constructed at the same operation (Mitrofanoff stoma) for life-long intermittent catheterisation. Children with a neuropathic bladder may also have severe constipation, and benefit from formation of an antegrade continence enema (ACE) stoma at the same time.

In augmentation cystoplasty, a segment of ileum is separated on its mesentery, detubularised, and anastomosed to the superior aspect of the bladder to increase the capacity of the bladder. The appendix is separated on its mesentery and anastomosed between the bladder and the abdominal wall to form the Mitrofanoff channel, with a specially constructed stoma from which urine will not leak.

Children require pre-operative bowel preparation, and are given clear fluids for 2 days pre-operatively. Renal function and plasma electrolytes should be assessed, and blood should be cross-matched. These children may have had frequent surgical interventions and may often be very anxious – premedication and access to a play specialist and/or psychologist may all be useful pre-operatively. These children are at high risk of latex allergy due to long-term intermittent catheterisation.

Anaesthesia considerations are similar to a standard laparotomy, and there may be significant adhesions and fluid shifts. Broad-spectrum antibiotics such as co-amoxiclav or benzylpenicillin, metronidazole and amikacin are required prior to incision and are continued post-operatively. Central access and blood transfusion are commonly required. Surgery usually takes 4–6 hours, and epidural analgesia is ideal, if feasible.

Intersex and genitoplasty

The topic of intersex is complex and full of controversy, and a full discussion of the subject is beyond the scope of this book. For the children and families faced with ambiguous genitalia there are difficult psychological problems and decisions. There are a number of causes of ambiguous genitalia, the most common of which is congenital adrenal hyperplasia (CAH or adrenogenital syndrome). The production of cortisol and aldosterone depends on a series of enzymatic steps regulated by hydroxylases. CAH results from a deficiency of 21-hydroxylase, which results in low levels of production of cortisol. This in turn causes the pituitary to produce large amounts of ACTH, stimulating the production of large quantities of androgenic steroids. These children may present as neonates with a salt-losing crisis. Female infants become virilised with clitoral hypertrophy and/or labial fusion and require a feminising genitoplasty in early life. These children will be treated with corticosteroids to reduce ACTH production and may also require mineralocorticoid replacement.

During the pre-anaesthetic visit, account must be taken of the difficult psychological aspects of this type of surgery. Expert advice should also be sought from the endocrine team about steroid cover and fluid management in the peri-operative period; hydrocortisone $1\,mg\,kg^{-1}$ will be required on induction and 6 hourly IV post-operatively until oral steroids can be recommenced. The dose should be reduced to the maintenance level after 1–4 days, depending on the nature of the surgery and the condition of the patient.

Anaesthesia involves tracheal intubation and controlled ventilation, and surgery usually takes place in the lithotomy position. Care should be taken with positioning to avoid nerve injury and pressure injury in the lower limbs.

Low-level bleeding may obscure the surgical view and can make surgery more difficult. Moderate hypotension can be helpful; the addition of clonidine $1–2\,mcg\,kg^{-1}$, either IV or as a caudal additive is helpful in this respect. The surgeon usually infiltrates with adrenaline 1:200 000 +/− local anaesthetic to reduce bleeding. A low lumbar epidural or caudal provides excellent intra-operative conditions, and an epidural provides excellent post-operative analgesia. The total dose of local anaesthetic given by any route (epidural or infiltration) should remain within safe levels (bupivacaine $2.5\,mg\,kg^{-1}$ maximum).

Renal failure

The common causes of renal failure in children vary with age:

Under 5 years

- Renal dysplasia
- Obstructive uropathy

Over 5 years

- Glomerulonephritis
- Nephrotic syndrome

Systemic effects of chronic renal failure

There are numerous systemic effects of chronic renal failure. Anaemia is common, and patients often have haemoglobin concentrations in the region of $6–7\,g\,dl^{-1}$. Anaemia results from a combination of reduced erythropoietin production, reduced red cell survival, and iron and folate deficiency. Coagulopathy may be present owing to platelet dysfunction, increased capillary fragility and thrombocytopenia secondary to bone marrow depression. Fluid and electrolyte abnormalities include fluid overload, hyperkalaemia, hypocalcaemia, hyperphosphataemia and either hyponatraemia or hypernatraemia depending on the type of renal disease. Acid–base abnormalities include metabolic acidosis and low plasma bicarbonate. There is an increased incidence of cardiac failure, pulmonary congestion and hypertension, and there is a risk of dysrhythmias. Other effects include peripheral neuropathy, encephalopathy and seizures. There is reduced immunity with an increased risk of infection.

Renal transplantation is the treatment of choice for end-stage renal failure. Renal dialysis may be required for a period prior to transplantation. Common indications for dialysis include fluid overload, electrolyte abnormalities and hypertension.

Renal transplantation

Renal transplantation is the most common form of solid organ transplantation in children. Graft survival is now about 95% at 1 year and 85% at 5 years.

The principles of good anaesthetic management for renal transplant include:

- Pre-transplant medical optimisation
- Careful pre-operative assessment
- Stable intra-operative haemodynamics
- Optimal perfusion of the newly transplanted kidney
- Good post-operative analgesia

Significant anaemia and coagulopathy should be excluded pre-operatively. Electrolyte imbalance should be treated and blood cross-matched. It is usual to do a chest X-ray to exclude respiratory pathology, and an ECG/echocardiogram if indicated.

The condition of the patient should be discussed with the renal team and the anaesthetist should be familiar with local protocols, such as antibiotic prophylaxis, fluid management and anti-rejection therapy. Pre-transplant dialysis may be required. If a vascular shunt is in place, IV or arterial access and blood pressure cuff should be avoided in that limb.

In infants the iliac vessels are very small, so the donor kidney is anastomosed to the aorta and inferior vena cava; renal transplantation is thus a major vascular procedure.

Induction and maintenance of anaesthesia is designed to maintain cardiovascular stability. Invasive monitoring with arterial line and CVP line is required. Epidural analgesia has been used successfully but is controversial because of the use of heparin

and the risk of coagulopathy. Many argue that the risks are small and an epidural confers greater haemodynamic stability. Optimal renal perfusion is achieved at a target CVP of $10–12\,cmH_2O$ and a haematocrit of 35–40%.

Before perfusion of the donor kidney most protocols call for furosemide $1\,mg\,kg^{-1}$, mannitol $1\,g\,kg^{-1}$ $+/-$ dopamine $5\,mcg\,kg^{-1}\,min^{-1}$. When the vascular clamps are released, hypotension is common as the new kidney fills with blood. Arrhythmias may also occur secondary to hyperkalaemia as the fluid used to preserve the transplanted kidney enters the circulation. Before the clamp is released it is important to ensure adequate filling, and it may be necessary to give blood and fluid to maintain a generous CVP. The problems of reperfusion of the grafted kidney are more pronounced in small children receiving large kidneys.

Post-operative ventilation is sometimes necessary if the donor kidney is large, or if aggressive fluid management has been required. Post-operatively, fluid balance should be managed by the renal team, with frequent estimation of plasma and urinary electrolytes. A typical regimen includes maintenance fluids with replacement of hourly urine losses and fluid boluses of isotonic fluid as required. Large volumes of hypotonic fluids must be avoided, particularly in children with polyuria associated with natriuresis. Good post-operative analgesia with morphine infusion, PCA or NCA or epidural analgesia is required, with the protocol tailored to renal function. Morphine should only be administered as boluses if the renal function is slow to recover. It may be necessary to treat hypertension, usually using hydralazine, nifedipine or labetalol or a combination of these drugs.

Survival after renal transplantation is 97% at 5 years and 94.5% at 10 years post-transplant. The most common causes of death are infection, secondary malignancy or cardiovascular event such as stroke.

Key points

- Minor urological surgery is common, and usually performed as day-case surgery. Provision of adequate post-operative analgesia using a combination of regional blocks and oral analgesia is essential.
- Antibiotic prophylaxis is essential in cystoscopy, major urological and reconstructive surgery.

- Major urological surgery requires close teamwork with the urologist to identify the extent of surgery, positioning and appropriate vascular access.
- Wilms' nephrectomy may be associated with major haemorrhage if pre-operative

chemotherapy has not been given, or if heminephrectomy is performed.
- Renal transplantation is a major vascular procedure in young children. Surgery involves close teamwork with the transplant surgeons and the nephrologists.

Further reading

Antal Z, Zhou P. Congenital adrenal hyperplasia: diagnosis, evaluation, and management. *Ped Rev* 2009;**30**: e49–e57.

Coupe N, O'Brien M, Gibson P, de Lima J. Anesthesia for pediatric renal transplantation with and without epidural analgesia – a review of 7 years experience. *Paed Anaes* 2005;**15**:220–8.

El-Hennawy AM, Abd-Elwahab AM, Abd-Elmaksoud AM, El-Ozairy HS, Boulis SR. Addition of clonidine or dexmedetomidine to bupivacaine prolongs caudal analgesia in children. *Br J Anaes* 2009;**103**: 268–74.

Howard RF, Lloyd-Thomas A, Thomas M *et al.* Nurse-controlled analgesia (NCA) following major surgery in 10,000 patients in a children's hospital. *Paed Anaes* 2010;**20**: 126–34.

Hughes IA, Houk C, Ahmed SF, Lee PA. Consensus statement on management of intersex disorders. *J Ped Urol* 2006;**2**:148–62.

Laine J, Jalanko H, Ronnholm K *et al.* Paediatric kidney transplantation. *Ann Med* 1998;**30**:45–57.

Llewellyn N, Moriarty A. The national pediatric epidural audit. *Paed Anaes* 2007;**17**:520–33.

Menzies R, Congreve K, Herodes V, Berg S, Mason DG. A survey of pediatric caudal extradural anesthesia practice. *Paed Anaes* 2009;**19**:829–36.

Rees L. Long-term outcome after renal transplantation in childhood. *Ped Nephrol* 2009;**24**:475–84.

Anaesthesia for hepatic surgery, including transplantation, in children

James Bennett and Peter Bromley

Introduction

Liver disease is rare in children, but its consequences may be devastating. Care for children with liver disease is usually provided in specialist centres, but children may present to non-specialist centres, so it is important that any anaesthetist treating children should be aware of the principles of management for this group of patients. Liver disease affects children from the neonate to the adolescent, and anaesthesia for children with liver disease can be one of the most challenging aspects of paediatric anaesthesia. This chapter will consider normal hepatic function, the pathophysiology of liver disease, common conditions that present to the anaesthetist working in a specialist unit, and a brief discussion of hepatic transplantation in children.

Anatomy

The liver is a large abdominal organ, typically 5% of the body weight of a neonate, falling to 2% by adolescence. It lies in the right upper quadrant and is effectively divided into left and right lobes and a smaller caudate lobe.

The blood supply to the liver consists of the portal vein and hepatic artery, which together comprise around 25% of the cardiac output. The portal vein provides two-thirds of the liver blood flow, but hepatic artery flow can increase to compensate for decreases in portal vein flow, even in the presence of advanced liver disease. The portal vein drains the intestines and receives flow from the superior mesenteric and the splenic veins. Thus the portal vein carries deoxygenated blood at relatively low pressure whereas the hepatic artery, being a branch of the coeliac trunk, carries oxygenated blood at systemic pressure. The vessels enter inferiorly via the porta

hepatis and divide repeatedly within the liver along with related bile ducts to form eight functional segments. These segments are not macroscopically apparent but have important implications for the surgeon operating on the liver.

The venous drainage of the liver is via the left, middle and right hepatic veins. The vessels are short and enter the inferior vena cava (IVC). The bile ducts leave the liver at the porta hepatis; left and right bile ducts join to form the common hepatic duct. The cystic duct from the gall bladder joins the common hepatic duct to form the common bile duct, which ultimately empties into the second part of the duodenum.

Microscopically the liver is divided into lobules organised around small branches of the portal vein, hepatic artery and the bile ducts in the portal tracts. Blood perfuses the lobules via sinusoidal vessels that ultimately drain into the hepatic veins.

Normal physiology and pathophysiology of liver disease

Some knowledge of liver physiology is essential for understanding the effects of liver disease. The liver is a complex organ with myriad functions; those that are important to the anaesthetist include:

- Synthesis
- Catabolism and excretion
- Intermediary metabolism – carbohydrates, protein, lipid, vitamins and cholesterol
- Immunological functions

Synthesis

All the coagulation factors (except factor VIII vWF which is derived from vascular endothelium) are synthesised in the liver. The synthesis of factors II, VII,

Core Topics in Paediatric Anaesthesia, ed. Ian James and Isabeau Walker. Published by Cambridge University Press. © 2013 Cambridge University Press.

IX and X is dependent on vitamin K. Bile is necessary for the absorption of the lipid-soluble vitamin K, and a loss of bile flow into the gut causes coagulopathy. The half-lives of factor V and VII are only a few hours, so coagulopathy can develop quickly.

Albumin forms the largest fraction of the protein output of the liver. Its half-life is long (20 days or so) so albumin levels change slowly in response to changes in liver function. Albumin is an important acid–base buffer, has oncotic effects and is an important determinant of the free fraction of many drugs, but the consequences of low albumin levels can be relatively minor. Other plasma proteins, including transport globulins and lipoproteins, are more crucial in maintaining health.

Bile and the bile salts play an important role in digestion, particularly of lipids.

Catabolism and excretion

Bilirubin is the breakdown product of haemoglobin. It is excreted in bile, and the appearance of jaundice can be the first sign of liver problems. Protein catabolism forms amino acids that provide a substrate for gluconeogenesis. Deamination of protein releases toxic ammonia, which is normally safely excreted via conversion to urea by the urea cycle enzymes. Ammonia accumulates in acute liver failure and is associated with hepatic encephalopathy, raised intracranial pressure and coma.

Failure of protein catabolism can be very disruptive; for example if insulin is not removed from the circulation, hypoglycaemia can result. Failure of regulation of other hormones can also be important.

Metabolism and excretion of xenobiotics, including drugs, is also vital. Most of these reactions are phase 1 reactions, carried out by cytochrome P-450 enzymes. Phase 2 reactions are conjugation processes such as glucuronidation to create water-soluble compounds that are then excreted in the urine. Some drugs, particularly larger molecules, are excreted in bile.

Intermediary metabolism

Carbohydrates

The liver plays a key role in carbohydrate metabolism and glucose homeostasis. Insulin release after meals promotes hepatic glucose uptake; glucose monomers are phosphorylated to glucose-6-phosphate and then polymerised into glycogen. When energy supplies are low, liver glycogen can be broken down into glucose-6-phosphate and then into glucose that is released into the circulation; the process does not consume any energy as the glucose has already been phosphorylated. Seventy-five per cent of the body's glycogen is stored in muscle, but this is only for 'local' use – muscle does not contain glucose-6-phosphatase, so glucose cannot be released from muscle glycogen. The liver can store only a limited amount of glycogen, and liver failure rapidly destroys the ability to maintain plasma glucose levels.

Protein

The liver is a major site of protein synthesis and catabolism. A wide range of essential proteins are synthesised, including albumin and the clotting factors, as described above. Protein catabolism produces amino acids that can be used in energy production via gluconeogenesis or ketone body formation. The handling of dietary protein depends on the liver. End-stage liver disease is commonly associated with marked muscle wasting, and this can be impossible to prevent despite determined nutritional care.

Lipid and cholesterol

The liver regulates the distribution of lipid and cholesterol by packaging these substances with apoproteins to form a range of lipoproteins that are essential for health. Lipids can be catabolised and the products directed into gluconeogenesis and the formation of ketone bodies.

Vitamins and trace elements

The liver is crucial in the synthesis, regulation and storage of many of these substances.

Immunological functions of the liver

A sizeable fraction of the cells in the liver (Kupffer cells, pit cells) have immunological functions and are important for the control of pathogens and tumour surveillance.

Chronic liver disease

In chronic liver disease there are repeated episodes of hepatic damage and regeneration, with fibrosis and eventual cirrhosis. This leads to portal hypertension and cholestasis, as well as loss of liver cell function. Cellular function is often well preserved until end-stage disease, and the severity of portal hypertension and cholestasis may vary according to the aetiology of the liver disease, and even between individuals suffering from the same disease.

Portal hypertension

Normal portal vein pressure is less than 15 cmH$_2$O. Increased portal vein pressure can lead to the formation of varices, and variceal bleeding. There may be ascites and pleural effusions. Hypersplenism may cause thrombocytopenia, or pancytopenia. Fluid shifts and other factors may contribute to the hepatopulmonary or hepatorenal syndromes.

Cholestasis

Obstruction to, or loss of, bile ducts as a result of fibrosis will cause jaundice with a conjugated hyperbilirubinaemia. Pruritus is common and may severely impair quality of life. Biliary obstruction may lead to cholangitis and systemic sepsis. The lack of bile flow into the gastrointestinal tract can cause malabsorption and steatorrhoea, leading to depletion of lipid-soluble vitamins A, D, E and K, coagulopathy due to loss of vitamin K-dependent clotting factors, and accumulation of drugs that are eliminated in bile.

Hepatocellular dysfunction

An early indicator of hepatocellular dysfunction is coagulopathy that is not fully corrected by vitamin K. Low albumin levels aggravate ascites, and peripheral oedema may develop. Drug volume of distribution and plasma protein binding may be altered. Drug metabolism may be impaired, either phase 1 or phase 2 conjugation processes. There may be loss of peripheral vascular resistance causing a high-output low-pressure circulation. Encephalopathy may occur secondary to raised ammonia levels, and there may be enhanced GABA-receptor effects and neuroinflammatory processes. Impaired immunity increases the likelihood and severity of sepsis.

Acute liver failure

Acute liver failure is defined by a period of less than 8 weeks between the onset of jaundice and the onset of encephalopathy. The presenting features are those of loss of hepatocyte function; there is no portal hypertension. There is a marked coagulopathy. There is a failure of glucose homeostasis and intravenous glucose is usually required, sometimes in large amounts. There is usually a metabolic acidosis and a high serum lactate. The clinical course is variable. Mild disease may recover completely, or may progress slowly over some weeks. Conversely, deterioration may be extremely rapid, causing death within a few days if the patient does not undergo liver transplantation. Acute liver failure is associated with high output cardiac failure, and acute renal failure is inevitable if the patient lives long enough. As encephalopathy progresses it is accompanied by cerebral oedema and raised intracranial pressure. Ascites is generally mild, if present. Bilirubin rarely reaches the high levels seen in some of the chronic cholestatic conditions. Death is usually from cerebral herniation, overwhelming sepsis, circulatory failure, or occasionally, catastrophic haemorrhage.

Liver function tests

The most important blood tests for the assessment of liver function are the coagulation parameters and albumin levels, both indicators of synthetic function. Excretory function can be assessed by the serum bilirubin level and the proportion of conjugated *versus* unconjugated bilirubin. A predominantly conjugated hyperbilirubinaemia implies biliary obstruction; a higher unconjugated fraction implies hepatic dysfunction, or that the conjugating capacity has been overwhelmed by haemolysis. The liver enzymes help to indicate the origin and nature of hepatocyte damage: aspartate transaminase (AST) is partially microsomal, whereas alanine transaminase (ALT) is exclusively cytosolic; a high AST/ALT ratio implies cell death (e.g. cirrhosis or tumour secondaries), whereas ALT will rise more in conditions where the cell membrane becomes 'leaky' (e.g. viral hepatitis). Alkaline phosphatase (ALP) and gamma glutamyltransferase (GGT) are both membrane-bound and do not 'leak' out. GGT is a marker of enzyme induction, and both ALP and GGT rise when there is biliary obstruction.

Special investigations and imaging

The liver is effectively imaged by ultrasound, and structural abnormalities of liver parenchyma, biliary tree and vasculature can be readily identified. Computerised tomography with and without contrast may be indicated to define the size of lesions and their relation to major vessels or to guide specific therapeutic options. Magnetic resonance imaging may give greater resolution of subtle tissue differences.

Oesophagogastroendoscopy may be indicated to identify oesophageal and gastric varices and thus portal hypertension. Percutaneous liver biopsy can be a valuable investigation, yielding diagnostic information not available from liver function tests. It is a painful procedure and requires general anaesthesia in most children, and it carries a significant risk of bleeding. Transjugular liver biopsy may be indicated in the presence of coagulopathy in acute liver failure.

Neonatal jaundice

Establishing a diagnosis in a baby with jaundice is important as some conditions, such as biliary atresia, have a good prognosis provided the baby receives early surgical treatment.

Physiological jaundice is common in neonates; it is worse in the breast-fed and premature baby, but usually disappears by 2 weeks. Persistent or worsening jaundice requires investigation. Haemolytic disease of the newborn is rare since the introduction of anti-D immunoglobulin to prevent the sensitisation of rhesus-negative mothers after a pregnancy with a rhesus-positive baby.

The differential diagnosis of neonatal jaundice includes:

- Physiological jaundice
- Haemolytic disease
- Biliary atresia (or possible choledochal cyst, although this is often asymptomatic, at least initially)
- Neonatal hepatitis
- Metabolic disorders
- Drug reactions (rare)

Pale stools and dark urine suggest bile is not entering the gut normally. Conjugated hyperbilirubinaemia suggests biliary obstruction while unconjugated hyperbilirubinaemia suggests physiological jaundice or haemolytic disease.

Anaesthesia and intensive care for children with liver disease

Common conditions in children with liver disease will be described. Procedures may be categorised as minor, intermediate and major. As a general rule of thumb, we suggest that the anaesthetist should 'upgrade' the intensity of the care given to a child with liver disease compared with a healthy child. For instance, for a child with liver disease having a hernia repair, consider using invasive monitoring, active warming, fluid therapy and an intensity of perioperative care that might be selected for a major procedure in a normal child. This might appear to be unnecessarily cautious, but surgery is high risk in this patient population and the child must be offered the best chance of a favourable outcome. If a child presents to a non-specialist unit, advice should be sought, and transfer to a specialist unit considered.

Hepatobiliary procedures

Hepatobiliary surgery can be divided into procedures for conditions of the biliary tree and for those of the liver itself, although there are obviously some features common to both.

Biliary atresia

Biliary atresia is a rare condition of unknown aetiology affecting roughly 1:14 000 live births in the United Kingdom. Around 25% of cases are associated with other anomalies, typically abdominal situs inversus, polysplenia and atrial septal defect. Absence of extrahepatic and intrahepatic bile ducts leads to cholestasis, progressive fibrosis and cirrhosis of the liver.

The affected neonate is usually born at term. Jaundice and pale stools soon become apparent and the infant fails to thrive. The presence of hepatomegaly suggests hepatic fibrosis. Investigation reveals a raised conjugated bilirubin, alkaline phosphatase and AST. Serum albumin and prothrombin time are usually normal in the early stages. Abdominal ultrasound reveals a contracted or absent gallbladder, and TEBIDA (Tc trimethyl-bromoiminodiacetic acid) scan demonstrates failure to excrete radioisotope from the liver into bowel. Liver biopsy demonstrates cholestasis, ductular plugging and bile duct proliferation.

Definitive diagnosis is with an operative cholangiogram to demonstrate absent bile ducts. Following confirmation of the diagnosis the surgical team will proceed to the Kasai portoenterostomy procedure. This involves excision of the fibrotic portion of the biliary tree and formation of a Roux-en-Y portoenterostomy to allow bile drainage. The Kasai procedure achieves some biliary drainage in 70% of infants. The outcomes are worse when performed in infants older than 8 weeks of age, or with advanced fibrosis or established cirrhosis.

Anaesthesia for the Kasai procedure

Careful pre-operative assessment is necessary for infants undergoing this operation. The full blood count may reveal anaemia, but the platelet count is usually normal as portal hypertension is unusual at this stage. The prothrombin time is generally normal provided the child has received supplementary vitamin K. The normal starvation guidelines can be applied, but the risk of hypoglycaemia should be remembered, and intravenous glucose infusion may be required.

Following the establishment of appropriate monitoring, induction of anaesthesia may proceed according to the anaesthetist's preference. The authors generally prefer a gaseous induction with sevoflurane. Following establishment of secure venous access, a non-depolarising muscle relaxant is administered, oral tracheal intubation is performed and a nasogastric tube placed. High ventilatory pressures and PEEP may be required owing to hepatosplenomegaly. Anaesthesia is maintained with a volatile agent, usually isoflurane, in a mixture of oxygen and air.

The role of epidural analgesia is debatable. The authors favour its use, as it promotes early feeding and avoids the risk of accumulation of morphine; however, there are concerns about sepsis in the epidural space as a result of systemic sepsis secondary to ascending cholangitis.

When forming the anastomosis between the Roux-en-Y and the porta hepatis the liver is retracted, potentially reducing venous return from the IVC. Thus good venous access in the upper limbs is necessary; the authors favour a central venous catheter for both access and measurement of central venous pressure. Arterial cannulation is generally unnecessary in the absence of associated cardiac abnormalities.

Babies with biliary atresia are very young and prone to hypothermia; this may be avoided by the use of warmed intravenous fluids and external warming devices. Extubation at the end of surgery and return to a high-dependency unit is normal. Antibiotic prophylaxis should be continued for 5 days to prevent post-operative cholangitis. Recurrent cholangitis, cirrhosis and portal hypertension may all occur despite adequate biliary drainage. Rotating courses of antibiotics are often necessary as prophylaxis for cholangitis, and nutritional support is useful to help with growth, which may be impaired secondary to a degree of malabsorption.

The outcome of infants with biliary atresia is variable. In the United Kingdom this surgery is performed in three designated centres allowing close monitoring and timely assessment for liver transplantation, should this become necessary.

Choledochal cysts

Choledochal cysts are localised cystic dilations of the common bile duct. The aetiology is obscure and the incidence is around 1:150 000 live births. Presentation in infancy is usually with obstructive jaundice and hepatomegaly. In the older child, right upper quadrant pain, cholangitis and hepatomegaly are more likely presenting features. Antenatal diagnosis is common and may be confirmed by ultrasound and magnetic resonance cholangiopancreatography (MRCP).

Choledochal cysts can lead to severe cholangitis, hepatic fibrosis, and cirrhosis, and there is a potential risk of malignancy in later life if left untreated. Surgical treatment is by excision of the cyst and formation of a Roux-en-Y anastomosis. Anaesthetic management is similar to that for infants with biliary atresia, but infants and children with choledochal cysts are generally more robust, and prognosis and recovery is usually very good.

Gallstone disease

Although considered a disease of adult life, gallstones can affect children with haemoglobinopathies, where haemolysis leads to the deposition of pigment stones, and children with disorders of cholesterol metabolism. It rarely affects infants. Presentation is most commonly with right upper quadrant pain, intermittent jaundice and pancreatitis. Surgical treatment is cholecystectomy, often with intra-operative cholangiography to exclude the presence of biliary obstruction due to residual stones in the bile duct. Laparoscopic cholecystectomy is popular because of less post-operative pain and shorter recovery time. This approach necessitates a significant pneumoperitoneum and often steep head-up tilt, which may cause some degree of haemodynamic compromise. Good vascular access is required. Routine anaesthesia is used, avoiding nitrous oxide owing to its potential to diffuse into gas-filled cavities. Analgesia is usually with intravenous paracetamol, a non-steroidal anti-inflammatory agent and titrated doses of morphine. Local anaesthetic infiltration to the sites of the laparoscopy ports may be useful. Shoulder-tip pain secondary to diaphragmatic irritation can be severe, but is usually relatively short lasting.

Laparoscopic cholecystectomy may be technically difficult and require conversion to an open procedure. Post-operative pain should be managed with morphine PCA or with epidural analgesia in this situation. The post-operative course may be complicated by pain, fluid shifts and ileus.

Hepatic tumours

Hepatoblastoma is the commonest liver tumour encountered in the paediatric population with an incidence of 0.77 per million. Hepatoblastoma is commonest in children under the age of 4 years, is associated with conditions such as Beckwith–Wiedemann syndrome and hemihypertrophy, and is more common in boys. It usually presents as an abdominal mass. Full blood count may reveal anaemia but liver function tests are often normal. α-Fetoprotein (AFP) is a useful diagnostic and prognostic marker. Abdominal ultrasound helps to differentiate hepatoblastoma from other abdominal tumours. CT and MRI scanning provide information about metastatic spread and the relationship of the tumour to vascular structures, and thus staging and surgical resectability. Treatment is with chemotherapy (cisplatin and doxorubicin) and surgical resection as guided by the SIOPEL (International Society of Paediatric Oncology) regimen. Children with unresectable hepatoblastoma may be suitable for liver transplantation. Doxorubicin toxicity may lead to cardiomyopathy, and all children should be assessed by routine echocardiography.

Anaesthesia for liver resection shares many similarities with that for liver transplantation (described below). Issues specific to hepatic resection are the risks of air embolus and hepatic insufficiency. In order to achieve clearance and reduce bleeding, surgical resection is usually by hemihepatectomy using a harmonic scalpel to divide the liver parenchyma along the planes of the functional anatomical segments. Entrainment of air into veins held open in the liver can lead to air embolus; this may be minimised by meticulous surgical technique and adequate fluid loading. However, excessive administration of fluid

leads to engorgement of the liver and increased bleeding. Clamping the portal vein and hepatic artery or vascular exclusion, with clamping of the vena cava, may reduce bleeding. This has the advantage of increased speed and reduced blood loss, but risks ischaemic damage to the remaining liver, leading to post-operative hepatic dysfunction.

Peri-operative hepatic dysfunction is suggested by a progressive base deficit and lactic acidosis. Adequate cardiac output must be maintained. Clotting factors are sometimes needed to support coagulation, and administration of N-acetylcysteine may be of value while the residual liver recovers. Children with hepatic dysfunction are best managed in the intensive care unit.

For children with uncomplicated hemihepatectomy it is our practice to use epidural analgesia, and to aim for early extubation and return to the high-dependency unit. Epidural analgesia may be high risk in the presence of coagulopathy due to post-operative hepatic dysfunction, so careful consideration should be given to the size of the tumour and expected difficulty of the resection.

Management of acute liver failure in children

Ten to fifteen per cent of liver transplants are carried out in patients with acute liver disease. The features of acute liver failure are different from chronic disease, and it is essential that prompt and effective treatment be offered.

The aetiology of acute liver failure varies with age. In the newborn, neonatal haemochromatosis is the most frequent diagnosis; in older children viral hepatitis and seronegative hepatitis are most likely but often no cause is found.

Acute liver failure is an emergency and requires rapid diagnosis and management. Early transfer to a specialist unit with transplantation facilities is essential. If moderately or severely encephalopathic, children should be admitted to the intensive care unit for elective ventilation and establishment of invasive monitoring.

The high mortality rate in acute liver failure is mainly from circulatory collapse, neurological deterioration and sepsis; it is essential that close attention be paid to haemodynamics and neurology. Hypotension is common and must be treated aggressively as cerebral autoregulation is impaired.

Intravascular volume must be maintained to ensure adequate organ perfusion in the face of high cardiac output and low systemic vascular resistance. Inotropic support, usually noradrenaline, is often required to maintain adequate perfusion pressure.

Sedation must be given so that the child tolerates the tracheal tube and mechanical ventilation. The child should be nursed with a 10° head-up tilt, and any tube ties should be kept loose to avoid obstruction of jugular venous drainage. Pupillary changes suggestive of worsening intracranial pressure should be treated with deep sedation (barbiturate coma has been used in this situation), adequate ventilation and intravenous mannitol. The role of intracranial pressure monitoring remains controversial, as there is a risk of provoking intracranial bleeding, particularly in the presence of a coagulopathy. Hypertonic saline and mild hypothermia appear promising treatments. Dextrose infusions may be required to avoid hypoglycaemia, and many centres start enteral feeding. Intravenous broad-spectrum antibiotics and antifungal agents should be given.

Survival in acute liver failure depends on rapid diagnosis and exemplary medical management, with timely liver transplantation if spontaneous recovery is not expected. Neurological deterioration suggestive of brain stem death, circulatory collapse unresponsive to increasing inotropic support and multi-organ failure are indicators of non-recovery. Liver transplantation is futile in these situations, and precious liver grafts must not be wasted.

Liver transplantation

Liver transplantation offers the hope of cure from debilitating and life-threatening symptoms of acute and chronic liver disease. Although first performed in the late 1960s, liver transplantation established itself as a viable therapy in the 1980s following the introduction of the immunosuppressant agent ciclosporin. Improved anaesthetic and surgical techniques and refinements in immunosuppression mean that children undergoing liver transplantation for chronic conditions can now expect a 1-year survival of over 90%. It is essential to differentiate between transplantation for acute and chronic liver disease, as the features and management of acute liver failure are distinct, as described above.

Common indications for liver transplantation are shown in Table 35.1.

Table 35.1 Age of onset of different diseases

Disease	Typical age
Neonatal haemochromatosis	Neonatal period
Biliary atresia	Infancy
Unresectable hepatoblastoma	3 years and under
Alagille syndrome	4 years and older
α-1-antitrypsin deficiency	6 years and older
Autoimmune hepatitis	10 years and older
Wilson's disease	10 years and older
Cystic fibrosis	Adolescence

Assessment of children for liver transplantation

In the United Kingdom, most liver transplants are performed at short notice with grafts from cadaveric donors, so it is useful if children can have an initial assessment around the time of listing for transplantation. The anaesthetist has an important role as part of the multidisciplinary team assessing all aspects of preparation for liver transplantation. The factors that are especially relevant are the features and severity of the liver disease itself, and the effects on other systems, with special regard to the cardiovascular, respiratory, renal and neurological systems.

Despite variation in severity and aetiology, there are some features of chronic end-stage liver disease and portal hypertension that are seen in most of these children. They are often malnourished and display poor growth, reduced muscle mass and thin subcutaneous tissue. The abdomen may be distended owing to ascites and hepatosplenomegaly. The skin may demonstrate jaundice, scratch marks from severe pruritis, bruising and dilated veins, particularly around the umbilicus.

Cardiovascular function and assessment

Cardiac output is typically raised and systemic vascular resistance is reduced. Fluid retention and peripheral oedema are common despite diuretic treatment. ECG and transthoracic echocardiography should be reviewed to exclude cardiac disease. Discovery of associated cardiac abnormalities allows risk stratification, which includes the risk of paradoxical air embolus during surgery in cases where there is the potential for right-to-left intracardiac shunting.

Decisions to treat cardiac abnormalities either surgically or by interventional cardiological techniques must be balanced by the extra risk of the procedure in a patient with liver disease.

Respiratory function

Moderate hypoxia and respiratory impairment are common and usually secondary to tense ascites and hepatosplenomegaly causing basal atelectasis. Pleural effusions are common. Chest infection may be present because of the immunological impairment associated with advanced liver disease.

Hepatopulmonary syndrome (HPS) can be a challenging condition. It is defined as hypoxia associated with liver disease, for which no other cause is apparent. The hypoxia is caused by a mixture of true shunting through pulmonary vessels and V/Q mismatch. The children may demonstrate clubbing and marked hypoxia, particularly on standing, but dyspnoea is uncommon. Investigation with contrast echocardiography or a Tc99 radiolabelled microalbumin scan may quantify the degree of shunting. Alarming levels of shunting may be discovered, and nocturnal or continuous oxygen therapy may be indicated. Although children with HPS often do well following liver transplantation, the hypoxia may worsen acutely and they may require higher inspired oxygen levels peri-operatively. The hypoxia typically gradually improves in the weeks and months after transplantation, and usually resolves completely with a well-functioning liver graft.

Renal function

Renal impairment is fairly common in advanced liver disease as a consequence of sepsis, diuretic therapy and hypovolaemia. The hepatorenal syndrome, HRS, is unusual in children.

Neurological assessment

Hepatic encephalopathy is difficult to treat and is a worrying sign (see Table 35.2). The cause remains elusive but raised serum ammonia and short-chain neuroactive polypeptides acting as false neurotransmitters are suspected; there may also be a neuroinflammatory component. Other causes of impaired conscious level include hypoglycaemia and impaired metabolism of sedative drugs.

Table 35.2 Grading of hepatic encephalopathy

Grade 0	Normal
Grade I	Minimal drowsiness but orientated; some impairment of cognitive functions, or reversal of day/night sleep pattern
Grade II	Drowsy, confused, mood swings
Grade III	Very drowsy, unresponsive to speech
Grade IV	Comatose

Anaesthesia for liver transplantation

If time allows, usual starvation protocols should be followed. If hypoglycaemia is a risk a dextrose-containing infusion should be commenced; otherwise oral intake of clear sugar-containing fluid is allowed up to 2 hours before induction. Coagulopathy should be corrected or partially corrected with fresh frozen plasma (FFP) and platelet transfusion, but fluid overload should be avoided. Hyponatraemia may be present as a consequence of high dose diuretics. The authors consider a serum sodium of $126 \, \text{mmol} \, l^{-1}$ as a minimum; lower values than this risk central pontine myelinolysis and should be treated.

Premedication is best avoided as the metabolism of sedative drugs may be impaired and starting times for surgery are often uncertain. Our practice is to induce anaesthesia with sevoflurane, or intravenous propofol 2–$5 \, \text{mg} \, \text{kg}^{-1}$ and fentanyl up to $2 \, \text{mcg} \, \text{kg}^{-1}$. A high initial dose of a non-depolarising muscle relaxant may be required to allow good intubating conditions, owing to increased volume of distribution in advanced liver disease and binding to acute phase proteins. Nasal intubation may provoke bleeding and should be avoided. The abdominal distension from ascites and hepatosplenomegaly often makes positive pressure ventilation difficult initially; PEEP, high inflation pressures and high inspired oxygen levels may be needed to avoid hypoxia. The situation usually improves following opening of the peritoneum and drainage of ascites.

Anaesthesia is maintained with isoflurane or desflurane in a mixture of oxygen and air, supplemented with an infusion of a short-acting opioid (e.g. remifentanil or alfentanil) and an atracurium infusion.

During the transplant procedure venous return may be reduced because of manipulation or clamping of the IVC, so intravenous cannulae and central catheters are sited in the upper body. Similarly, the infrarenal aorta may be clamped when forming an arterial conduit to the graft, so radial artery cannulation is preferred. Generally one or two peripheral cannulae and a multiple-lumen central venous catheter provide adequate vascular access for pressure monitoring and infusion of inotropes and other drugs. High-risk cases warrant the placement of a wide-bore sheath in a central vein to allow rapid transfusion. Coagulopathy and thrombocytopenia increase the risk of central venous cannulation and ultrasound guidance is recommended.

Children undergoing liver transplantation are susceptible to intra-operative hypothermia because of their small size, malnourished state and peripheral vasodilation, which may be exacerbated by rapid transfusion, loss of ascites and implantation of a cold liver graft. The ambient temperature of the theatre should be raised, and the child should be placed on a warming mattress and covered with clear PVC drapes to prevent wetting and subsequent cooling. Transfused fluids and surgical wash should be warmed, and inspired gases humidified. Care should be taken to prevent pooling of ascitic fluid on the child's skin. Core and peripheral temperature should be monitored.

The major fluid shifts and alterations in cardiac output that occur during liver transplantation have profound effects on haemodynamics, making cardiac output measurement useful. The pulmonary artery catheter is rarely used in children. Transoesophageal echocardiography (TOE) offers a dynamic assessment of ventricular filling, cardiac output and ejection fraction, and it can be used even in small children. PiCCO, which provides a continuous measurement of cardiac output and stroke volume from pulse contour analysis, or LiDCO, a similar device providing continuous cardiac output measurement by analysis of the arterial pressure waveform and dilution of lithium ions, are alternatives.

Intravenous fluid management is initially with crystalloids such as dextrose saline (5%/0.45%). Ascitic losses, bleeding and alterations in venous return may necessitate transfusion of further intravenous fluid, colloid and blood products. Regular blood glucose, electrolyte and haematocrit measurements can direct the type of infused fluid. Rapid changes in coagulation occur as a result of transfusion, dilutional coagulopathy and loss of liver function. Transfusion of coagulation factors and platelets is guided by

prothrombin time, activated partial thromboplastin time and thromboelastography. Appropriate analysers should be situated in or very close to the theatre.

The liver transplant procedure is classically divided into three phases: dissection, anhepatic and reperfusion. The dissection phase is from incision to occlusion of the hepatic artery and portal vein, which is the start of the anhepatic phase. The anhepatic phase ends when blood first reperfuses the transplanted liver via the portal vein.

Dissection phase

Division of adhesions, venous collaterals and varices may result in considerable loss of blood, and large volumes of fluid may also be lost as ascites. Transfusion should be guided by filling pressures, haematocrit and coagulation studies. Despite intensive preventive measures, hypothermia and coagulopathy are common. Manipulation of the liver may cause kinking of the IVC, which reduces venous return and cardiac output. Hypocalcaemia may be aggravated by the citrate load secondary to FFP transfusion and should be treated with an infusion of calcium ions. Intra-operative cell salvage reduces the requirement for donor blood.

Anhepatic phase

This phase is characterised by a sustained reduction of venous return and absence of liver function. Although surgical techniques vary, the IVC and portal vein are often clamped, which leads to reduced cardiac output and hypotension, often accompanied by a compensatory tachycardia. Treatment is with inotropic support and cautious fluid administration to avoid excessive right-sided pressures at reperfusion. Clamping of the portal vein may lead to congestion of the intestines and is associated with intestinal perforation and bacterial translocation.

Absent hepatic function leads to profound metabolic changes. Implantation of the ice-cold liver graft reduces core temperature, requiring adjustment of warming devices. Hypoglycaemia is likely and may be profound, necessitating adjustment of the dextrose infusion. A progressive metabolic acidosis develops. Sodium bicarbonate or other acid-buffering solutions should be withheld unless the acidosis becomes so severe that it causes inotrope-resistant hypotension, hyperkalaemia, or other dangerous effects. Severe hyperkalaemia at reperfusion carries a risk of cardiac arrhythmias, and buffers, calcium, furosemide and dextrose/insulin may be needed.

Towards the end of the anhepatic phase the liver graft is flushed to wash out potassium, preservation medium, heparin, metabolites, inflammatory mediators, cell debris and air. Crystalloid, colloid or the patient's blood may be used. Careful attention should be paid to the serum potassium, calcium and acidosis prior to reperfusion, and intravenous fluid and inotrope infusions should be prepared.

Reperfusion phase

Unclamping of the IVC leads to a sudden increase in venous return to the heart. The portal vein is unclamped slowly. The characteristic features of reperfusion are systemic hypotension, increased cardiac output and pulmonary vasoconstriction. The mechanisms of this reperfusion syndrome are obscure but endogenous mediators are implicated. The reperfusion syndrome is usually transient, but may be profound, requiring fluid and inotropic support, usually noradrenaline or adrenaline. Often the simplest and most successful strategy is to use the minimum therapy required to support a viable circulation until the transient reperfusion phenomena start to wear off, which may be no more than a few minutes. Liver grafts from older and unstable donors may be associated with a more profound reperfusion syndrome. Reperfusion coagulopathy is common; heparinase thromboelastography sometimes reveals fibrinolysis, requiring treatment with clotting factors and aprotinin or other anti-plasmin agents. Over-transfusion should be avoided to prevent congestion of the graft, excessive volume loading of the heart, and worsening of bleeding.

The surgical team then commence arterialisation of the graft, which requires good systemic arterial blood pressure. In infants undergoing a split liver transplant, an aortic conduit is often required, necessitating temporary aortic clamping.

Following completion of the arterial anastomosis the biliary anastomosis is performed (usually with a Roux-en-Y), and the abdomen is closed. If the liver is oedematous or oversize, a temporary abdominal wall prosthesis can be used. Abdominal closure is completed (in stages, if necessary) over the first week or so post-transplantation.

Types of liver grafts

The imbalance between the number of children awaiting liver transplantation and the availability of size-matched donor livers has led to innovative surgical techniques to provide more liver grafts and to reduce waiting-list times and mortality. Reduced-size grafts and split liver grafts allow adult cadaveric livers to be used even for small infants. Living-related grafts have the advantage of allowing scheduling of the liver transplant operation, but the risk of morbidity and mortality to the donor should be considered carefully.

Outcomes and complications after liver transplantation

Liver transplantation is one of the most physiologically challenging procedures performed in children. Given the fact that children undergoing transplantation can be extremely sick, it is perhaps surprising that after an uncomplicated procedure, most children can be discharged from intensive care within 24 hours, and from the ward in 7–10 days or even less. However, disastrous complications can occur, resulting in peri-operative mortality. Five-year survival rates of 80–90% are achievable for chronic liver disease, but nearer 60–70% for acute liver failure. With meticulous surgical technique and close attention to the treatment of coagulopathy, early returns to theatre for bleeding are rare. Complete normalisation of clotting parameters is not necessary and may even be undesirable; prothrombin times or INR less than twice normal is generally acceptable.

- Early graft failure is rare and may necessitate urgent retransplantation, often within 48 hours or even sooner.
- Early graft loss (within the first few days or weeks) is usually due to vascular problems (artery or portal vein thrombosis).
- Graft perfusion may be compromised if abdominal closure is too tight (abdominal compartment syndrome) or if the patient is allowed to become hypovolaemic, or if there is excessive use of vasoconstrictors.
- Grafts may be lost or the patient may die in the first month or two because of infective complications.
- Later complications include problems with immunosuppressive therapy leading to graft rejection or malignancy, particularly post-

transplant lymphoproliferative disorder (PTLD). Problems with biliary or venous drainage may require further surgery or radiological intervention.

Overall a retransplantation rate of about 10% can be expected. Good communication and collaboration and an experienced multidisciplinary team are needed to achieve the best results from this potentially very challenging procedure. The rewards can also be great, as transplantation provides a realistic hope of near-normal growth and development for children who are desperately ill with end-stage liver disease.

Key points

- Jaundice is relatively common in the neonatal period and is usually benign, but warrants investigation to detect serious but treatable conditions.

- Chronic liver disease is characterised by portal hypertension, jaundice and relatively preserved synthetic function until end-stage.
- Acute liver disease is characterised by hypoglycaemia, coagulopathy, acidosis, raised intracranial pressure and high-output low-resistance circulatory failure.
- Liver transplantation provides the hope of cure from the symptoms of liver disease with excellent survival for many indications.
- Significant liver disease is best treated in specialist units, and so prompt referral is recommended.

Further reading

Holcomb GW, Murphy PJ, Ostlie DJ, eds. *Ashcraft's Pediatric Surgery*, 4th edition. Elsevier/Saunders. 2010.

Kelly D, ed. *Diseases of the Liver and Biliary System in Children*, 3rd edition. Blackwell Publishing. 2008.

Chapter 36

Anaesthesia for radiology in children

Jane Herod

Radiology is a rapidly expanding service in paediatrics, often requiring general anaesthesia. Paediatric interventional radiology is a new speciality, and radiologists are able to perform an increasing number of procedures to facilitate treatment for some of the sickest patients in the hospital. Examples include tumour biopsy, embolisation of arteriovenous malformations, delivery of intra-arterial chemotherapy, and insertion of tunnelled central lines for chemotherapy or long-term inotropic support for cardiac failure patients.

The radiology suite is an 'unfriendly' environment for the anaesthetist, with access to the patient often limited by long distances and bulky X-ray equipment, and procedures may occasionally be performed with dimmed lights. Scrupulous attention must be paid to patient positioning, security of lines and tubes and maintenance of normothermia during long procedures. Constant vigilance with respect to both the patient's needs and the demands of the radiologist are required. Good communication and teamwork between the radiology team and the anaesthetist are essential to ensure patient safety in this challenging but rewarding area of work. This chapter will describe anaesthesia for interventional radiology, including neuroradiology, computerised tomography (CT) and magnetic resonance imaging (MRI).

Vascular access
Long-term vascular access

This is one of the mainstays of the interventional radiologist. Children require long-term vascular access for the administration of chemotherapy, parenteral nutrition or inotropes, or for short-term access for courses of antibiotics, or antiviral or antifungal medication. A cuffed Hickman line or Portacath is inserted, depending on the treatment required and patient or parental preference. Lines are required for the duration of treatment and may remain in place for years unless they become infected.

It is important to assess children carefully preoperatively, as candidates for central access are rarely fit and healthy. Children with cardiomyopathy or severe pulmonary hypertension (right ventricular pressure approaching systemic pressure) are at particular risk of cardiac arrest under anaesthesia. The risks and benefits of the procedure should be carefully considered and a back-up plan formulated in case of complications.

Anterior mediastinal mass

Children presenting with a haematological malignancy, neuroblastoma or intrathoracic germ cell tumour may have an anterior mediastinal mass (seen in up to 50% of children with non-Hodgkin's lymphoma). This may cause airway compression, or SVC obstruction or vascular compression, which may result in cardiovascular collapse on induction of anaesthesia. Worrying symptoms and signs include stridor, wheeze, orthopnoea, facial swelling or history of cardiovascular collapse. Review of the preoperative chest X-ray and CT scan is essential to look for a widened mediastinum, compression of the great vessels, tracheal or mainstem bronchus, or pericardial or pleural effusion (see Figures 36.1 and 36.2).

It may be preferable to start treatment and delay line insertion for a few days in children with a new diagnosis of lymphoma and severe respiratory symptoms to reduce the risk of anaesthesia. This requires close liaison with the oncologist as treatment will shrink lymph nodes rapidly and may make diagnosis impossible.

For induction of anaesthesia, children with an anterior mediastinal mass should be placed in a position of comfort (often on the side), and spontaneous respiration should be maintained if possible. If a muscle relaxant is given and thoracic tone reduced, be prepared for distal airway obstruction; this should be managed by application of CPAP, repositioning, and intubation with a long tracheal tube. Some advocate the use of a rigid bronchoscope to regain airway patency. It is sensible to obtain vascular access in the lower limbs prior to induction if the SVC is obstructed, and intravenous fluids and resuscitation

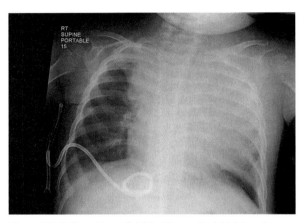

Figure 36.1 Chest X-ray of child with non-Hodgkin's lymphoma associated with a large anterior mediastinal mass.

drugs should be available in case of vascular compromise when the child is anaesthetised.

Tumour lysis syndrome

Children with lymphoma or high-count acute lymphoblastic leukaemia (ALL) are at risk of tumour lysis syndrome 12–72 hours after starting chemotherapy, owing to massive release of intracellular metabolites. These children require hyperhydration and treatment with allopurinol or rasburicase to preserve renal function and prevent deposits of uric acid or calcium phosphate in renal tubules. The main chemotherapy drug used for lymphoma is dexamethasone, so children with a new diagnosis of lymphoma or leukaemia should not receive dexamethasone as an antiemetic, as this may inadvertently precipitate tumour lysis syndrome.

Other types of lines for vascular access

For children requiring intermediate-duration vascular access (6 weeks to 6 months), a non-cuffed line such as a peripherally inserted central catheter (PICC) is inserted, usually via an antecubital fossa vein, or, in infants and small children, tunnelled over the chest wall and inserted into the internal jugular vein.

The other types of vascular access lines inserted in the radiology suite are dialysis catheters, either temporary (Vascath®) or long-term (Permacath®). These are large-bore catheters, which are 'locked' with heparin 1000 IU ml^{-1} to prevent line thrombosis and

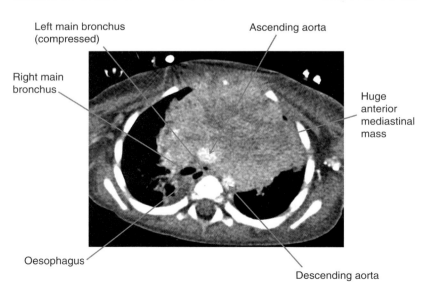

Figure 36.2 CT scan of child with non-Hodgkin's lymphoma associated with a large anterior mediastinal mass.

Left main bronchus (compressed)
Right main bronchus
Oesophagus
Ascending aorta
Huge anterior mediastinal mass
Descending aorta

occlusion. The dead space of the line is always printed on the line, and this volume must be aspirated and discarded prior to use to prevent unintentional heparinisation of the patient.

Positive pressure ventilation is usually required to decrease the risk of venous air embolism during central vein puncture in all tunnelled line insertions. If a PICC line is inserted in older children then a spontaneous ventilation technique may be acceptable as the line insertion utilises an arm vein only. A platelet count above $50 \times 10^9 l^{-1}$ and normal coagulation are required; children with a coagulopathy may require blood products to cover line insertion.

Portacaths and cuffed lines are removed under general anaesthesia, but non-cuffed lines may be removed on the ward. Children with acute myeloid leukaemia (AML), non-Hodgkin's lymphoma, Wilms' tumour, neuroblastoma or bone tumours may have received intensive chemotherapy with anthracyclines (doxorubicin, daunorubicin or epirubicin). They are at risk for anthracycline-induced cardiomyopathy, which may be subclinical. These children require thorough pre-operative assessment, and a recent echocardiogram should be reviewed.

Biopsy of solid organs or tissues
Liver biopsy
Diagnostic liver biopsy may be required to determine the nature of acute or chronic liver disease. A Tru-Cut biopsy needle is inserted into the liver under ultrasound guidance, and several core samples are taken using the same tract. The following precautions are taken to reduce the risk of bleeding:

- Platelet count must be at least $100 \times 10^9 l^{-1}$;
- Coagulation must be normal;
- A collagen gel foam plug is inserted in the biopsy tract at the time of the procedure.

The patient is usually positioned on their side with a bolster placed underneath them in order to open up the gap between the lower end of the rib cage and the iliac crest. Spontaneous ventilation with an LMA is acceptable. Patients should be observed carefully over the next 6 hours for signs of ongoing blood loss (pain, tachycardia, hypotension). If the clotting is grossly deranged and the risk of ongoing blood loss from the biopsy site is deemed to be great, then a biopsy may be taken via a catheter inserted into the internal

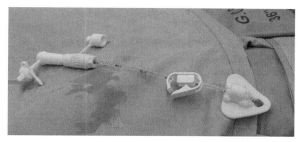

Figure 36.3 Percutaneous endoscopic gastrostomy tube (PEG). A Freka® PEG feeding tube is shown.

jugular vein and passed into the liver via the hepatic vein. If bleeding from the liver does occur, it is contained within the venous circulation.

Renal biopsy
Renal biopsy of a native kidney may be required in order to establish a diagnosis or monitor disease progression or, post-transplant, to help confirm or rule out rejection. To biopsy a native kidney, the patient is positioned on their side with a bolster placed underneath them, as for liver biopsy. Following renal transplantation the kidney is in the iliac fossa so the patient can remain supine.

Tumour biopsies
The same principles apply as for liver and renal biopsies. The site of the tumour determines the anaesthetic technique and positioning. Biopsies may be either ultrasound or CT guided. The latter can be quite a logistical feat, as the patient may need to be positioned prone in the CT scanner for the radiologist to locate and biopsy the tumour. All patients must be closely observed post-biopsy for signs of ongoing blood loss.

Gastrostomy
Percutaneous gastrostomy insertion is another procedure that is being performed more commonly in the radiology suite (see Figure 36.3). The major advantage of fluoroscopic control over the traditional endoscopic method is that the patient can be given a barium meal the day before to outline the colon, which reduces the risk of inadvertent colonic puncture.

A nasogastric tube is inserted under fluoroscopic control, and the stomach is inflated with air to aid distension and ease of percutaneous puncture. A dose of glucagon (40 mcg kg^{-1} IV) is given to cause gastric paresis. Once the stomach has been punctured a catheter over a wire is passed retrograde up the oesophagus and out of the mouth. A thread is then passed via the catheter and the gastrostomy tube is attached to this thread. The thread is used to pull the gastrostomy back down through the mouth and oesophagus so that the flange is in the stomach and the tube protrudes from the abdominal wall. The position is confirmed fluoroscopically.

As with any percutaneous gastrostomy, there is a risk of contamination of the abdominal cavity with gastric contents, so prophylactic antibiotics (co-amoxiclav or metronidazole) are given before the start of the procedure. The stomach is usually rested for 6–24 hours after gastrostomy insertion, so post-operative intravenous maintenance fluids are required.

Oesophageal dilation

There are two main groups of children who present to the radiology suite for oesophageal dilation: those with a stricture following surgical repair of oesophageal atresia and those with a stricture secondary to other scarring processes, such as dystrophic epidermolysis bullosa (DEB), or, less commonly, ingestion of caustic soda.

DEB is a hereditary skin disease that is characterised by painful blistering when skin or other stratified squamous epithelial membranes are exposed to shearing forces. Direct pressure does not cause new bullae to form, only shearing forces. Swallowing food boluses results in chronic bullae in the oropharynx and oesophagus, with subsequent scarring and stenosis.

Oesophageal dilation involves passing a wire, usually via the mouth, across the stricture under fluoroscopic control, followed by balloon inflation. Patients with the most severe form of DEB may have limited mouth opening owing to oral strictures, and intubation may be very difficult. These patients usually have a gastrostomy *in situ* and a retrograde technique may be used.

Anaesthesia for patients with DEB can be very challenging, and the following precautions should be taken:

- Intravenous access is often difficult because of multiple dressings. Access should be secured with a non-adhesive silicone dressing such as Mepitel®.

- ECG electrodes should not be stuck to the patient. Placing the electrodes on pieces of defibrillator pad on the skin makes good electrical contact.
- An adhesive pulse oximeter should be placed on a digit over a covering of plastic food wrap, and not straight onto skin.
- The blood pressure cuff should be padded.
- If the patient is intubated the tracheal tube should be tied using plastic food wrap, rather than taped in place.
- The facemask should be lined with paraffin gauze. Gloves should be worn, and it is sensible to protect pressure points on the chin and jaw with paraffin gauze.
- The eyes should be covered with gel pads, and artificial tears may be used to protect the cornea.
- A well-lubricated LMA may be used if a retrograde technique is used, but mouth opening is often too limited for LMA insertion.
- Great care is needed in transferring the patient onto the X-ray table, using a straight lift rather than a slide.

Even when the utmost care has been taken, anaesthesia is often associated with new bullae formation, and it is sensible to warn the family that this may occur.

Airway procedures
Bronchoscopy, bronchogram, tracheal dilation or insertion of airway stents

Patients may come to the radiology suite for bronchoscopic, radiographic and intraluminal ultrasound assessment of the airway as part of the management for both congenital and acquired tracheal stenosis, tracheomalacia or bronchomalacia (see Figure 36.4). Direct bronchoscopy is useful to document the nature and extent of tracheal disease and the presence of abnormal complete tracheal rings. A dynamic contrast bronchogram is required to delineate distal tracheobronchomalacia and define the level of CPAP required to keep the airway patent. Both bronchoscopy and bronchogram are vital parts of the surgical work-up and post-operative follow-up for patients with tracheobronchial abnormalities. Balloon dilation or insertion of intraluminal stents may be required at suture lines or in the presence of residual stenosis. Granulation

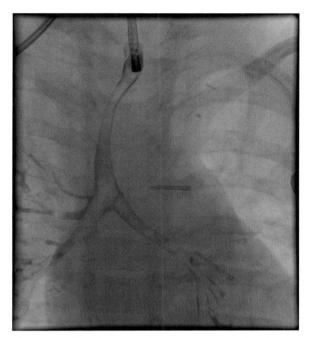

Figure 36.4 Bronchogram to demonstrate congenital tracheal stenosis.

Table 36.1 Guide for size of fibre optic bronchoscope suitable for different-sized tracheal tubes

Scope diameter	Minimum internal diameter of tracheal tube (mm)
Olympus 2.2 (no suction channel)	2.5
Storz 2.8	3 (tight) 3.5 acceptable
Olympus 3.8 Storz 3.7	4 (tight) 4.5 acceptable

tissue in the airway may also be managed with stenting.

Patients with congenital tracheal stenosis may have an underlying cardiac abnormality, and an echocardiogram is required as part of their pre-operative work-up.

Our preferred anaesthetic technique for bronchoscopy is spontaneous ventilation via LMA so that dynamic assessment of the airway can be made during the respiratory cycle, particularly if tracheobronchomalacia is suspected. A pressure manometer inserted into the Ayres T-piece circuit will give an indication of opening pressures required to overcome inspiratory collapse due to tracheobronchomalacia. This method using an LMA may not always be possible, for instance in neonates or those already ventilated, in which case a bronchoscope of appropriate size may be passed via a tracheal tube (see Table 36.1).

An angle piece with a self-sealing valve (see Chapter 22, Figure 22.1) is used so that there is no or minimal leak of anaesthetic gases when the bronchoscope is passed down the LMA. Atropine 20 mcg kg^{-1} IV may be given to dry secretions. Topical lidocaine (3 mg kg^{-1}) to the larynx and between the cords prior to endoscopy reduces coughing, although this has the disadvantage of preventing the child from drinking

for 2 hours post-procedure. Passing the bronchoscope through the vocal cords rarely causes coughing/spasm in patients if the child is relatively deep (end-tidal sevoflurane concentration of around 4%). The child may cough if the bronchoscope 'tickles' the carina, and a bolus of 1–2 mg kg^{-1} of propofol is usually enough to prevent or treat this. Transient apnoea associated with the propofol bolus can be overcome by assisting ventilation until spontaneous respiration returns.

A dynamic assessment of the airway is made with the child breathing spontaneously prior to airway stent insertion or balloon dilation. A bolus of propofol is administered just before the balloon is inflated so that the child is apnoeic and does not cough. This technique allows spontaneous ventilation to return rapidly after the procedure, so that the dynamic assessment of the airway can be repeated (see Figures 36.5 and 36.6).

Transbronchial lung biopsy

Following lung transplantation, patients undergo regular bronchoscopy to assess the bronchial anastomoses, to undertake a broncheoalveolar lavage (BAL) for microbiology, and to obtain a biopsy to look for signs of rejection. The bronchoscope is passed through an LMA as above and the biopsy forceps are passed down a side channel under X-ray control; three to four biopsies are taken from distal lung tissue. A spontaneous breathing technique can be utilised as above, but as dynamic airway assessment is not necessary the patient can be paralysed and ventilated via the LMA; this avoids the need to spray the larynx and the carina.

Transbronchial biopsy should not be undertaken in the presence of abnormal coagulation as intrapulmonary

(a)

(b)

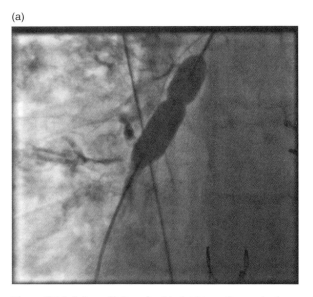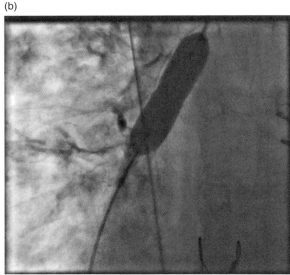

Figure 36.5 Balloon dilation of residual stricture after repair of congenital tracheal stenosis. (A) Bronchial waist on balloon. (B) Bronchial waist abolished after dilation.

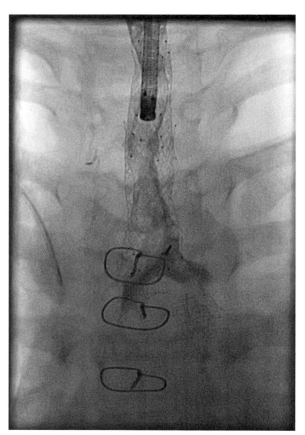

Figure 36.6 Tracheal stent *in situ* for residual stricture in severe congenital tracheal stenosis.

haemorrhage can then be troublesome. Pneumothorax is a rare complication and should be excluded radiographically at the end of the procedure.

Visceral angiography

Access for most angiographic procedures is via a femoral artery. It is often best to paralyse and ventilate the patient as repeated periods of apnoea may be required after injection of contrast, and small movements, even those associated with respiration, cause significant artefacts.

Conventional X-ray contrast (iodine-based Omnipaque® 240 mg I ml^{-1}) is used. As with all contrast media there is a small risk of prior sensitisation, and a full allergy history should be taken during preoperative assessment in case an alternative is required. A cumulative dose of 5 ml kg^{-1} is the usual maximum, although up to 7 ml kg^{-1} may be given safely. Radiographic contrast media are usually osmotic diuretics, and intravenous fluids should be given during the procedure. 'In–out' catheterisation may be required at the end of the procedure if the bladder is distended. Occasionally, carbon dioxide gas (1 ml kg^{-1} to the nearest 5 ml aliquot) is used as a contrast medium in order to keep the dose of iodinated contrast medium to a minimum. Hyoscine butylbromide (0.3 mg kg^{-1} IV) is useful to counteract spasm of the gastrointestinal tract prior to enteric angiography.

The arterial sheaths used for angiography are relatively large, and it is helpful if the child does not cough vigorously during emergence as this will lead to haematoma formation. For this reason, some advocate topical lidocaine to the cords prior to intubation, and plan for deep extubation at the end of the procedure.

Renal vein sampling and angioplasty

Approximately 10% of children with secondary hypertension have renovascular disease that results from one or more lesions that impair renal blood flow. This is usually secondary to fibromuscular dysplasia of the renal vessels, which is often bilateral. Patients may be taking multiple anti-hypertensive agents and may have evidence of left ventricular hypertrophy or even hypertensive cardiomyopathy on pre-operative echocardiogram or ECG. There is a common association between renal artery stenosis and disease in other vascular beds, and 20–25% of these patients have cerebral vascular involvement. Cerebral angiography is often performed at the same time as renal imaging.

Children who have severe hypertension resistant to medical treatment may benefit either from angioplasty, or from surgical resection or stenting of a stenosed renal artery. Selective renal vein angiography and sampling allows measurement of local renin secretion to identify those who may benefit from this intervention. It may also be of diagnostic value, and helps differentiate these children from those with hypertension due to nephropathy or vesico-ureteric reflux.

Angiographic treatment alone (stenting or balloon dilation) results in improvement in blood pressure control in approximately half of these patients, although re-stenosis may require further treatment. This is especially true when a stent is inserted. Those with severe disease involving the aorta require surgical repair with a GoreTex® graft, but they may develop stenosis at the graft site, which will also benefit from angiographic dilation.

Good control of blood pressure pre-operatively is difficult in these children, despite the use of combination therapy. Treatment may be compromised by poor compliance, or limitation of dose owing to adverse drug side effects.

As with all angiographic procedures, the patient must be completely still during the procedure, and multiple episodes of breath holding are required. The child should therefore be intubated and ventilated.

A loading dose of heparin (75–100 IU kg^{-1}) is given prior to balloon inflation if angioplasty is undertaken.

The major complication of any angioplasty is vessel rupture, and vascular surgical support should always be readily available before this procedure is undertaken.

Pancreatic venous sampling

The most frequent cause of prolonged severe hypoglycaemia in infancy is congenital hyperinsulinism, usually secondary to one or more insulin-secreting lesions within the pancreas. This is treated surgically by partial pancreatectomy after localisation of the tumour by pancreatic arterial stimulation and venous sampling.

Pancreatic venous sampling of insulin is usually performed under general anaesthesia in children, but may be performed under sedation in the adult population. Both venous and arterial catheters are inserted and timed samples are taken from the right hepatic vein after injection of calcium gluconate into pancreatic arteries that supply different parts of the pancreas. Diagnosis requires at least doubling of the insulin level sampled from the hepatic vein.

High levels of endogenous catecholamine released because of stress such as intubation may cause a rise in blood glucose concentrations, which in turn can interfere with the interpretation of test results. Deep anaesthesia is therefore ideal. Theoretically, using high concentrations of volatile agents may also interfere with test results, as volatile agents block calcium channels, which in turn reduces insulin release. A balanced anaesthetic to maintain heart rate and BP to within 20% of baseline may be achieved using remifentanil (0.5–1.5 mcg kg^{-1} min^{-1} IV) and volatile anaesthesia with end-tidal concentration of 0.5 MAC.

These infants usually require a glucose infusion to prevent profound and dangerous hypoglycaemia due to their insulinoma. The amount of glucose required may be quite substantial, and they commonly require a tunnelled PICC or Hickman line so that glucose 20% or more can be given to maintain normoglycaemia. Regular blood sugar measurement should be taken throughout any intervention, and the glucose infusion rate altered accordingly.

Extracranial sclerotherapy

This is used to treat cutaneous or peripheral lymphangiomas, either simple or macrocystic-type (cystic hygromas), or vascular arteriovenous malformations

(AVM). A sclerosing agent, either the sclerosant OK432 (picibanil) for lymphatic and cystic hygromas, or micro-beads for AVMs, is injected under ultrasound or fluoroscopic guidance into the malformation. A course of sessions is usually required. This may be as a prelude to surgical excision if required. In head and neck lymphangiomas approximately 90% show improvement after sclerotherapy and 40% of lesions show complete regression. The anaesthetic technique will be dependent on the site of the lesion. Spontaneous ventilation is usually adequate for extracranial lesions (see below).

Patients with malformations on the face or oral area require a single dose of prophylactic antibiotics (co-amoxiclav or teicoplanin and an aminoglycoside for penicillin allergic patients). A single dose of dexamethasone 250 mcg kg^{-1} IV up to 8 mg should be given to reduce inflammation in patients with facial or oral lesions.

Sclerotherapy may be quite painful postoperatively, and patients may require opioid analgesics such as oral morphine in addition to regular paracetamol and NSAIDs such as ibuprofen or diclofenac.

Neuroradiological interventions

Cerebral angiography

Children may require cerebral angiography and/or embolisation of intracranial congenital AVMs and shunts. These are often first diagnosed after an intracranial bleed. The initial visit to the angiographic suite may be during the acute phase while intubated and ventilated in the intensive care unit, possibly while requiring inotropic support to maintain cerebral blood flow.

There are three methods of embolising cerebral AVMs: coils, microparticles or glue. In children the use of coils is uncommon as most large, rapidly shunting AVMs are thin-walled and may rupture when coiled. Thus the vast majority of malformations, shunts and tumours are embolised using either microparticles or glue. Microparticles are usually employed in tumours and glue in the embolisation of AVMs, although some operators may use microparticles for AVMs that have a small shunt component. Where there is a large arteriovenous (AV) shunt, such as Vein of Galen aneurysmal malformation, then glue is always used. Glue used for

embolisation starts to polymerise when it comes into contact with blood.

The extent of glue dispersion depends upon three variables: the concentration of glue, the speed of injection and the flow velocity within the AV shunt. This last factor is affected by the nature of the lesion and where, in relation to the lesion, the neuroradiologist can place the microcatheter. The process of glue polymerisation is exothermic, so dexamethasone (200–250 mcg kg^{-1} IV) should be given to reduce inflammation and reduce the risk of 'peri-glue' oedema.

Cerebral angiography carries a small risk of stroke and blindness, which is increased when a lesion is embolised. The neuroradiologist looks specifically for signs of retinal 'blush' during angiography as embolisation near the origin of the ophthalmic artery would cause permanent visual loss.

There are three possible major intracerebral complications if glue has been used:

- The microcatheter tip may be retained within the glue.
- Proximal spread of glue may occur because of invagination of the 'glueoma' when the embolisation catheter is removed.
- A vessel is torn when the catheter is removed. This may occur if the catheter has become lodged within the glue ball stuck to the vessel wall, and may result in cerebral haemorrhage.

The second two complications are fortunately very rare but contribute to the risk of stroke during the procedure. Cerebral haemorrhage may require further embolisation or surgery such as ventricular drain insertion. Retention of the microcatheter tip within the glue mass does not usually cause a problem as the catheter becomes epithelialised with time.

The main systemic risk of cerebral embolisation is that of migration of the embolising material into the extracranial venous circulation and the pulmonary bed. The anaesthetist should look for signs of systemic spread such as a fall in end-tidal CO_2 or a fall in oxygen saturation. Fortunately, these pulmonary emboli are very small and the effect is not usually long-lasting.

Vein of Galen aneurysmal malformation

Large AV shunts often present with signs of high-output right heart failure rather than an intracranial bleed. This is due to the rapid recirculation of blood from the arterial circulation through the AV shunt

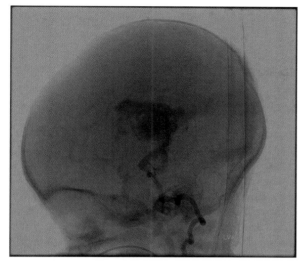

Figure 36.7 Vein of Galen aneurysmal malformation.

back to the right heart without passing through the systemic vascular bed. The vein of Galen aneurysmal malformation (VGAM) is a rare but important cause of high-output cardiac failure presenting in neonates (see Figure 36.7).

The VGAM is a heterogeneous collection of rare midline intracranial choroid AV vascular malformations. A VGAM consists of multiple AV shunts draining into a dilated median prosencephalic vein of Markowski, a persistent embryonic vein that is normally absent in adults. The normal vein of Galen is formed by the junction of the internal cerebral veins, and passes between the corpus callosum and pineal gland to form the straight sinus as it joins with the inferior sagittal sinus. A VGAM is anatomically different to an AV malformation where the venous drainage is into a dilated, but already formed, vein of Galen.

Without treatment VGAMs are invariably fatal. Advances in cerebral angiography with early embolisation have improved outcomes significantly, so that in some series, 74% of those who are treated are neurologically normal at follow-up.

Babies presenting with VGAMs have a massive intracranial AV shunt. They usually present in the neonatal period with signs of poor systemic perfusion, pulmonary hypertension and right heart failure. The systemic vascular resistance is higher than AV shunt resistance; thus blood leaving the left side of the heart goes preferentially to the carotid arteries, through the AV shunt and back to the right heart to cause volume overload and subsequent right heart failure. Increased pulmonary blood flow may result in pulmonary hypertension (PHT), particularly in the newborn period, and right ventricular pressure may approach or exceed systemic values.

Diagnosis is made by eliminating cardiac causes of failure, and by demonstration of the AVM on cranial ultrasound. A loud bruit may also be heard over the anterior fontanelle. Occasionally a VGAM can be diagnosed antenatally if a third-trimester scan is done.

Babies presenting in the first few days of life with poor systemic perfusion and cardiac failure require pre-intervention ventilation and inotropic support in the NICU. Milder cases of cardiac failure presenting in the first few weeks of life usually respond to diuretics.

Close cooperation with the neuroradiologist is essential. If the arterial pressure is high during an embolisation run, the glue may spread further than intended, thus unintentionally embolising other areas of the brain. The neuroradiologist will usually ask for a drop in systemic blood pressure to about two-thirds of awake values. Fentanyl 1–2 mcg kg^{-1} and sevoflurane 2–3 MAC is usually sufficient if the patient is fully paralysed. The diastolic BP is often very low and starts to normalise once the AV shunt is embolised. Tachycardia often becomes less pronounced as systemic blood flow increases, although this may not be as obvious in the anaesthetised patient.

Most neonates are kept sedated, intubated and ventilated in NICU after embolisation. Closure of the AV shunt will cause a sudden increase in cerebral (rather than shunt) perfusion, as well as increased systemic perfusion. These factors may result in reperfusion injury and there is a risk of post-embolisation cerebral bleed. Although right-sided heart failure may start to improve post-embolisation, an element of left-sided heart failure often develops, as the left ventricle now has to work much harder.

Blood pressure must be carefully controlled post-embolisation, and an agent such as glyceryl trinitrate (GTN) or sodium nitroprusside (SNP) may be required if simple sedation is not sufficient. Some neuroradiologists heparinise patients post-embolisation to prevent retrograde blood clots resulting in ischaemic stroke. Heparin should only be started if there has been no bleeding during or after the embolisation procedure. A CT scan is routinely performed at the end of the procedure to determine whether this is a safe course of action.

As there are potentially huge changes in both cerebral blood flow and physiology, the AV shunt is usually closed in stages in the first 2–3 months of life. Children for repeat embolisation are not usually as sick and may no longer require anti-failure medication. Post-embolisation management of these patients, including admission to NICU for ventilation post-procedure depends on the residual AV shunt and operator preference.

Ophthalmic artery chemotherapy

Selective catheterisation of the ophthalmic artery for intra-orbital chemotherapy is a relatively new but expanding area of interventional neuroradiology.

This is currently reserved as second-line treatment for children with retinoblastoma who have relapsed during or after conventional systemic chemotherapy and cryotherapy. It avoids the need for radiotherapy during a critical time of brain development with the attendant risks of secondary malignancy and developmental delay. Initial results are encouraging, and with more experience this treatment option may become more widely available for other patients.

A micro-catheter is placed directly into the ophthalmic artery, and once it is in place, the chemotherapy agent melphalan is slowly infused into the orbit over a period of at least 20 minutes. Response to treatment is assessed 2–3 weeks later by formal examination under anaesthesia, and if responding, the child will receive further treatments, up to a maximum of four.

Standard cerebral angiography is performed, but there are some additional special considerations:

- The eye is at risk from arterial thrombosis, so a loading dose of heparin (75 IU kg^{-1}) is given after femoral access has been obtained.
- Dexamethasone (250 mcg kg^{-1}) is given to reduce orbital and peri-catheter oedema.
- Chemotherapy is very emetogenic, so a dose of ondansetron (150 mcg kg^{-1}) is given.

The procedure may also stimulate an unusual 'oculo-cardiac' reflex, similar to that seen with ocular procedures such as strabismus surgery. The reaction is unpredictable, but can be quite extreme. The first sign is sudden reduction in lung compliance and fall in tidal volume. The end-tidal CO_2 trace is similar to that seen in a patient with bronchospasm, although this is not heard on auscultation, and is probably due to acute pulmonary venous congestion. The reaction is accompanied by a fall in oxygen saturation and hypotension, which may be profound. Screening with fluoroscopy

shows the heart appears to be poorly contracting ('myocardial stun'), although the heart rate does not usually fall initially. Bradycardia may occur a few minutes later. The child should be treated with atropine (5–10 mcg kg^{-1} IV), and a bolus of isotonic fluid (10 ml kg^{-1} IV) may be required. Resistant hypotension should be treated with adrenaline (1–2 mcg kg^{-1} IV).

This reaction is seen when the micro-catheter is flushed, prior to chemotherapy injection. It is only seen on repeat administration of intra-arterial chemotherapy, never the first. The exact mechanism is unclear, but is thought to be due to sensitisation of the ciliary ganglion, the parasympathetic ganglion located in the posterior orbit. Thermal or mechanical stimulation during a repeat procedure results in this unusual phenomenon. Prophylactic IV atropine and slow injection of intra-ophthalmic contrast seems to reduce the severity of the reaction.

Anaesthesia for CT

CT is used as a diagnostic modality and to monitor treatment in children. It is particularly useful to delineate bony or vascular anatomy with 3D reconstruction, to image the lungs or identify intracranial bleeding. High-quality scans require the child to remain still to reduce motion artefacts, with breath-holds required for cardiac CT. CT scans are quick (although the dose of radiation is high), and the majority of children do not require anaesthesia. Babies may be managed with 'feed and wrap' and older children will lie still in the scanner, but sedation is generally used for younger children (see Chapter 17). Anaesthesia is required for CT guided biopsy, cardiac CT (frequent breath-holds), and those children unsuitable for sedation, for instance children with airway problems. Particular issues relate to anaesthesia in remote locations, with the added challenge of limited space in the scanner, and limited access during the scan. Monitors must be visible from the control room, although the anaesthetist may stay in the scanner if wearing appropriate radiation protection.

Anaesthesia for magnetic resonance imaging

Magnetic resonance imaging (MRI) is particularly useful for providing high-quality images of soft tissue, and is the technique of choice in neurological, cardiovascular, oncology and musculoskeletal imaging. The imaging is based on the physical behaviour of protons in hydrogen atoms in water and phosphorus in ATP when placed in externally applied magnetic fields. MR scanners therefore contain very strong magnets, between 0.2 and 3 tesla, and specific safety precautions are required to prevent ferrous objects from being sucked into the scanner. The presence of ferromagnetic implants, including pacemakers, is an absolute contraindication to MRI scanning. The scanners generate weak signals, and it is important to shield external radiofrequency sources such as from monitors.

MR scans are often long, between 30 minutes and 2 hours, depending on the area of interest, and the child must remain still during acquisition of images. The child is relatively inaccessible during the scan, and additional precautions need to be taken because of the magnet. Many older children will be able to manage by watching videos or with sedation, but fortunately, MR-compatible anaesthesia machines and monitors are now available, which means that safe anaesthesia can be undertaken when required.

Induction of anaesthesia should take place in an anaesthetic room adjacent to the MR room, after metal checks have been completed. A repeat metal check should take place just before moving the child into the scanner. A spontaneously breathing technique with LMA is suitable for most scans, although small infants should be intubated as access is limited. Children undergoing cardiac MR require frequent breath-holds and should also be intubated and ventilated. Specific MR-compatible ECG electrodes, cables, saturation and blood pressure cuffs should be used. In an emergency, the child should be taken out of the scanner back to the anaesthetic room, as metal objects such as laryngoscopes and stethoscopes cannot be taken into the scanning room. Ward infusion pumps may malfunction close to the magnet, and MR compatible pumps will need to be used in the scanner. These must still be kept outside the immediate vicinity of the magnet (the 50 gauss line). Unstable patients requiring inotropic support may not be suitable for MR scanning for this reason.

Key points

- Interventional radiology is a rapidly expanding area in paediatric anaesthesia, with a range of complex procedures now being possible for some of the sickest patients in the hospital.
- Limited access due to X-ray equipment and dimmed lighting requires constant vigilance.

- Scrupulous attention to detail is required, including choice of anaesthetic technique, patient positioning and monitoring.
- Good communication and teamwork are essential to ensure patient safety during radiological procedures. Although both technically and environmentally challenging, overcoming these obstacles makes this a very rewarding area in paediatric anaesthesia.
- Special precautions are required for safe anaesthesia in MRI.
- Children with lymphoma or high-count acute lymphoblastic leukaemia are at risk of tumour lysis syndrome 12–72 hours after starting chemotherapy and should not be given dexamethazone.
- Special precautions are required for safe anaesthesia in MRI.

Further reading

Acevedo J, Shah RK, Brietzke SE. Nonsurgical therapies for lymphangiomas: A systematic review. *Otolaryngology – Head and Neck Surgery* 2008;**138**:418–424.

Cucchiaro G, Markowiz SD, Kave R *et al.* Blood glucose control during selective arterial stimulation and venous sampling for localization of focal hyperinsulinism lesions in anesthetized children. *Anes Analg* 2004; **99**:1044–8.

Goonasekera CD, Shah V, Wade AM, Dillon MJ. The usefulness of renal vein renin studies in hypertensive children: a 25-year experience. *Ped Nephrol* 2002;**17**(11):943–9.

Herod J, Denver J, Goldman A, Howard R. Epidermolysis bullosa in children: pathophysiology, anaesthesia and pain management. *Ped Anes* 2002;**12**:388–97.

King DR, Patrick LE, Ginn-Pease ME, McCoy KS, Klopfenstein K. Pulmonary function is compromised in children with mediastinal lymphoma. *J Ped Surg* 1997;**32**(2):294–300.

Lasjunas P, Chng SM, Sachet M *et al.* The management of Vein of Galen aneurysmal malformations. *Neurosurgery*: 2006;**59**(5):S3-184–S3-194.

Shroff R, Roebuck DJ, Gordon I *et al.* Angioplasty for renovascular hypertension in children: 20-year experience. *Pediatrics* 2006;**118**:268–75.

Stuart G. Understanding magnetic resonance imaging. Anaesthesia tutorial of the week no 177. http://totw. anaesthesiologists.org/2010/05/03/understanding-magnetic-resonance-imaging-177 (accessed 22 July 2012).

Chapter 37

Anaesthesia for oncology and other medical procedures in children

Michael Broadhead and Isabeau Walker

Introduction

There has been a rapid increase in demand for anaesthesia services outside the operating room in the past decade, and anaesthesia in remote locations is now a routine part of paediatric practice. Anaesthesia is required for painless procedures such as CT or MRI where the child must remain immobile, or for minor procedures that are painful or uncomfortable, such as lumbar puncture (LP), bone marrow aspiration (BMA) or endoscopy.

Anaesthetists have a key role to play to make sure that these procedures can be undertaken safely, efficiently and without pain or distress for the child. A positive experience will colour the child's future attitude towards hospital care – a bad experience will also have a lasting effect. This chapter will consider the general principles for provision of remote anaesthesia, and specific requirements for anaesthesia for oncology patients, muscle biopsy and joint injections. The development of safe sedation services and endoscopy for children is described in Chapter 17, and anaesthesia for radiology is covered in Chapter 36.

General principles: anaesthesia in remote locations

Children undergoing minor medical procedures are frequently admitted as day cases. Procedures may be undertaken in the main operating theatre on an ad hoc basis, but it is probably more efficient, and more pleasant for the child and family, to base their care in a dedicated day unit or day-case list. A stand-alone medical procedure unit is ideal for high-volume, rapid turnover services such as oncology or gastroenterology.

It is important that in all these situations, the same standards of care are provided as in the main operating suite:

- The service should be consultant led and ideally consultant delivered, with appropriate supervision of trainees.
- There should be clear policies covering patient selection and preparation, and a forum to discuss high-risk patients at a multidisciplinary team meeting. Children with an abnormal airway, congenital heart disease, pulmonary hypertension, cardiomyopathy, mucopolysaccharidosis or children with unstable disease, ASA III or above, should be discussed as to their suitability for treatment in a remote location. Additional support and planning will be required for high-risk patients.
- There should be appropriately trained theatre staff, including a trained anaesthetic assistant, and a fully equipped recovery room with trained staff. Emergency drills should be practised regularly.
- The theatre should have piped medical gases, suction, air exchange and electrical safety standards as for any operating room.
- Full anaesthesia monitoring should be available, according to national guidelines.
- There should be full access to appropriate anaesthetic equipment, disposables and anaesthetic drugs. Service contracts for equipment and pharmacy support should be the same as for the main operating theatre.
- There should be regular audit of patient outcomes, training of staff, and feedback from parents about the quality of the service.

Paediatric oncology

Cancer affects around 1:600 children under the age of 14 years in the United Kingdom, with around 1500 new cases diagnosed each year. It is the most common cause of death in children aged 1–14 years in the UK. There has been an apparent 43% increase in cancer incidence from 1996 to 2005, most likely related to improved cancer diagnosis and registration. Outcomes have improved markedly over the same period of time, owing to more intense treatment regimens with improved support and rescue therapies. The corollary of this is that there are more children surviving with long-term side effects from cancer treatments.

Cancer is 20% more common in boys than girls, with most tumours presenting in children less than 5 years of age. The most common diagnoses are leukaemia, CNS tumours and lymphomas; the overall 5-year survival rate is 78%, but survival varies greatly according to diagnosis (see Table 37.1). Brain and CNS tumours account for most deaths, and retinoblastoma has the best survival rate (99% cure).

Diagnosis in children is often delayed as childhood cancer is rare and slow to be considered. The child may have non-specific symptoms such as weight loss and listlessness, and then develop signs such as:

- Bruising and petechial haemorrhage, lymphadenopathy or bone pain (haematological malignancy);
- Abdominal distension or pain (Wilms' tumour (nephroblastoma), or neuroblastoma);
- Headache with ataxia (posterior fossa tumour).

Spread to distant sites and bone marrow is common at presentation. The parents are often devastated when the diagnosis is made, and the child frightened, upset and unwell.

One of the major achievements of paediatric cancer treatment, and one of the factors that has led to improvements in outcome, has been the centralisation of care and the development of international research registries. The UK Children's Cancer and Leukaemia Group (CCLG) is the national association for the treatment of cancer in children and young people. More than 70% of children with cancer in the United Kingdom are registered as part of a national or international clinical trial. The CCLG is also a registered charity and provides support and information for children and their families. There are currently 21 specialist centres with multidisciplinary teams undertaking the treatment of cancer in children in the United Kingdom, with 'shared-care'

Table 37.1 UK children's cancer incidence and 5-year survival rates

	Incidence Children <14 years (% all cases)	Five-year survival (%)
Leukaemia	31	
Acute lymphoblastic leukaemia		88
Acute myeloid leukaemia		64
CNS tumours	25	
Astrocytoma		81
Ependymoma and choroid plexus tumours		67
Embryonal CNS tumours		56
Other gliomas		44
Lymphoma	10	
Hodgkin's lymphoma		95
Non-Hodgkin's lymphoma		83
Soft tissue tumours	7	
Rhabdomyosarcoma		63
Neuroblastoma	6	64
Nephroblastoma	6	85
Retinoblastoma	3	99
Bone tumours	4	
Ewing sarcoma of bone		64
Osteosarcoma		54
Germ cell tumours	3	
Melanoma / epithelioma	3	
Hepatic tumours	1	

Source: UK National Registry of Childhood Tumours 2001–2005, from Cancer Research UK Childhood Cancer – Great Britain and UK.
http://publications.cancerresearchuk.org/downloads/product/CSCHILD10childhood.pdf

with non-specialist centres. Treatment is continued over several months or years, and shared care allows children to stay as close to home as possible.

Anaesthesia may be required at many stages of the care of children with malignancy, for instance BMA, LP or biopsy for diagnosis or staging, routine scans, line insertion or definitive surgery. The anaesthetist must be aware of how the condition affects the child, the effects of treatment, and whether the child has undergone surgery, radiotherapy or chemotherapy, or a combination of these. Children with cancer require repeated anaesthetics – some may be relatively well, receiving long-term maintenance chemotherapy, but some may be acutely unwell as a result of their treatment or a complication of treatment.

Treatment of specific conditions

Current approaches to cancer treatment depend on clinical features and biological characteristics of the tumour, response to treatment, and extent of residual disease (see Table 37.2). An aggressive approach is used to chemotherapy, which requires close monitoring with repeated scans and BMAs.

Chemotherapy is given in cycles to increase efficacy and allow time for recovery. It is given either orally (PO) or IV, with intrathecal chemotherapy given to treat overt or potential CNS disease.

Standard-risk acute lymphoblastic leukaemia (ALL)

Treatment of standard-risk childhood acute lymphoblastic leukaemia has a relatively good prognosis, so the aim is to limit exposure to drugs associated with late toxic effects. Children receive induction therapy over 4 weeks to induce remission in blood and bone marrow (steroids and vincristine), with treatment of CNS disease (intrathecal methotrexate), possible intensification blocks to remove residual cells (methotrexate or asparaginase), and a maintenance phase of daily 6-mercaptopurine (6-MP) PO, with weekly methotrexate PO, and 6-weekly intrathecal methotrexate to prevent CNS recurrence. This treatment continues for 2–3 years.

High-risk ALL

High-risk ALL includes presentation <1 year of age, those presenting with high white cell count or CNS disease at diagnosis, those with chromosomal

Table 37.2 Treatment for children's cancers

Cancer	Treatment
Acute lymphoblastic leukaemia	Steroids, chemotherapy, donor stem cell or bone marrow transplant if relapse
Acute myeloid leukaemia	Chemotherapy, donor stem cell or bone marrow transplant if relapse
Hodgkin's lymphoma	Surgery (stage 1 disease), chemotherapy, radiotherapy
Non-Hodgkin's lymphoma	Chemotherapy, radiotherapy, donor stem cell or bone marrow transplant if relapse
Brain and CNS tumours	Surgery, chemotherapy, radiotherapy for children >3 years
Neuroblastoma	Surgery, chemotherapy, stem cell transplant, monoclonal antibody
Retinoblastoma	Surgery, laser, cryotherapy, chemotherapy, radiotherapy
Nephroblastoma	Surgery, chemotherapy, radiotherapy
Osteosarcoma	Surgery, chemotherapy, radiotherapy
Rhabdomyosarcoma	Surgery, chemotherapy, radiotherapy

abnormalities such as the Philadelphia chromosome, or with poor response to induction treatment with increased minimal residual disease (MRD) in bone marrow. These children are treated with more intensive chemotherapy regimens associated with increased short- and long-term side effects, as for AML (see below). Stem cell transplantation may be offered when the child is in first remission or presents with recurrent disease. Radiotherapy may be used for children presenting with CNS or testicular disease.

Acute myeloid leukaemia

Acute myeloid leukaemia (AML) has a lower cure rate; treatment involves high dose induction and intensification chemotherapy that may induce prolonged marrow suppression requiring in-patient stay, with associated episodes of febrile neutropenia or mucositis. Stem cell transplantation is often used for children with high-risk disease.

Solid tumours

For solid tumours such as Wilms' or neuroblastoma, tumour staging is carried out at diagnosis with CT/ MRI, bone marrow and tumour biopsy. Current UK practice is to reduce tumour size and vascularity with several courses of chemotherapy prior to definitive surgery, followed by further courses of chemotherapy or radiotherapy (see Chapter 20).

Tumours associated with anterior mediastinal mass

Children presenting with T-cell ALL, lymphomas, neuroblastoma or intrathoracic germ cell tumour may present with a mass in the anterior mediastinum. This may result in airway compression, SVC obstruction or cardiorespiratory collapse in severe cases.

Anaesthesia is required for tumour staging and line insertion. Induction of anaesthesia is particularly high risk for children with an anterior mediastinal mass. Complications have been reported in up to 20% of cases, mainly relating to respiratory compromise (desaturation). Features suggesting increased risk include:

- History of cardiovascular collapse
- Stridor
- Orthopnoea
- Wheeze
- Upper body oedema
- Compression of major vessels or airway on CT

Timing of procedures such as diagnostic BMA, LP and line insertion should be made after discussion with the oncology team. A possible option is to start chemotherapy and monitor symptoms. Biopsies need to be undertaken within 5 days of starting treatment if an accurate tissue diagnosis is to be obtained.

Bone marrow transplantation

Bone marrow transplantation is used to treat high-risk malignant disease such as relapsed ALL or AML, or non-malignant disease such as aplastic anaemia, severe combined immune deficiency, sickle cell anaemia or inborn errors of metabolism. Stem cells

may be obtained from the patient (autologous transplant), or from a matched related or unrelated donor (allogeneic transplant). Autologous transplant is used as 'rescue' after high-dose chemotherapy, and allogeneic transplant is used for treatment of malignant or non-malignant disease.

Autologous stem cells may be obtained from bone marrow harvest or peripheral blood (PBSC). PBSC are harvested by apheresis after granulocyte colony stimulating factor (G-CSF) is given to increase the stem cell count in peripheral blood. Allogeneic stem cells may be obtained from bone marrow, peripheral blood or cord blood. Children donating bone marrow to a sibling require general anaesthesia. The child is placed in the prone position and a volume of approximately $10 \, ml \, kg^{-1}$ marrow is collected under aseptic conditions. Intravenous fluids and multimodal analgesia are required. The relative risks and benefits of the procedure to the healthy donor should be considered.

The recipient receives 'conditioning' chemotherapy and/or total body irradiation prior to transplant, followed by reinfusion of harvested stem cells. Conditioning may result in complete ablation of the recipient bone marrow to remove residual cancer cells, but less aggressive regimens associated with fewer complications are currently being investigated, particularly for non-malignant conditions. The child will require intensive supportive therapy after conditioning and until engraftment occurs, and will be extremely vulnerable to infection. Full barrier precautions should be used when treating these patients.

Graft versus host disease

Graft versus host disease (GvHD) is the term given to the immunological reaction of donor cells introduced to an immunocompromised host. It is usual after allogeneic bone marrow transplantation, and is an indication that engraftment is taking place. It may be useful to clear residual cancer cells. GvHD may also be seen after transfusion of non-irradiated blood to an immunocompromised patient (transfusion-related GvHD, see below).

Acute GvHD occurs within 100 days of transplant and is associated with generalised skin rash, hepatitis and diarrhoea. Severe GvHD has a high mortality. Chronic GvHD occurs later with a more indolent course with characteristics of a chronic autoimmune disease affecting multiple organ systems, including skin, liver and gastrointestinal tract.

Severe GvHD should ideally be prevented, for instance by improved matching of donor and recipient, by less severe recipient conditioning regimens, and also by avoiding non-irradiated blood in vulnerable patients. Treatment is supportive, including immunosuppression (e.g. steroids, tacrolimus, ciclosporin, mycophenolate (MMF)) or immunotherapy. Children with severe GvHD usually require admission to PICU.

Side effects of chemotherapy treatment

Cytotoxic agents commonly induce bone marrow suppression, hair loss, and nausea and vomiting. A number of agents also have other specific side effects, described in Table 37.3. Children with bone marrow suppression require support with platelet and red cell transfusions, and they may require broad-spectrum antibiotics and removal of a central venous line during a period of febrile neutropenia. G-CSF may be given to aid recovery from neutropenia, and allows more intense chemotherapy to be given in high-risk disease. Some specific complications of treatment relevant to the anaesthetist are described below.

Steroids and tumour lysis syndrome

Steroids are the mainstay of treatment in ALL, but they are given in short courses, so adrenal suppression is rarely a problem.

Tumour lysis syndrome results from the massive release of intracellular metabolites. It is seen in the first 12–72 hours of the start of treatment in children with high tumour load or high proliferative rate, or those where tumours are very chemo-sensitive. Anaesthetists should be aware that tumour lysis syndrome may be triggered by dexamethasone given as an antiemetic to a child in an at-risk category; dexamethasone must be avoided in this situation.

Children at risk of tumour lysis syndrome include those with:

- High-count ALL
- AML
- Hodgkin's lymphoma, non-Hodgkin's lymphoma, Burkitt's lymphoma

Tumour lysis results in hyperuricaemia, hyperkalaemia, hyperphosphataemia, hypocalcaemia and uraemia,

Table 37.3 Commonly used agents and side effects of treatment

Drug	Conditions treated	Common side effects of drug
Vincristine	ALL	Myelosuppression, syndrome of inappropriate antidiuretic hormone (SIADH), peripheral neuropathy, mucositis
Anthracyclines (daunorubicin, doxorubicin, epirubicin)	Acute leukaemia, sarcoma, Wilms' tumour, neuroblastoma, Hodgkin's disease	Myelosuppression, cardiomyopathy, arrhythmias
Cyclophosphamide	Non-Hodgkin's lymphoma, neuroblastoma, sarcoma, conditioning prior to bone marrow transplant	Myelosuppression, cardiomyopathy, arrhythmias, haemorrhagic cystitis
Ifosfamide	Non-Hodgkin's lymphoma, sarcoma, bone tumours	Myelosuppression, Fanconi's syndrome, renal failure
Cisplatin	Neuroblastoma, germ cell tumour	Seizures, hypomagnesaemia, renal failure
L-Asparaginase	ALL	Coagulopathy, allergic reaction, pancreatitis
Nitrosureas		Pneumonitis, renal failure
Bleomycin	Hodgkin's disease, germ cell tumours	Allergic reactions, pulmonary fibrosis, Reynaud's
Methotrexate	ALL	Myelosuppression, mucositis, pneumonitis, renal failure
Actinomycin D	Wilms' tumour, sarcoma	Coagulopathy, liver failure, acute respiratory distress syndrome
Busulfan	Conditioning prior to bone marrow transplant	Hepatic veno-occlusive disease, seizures

and is associated with deposits of uric acid or calcium phosphate in the renal tubules. Children present with nausea and vomiting, muscle cramps, renal impairment, seizures or arrhythmias. Children who are at risk should be closely monitored and treated with hydration and rasburicase, which promotes the metabolism of uric acid to soluble metabolites, or allopurinol, which reduces the formation of uric acid.

Mucositis

Mucositis is painful inflammation and ulceration of all mucous membranes, seen in all children receiving high-dose chemotherapy, 50% of children receiving head and neck radiotherapy, and 5–10% of children receiving standard chemotherapy. Severe mucositis may limit therapy. Treatment is symptomatic with intravenous fluids and total parenteral nutrition (TPN) if required. Abdominal pain should be treated with IV morphine PCA or NCA, with added ketamine if required.

Vincristine

Vincristine is neurotoxic; children are monitored for possible sensory or motor neuropathy, and doses adjusted accordingly.

Vincristine and other vinca alkaloids such as vinblastine and vindesine are universally fatal if given intrathecally. There have been more than 50 deaths reported internationally involving accidental intrathecal administration of vinca alkaloids, often with systems errors and human factors identified as the root cause. Administration of chemotherapy in the United Kingdom is now tightly regulated, and can only be given by registered individuals with appropriate training, in designated areas, and following specified checks. Intrathecal and intravenous agents are given on different days, and vincristine is often prepared in intravenous mini-bags to prevent accidental intrathecal administration. Non-Luer spinal needles that are incompatible with intravenous Luer connections are being introduced into clinical practice to prevent such accidents in future.

Anthracyclines and other agents associated with cardiac toxicity

Anthracyclines (doxorubicin, daunorubicin, epirubicin) are commonly used in children with the following conditions:

- AML
- Non-Hodgkin's lymphoma (NHL)
- Wilms' tumour
- Neuroblastoma
- Bone tumours

Anthracyclines are cardiotoxic, particularly when given in high dose. Risk factors for anthracycline cardiotoxicity include treatment for relapsed disease, high cumulative dose ($>300\,\mathrm{mg\,m^{-2}}$), associated radiotherapy, and if there have been signs of early cardiac toxicity. All children are monitored with routine echocardiograms during treatment and long-term follow-up. Mortality associated with overt cardiomyopathy is high (50%), and many of these children will be candidates for cardiac transplantation. Subclinical cardiomyopathy is common (a degree of cardiac impairment has been reported in up to 65% of such children) and may become be un-masked at times of increased demand, such as puberty, pregnancy or intercurrent illness, and possibly during anaesthesia and surgery. A high index of suspicion should be maintained when anaesthetising these children, and a recent echo should be available.

Cyclophosphamide is associated with cardiomyopathy or cardiac arrhythmias when used in high dose to induce bone marrow ablation (conditioning) prior to bone marrow transplant. Fluorouracil is occasionally associated with cardiac toxicity.

Bleomycin

Bleomycin is used in the treatment of children with Hodgkin's lymphoma and germ cell tumours. It is associated with an inflammatory pneumonitis and progressive pulmonary fibrosis, particularly when given in high doses. Risk factors for bleomycin toxicity include increasing age (toxicity rarely seen in children), increasing dose, radiotherapy, and renal impairment.

Bleomycin is used to induce fibrosis in animal models of pulmonary fibrosis, and is deactivated in the lungs by pulmonary hydroxylases. The role of oxygen in promoting bleomycin toxicity is controversial, with evidence mainly from case reviews. Hyperoxia should be avoided after recent exposure to bleomycin and if there is evidence of pre-existing pulmonary disease. It is sensible to use the lowest possible inspired oxygen during anaesthesia.

Table 37.4 Minimum platelet count for oncology procedures

Procedure	Platelet count (×10⁹ l⁻¹)
Line insertion	100
LP	50
Trephine	20
BMA	No minimum count specified

Table 37.5 Alternative anaesthesia protocols for short oncology procedures such as BMA, LP or trephine

Propofol 3–5 mg kg⁻¹ IV + remifentanil 1 mcg kg⁻¹ IV bolus Repeat propofol 1–2 mg kg⁻¹ IV if required
Propofol 3–5 mg kg⁻¹ IV + alfentanil 5 mcg kg⁻¹ IV bolus Repeat propofol 1–2 mg kg⁻¹ IV if required

Anaesthesia for LP and BMA

In our institution, oncology procedures are undertaken on dedicated lists, usually in the dedicated procedure unit, with a senior nurse acting as a list coordinator to book patients, coordinate review by the oncologists and prepare children with up-to-date blood counts. It is our preference to provide general anaesthesia for these short painful procedures, rather than deep sedation or local anaesthesia alone.

From an anaesthesia perspective, the child requires careful assessment, particularly if newly diagnosed, receiving high-dose chemotherapy or suffering from acute GvHD. Active sepsis should be excluded. Children on long-term maintenance chemotherapy are generally well and often develop their own particular 'routine', which is helpful for the anaesthetist to follow.

Commonly accepted minimum platelet counts for procedures are shown in Table 37.4.

BMA and LP are quick procedures and ideally suited to TIVA with propofol, with assisted/spontaneous ventilation with a facemask. This technique facilitates early discharge home (see Table 37.5 for suggested protocol). Supplementary local anaesthesia and IV paracetamol are indicated if bone marrow trephine is performed.

Children usually have an in-dwelling central line, which may be used for anaesthesia provided full aseptic precautions are taken when accessing the line. *It is the responsibility of the anaesthetist to ensure that the line is flushed after use to remove residual anaesthesia drugs.*

Anaesthesia for radiotherapy

Targeted radiotherapy is used as a primary therapy or to clear microscopic disease in children with CNS tumours, Hodgkin's lymphoma, Wilms' tumour, neuroblastoma and sarcoma of bone and soft tissue.

Radiotherapy is delivered in fractionated daily doses over 6 weeks; side effects are localised to the area of treatment, and may include redness and blistering of the skin, mucositis, neurocognitive impairment and pituitary damage. Damage to normal tissue is minimised by use of three-dimensional targeted beams (3D conformational radiotherapy, 3D CRT), and modulating the intensity of the beams (intensity modulated radiotherapy, IMRT). Proton beam radiotherapy enables treatment to be targeted at a precise depth, ideal for cranial irradiation in children. It is only currently available in the United States, but units are planned in the United Kingdom. Radiotherapy units are usually based in adult hospitals, and special arrangements may need to be made for paediatric patients.

Each treatment typically takes 10–45 minutes. The child must remain by themselves in the treatment room and is required to wear an immobilisation device. With careful preparation and play therapy, treatment can often be performed without sedation in children >8 years (and some younger children). When required, a propofol-based anaesthetic is ideal with an LMA for airway control. As for any anaesthesia service for children, trained staff and full monitoring are required. The anaesthetist cannot stay with the child during treatment, and output from the monitors must be relayed to the control room.

Rare 'non-malignant' medical conditions

Haemophagocytic lymphocytic histiocytosis

Haemophagocytic lymphocytic histiocytosis (HLH) is a rare disease presenting in infancy associated with high mortality. It is caused by activation of normal macrophages and T-lymphocytes which results in an overwhelming inflammatory response with release of cytokines and phagocytosis of normal cells by activated macrophages. It is inherited as an autosomal recessive condition, but secondary HLH may occur in older children after systemic infection, immune deficiency or associated with underlying malignancy. Typical presentation is with fever, skin rash, hepatosplenomegaly and pancytopenia. CNS involvement including seizures is common. Skin, lymph node, liver and bone marrow biopsy confirm diagnosis. Treatment is with supportive therapy followed by bone marrow transplantation.

Langerhans cell histiocytosis

Langerhans cell histiocytosis (LCH) is a rare condition, previously known as histiocytosis X. It is a proliferative disorder of epidermal Langerhans cells, typically associated with lytic lesions in bone, with skin involvement in many cases. Controversy exists as to whether LCH is an inflammatory or malignant condition, but recent evidence suggests that it is a distinct myeloid neoplasm. There is a spectrum of disease, with three typical presentations:

- Eosinophilic granuloma. One or more bone lesions, classically in the skull, but may affect other sites, including vertebra or femur. Recurrent mastoiditis and otitis media may occur because of destruction of the mastoid bone. Diabetes insipidus may occur because of destruction of the sella turcica.
- Hand–Schüller–Christian disease. Multifocal disease with classical triad of bony defects of the skull, exophthalmos and diabetes insipidus. Mucocutaneous and systemic involvement may occur.
- Letterer–Siwe disease. Fulminant disorder associated with generalised skin rash, fever, hepatosplenomegaly, lymphadenopathy, bone lesions and marrow infiltration.

Diagnosis is by imaging, skin or bone marrow biopsy. Isolated LCH of bone may be treated by surgical curettage and local injection of steroid. Mild systemic LCH is treated by chemotherapy, particularly where LCH involves vulnerable sites such as the skull or there is a risk of fracture; multisystem disease is treated by chemotherapy, but may be associated with up to 20% mortality. Children with diabetes insipidus should continue desmopressin (DDAVP) in the perioperative period.

Severe combined immune deficiency

Severe combined immune deficiency (SCID) is associated with life-threatening infection, dermatitis, diarrhoea and failure to thrive. SCID results from one of a range of gene defects causing impairment of T-cell, B-cell and NK-cell function. It is inherited as an autosomal recessive condition, X-linked or may be sporadic. A subgroup of children with immune deficiency and DiGeorge syndrome have a hypoplasia of the thymus with absent T-cells (associated with chromosome 22q11 deletion).

Children with SCID present with severe opportunistic infection in the first 3 months of life, which may be bacterial, viral or fungal, for example *Candida* or *Aspergillus*. Without treatment, SCID is usually fatal by 2 years of age. Allogeneic bone marrow transplantation is ideally performed before the age of 6 months to avoid the effects of repeated infections. Children with SCID or other conditions associated with immune deficiency must not receive live vaccines. They must only receive irradiated blood products to prevent GvHD from immunocompetent lymphocytes in donor blood or blood products.

Neuromuscular disorders and myopathy

Muscle biopsy may be required as a diagnostic procedure in children with suspected neuromuscular disorders or in children with mitochondrial myopathy. Muscle is taken from the anterolateral aspect of the thigh, either as a needle biopsy, or excised as a small strip. It is a short painful procedure, usually requiring general anaesthesia, although it can be performed under regional block in older children.

The choice of anaesthesia for muscle biopsy may be difficult. Volatile agents may cause anaesthesia-induced rhabdomyolysis (AIR) in patients with one of the muscular dystrophies, or may trigger malignant hyperthermia (MH) in susceptible patients. Conversely, TIVA using propofol may cause propofol-related infusion syndrome (PRIS), particularly if the child has a mitochondrial disorder. PRIS is associated with metabolic acidosis, lipidaemia, bradycardia, rhabdomyolysis and heart failure.

Suxamethonium must not be used in any patient with abnormal muscle, as fasciculations may cause hyperkalaemic cardiac arrest. Non-depolarising muscle relaxants should be avoided or used in reduced dose in a child who has a myopathy.

Children presenting for muscle biopsy usually fall into four main categories:

- *The child presents for investigation as a 'floppy baby'.* It is best to use a volatile anaesthetic rather than use TIVA, which may not be a familiar technique in this age group and may induce significant hypotension.

- *An older child is being investigated for MH or suspected central core disease.* A trigger-free anaesthetic must be given. Central core disease is associated with a mutation of the RyR1 gene and an abnormality of the intracellular ryanodine receptor. It is inherited as an autosomal dominant, but sporadic cases occur. Children present with hypotonia from birth, with truncal weakness, delayed motor milestones, muscle cramps, mild facial weakness, contractures and scoliosis. The disease is slowly progressive, but children generally walk. There is a characteristic appearance on biopsy, and a genetic test from a blood sample is also available.

- *A boy with raised creatinine kinase (CK) is being investigated for failure to walk, aged 3–4 years.* The likely diagnosis is Duchenne muscular dystrophy (DMD). TIVA with propofol should probably be given as volatile agents may trigger AIR and hyperkalaemic cardiac arrest, usually in recovery when the child starts to move again. There is usually a family history in a boy with DMD, with characteristic hypertrophic calves and global hypotonia. A raised CK should act as a 'red flag' for the anaesthetist. Volatile agents have been used uneventfully in this group of patients, but are best avoided, particularly in the young DMD patients when they still have significant muscle mass. If it is not possible to obtain venous access in these patients, it is acceptable to use a volatile agent for induction, then switch to TIVA.

- *The child is suspected to have a mitochondrial myopathy.* Prolonged high-dose propofol infusion should be avoided. Mitochondrial myopathies are associated with abnormalities of electron train transport or oxidative phosphorylation. Mitochondrial disorders may be associated with myopathy, encephalopathy, epilepsy, lactic acidosis or gastrointestinal disorders. Mitochondrial myopathies are not associated with MH, and volatile agents are safe. The child should

also be given dextrose-containing intravenous fluids to avoid lactic acidosis.

A careful history should be taken, and the case discussed with the referring team with respect to their 'best guess' diagnosis, so that the risks and benefits of each different technique can be decided. It may be logical to use TIVA as the default technique for all patients (except babies); it avoids the risk of MH or rhabdomyolysis, and since muscle biopsy takes less than 15 minutes, the exposure to propofol will not be long enough to develop PRIS in children with mitochondrial myopathies.

Anaesthesia may be given by intermittent bolus injection, and the airway controlled with an LMA – mix propofol 200 mg with alfentanil 1 mg in a 20 ml syringe and give propofol $3–5\,mg\,kg^{-1}$ for induction, with increments as required.

Juvenile arthritis

Juvenile idiopathic arthritis (JIA) is an autoimmune condition associated with painful swollen joints that may affect children from around 6 months of age. There are a number of different types of JIA, including:

- Systemic JIA. Associated with fevers, rash, lymphadenopathy and splenomegaly. Inflammation and stiffness may affect any joint.

- Oligoarthritis. Pain, stiffness and swelling affecting the wrists and knees.

- Polyarticular arthritis. Affects small joints of the hands, weight bearing joints and the neck, more common in girls than boys. Fifteen per cent of children are rheumatoid factor positive, and may develop joint damage and erosions.

- Psoriatic arthritis. Associated with psoriatic rash and/or family history of psoriasis.

The treatment of JIA is analgesia (NSAIDs), physiotherapy and exercise. Children who do not respond may be treated with oral methotrexate. Injections of steroid help to reduce pain and disability associated with an acute exacerbation. These procedures are usually undertaken as day cases. Joints to be injected should be clearly marked, and an image intensifier should be available. For large joints, the steroid may be combined with local anaesthetic to reduce postoperative pain. Injections into multiple small joints are more painful, and morphine may be required.

Key points

- The demand for anaesthesia services outside the main theatre is rising; the same standard of care should be available in all areas.
- Children receiving chemotherapy may be unwell if newly diagnosed or receiving high-dose chemotherapy or suffering from sepsis, or they may be in good health if receiving long-term maintenance treatment. High-dose anthracyclines may cause cardiomyopathy.
- The choice of anaesthetic for undiagnosed muscle biopsy is difficult. TIVA is preferred in older children to prevent anaesthesia-induced rhabdomyolysis and reduce the risk of MH. PRIS is unlikely after a short procedure. Volatile agents are safer in babies.

- Children undergoing joint injections are managed as day cases; adequate analgesia is required.

Further reading

Culshaw V, Yule M, Lawson R. Considerations for anaesthesia in children with haematological malignancy undergoing short procedures. *Paed Anes* 2003;**13**:375–83.

Kinder Ross A. Muscular dystrophy versus mitochondrial myopathy; the dilemma of the undiagnosed child. *Ped Anes* 2007;**17**:1–6.

McFadyen JG, Pelly N, Orr RJ. Sedation and anesthesia for the pediatric patient undergoing radiation therapy. *Curr Opin Anesthesiol* 2011;**24**:433–8.

38

Principles of paediatric resuscitation

Jonathan Smith

Introduction

Cardiac arrest in a child is very stressful for everyone concerned but fortunately these events are rare. Recent advances have shown that good-quality resuscitation can lead to improved outcomes. Paediatric resuscitation is considered a core skill for anaesthetists, so it is important to practise and refine these skills on a regular basis, both as an individual and as a team within the workplace. This chapter will describe the principles of resuscitation for the following age groups: 'infants' (0–12 months), 'children' (1–11 years) and 'adolescents' (12–18 years). Resuscitation sequences in adolescents are the same as for adults.

Epidemiology of cardiorespiratory arrest in children

Cardiorespiratory arrest in a child is usually secondary to an underlying illness associated with respiratory and/or circulatory failure. In contrast to adults, primary cardiac arrest in a child of any age is rare. The typical picture is one of worsening tissue hypoxia and acidosis over time, leading to bradycardia and then asystole. Paediatric resuscitation guidelines differ slightly from adult guidelines to reflect the underlying aetiology of cardiac arrest in children.

Overall the incidence of out of hospital cardiac arrest (OHCA) in children and adolescents is much lower than in adults, and their probability of survival to discharge is greater. In infants, the rate of OHCA and survival to discharge is similar to adults, mainly owing to cases of sudden infant death syndrome (SIDS). Children who suffer an in-hospital cardiac arrest are twice as likely to survive as adults. The most common arrest rhythm in paediatrics is asystole (40%), then pulseless electrical activity (24%) and finally ventricular fibrillation or pulseless ventricular tachycardia (14%).

Basic life support (BLS) in children

Bystander cardiopulmonary resuscitation (CPR) more than doubles patient survival rates but is performed on only 30% of children who have suffered an OHCA. This lack of bystander response may be due to a fear of doing harm, but it is clear that any form of resuscitation (including compression or ventilation-only techniques) is better than no CPR. Resuscitation guidelines have therefore been simplified to avoid confusion and hopefully increase bystander CPR rates. Conventional CPR (ventilation with compression) has been shown to be more effective than compression-only CPR in children (see Figure 38.1).

The 'SAFE' approach

The SAFE approach is used (Shout for help; Approach with care; Free from danger; Evaluate ABC).

Responsiveness

Responsiveness should be assessed by placing one hand firmly on the child's forehead (to immobilise the neck) and then gently stimulating the child while asking, 'Are you all right?' Small children and those who are scared or in pain are unlikely to respond meaningfully to direct questions, but may open their eyes or make some sound.

Core Topics in Paediatric Anaesthesia, ed. Ian James and Isabeau Walker. Published by Cambridge University Press. © 2013 Cambridge University Press.

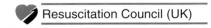

2010 Resuscitation Guidelines

Resuscitation Council (UK)

Paediatric Basic Life Support
(Healthcare professionals with a duty to respond)

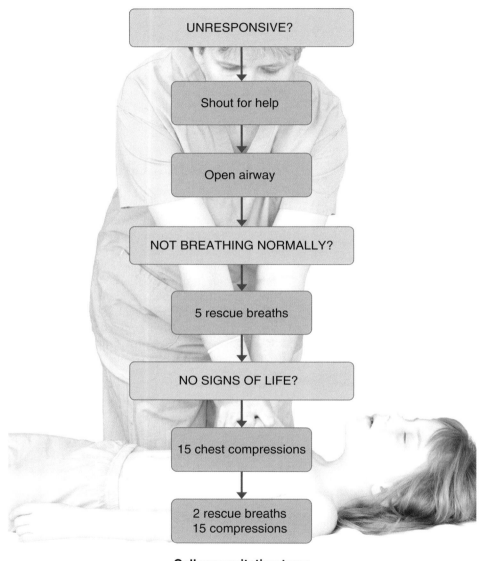

UNRESPONSIVE?

Shout for help

Open airway

NOT BREATHING NORMALLY?

5 rescue breaths

NO SIGNS OF LIFE?

15 chest compressions

2 rescue breaths
15 compressions

Call resuscitation team

October 2010

5th Floor, Tavistock House North, Tavistock Square, London WC1H 9HR
Telephone (020) 7388-4678 . Fax (020) 7383-0773 . Email enquiries@resus.org.uk
www.resus.org.uk . Registered Charity No. 286360

Figure 38.1 Paediatric basic life support. See plate section for colour version.

Airway (A)

The airway needs to be open for any resuscitation attempts to succeed. Conscious children who are having difficulty breathing will find a position that best maintains their airway. Further airway manoeuvres are avoided in these children and they should be transferred to an area where advanced airway equipment is available. If the child is unresponsive they should be placed supine and the mouth inspected visually for any foreign body. A blind finger sweep is not recommended in children as it may impact a foreign body further into the airway. If no trauma is suspected a *chin lift* manoeuvre is then performed. Chin lift is performed by placing one hand on the child's forehead, and extending the head on the neck (to a *neutral* position in infants and a *sniffing* position in children) while lifting the chin upwards with the other hand. The airway is then assessed by the rescuer who places their ear to the mouth and nose of the child while looking at their chest. The rescuer then:

- *Looks* (for chest or abdominal movement);
- *Listens* (for breath sounds); and
- *Feels* (for breath) for up to 10 seconds.

If there is chest or abdominal movement but no breath is felt or heard then a *jaw thrust* manoeuvre can be tried. This is the preferred airway manoeuvre in cases of suspected trauma and it is performed by lifting the jaw forward by pushing upwards with the fingers from behind the mandible. There should be minimal movement of the cervical spine during this manoeuvre.

Breathing (B)

Breathing should be assessed within 10 seconds of the airway being open, and may be adequate, gasping or inadequate. If there is any doubt then *five rescue breaths* should be delivered. This is different from the adult guidelines and takes into account that children are more likely to be hypoxic in the peri-arrest phase. The timely delivery of rescue breaths may be enough to prevent asystole in a child with bradycardia due to hypoxia.

The airway should be maintained as described above and the rescue breaths delivered either by mouth-to-mouth, mouth-to-mouth-and-nose (using a face shield if available), mouth-to-mask, or using an Ambu bag and mask (BVM). There should be no

delay. Rescue breaths should be 1–1.5 seconds in length and be of sufficient pressure to make the chest rise. If the rescue breaths fail to make the chest rise then the airway should be reassessed, an alternative manoeuvre performed to open the airway and a foreign body excluded.

Circulation (C)

The circulation should be assessed for up to 10 seconds after the rescue breaths have been delivered. A *central* pulse should be palpated and a search made for any *signs of life* such as breathing, coughing or movement. In children the carotid artery should be palpated, in infants either the brachial or femoral pulses should be assessed. *Chest compressions* should be started if there is *no pulse, a pulse of less than 60 with poor perfusion, or no signs of life.*

Chest compressions are performed one finger's breadth above the xiphisternum in all ages. The aim is to deliver compressions at least one-third the depth of the child's chest. In infants the lone rescuer should use two fingers to compress the chest, but if there are two rescuers then one should 'encircle' the chest with both hands placing both thumbs on the sternum while the other rescuer maintains the airway and performs ventilations.

- *Compression rates and ratios* have been standardised for all age groups. The aim of this is to simplify the resuscitation guidelines and encourage bystander CPR. The phrase '*Push hard and fast*' should be used when describing how to perform chest compressions as evidence shows that most people push too gently. It is essential to minimise interruptions to compressions and to ensure full chest recoil after each compression by releasing the pressure totally.
- Healthcare professionals performing CPR on children are recommended to perform chest compressions at a rate of *100–120 compressions per minute* with a ratio of *15 compressions to 2 breaths (30:2 in adults)*.
- Lay rescuers should perform CPR with a ratio of 30 compressions to 2 ventilations in both adults and children.

Once the child's trachea is intubated, continuous chest compressions should be performed at a rate of 100–120 per minute and the child should be ventilated at a rate of 10–12 breaths per minute.

Foreign body airway obstruction

Foreign body airway obstruction (see Figure 38.2) should be suspected if a child develops sudden onset of respiratory distress associated with coughing, gagging or stridor. The episodes are often witnessed and associated with a history of eating or playing with small items. A blind finger sweep should *never* be used in this situation, but the mouth should be carefully inspected to see if any foreign body can be hooked out with the finger.

The following sequence of events should be followed

- If there is an *effective cough* then the child should be observed until the obstruction is relieved.
- A conscious child with an *ineffective cough* should be treated with 5 back blows alternating with 5 chest thrusts (infants) or 5 abdominal thrusts (child >1 year). If possible the child should be held in a head-down position (over the rescuer's knees) during the thrusts to encourage the obstruction to move away from the larynx.
- An *unconscious child* should be placed supine and any obvious obstruction removed from the mouth. Five rescue breaths should be performed. If there is no chest movement then chest compressions should be commenced in the hope that the increase in intrathoracic pressure will expel the obstruction. BLS should be performed for 1 minute and then the emergency medical services contacted.

Emergency medical services

For children in cardiopulmonary arrest, emergency medical services (EMS) should be contacted after 1 minute of CPR. Most children collapse from a respiratory cause so the priority should be *airway* and *ventilation*. Adult resuscitation guidelines recommend alerting the EMS before commencing CPR as the priority is early defibrillation. This is only appropriate in children who are seen to collapse suddenly or who have a known cardiac condition and no preceding respiratory distress. In these scenarios the cause of the arrest is more likely to be an arrhythmia and early defibrillation will improve survival.

Automatic external defibrillators

Automatic external defibrillators (AEDs) are increasingly available in public places. Studies have shown AEDs to be very accurate when analysing rhythms in children. Currently the recommendations are to use a standard adult AED for a child over 8 years old. An AED with a paediatric dose attenuator should be used on children aged 1–8 years. Paediatric dose attenuators are a set of adhesive pads that limit the defibrillation energy to 50 J. There is a picture of a child on the packet and the leads often have a plug shaped as a teddy bear. Currently there is no evidence for or against the use of AEDs in children less than 1 year old. However, if faced with a pulseless infant who is not responding to CPR, the potential benefit of delivering a shock from an AED (if instructed to do so) outweighs the risks.

Improving BLS

High-quality BLS increases myocardial, cerebral and systemic perfusion. The key aims are to:
- Push hard
- Push fast
- Minimise interruptions
- Allow full chest recoil
- Avoid over-ventilation

Unfortunately, slow, shallow compressions (with many pauses) and over-ventilation are common during many arrests. Intensive training and feedback using force sensors and accelerometers can improve technique. Mechanical aids such as an 'active compression–decompression device' and an 'inspiratory impedance threshold device' are currently being evaluated. Both of these devices enhance negative intrathoracic pressure during the decompression phase to increase coronary, cerebral and systemic perfusion.

Advanced life support in children

Basic life support in the form of CPR should be continuous and of good quality. Trained healthcare professionals should institute advanced life support (ALS) measures such as a definitive airway, positive pressure ventilation with supplemental oxygen, cardioversion, intravenous (IV) access, drug administration, further monitoring and definitive treatments (see Figure 38.3).

Monitoring

Monitoring is an important part of ALS. In most cardiac arrest situations, monitoring is applied whilst an initial assessment is made. Minimal monitoring

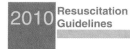
2010 Resuscitation Guidelines

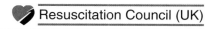
Resuscitation Council (UK)

Paediatric choking treatment algorithm

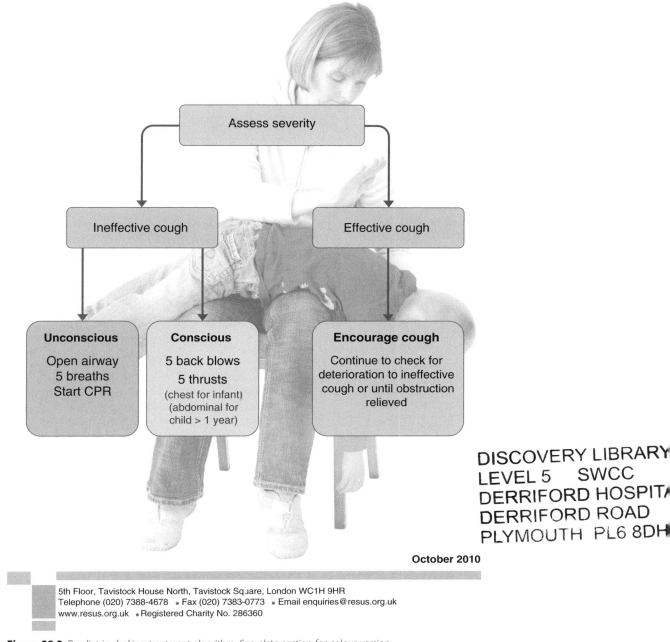

October 2010

5th Floor, Tavistock House North, Tavistock Square, London WC1H 9HR
Telephone (020) 7388-4678 • Fax (020) 7383-0773 • Email enquiries@resus.org.uk
www.resus.org.uk • Registered Charity No. 286360

Figure 38.2 Paediatric choking treatment algorithm. See plate section for colour version.

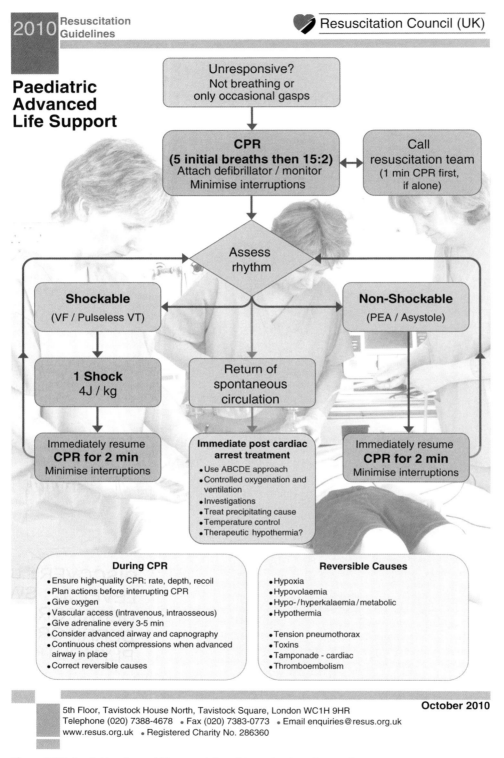

Figure 38.3 Paediatric advanced life support. See plate section for colour version.

that should be available includes: *electrocardiogram (ECG), pulse oximetry, end-tidal CO$_2$* and *blood pressure*. It is vital that the placement and interpretation of monitoring does not interfere with the continuous performance of good BLS.

Advanced airway manoeuvres

Advanced airway manoeuvres include the insertion of airway adjuncts such as oral or nasopharyngeal airways, laryngeal mask airway (LMA) insertion and tracheal tube placement.

- *Oropharyngeal (Guedel)* and *nasopharyngeal airways* are sized by holding the airway against the child's cheek. The oral airway should reach from the child's mouth to the angle of their jaw, while the nasal airway should reach from the nose to the tragus of the ear. Nasal airways should be used with caution where there is a history of trauma as there is a risk of disrupting a basal skull fracture.
- *Laryngeal mask airways* are particularly helpful in relieving upper airway obstruction caused by abnormalities such as micrognathia, macroglossia and craniofacial dysmorphism. However, the LMA cannot be used if airway reflexes are intact, and does not protect the airway or allow high-pressure ventilation. It is best used as a temporary measure.
- *Tracheal intubation* with an oral tube is the 'gold standard' advanced airway manoeuvre. The airway is secured and protected, and positive pressure ventilation with PEEP is facilitated.

Tracheal intubation in resuscitation

Tracheal tubes are sized according to their internal diameter (ID) in millimetres (mm). The following is a guide to size of tracheal tube in resuscitation:

- Neonates 2.5–3.5 mm ID
- Infants 4.0–4.5 mm ID
- Children over 1 year: (Age in years/4) + 4 mm ID

If the child's age is unknown the correct size of tube can be estimated using a resuscitation tape such as the Broselow tape. Alternatively, simply choose a tube with outer dimension the same as the child's little finger.

Traditionally uncuffed tracheal tubes have been used for children below the age of 8 years. Cuffed tubes should be used with caution in neonates because of the risk of subglottic stenosis. Cuffed tubes above 4.0 mm ID have some advantages over uncuffed tubes in resuscitation. Repeated laryngoscopy and intubation due to incorrect initial tube size can be avoided, and a cuffed tracheal tube offers the ability to deliver higher ventilatory pressures and PEEP in cases with poor lung compliance or pulmonary oedema.

Prolonged attempts at tracheal intubation can be traumatic, cause hypoxia and result in significant pauses in chest compressions. A time limit of 30 seconds should therefore be adhered to and repeated attempts avoided. *Good ventilation with a BVM is preferable to multiple prolonged attempts at tracheal intubation.*

Correct tracheal tube placement must be confirmed by the following:

- Direct visualisation of the tracheal tube passing through the vocal cords
- Presence of end-tidal CO$_2$ (there must be pulmonary blood flow present)
- Bilateral symmetrical chest movement and breath sounds
- Misting of the tube during expiration
- Improvement of oxygen saturation and heart rate
- Lack of gastric distension and air entry on inspiration
- Chest X-ray (tracheal tube tip between clavicles)

A combination of the above is needed to confirm the placement of the tracheal tube. If there is any doubt then the tube should be removed and BVM ventilation re-established.

Children with a tracheostomy

Children with tracheostomies are increasingly cared for in the community. A tracheostomy-dependent child may present acutely to their local hospital in great distress. It is essential to confirm that the airway is patent.

Persistent hypoxia despite a tracheal tube or tracheostomy *in situ*

This scenario can be faced in the emergency department, ambulance, during transfer, in the ward, intensive care unit or operating theatre. The key is to rapidly exclude a problem with the current airway. 'DOPES' is a useful acronym:

- **D**isplacement of the tube
- **O**bstruction of the tube

- **P**neumothorax
- **E**quipment failure
- **S**tomach (gastric distension)

Needle cricothyroidotomy

The scenario *'can't ventilate/can't intubate'* is fortunately very rare, and has been historically described in association with acute epiglottitis (fortunately epiglottitis is now uncommon since the introduction of *Haemophilus influenzae* b immunisation).

Once in the situation of being unable to ventilate and unable to intubate, the priority is to provide oxygen to the lungs. The quickest procedure is a needle cricothyroidotomy, which should be performed as described below:

- Place the patient supine with a roll under the shoulders;
- Attach a cricothyroidotomy needle (or large-bore cannula) to a 5 ml syringe;
- Identify the cricoid membrane between the thyroid and cricoid cartilages (or the space between the upper tracheal rings in an infant);
- Clean the neck with alcohol swabs;
- Stabilise the trachea with one hand;
- Insert the cannula in the midline at an angle of 45° caudal while aspirating.

Once air is aspirated, advance the cannula into the airway and dispose of the needle. The hub of the cannula should be attached to an oxygen supply that *must* incorporate an *open three-way tap, side port or Y-piece.*

- Set an oxygen flow rate (in litres per minute) equivalent to the child's age in years.
- To ventilate, occlude the open port for 1 second and observe the child's chest for movement.
- Allow passive exhalation by releasing the port for 4 seconds.
- Increase the oxygen flow by 1 litre per minute if the child's chest does not move.
- Re-assess the child's oxygenation.
- Secure the cannula and check the neck for air-leaks and surgical emphysema.

It is important to note that this technique will provide short-term oxygenation only; the minute volume achieved is minimal and carbon dioxide clearance will be inadequate. A definitive airway should be achieved as soon as possible, either by tracheal intubation or tracheostomy. A surgical airway may be the better first option.

Ventilation during ALS

Breathing is supported by positive pressure ventilation. Once the trachea has been intubated (or an LMA placed), continuous chest compressions can be given at a rate of $100–120 \, min^{-1}$, with the accompanying ventilation at a rate of $10–12 \, min^{-1}$. The pulmonary blood flow is very low during cardiopulmonary arrest so less ventilation is needed. Over-ventilation has been identified as a cause of decreased myocardial, cerebral and systemic perfusion during CPR.

Supplemental oxygen should be given at a concentration of 100% if the child is receiving CPR. If there is a perfusing rhythm, oxygen should be delivered to keep the oxygen saturation 94% or above. Hyperoxia in the post-resuscitation phase has been shown to be detrimental.

Circulation during ALS

Perfusion during CPR is totally dependent on chest compressions. The critical elements are to push hard and fast. Coronary perfusion pressure is dependent on aortic root pressure. It takes six to eight compressions to reach a perfusing aortic root pressure, which is lost immediately if the compressions stop. Allowing full chest recoil encourages venous return and hence systemic perfusion.

Cardiac rhythms in cardiopulmonary arrest

ECG monitoring should be commenced as soon as possible to identify the underlying rhythm. There should only be brief pauses in CPR to allow rhythm analysis. The common cardiac arrest rhythms are divided into 'non-shockable' and 'shockable' rhythms.

Non-shockable rhythms

- *Bradycardia* – heart rate is less than 60 beats $minute^{-1}$. CPR should be started. This is most commonly seen in response to hypoxia and will progress to asystole unless oxygenation is improved.
- *Asystole* – no electrical activity of the heart. The ECG is a flat line. Both leads and gain should be checked on the monitor to exclude disconnection and fine ventricular fibrillation (VF). This is the

most commonly seen rhythm in pulseless children as hypoxia causes bradycardia which progresses to asystole.

- *Pulseless electrical activity (PEA)* occurs when normal electrical complexes are present on the ECG but there is no palpable pulse.

The treatment of the non-shockable rhythms is continuous, good-quality CPR with adrenaline being given every 3–5 minutes.

There may be an identifiable and rapidly treatable cause of the PEA/asystole such as: *hypoxia, hypovolaemia, hypothermia, hyper/hypokalaemia, tension pneumothorax, pericardial tamponade, toxic substances, thromboembolic events.* These are known as the 4 Hs and 4 Ts and should be actively sought and treated as necessary (Figure 38.3).

Shockable rhythms

- *Ventricular fibrillation*
- *Pulseless ventricular tachycardia (VT)*

Shockable rhythms are relatively rare initial arrest rhythms in children. These rhythms should be suspected if there is a history of sudden collapse, hypothermia, previous cardiac disease or tricyclic poisoning. VF is characterised by chaotic complexes that are irregular in both their amplitude and rate. Pulseless VT is characterised by a tachycardia of wide complexes that are of similar shape and occur at regular intervals.

Rapid defibrillation is the treatment of choice and if delivered promptly survival from these rhythms is much more likely than from asystole or PEA.

Defibrillation

Defibrillation can be performed with either an AED device or a manual defibrillator. AEDs have been discussed above. Manual defibrillators with a set of adult and paediatric paddles (8–12 cm and 4.5 cm respectively) should be available in all areas where children are treated. Modern machines will come with a set of sticky pads that will save time, as they only have to be placed once at the start of the resuscitation. The paddles or pads should be placed with one under the clavicle to the right of the sternum and the other over the apex of the heart in the mid-axillary line. If there are no paediatric paddles or pads available for an infant, then adult ones can be used, one placed on the infant's back, the other on the left side of the chest.

Continuous CPR should be performed while the defibrillator is being prepared. An asynchronous shock of $4\,J\,kg^{-1}$ should be delivered and CPR restarted immediately. There should be no pulse check or rhythm analysis immediately post-shock. Even if the heart is cardioverted to a potential perfusing rhythm the myocardium will be 'stunned' and the right ventricle distended with blood. Restarting CPR immediately will maintain coronary perfusion pressure and aid ventricular emptying. CPR should be performed for 2 minutes before a rhythm check is done. Subsequent shocks should be given at $4\,J\,kg^{-1}$. Adrenaline $(10\,mcg\,kg^{-1})$ and amiodarone $(5\,mg\,kg^{-1})$ are both given prior to the fourth shock. Adrenaline $(10\,mcg\,kg^{-1})$ is subsequently given every 3–5 minutes until there is return of a spontaneous output. Amiodarone $(5\,mg\,kg^{-1})$ is repeated after the fifth shock if the child is still in a shockable rhythm.

Other cardiac arrhythmias in children

Supraventricular tachycardia (SVT) should be suspected in any child with a narrow complex tachycardia of 220 beats min^{-1} or above. If the child is showing signs of very low cardiac output, then immediate synchronised cardioversion with 0.5–$2\,J\,kg^{-1}$ is indicated. Stable children in SVT should be treated with a vagal stimulus such as the Valsalva manoeuvre (pressing on the eyes is no longer recommended), adenosine or amiodarone (see below).

Intravenous access in cardiopulmonary arrest

Intravenous access may be very difficult in critically ill children owing to peripheral vasoconstriction; venous cannulation should only be attempted if there is an obvious vein.

Intraosseous (IO) access provides rapid access for administration of fluids and drugs. Suitable sites include the tibia, femur and humerus. Mechanical devices such as the EZ-IO® are available for use in children. A range of basic blood tests can be performed on samples obtained from an IO needle but the laboratories must be informed that the sample is from an IO needle (see also Chapter 13). Definitive venous access should be secured as soon as the child is stable.

Tibial IO insertion technique is as follows:

- Identify the insertion site 2–3 cm below the tibial tuberosity, avoiding the same side as fractured bones.
- Clean the skin.
- Insert the needle at 90° to the skin. Avoid holding the leg from directly behind as there is a risk of needle injury to the operator.
- Advance the needle using firm pressure until a 'give' is felt (use a 'twisting' action if using a manual insertion technique).
- Remove the central trocar. The needle should feel firm in the bone and stand straight with minimal support.
- Attach a 5 ml syringe and aspirate blood. (A glucose stick test should be performed and any bloods required sent.)
- Flush and secure the needle.

Drugs used in cardiopulmonary resuscitation

Medications required during cardiac arrest can be given IV, IO or via the tracheal tube. It is good practice to have an aide-memoire for the commonly used drug doses clearly visible in all resuscitation areas.

Drug doses are calculated on a per kg basis. For children 1 year or above, weight can be estimated using the formula below:

- Weight in kg = (age in years + 4) × 2

For infants, estimated weights are:

- Term baby 3.5 kg
- 6 month old 7 kg
- 1 year old 10 kg

If the child's age is unknown then a Broselow tape can be used.

- *Adrenaline (epinephrine)* is the primary drug used in cardiopulmonary resuscitation. It is an α-adrenoreceptor agonist and causes vasoconstriction and hence increases diastolic pressure and improves coronary artery and cerebral perfusion. Myocardial contractility is improved by its β-adrenoreceptor actions. Adrenaline increases the amplitude of VF and makes successful defibrillation more likely. Adrenaline should be given IV or IO as a dose of $10 \, mcg \, kg^{-1}$ ($0.1 \, ml \, kg^{-1}$ of 1:10 000 solution). If the tracheal tube is used, $100 \, mcg \, kg^{-1}$ should be given distally via a suction catheter. All doses

should be flushed in with normal saline. High-dose adrenaline is not recommended unless there is a clear history of β-blocker overdose. Adrenaline should be given every 3–5 minutes while CPR is being performed.

- *Fluid bolus* of $20 \, ml \, kg^{-1}$ of warmed normal saline. Hypovolaemia should be considered and fluids given in all children with PEA.
- *Amiodarone* is the antiarrhythmic of choice in children. It should be given as a dose of $5 \, mg \, kg^{-1}$ IV or IO after the third and fifth DC shock in cases of pulseless VF/VT.
- *Atropine* is indicated only if arrest has been preceded by a vagal stimulus such as tracheal suctioning. The dose is $20 \, mcg \, kg^{-1}$ IV or IO and $30 \, mcg \, kg^{-1}$ via the tracheal tube. A minimum dose of 100 mcg should be given.
- *Sodium bicarbonate* should only be considered if there is a documented severe metabolic acidosis despite having established effective chest compressions and ventilation. It can be helpful in cases of hyperkalaemia and in tricyclic overdose.
- *Adenosine* is indicated in supraventricular tachycardia without shock. The dose is $100–500 \, mcg \, kg^{-1}$ followed by a rapid flush of normal saline to deliver the drug to the heart.

Putting it all together

Continuous good-quality CPR should be performed on all children in cardiopulmonary arrest. Pauses in chest compressions should be minimised. Ventilation with 100% oxygen should be established rapidly as most children arrest secondary to hypoxia.

Once ECG monitoring is established either the shockable or non-shockable algorithm should be followed (Figure 38.3).

Non-shockable (asystole/PEA):

- Check electrode position and gain.
- IV/IO access, airway and oxygen should be confirmed.
- Compressions should be continuous after tracheal intubation.
- Adrenaline $10 \, mcg \, kg^{-1}$ should be given every 4 minutes.
- 4 Hs and 4 Ts should be considered and treated.

Shockable (VF/pulseless VT):

- A shock of $4 \, J \, kg^{-1}$ should be given every 2 minutes.
- CPR should be resumed immediately post-shock.

- A pulse check is done after 2 minutes of CPR *only* if there is a rhythm change.
- IV/IO access, airway and oxygen should be confirmed.
- Adrenaline 10 mcg kg^{-1} should be given after the third shock and then every 3–5 minutes (2 shocks).
- Amiodarone 5 mg kg^{-1} should be given after the third and fifth shocks.
- 4 Hs and 4 Ts should be considered and treated.

Cardiac arrest in special circumstances

Hypothermia is common following drowning and in trauma cases when the time to rescue the child has been prolonged. At core temperatures below 30 °C, arrhythmias are more common and may be refractory to defibrillation. Active core rewarming should be initiated at the same time as CPR. For a child in VF/VT, three initial shocks should be given, but after that, no drugs or further shocks should be administered until the core temperature reaches 32 °C. Hypothermic patients may be hypovolaemic and require fluid resuscitation with re-warming. Successful outcomes have been reported after very prolonged periods of CPR in children with hypothermia.

Torsade de Pointes is a form of polymorphic ventricular tachycardia that is refractory to defibrillation. The treatment is IV magnesium 25–50 mg kg^{-1} (max dose 2 g).

Extracorporeal life support (ECMO) can be used in cases where there is a reversible underlying disease process. Examples include post-cardiac surgery, cold water drowning and acute drug poisoning.

Prognostic and family considerations

After 20 minutes of unsuccessful CPR the team leader should consider stopping the resuscitation.

Poor prognostic factors include:

- Out of hospital arrest
- Prolonged interval from collapse to initiation of CPR
- Sepsis
- Blunt trauma

Good prognostic factors include:

- Witnessed arrest with bystander CPR
- Short periods of CPR
- Arrest with hypothermia or immersion in cold water
- Toxic drug exposure

Parental presence at the resuscitation helps the family come to terms with their loss if the child dies. A dedicated member of the resuscitation team should be allocated to accompany the parents and explain what is happening, answer any questions and ensure that they do not interfere with the resuscitation process.

Post-resuscitation care

Ventilation should be continued with an inspired oxygen concentration titrated to give an SpO$_2$ of 94–98%. Normocapnia should be maintained and hyperventilation avoided unless there is an acute rise in intracerebral pressure.

Invasive monitoring should be instituted and the circulation should be supported with fluids and inotropic agents as required. There are no recommendations for any individual drugs or combinations.

Temperature management after resuscitation from cardiac arrest is important. Many children develop a fever post-resuscitation, and this should be treated with the aim of maintaining a core temperature of 32–34 °C for the first 12–24 hours. Children who are in coma should also be cooled to a core temperature of 32–34 °C for 24 hours after return of spontaneous circulation. Children with hypothermia should be actively warmed at a rate of 0.25–0.5 °C h^{-1} until a core temperature of 32 °C is reached.

Glycaemic control should aim to avoid hyperglycaemia and dextrose containing fluids should be avoided. Tight glycaemic control with insulin is not recommended in children owing to the risk of inadvertent hypoglycaemia.

Newborn life support

Most newborn babies respond well to having their umbilical cord clamped and the stimulation of being dried and covered in warm towels. If there has been a period of hypoxia *in utero* the baby enters a period of 'primary apnoea', which if untreated is followed by 'whole-body gasping' at a rate of about 12 breaths min^{-1}. Without effective intervention the baby enters 'terminal apnoea' and eventually the circulation will fail. In a term baby the whole process takes about 20 minutes.

With any newborn, the priority is to provide warmth, stimulation and, if there is no response, to inflate the lungs. The sequence is as shown in the algorithm (Figure 38.4) and described below:

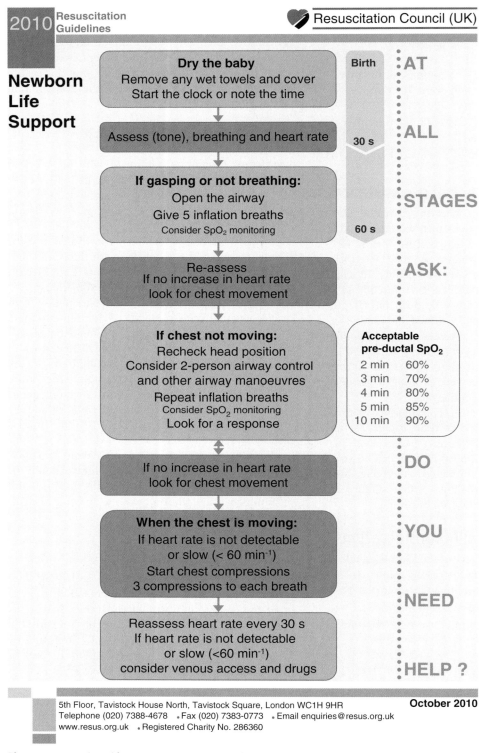

5th Floor, Tavistock House North, Tavistock Square, London WC1H 9HR
Telephone (020) 7388-4678 • Fax (020) 7383-0773 • Email enquiries@resus.org.uk
www.resus.org.uk • Registered Charity No. 286360

October 2010

Figure 38.4 Newborn life support. See plate section for colour version.

- Clamp the cord and dry the baby with warm towels. Then remove the wet towels and cover with dry ones.
- Preterm babies (less than 28 weeks gestation) should be covered with food wrap and placed under a radiant heater.
- Assess the colour, tone, breathing and heart rate. This should be repeated every 30 seconds throughout the resuscitation.
- *Airway* should be opened by placing the head in a neutral position. A roll may be needed under the shoulders. If the baby is floppy then jaw thrust or an oropharyngeal airway may be needed.
- *Breathing* should have started spontaneously with the stimulation of being dried. If not adequate then *5 inflation breaths* should be given over 2–3 seconds each at a pressure of 30 cmH$_2$O. It is important to confirm chest movement during each breath. If effective these breaths will clear the amniotic fluid from the lungs.
- The *heart rate* should be above 100 min^{-1} if the inflation breaths are successful. If the heart rate is below 100 min^{-1} and not responding then the airway manoeuvres and rescue breaths should be repeated to ensure chest movement.
- *Chest compressions* are rarely needed but should be started if the heart rate is less than 100 min^{-1} despite effective rescue breaths. The technique of choice for babies is to encircle the chest with both hands; the thumbs compress the lower third of the sternum while the fingers hold the baby from behind. The *ratio of chest compression to ventilation is 3:1*, which reflects the importance of ventilation in newborn resuscitation.
- *Adrenaline* at a dose of 10 mcg kg^{-1} is required rarely and should be given IO.
- *Fluid* as a bolus of 10 ml kg^{-1} of normal saline should be given if there is a history of blood loss.
- *Oxygen* should be given if the baby's condition does not improve rapidly when the baby is ventilated with air.

Teaching paediatric life support skills

Paediatric cardiac arrest is a relatively rare event and there are limited opportunities to practise the skills needed.

There are a number of life support courses run by organisations such as the Resuscitation Council of the United Kingdom, and the Advanced Life Support

Group, that teach a structured approach to the sick child and guidelines based on the latest evidence. A key part of these courses is the opportunity to practise 'scenarios' as part of a team.

- Ongoing practice is required between attending the life support courses to retain knowledge and technical skills.
- Practising as a team is also important, as communication errors are common during arrest situations.
- *'Just in place'* training can allow teams to practise within their own environment and is less time-consuming and expensive than attending a course.
- *'Just in time'* training can allow teams to refresh their skills and knowledge while waiting for a case to arrive.

Key points

- Cardiac arrest in a child is usually secondary to underlying causes – consider 4Hs and 4Ts.
- High-quality basic life support improves outcomes – 'push hard and push fast', minimise interruptions and allow full chest recoil after each compression.
- Post-resuscitation care is important. Avoid hyperoxia and hyperventilation, and cool to 32–34 °C.

Further reading

Advanced Life Support Group. *Advanced Paediatric Life Support. The Practical Approach'*, 5th edition. Wiley-Blackwell. 2005.

de Caen AR, Kleinman ME, Chameides L *et al.* Part 10: Paediatric basic and advanced life support. 2010 International Consensus on Cardiopulmonary Resuscitation and Emergency Cardiovascular Care Science with Treatment Recommendations. *Resuscitation* 2010;**81**(1)(Suppl.):e213–e259.

Department of Health. *The Acutely or Critically Sick or Injured Child in the District General Hospital – A Team Response.* Department of Health. 2006. http://www.dh.gov.uk/en/Publicationsandstatistics/Publications/PublicationsPolicyAndGuidance/DH_062668

Topjian AA, Berg R, Nadkarni VM. Pediatric cardiopulmonary resuscitation: advances in science, techniques, and outcomes. *Pediatrics* 2008;**122**:1086–98.

Trauma in children

Karl C. Thies and Ben Stanhope

Introduction

The World Health Organisation (WHO) has identified trauma as the leading health problem of the twenty-first century, claiming more productive life years than infectious, neoplastic or cardiovascular disease. Trauma is the primary cause of death in children above the age of 1 year. In the United Kingdom, 10% of all trauma fatalities occur in children less than 16 years old, and about 2500 children suffer major injury per year. The economic impact of major trauma in children and adolescents should not be underestimated and includes the 'loss' of educational investment, the cost of rehabilitation and care for temporary or permanent disability, and the care for families after the loss of a child.

Socioeconomic background appears to be the most significant risk factor for children who die from trauma. Children of parents who are long-term unemployed are 13 times as likely to die from unintentional injury as are children of parents with higher managerial and professional jobs. Prevention has proven to be highly effective in reducing trauma mortality. If Scotland matched Sweden in death rates for children and adolescents from unintentional injury, more than 40% of the lives lost would be saved.

Good trauma care and secondary injury prevention can decrease mortality by up to 30%. This depends on an intact 'chain of survival', commencing at the scene of injury through to the place of definitive treatment and further into early rehabilitation. Suboptimal outcomes may result from delayed access to definitive treatment, underestimation of injury severity, airway management problems and inexperienced trauma teams.

Several factors exacerbate these problems in paediatric trauma care:

- Major paediatric trauma is characterised by low incidence and high acuity. As such, even large paediatric centres have limited exposure and experience from which to develop competence in managing major trauma.
- The centralisation of paediatric care imposes long journey times to paediatric trauma centres.
- A large proportion of trauma patients presenting to paediatric centres are adolescents; paediatric trauma centres must provide the same infrastructure and expertise as needed for adult trauma.

Patterns of injury

Patterns of injury in children depend on age (Figure 39.1). The majority of injuries are traumatic brain and limb injuries. Thoracic and abdominal injuries occur less frequently but carry a high mortality, especially if combined with other injuries (Figure 39.2).

Trauma networks

The 2007 UK National Confidential Enquiry into Patient Outcome and Death (NCEPOD) report 'Trauma: Who cares' highlighted the issues of paediatric trauma care. The ideal service configuration is a regional network model consisting of a group of trauma centres, their number and location determined by the local population distribution. Children with major injuries should be taken directly to a paediatric trauma centre, bypassing the nearest hospital if necessary. This approach requires efficient coordination among all partners within the network, particularly hospitals and the ambulance service, and

Core Topics in Paediatric Anaesthesia, ed. Ian James and Isabeau Walker. Published by Cambridge University Press. © 2013 Cambridge University Press.

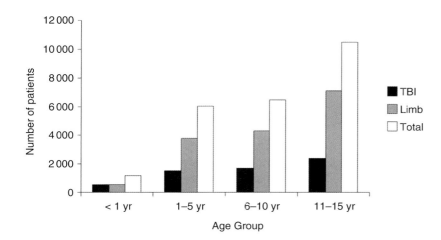

Figure 39.1 Injury pattern in children by age. TBI – traumatic brain injury.

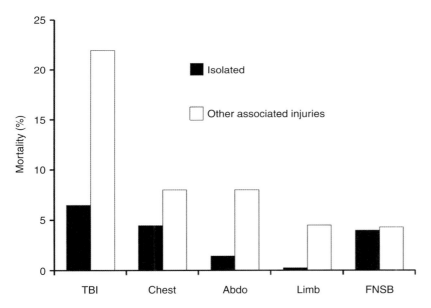

Figure 39.2 Paediatric trauma mortality by body part. TBI – traumatic brain injury; FNSB – face, neck, spine and burns.

the availability of a rapid medical response team to support the ambulance service, which may face extended on-scene care and prolonged journey times.

Trauma care – team care

A crucial link in the 'chain of survival' is a multi-specialty hospital team, responsible for the initial assessment and management of the trauma patient. Contemporary trauma care is a well-defined series of team processes running simultaneously rather than sequentially. Coordination of such a team therefore requires leadership, competent team members, clear task allocation and excellent cooperation. These factors are as important as the adequate performance of separate skills and the implementation of evidence-based guidelines. Given the low frequency of major trauma in children, paediatric trauma teams should receive continuous training and should rehearse regularly to enable all team members to fulfil their roles.

Clinical governance

Standard operating procedures (SOP) and local guidelines should be in place to allocate responsibilities and organise the complex multi-specialty care

Table 39.1 Facilities and equipment required in the paediatric trauma bay

- Dedicated large trauma resuscitation bay or theatre
- Fully equipped anaesthetic workplace
  - Airway equipment for all age groups including equipment for difficult airway management (supraglottic airways: LMA, laryngeal tube)
  - Ventilator
  - Suction equipment
  - Immediate access to anaesthetic and resuscitation drugs
  - Comprehensive monitoring: SpO_2, capnography, NIBP, IBP, ECG, CVP, temperature
- All sizes of intravenous, central venous, intraosseous and arterial cannulae
- Sonography machine to facilitate vascular access
- Patient warming equipment (forced air warming)
- Fluid/blood warmer
- Immediate access to blood products (O-negative PRBC)
- Bedside laboratory testing: blood gas, haemoglobin
- Immediate access to CT scanner, ideally in the ED

IBP, NIBP: invasive and non-invasive blood pressure monitoring. PRBC, packed red blood cells.

process. Immediate team debriefings and regular multi-specialty trauma audit meetings help to ensure the quality of care. TARN (Trauma Audit and Research Network) membership is mandatory in the United Kingdom and enables the participating hospitals to compare their performance. NCEPOD recommends appointing a director for trauma and establishing a multi-specialty trauma steering group in hospitals receiving major trauma.

Facilities and equipment

Emergency departments (ED) should have a dedicated trauma resuscitation bay that provides enough space to host a complete anaesthesia work place and allow the trauma team easy access to the patient from all sides, with appropriate lighting and surgical equipment to carry out urgent procedures. Space will also be required for a sonography machine and X-ray equipment (Table 39.1).

Role of the anaesthetist

Expertise in vital function care makes the anaesthetist an indispensable member of the trauma team, and anaesthetists have an increasing role in pre-hospital

care and retrieval to support rapid medical response teams. Anaesthetists make effective trauma team leaders as they have an overview of the whole care process from admission through to diagnostics, surgery and ICU.

Paediatric trauma resuscitation
Preparation

Before the patient arrives the anaesthetist should liaise with the trauma team leader (TTL) who usually holds a team briefing in the ED. Important information for the anaesthetist includes:

- Patient age
- Mechanism of injury
- Presence of airway problems, shock or uncontrolled haemorrhage
- Level of consciousness, or history of loss of consciousness

If the briefing indicates that the severity of the injuries might exceed his/her resources, the anaesthetist should call for back-up. Uncontrolled haemorrhage, airway injuries and ongoing CPR often require a 'reinforced' trauma team. If the briefing reveals that immediate surgical intervention is likely (penetrating chest injuries, uncontrolled external haemorrhage), theatres should be informed immediately.

Resuscitation and anaesthesia drugs should be prepared according to the age of the patient, and an equipment check should be carried out. Before patient arrival all team members should take universal precautions and put on tabards or similar to indicate their roles in the team.

The primary survey

The purpose of the primary survey in trauma is to identify and treat injuries that pose an immediate threat to life using the established ABCDE system. The role of the anaesthetist in trauma resuscitation is to assess and establish adequate oxygenation and ventilation, to help stabilise the circulation and to treat hypothermia (Table 39.2). The primary survey is carried out systematically and simultaneously by the whole trauma team, under supervision of the TTL (Table 39.3).

Cervical spine, chest and pelvic X-rays and, where indicated, sonography (Focused Assessment with

Table 39.2 Role of the anaesthetist in trauma resuscitation

Primary tasks
- Establishing patient contact; assessment of LOC, airway patency
- Airway assessment
- Airway interventions
- General anaesthesia, pain management

Secondary tasks
- Support in vascular access
- Central venous access for massive transfusion
- Arterial access
- Fluid and transfusion management
- Hypothermia prevention and treatment

Table 39.3 Primary trauma survey

Timing of the primary survey	
Within 5 seconds	*Initial assessment to identify* • Altered level of consciousness (**final common pathway for all vital functions**) • Complete airway obstruction • Massive external haemorrhage • Shock • Cardiac arrest
Within 1 minute	*Immediately life-saving interventions ('ABC')* • Establishing oxygenation and ventilation with basic airway manoeuvres • Compression of massive external haemorrhage
Within 10 minutes	*Very urgent interventions* • Chest decompression • Pelvic compression splint • Large-bore vascular access and bloods sent for laboratory examination • Commence monitoring • Analgesia, anaesthesia and definitive airway • Immobilisation of the cervical spine • Fluid therapy, transfusion of blood products • Sonography • Undressing the patient • Complete primary survey • Chest and pelvic X-ray
Within 30 minutes	*Urgent tests and interventions* • Urinary catheter • CT scan • Focused X-rays
Within 3 hours	• Completion of diagnostics and therapy • Special investigations and X-rays • Operative care • Intensive care

The **secondary survey** is carried out after all life-threatening injuries are under control or ruled out.

Sonography in Trauma, FAST) also form part of the primary survey, although many trauma centres now replace these by performing whole-body CT scans. There is evidence that a whole-body CT scan carried out on admission decreases mortality in major trauma.

A standard 'trauma panel' of blood investigations is taken, comprising full blood count (FBC), group-and-save or cross-match, clotting profile, U&Es and LFTs including amylase and lipase. A pregnancy test should be performed in all female patients of child-bearing age.

Pain treatment during the primary survey is essential for ethical and for medical reasons. Physical examination and procedures carried out in the awake child can be painful. Verbal and non-verbal communication with the patient needs to be maintained at all times, and all procedures need to be explained in order not to lose the patient's cooperation. Small aliquots of opioids (fentanyl 0.5 mcg kg^{-1}, morphine 25 mcg kg^{-1}) can be titrated to effect, or IV ketamine (0.5 mg kg^{-1}) can be given. Be aware, however, that even low doses of analgesic drugs can impair ventilation in the severely compromised patient. Ketamine may adversely affect neurological assessment.

Airway management, anaesthesia and ventilation

In the trauma team the anaesthetist is almost invariably in charge of assessment and management of the airway. In addition, because of their positioning at the head of the patient, the anaesthetist will also be in charge of controlling and protecting the patient's

Table 39.4 Causes of hypoxaemia and hypoventilation in trauma patients

Upper airway obstruction
- Decreased level of consciousness, loss of pharyngeal muscle tone
- Maxillofacial injuries
- Blood, vomitus

Central hypoventilation
- Traumatic brain injury
- Intoxication

Chest injury
- Lung contusion
- Pneumothorax
- Haemothorax

Direct airway trauma

cervical spine. They therefore assume leadership of any logroll procedure carried out during full exposure and secondary survey of the patient.

Common airway and ventilation problems in trauma

Airway and ventilation problems are common in severely injured children.

These may be a consequence of the injury (Table 39.4) or of attempts at airway support and ventilation in the field or during transport, and may be due to the following.

- Upper airway obstruction:
  - o Decreased level of consciousness and loss of pharyngeal muscle tone
  - o Blood or secretions in the upper airway
- Impaired ventilation due to gastric distension and diaphragmatic splinting:
  - o Aerophagia in the distressed child
  - o Facemask ventilation
- Airway complications in children arriving already intubated:
  - o Unrecognised oesophageal intubation
  - o Endobronchial intubation
  - o An undersized tracheal tube leading to ineffective ventilation

Basic airway management

During handover from the pre-hospital team, the anaesthetist establishes contact with the patient, and checks airway patency and conscious level.

- All trauma patients should receive high flow oxygen, which can be given via facemask or nasal prongs.
- If there is any sign of airway obstruction the airway should be cleared with basic manoeuvres first:
  - o The upper airway should be suctioned carefully with a soft catheter to avoid mucosal lacerations and reflex vomiting.
  - o The airway should be cleared using jaw thrusts or inserting an oropharyngeal airway if reduced consciousness.
  - o Cervical collars should be loosened if they impair airway access.
- In children who arrive with a tracheal tube in place, confirm correct tube position and size immediately by auscultation and capnography.
- The stomach should be decompressed with a large-bore orogastric or nasogastric tube if possible.

Immobilisation of the spine should be maintained at all times until a spinal injury is ruled out. Check for any overt haemorrhage during this time. Untreated large scalp lacerations are notorious for causing significant blood loss in children, and all findings need to be reported to the TTL immediately.

Monitoring

Oxygen saturation is the most important parameter to be monitored, and a pulse oximeter should be applied immediately. In the haemodynamically compromised child the signal can be weak and the readings unreliable. Capnography is essential in the intubated patient. Non-invasive blood pressure (NIBP) monitoring in shock can give false readings of the systolic and diastolic blood pressure, whereas the mean pressure better reflects invasive BP readings. It is important to use an adequately sized cuff to avoid over- or under-estimation of the BP. ECG monitoring is essential, because it is the most reliable indicator of the heart rate.

Tracheal intubation and general anaesthesia

Initial airway control can usually be achieved with basic measures, but the majority of severely traumatised children require early tracheal intubation and controlled ventilation. The indications for tracheal intubation are listed in Table 39.5.

Table 39.5 Indications for tracheal intubation

- **All patients requiring airway support on admission**
- Hypoxaemia
- Shock
- Severe head injury
- Severe chest injury
- Multiple trauma

Table 39.7 Modified children's Glasgow Coma Scale

Glasgow Coma Scale – age <4 years	Score
Eye opening:	
Spontaneously	4
To verbal stimuli	3
To pain	2
No response	1
Verbal response:	
Alert, babbles, words to usual ability	5
Fewer than usual words, spontaneous irritable cry	4
Cries only to pain	3
Moans to pain	2
No response to pain	1
Motor response:	
Obeys verbal command	6
Localises to pain	5
Withdraws from pain	4
Abnormal flexion to pain (decorticate)	3
Abnormal extension to pain (decerebrate)	2
No response	1

The decision to intubate is made by the TTL and the anaesthetist, and needs to be communicated to the whole team. The anaesthesia team can prepare for intubation while the primary survey is proceeding. Intubation should always be performed under general anaesthesia to avoid intracranial pressure (ICP) peaks and intubation trauma caused by coughing, bucking and vomiting.

General anaesthesia makes a neurological assessment of the patient impossible; it is the anaesthetist's responsibility to make sure that a brief neurological assessment is carried out before anaesthesia is given (Table 39.6). A decreased Glasgow Coma Scale (GCS) score is a strong predictor of mortality in children and adolescents (Table 39.7).

Table 39.6 Brief neurological assessment before induction of anaesthesia

- Glasgow Coma Scale
- Pupil size and reactivity to light
- Motor response and sensation in all four quadrants

Anaesthetic drugs

The choice and dosage of the drugs used for induction and maintenance depend on the cardiovascular and neurological condition of the child. Most anaesthetic drugs, analgesics and sedatives attenuate the compensatory vasoconstriction in shock and may cause a marked fall in blood pressure in a hypovolaemic child. The reduced volume of distribution and the decreased protein binding of anaesthetic drugs in shock leads to an increased effect-site drug concentration if standard doses are used, exacerbating the circulatory depressive effects even further. Drugs that decrease myocardial contractility or cause vasodilation should be avoided until the circulation is stabilised. These include histamine-releasing drugs such as morphine and the benzyl isoquinolones such as atracurium.

Induction

- *Ketamine* is the preferred induction agent in shock, because it produces analgesia and amnesia without affecting compensatory vasoconstriction. For induction of anaesthesia, ketamine 1 mg kg^{-1} can be given repeatedly until the patient becomes unresponsive. In traumatic brain injury, ketamine reduces raised intracranial pressure (ICP) whilst maintaining cerebral perfusion pressure (CPP), provided normoventilation is maintained.
- *Propofol* and *thiopentone* are less suitable in the severely compromised child because of their cardiovascular side effects.
- *Etomidate* provides excellent cardiovascular stability, but causes long-lasting suppression of the adrenal cortex, probably affecting the physiological endocrine response to trauma.
- *Morphine* and other histamine-releasing opioids can cause significant hypotension in hypovolaemic patients. Synthetic opioids including fentanyl, alfentanil and sufentanil exhibit some cardiovascular stability. However, they have to be titrated slowly and carefully, because they act as sympatholytics, which may

suppress the stress-induced catecholamine response, and may lead to severe hypotension.

- *Nitrous oxide* has no place in anaesthesia for major trauma, because of its cardiovascular side effects, its effect on cerebral blood volume and its tendency to diffuse rapidly into air-filled cavities, which can convert a pneumothorax into a tension pneumothorax.
- *Rocuronium* 1.5 mg kg^{-1} produces satisfactory muscle relaxation after 60 seconds without significant cardiovascular side effects, and has largely replaced suxamethonium.
- *Atracurium* and *cis-atracurium* have a longer onset time, release histamine and are not immediately reversible. They are therefore not ideal for use in trauma resuscitation.

Maintenance

- *Ketamine* can also be given for maintenance, infused at a dose of 5–10 mg kg^{-1} h^{-1}. Once haemorrhage is under control and the blood volume is re-established, volatile agents and opioids can be introduced and ketamine discontinued.
- *Isoflurane* or *sevoflurane* cause dose-dependent vasodilation and can be useful in treating persisting vasoconstriction. Active warming is necessary to compensate for associated heat loss and pre-existing hypothermia. There is no place for sevoflurane in the induction of anaesthesia in the hypovolaemic child.

Equipment

Airway management in trauma may be difficult and a failed intubation protocol needs to be part of the regular paediatric trauma training. Appropriate equipment needs to be prepared prior to induction, including at least one type of supraglottic device. Severely injured children are prone to aspiration of gastric contents, and adequate precautions need to be taken. A high-performance suction device may be life-saving in case of regurgitation or haemorrhage into the upper airway. Cuffed tracheal tubes allow high-pressure ventilation, which can be helpful in children with chest injury. Cuff pressure monitoring is mandatory to avoid tracheal lesions. Surgical airways are rarely required in children. Nevertheless, a pre-packed set for surgical airway access should be available.

Rapid sequence induction

Pre-oxygenation is essential because children with major trauma often have a decreased functional residual capacity (FRC) and desaturate rapidly, owing to shallow breathing, reduced tidal volume, atelectasis or direct chest injury (lung contusion).

- The C-spine must be kept immobilised during airway interventions. However, the priority in resuscitation is oxygenation and ventilation. The cervical collar may be removed to apply jaw-thrust or to reposition the head to optimise airway patency and prevent hypoxaemia. C-spine immobilisation must then be maintained with manual in-line stabilisation.
- Cricoid pressure distorts the anatomy of the upper airway and can make intubation difficult, and there is no evidence that is beneficial in paediatric RSI. We therefore recommend releasing cricoid pressure if it impairs the operator's view of the glottis, and it should be avoided altogether if a C-spine injury or laryngeal trauma is suspected (swelling, local crepitus, hoarse voice).
- The tracheal tube position must be confirmed by auscultation and capnography immediately after intubation.

Blood in the upper airway

Severe head injury or maxillofacial injury can result in ongoing haemorrhage into the upper airway leading to airway obstruction, aspiration or difficult intubation. Constant oropharyngeal suction should be applied to obtain an acceptable view under such circumstances.

- If the laryngeal inlet cannot be visualised and the patient is breathing spontaneously, air bubbles might indicate the position of the glottis. An assistant can be asked to compress the patient's chest to provoke air bubbles if the patient is paralysed.
- If tracheal intubation fails, a suction catheter can be left in the oropharynx, while PEEP is maintained with a soft-cuffed facemask, allowing constant suction while maintaining oxygenation.
- A soft nasopharyngeal airway can be life-saving if an oropharyngeal airway is not relieving airway obstruction sufficiently. The nasopharyngeal airway must be inserted with great care in a vertical direction, following the base of the nasal

cavity, to prevent inadvertent perforation of the cribriform plate (very rare).

- A supraglottic device (LMA or other) can be inserted to protect the lower airway from aspiration of blood.
- If there is bleeding from the nose, haemostasis can be achieved by inserting appropriately sized urinary catheters through the nose, inflating the balloon in the nasopharynx and applying traction. Anterior nasal packs complete haemostasis.
- An immediate surgical airway is required if oxygenation cannot be maintained.

Ongoing problems after tracheal intubation

After intubation the correct position of the tracheal tube needs to be confirmed immediately. The compliance of the respiratory system should then be assessed. Pressure-controlled ventilation at peak pressures of 15 cmH$_2$O should deliver normal tidal volumes. Inadequate tidal volumes can be caused by light anaesthesia, lack of muscle relaxation or other causes:

- *Aspiration* of blood or gastric contents is common in trauma, and tracheal suction should be applied immediately after intubation.
- Inadvertent *endobronchial intubation* is common in children and can lead to hypoxaemia and hypercapnia. Airway pressures are usually high, and if not detected, complete contralateral lung collapse and severe hypoxaemia can result.
- A simple pneumothorax can convert into a *tension pneumothorax* after institution of positive pressure ventilation. In children with chest injury there should be a high index of suspicion for pneumothorax, even if there are no rib fractures, and immediate chest decompression should be performed. Signs of tension pneumothorax include:
  - Ipsilateral decreased breath sounds
  - Ipsilateral decreased chest movement
  - Ipsilateral hyperresonant percussion
  - High airway pressure
  - Cardiovascular collapse
- Signs of *airway disruption* include rapidly developing surgical emphysema of the neck after institution of positive pressure ventilation.
- Progressive *mediastinal emphysema* is a life-threatening condition, and a flexible tracheo-

Table 39.8 Classification of shock in trauma

Haemorrhagic shock
- Intra-abdominal haemorrhage (e.g. liver rupture)
- Intrathoracic (e.g. penetrating chest injury)
- Retroperitoneal (e.g. pelvic fracture)
- External haemorrhage

Cardiogenic shock
- Blunt thoracic injury

Obstructive shock
- Tension pneumothorax (including secondary to PPV)
- Cardiac tamponade (penetrating chest injury)

Neurogenic shock
- Spinal cord injury
- Massive TBI

bronchoscopy needs to be carried out immediately to identify the lesion for further surgical planning. Prophylactic bilateral chest drains are indicated to prevent tension pneumothorax. An emergency mediastinostomy should be discussed with the surgeon.

- In haemorrhagic shock, positive pressure ventilation and PEEP can compromise venous return leading to *circulatory collapse*. These patients require immediate transfusion and probably inotropic support.

Management of shock

Circulatory shock after major trauma is in most cases due to haemorrhage (but see tension pneumothorax above). Other forms of circulatory shock are rare in paediatric trauma victims (Table 39.8).

Children compensate effectively for blood loss owing to a relatively greater ability to increase systemic vascular resistance and heart rate. The signs of early haemorrhagic shock are subtle in children, and the onset of decompensation is abrupt. Hypotension is therefore a late and pre-terminal sign (Table 39.9).

Assessment of the circulation

There is no single clinical measurement that can be used reliably for assessment of blood loss.

- *Blood pressure* and *heart rate* are unreliable because they are affected by other factors such as anxiety, pain and concomitant traumatic brain injury (TBI). They further depend on the type of

Table 39.9 Normal values in children

Age	Weight (kg)	Heart rate (beats min^{-1})	RR (breaths min^{-1})	Systolic BP (mmHg)
3–6 months	5–7	100–160	30–40	70–90
1 year	10	100–160	30–40	70–90
2 years	12	95–140	25–30	80–100
3–4 years	14–16	95–140	25–30	80–100
5–8 years	18–24	80–120	20–25	90–110
10 years	30	80–100	15–20	90–110
12 years	40	60–100	12–20	100–120

injury; blunt injuries with extensive tissue injury cause a more pronounced sympatho-adrenergic response resulting in a higher blood pressure and less tachycardia than exsanguinating penetrating injuries.

- In the awake patient, systolic blood pressure and heart rate can remain normal until more than 30% of the blood volume is lost.

- More useful clinical signs are *capillary refill time* (CRT, normal <2 seconds), *skin colour*, *temperature* and *level of consciousness*. Loss of up to 25% blood volume will be associated with a slight increase in CRT and cool peripheries; the child may also be slightly agitated. As blood loss increases, so does the CRT. The peripheries will become cold and mottled and the child increasingly lethargic. When more than 40% of the blood volume is lost, peripheral perfusion will be absent, there will be no discernible capillary refill and the skin will look cold and waxy, and *pulse oximetry* signals will be lost.

- *Bradycardia* in shock usually precedes cardiac arrest.

- *Metabolic acidosis* is the single most reliable indicator of shock and can be used to guide fluid resuscitation.

- *Serum lactate* is also valuable, but has a slower response time than a base deficit and can be affected by lactate-containing IV solutions.

- An arterial line should be placed early during resuscitation. The arterial waveform provides continuous information about blood pressure and vascular filling. *Narrow arterial pressure waveforms* and *systolic respiratory pressure variation* indicate hypovolaemia and can be used to guide fluid replacement.

- The *central venous pressure* is decreased in hypovolaemia and exhibits pronounced respiratory swings. However, the CVP only gives reliable information on the filling of the cardiovascular system as long as right ventricular function is not impaired and intra-thoracic pressures are not increased.

- The *SVC oxygen saturation* (SCVO$_2$) can be used as a substitute for mixed venous saturation and may be useful to assess the severity of blood loss.

- Apart from detecting free intra-abdominal fluid *FAST* can be used to assess the filling of the IVC and ventricular function and filling via the subxiphoid window.

- An excellent monitoring and diagnostic device in the anaesthetised patient is *transoesophageal echocardiography* (TOE). As well as assessing ventricular filling, TOE can be used to identify other causes of shock such as pericardial tamponade, myocardial contusion or valve rupture and haemothorax. TOE can help to optimise cardiac pre- and afterload in shock but clearly requires an experienced operator.

Damage control resuscitation

The combination of *metabolic acidosis* and *hypothermia* leads to severe *coagulopathy* and hence further blood loss that triggers a vicious cycle, intensifying acidosis and hypothermia. In severe trauma, 'damage control resuscitation' aims at breaking this cycle early, by addressing all three factors simultaneously:

- Fluid resuscitation and *transfusion of blood products and clotting factors* to re-establish tissue oxygenation and blood clotting.

- *Haemorrhage control* by hypotensive resuscitation (see below) and early surgical intervention, targeting haemostasis but not necessarily definitive repair (damage control surgery).

- Concurrent with these processes, *hypothermia treatment* to control *coagulopathy* and to *decrease oxygen demand.*

Definitive surgical repair may be carried out 12–24 hours later, after tissue oxygenation, blood clotting and normothermia have been re-established.

Vascular access

Exsanguination is the major cause of preventable death in major trauma, and therefore large-bore vascular access must be established early on during resuscitation.

- If peripheral IV access cannot be obtained within 90 seconds, intraosseous cannulation should be performed. Modern intraosseous systems such as EZ–IO® allow rapid vascular access without being too painful. Intramuscular ketamine can be given prior to insertion. The most common site used for intraosseous access is the tibial tuberosity. Alternatively, the anterolateral surface of the femur or the tibia proximal to the medial malleolus can be used. Fractured extremities should be avoided, particularly those with fractures proximal to the site of entry. The flow rate through an intraosseous needle is limited compared with large-bore venous access.

- If large-bore venous access cannot be accomplished immediately, the patient should be anaesthetised first and a large-bore central line (eg. cardiac catheter introducer sheath) should be sited subsequently.

- Alternatively a narrow-bore peripheral venous access can be converted via Seldinger technique to a large-bore line (Emergency Infusion Device®, Arrow) (Figure 39.3).

- CVP monitoring is strongly recommended if a rapid infusion system is being used.

- Femoral venous access is technically easy and has a lower rate of serious complications than other sites, but care is required if massive transfusion is necessary as the insertion site is difficult to check during surgery. In severe abdominal injury with rupture of the large veins, fluid administration via the femoral route is ineffective.

- Access to the internal jugular vein is useful as it is easily accessible with sonography, and the

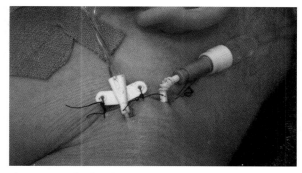

Figure 39.3 Shock catheter in the external jugular vein next to a central venous line in the internal jugular vein in a 2 year old.

patient's head can be kept in neutral position during insertion. Subclavian access is an alternative, but bears a higher risk of complications especially under resuscitation conditions.

- Arterial access is indicated in all severely injured children.

If time permits, central venous and arterial access should be placed early during resuscitation. However, in no case should this delay urgent resuscitative measures. *It is possible to treat massive blood loss using one large-bore peripheral access only.*

Fluid management and blood product in massive haemorrhage and trauma-induced coagulopathy (TIC)

Balanced electrolyte solutions are first-line treatment of hypovolaemia and should be administered in 10 ml kg^{-1} IV boluses. Infusion of large amounts of *normal saline* can lead to hyperchloraemic acidosis, which may contribute to coagulopathy and complicates the differential diagnosis of a metabolic acidosis. *Hartmann's solution* contains only 135 mmol l^{-1} of sodium, making it slightly hypo-osmolar, potentially exacerbating cerebral oedema in patients with TBI. Glucose-containing solutions have no place in fluid resuscitation. Other commercially produced solutions are available (such as Plasmalyte A®), which more closely resemble plasma electrolyte composition and avoid the problems of hypo-osmolarity and hyperchloraemic acidosis.

Colloids are second-line treatment for hypovolaemia. Newly available starch solutions such as 6% HES 130/0.4 have the advantage of causing less renal impairment and coagulopathy compared with previous preparations. Newer formulations of starch and

Table 39.10a Blood component therapy for controlled haemorrhage

Component	Indication	Volume
Red cell concentrate	• Transfusion trigger could be a Hb between 8 and 10 g dl^{-1} blood depending on patient condition (TBI)	4 ml kg^{-1} packed cells raises the haemoglobin by 1 g dl^{-1}
Platelet concentrate	• Platelet count <50 × 10^9 l^{-1} (single organ system injury) • Platelet count <100 × 10^9 l^{-1} (two organ systems or TBI)	Child <15 kg: 10–20 ml kg^{-1} Child >15 kg: One standard pool
Fresh frozen plasma	• Significant haemorrhage • INR >1.5 (PT or PTT)	10–20 ml kg^{-1}
Cryoprecipitate	• Significant haemorrhage • Plasma fibrinogen < 2 g l^{-1}	Child <15 kg: 5 ml kg^{-1} Child 15–30 kg: 5 units Child >30 kg: 10 units

gelatin solutions contain physiological electrolyte concentrations, reducing the risk of electrolyte imbalance.

Massive haemorrhage is defined as:

• Loss of 50% of the circulating blood volume within 3 hours; or
• Ongoing blood loss of 2 ml kg^{-1} min^{-1} (150 ml min^{-1} in an adult).

In the treatment of uncontrolled haemorrhage, balanced electrolyte solutions and colloids both aggravate trauma-induced coagulopathy (TIC), which increases mortality. Therefore early use of packed red blood cells (PRBC) in combination with fresh frozen plasma (FFP) is necessary. Longstanding European clinical practice and recent experience from the UK defence service show that early transfusion of FFP in haemorrhagic shock increases survival. If there is ongoing haemorrhage, PRBC, FFP and platelets should be transfused in a ratio of 'one to one' (Table 39.10a, b). But even this regimen cannot reliably prevent TIC, because the delivered haematocrit and clotting factor activity would be only 30% and 65% respectively.

TIC is a complex phenomenon caused by various factors, which are:

• Major blood loss and dilution of clotting factors
• Low platelet count
• Hypothermia and acidosis
• Activation of the fibrinolytic system triggered by tissue hypoxia and tissue damage

Hyperfibrinolysis appears to be present in more than 25% of all major trauma patients and is correlated to the severity of the injuries. As a result fibrinogen levels are low leading to impaired clot formation

Table 39.10b Blood component therapy for uncontrolled haemorrhage

• **Hypotensive resuscitation** (not in TBI) until blood loss is under control
• Give **RBC** concentrate and **FFP** in a one-in-one ratio to maintain sufficient arterial pressure and CVP
• One adult unit of **platelets** or five random units (250 × 10^9 platelets) for every five units of RBC/FFP
• Maintain fibrinogen level above 2 g l^{-1} with cryoprecipitate
• Continuous **invasive arterial** and **CVP** monitoring if possible
• Maintain normal **Ca^{++}** level
• Consider **Factor VIIa** (80 mcg kg^{-1}) if life-threatening and diffuse oozing persists despite standard therapy

and poor clot stability. Fibrinogen levels of less than 2 g l^{-1} require treatment with either cryoprecipitate or fibrinogen concentrate.

The recently published CRASH 2 Trial revealed that administration of the antifibrinolytic *tranexamic acid* (TXA) in bleeding trauma patients decreases the relative risk of death by 30% if given no later than 3 hours after the injury. In adult patients the recommendation is to give 1 g of TXA over 10 min as soon as possible and to give another 1 g over 8 hours. However, TXA should not be started later than 3 hours after the injury because the relative risk of death then is increased.

Children should receive a loading dose of 15 mg kg^{-1} over 10 minutes and then 2 mg kg^{-1} h^{-1} for at least 8 hours or until bleeding stops.

If oozing persists, infusion of *Factor VIIa* may be considered, but is controversial. *Thrombelastography* is a useful bedside test for guiding replacement of clotting factors and platelets. In order to prevent TIC, however, the decision to replace clotting factors often has to be made before the results are available.

Hypocalcaemia is a common problem in massive transfusion. It can cause myocardial dysfunction and ECG changes and worsen coagulopathy. Therefore plasma calcium concentration should be monitored frequently and corrected as necessary.

Hypotensive resuscitation

In adult patients with uncontrolled haemorrhagic shock it is common practice to maintain the systolic blood pressure at 80 mmHg until haemostasis is achieved. This approach increases survival by limiting blood loss and maintaining perfusion of the vital organs at the same time. Evidence in children is limited, but blood pressure should be maintained in the low-normal range, except where there is TBI when blood pressure of at least normal levels must be maintained to ensure adequate cerebral perfusion.

Vasopressors and inotropes in hypovolaemic shock

If hypotension is severe and not responding to fluid therapy, vasopressors such as noradrenaline or other alpha-agonists can be given temporarily within the concept of damage control resuscitation. If hypotension is refractory to alpha-agonists vasopressin can be tried, but there is no evidence that this approach increases survival. When vasopressors are used to treat shock, patients often need inotropic support as well. Invasive monitoring is necessary to guide treatment.

Endpoints of resuscitation

The endpoints of resuscitation in shock are not well defined in children. As a general recommendation in anaesthetised adults we would aim for:

- Normal blood pressure once the haemorrhage is under control
- Haemoglobin of $10 \, \text{g} \, \text{dl}^{-1}$
- CVP of 8–10 cmH$_2$O
- Improving base deficit and lactate levels (lactate can remain high, despite adequate resuscitation, if lactate-containing IV solutions have been given)
- Normal clotting
- Adequate urine output. This is a reliable indicator of fluid resuscitation, but has a slow response time and is reduced by high intra-abdominal pressure and hypothermia

- Good ventricular filling and contractility as shown by TOE

Hypothermia

Hypothermia is a common finding in severe trauma, particularly in children, and is associated with a significantly increased incidence of multiple organ dysfunction. There is evidence that hypothermia is an independent predictor of mortality in major trauma, owing to:

- Decreased platelet function
- Decreased clotting factor activity
- Increased oxygen demand (up to five-fold)

Treatment of hypothermia must start on arrival of the patient. Forced air-warming devices, overhead heaters, warmed IV solutions and blood products and high room temperature are used to prevent or treat hypothermia.

Specific injuries in children
Traumatic brain injury

Sixty per cent of all severely injured children suffer isolated traumatic brain injury (TBI), which is the leading cause of death and permanent disability in paediatric and adult trauma. Survivors of childhood TBI exhibit functional difficulties persisting into adulthood. Common findings include poor school performance, employment difficulties, poor quality of life and increased mental health problems.

Best outcomes after TBI require rapid access to definitive care and minimisation of 'secondary injury', including avoidance of hypoxaemia, hypotension, and hypo- or hypercapnia. Twenty per cent of all children with TBI require emergency craniotomy for evacuation of sub- or extradural haematoma. This should be undertaken within an internationally accepted target of 4 hours of the injury.

ICP management

ICP monitoring is indicated in all patients with TBI and a GCS ≤8. The threshold for ICP monitoring should be low if non-neurosurgical interventions or prolonged ventilation and sedation are necessary. The ICP can be measured at subarachnoid, epidural and intraventricular level, the latter allowing also for emergency drainage of cerebrospinal fluid (CSF). ICP readings above 20 mmHg require treatment.

Bradycardia and hypertension are signs of increased intracranial pressure (Cushing reflex) and imminent uncal herniation and require immediate intervention. Deepening of the anaesthesia/ sedation and administration of IV mannitol (0.5–1.0 g kg^{-1}) or hypertonic saline (3% or 7.5%) can be used to decrease the ICP. Mannitol induces diuresis, and any resulting intravascular volume depletion and hypotension must be avoided. Mannitol can diffuse into injured areas of the brain where the blood–brain barrier is dysfunctional, causing a rebound increase in cerebral oedema. Hypertonic saline avoids these problems and reliably decreases ICP in TBI patients, although there is limited evidence for use in children.

There are insufficient data to support a treatment standard regarding the cerebral perfusion pressure (CPP) in children. However, a CPP below 40 mmHg is consistently associated with a higher mortality. It therefore seems reasonable to avoid a CPP below 40 mmHg in children.

Anaesthesia for TBI

Patients require early intubation to restore oxygenation of the brain. The induction and maintenance of anaesthesia should aim at maintaining oxygenation and cerebral perfusion pressure and avoiding elevation of ICP.

The following factors need to be taken into consideration:

- *Hypoxaemia* in patients with TBI is associated with poor outcome.
- *Hyperventilation* leads to cerebral vasoconstriction, hypoperfusion and subsequent infarction.
- *Hypoventilation* increases intracranial blood volume and can raise ICP.
- Capnometry is thus mandatory and essential to adjust the ventilation. Repeated arterial blood gas analyses should be used to validate the end-tidal CO_2 readings, which can differ significantly from the arterial readings especially in patients with concomitant chest injury.
- *Hypotension* is associated with poor outcome after TBI and requires immediate treatment. Fluid resuscitation is the first line treatment, but if this fails to produce a high-normal blood pressure, vasopressors should be given. These should be administered through a central line.

Ideally arterial and central lines should be placed as soon as possible in order to guide fluid management and to obtain serial blood gas samples. However, this should not delay urgent neurosurgical interventions. If necessary, emergency craniotomies can be carried out using large-bore peripheral venous access only. During transport and CT scanning the patient should be fully monitored. It is important to obtain a full scan of the cervical spine when the cranial CT is done, to look for C-spine injuries. In order to avoid involuntary movements and removal of lines or dislocation of the tracheal tube, the patient should be paralysed. A urinary catheter should be inserted to monitor urine output, which can be excessive after application of mannitol. Increased urine output can also be a sign of diabetes insipidus due to high ICP.

Blood should be available in theatres because blood loss, especially in subdural haematomas, can be significant. Meticulous surgical haemostasis is required for scalp vessels to prevent unnecessary blood loss during the operation. In young children with open cranial sutures, the blood loss from an intracranial haematoma can be so large that blood transfusion becomes necessary.

Decompression of a space-occupying haemorrhage can cause severe temporary blood pressure drops (inverse Cushing reflex). With an extradural haematoma this will occur with the first burr hole; with a subdural haematoma this will occur on incision of the dura. A fluid bolus and a vasopressor should therefore be at hand.

During surgery, there should remain a high index of suspicion regarding other injuries. Note that high airway pressure and CO_2 retention could be signs of an undetected pneumothorax. An unexplained fall in blood pressure could be a sign of an intra-abdominal or pelvic injury.

The decision as to whether to extubate a child after an emergency craniotomy depends on the type and extent of the brain injury and the concomitant injuries. Subdural haematomas are usually associated with a significant lesion of the underlying brain tissue and patients will often develop cerebral oedema, which if diffuse carries a high mortality rate. These patients should remain sedated and ventilated with ICP monitoring. Patients with isolated extradural haematoma often can be extubated at the end of the procedure without significant problems.

Thoracic trauma

Serious chest injuries in children are rare, but can present without visible external signs and are associated with significant morbidity and mortality. The high flexibility of the paediatric ribcage explains why even fatal chest injuries can occur without any bony lesions. *Rib fractures* occur only if exceptional force is involved and if present should raise suspicion regarding further underlying serious injuries. Chest X-ray is the first imaging modality for thoracic trauma in children, but if there is suspicion of an intrathoracic injury a chest CT should be obtained. Thoracic injuries in children rarely require surgical intervention, apart from placing a chest tube for a pneumothorax.

Lung contusions can be identified on plain X-ray. Patients with severe lung contusions require early intubation and mechanical ventilation; PEEP is often required to maintain oxygenation. Lung compliance is reduced in major chest injury and may lead to elevated airway and intrathoracic pressures and hypotension in hypovolaemic patients. *Pneumothoraces* are easily detected with FAST and should be drained before institution of positive pressure ventilation. Anterior pneumothoraces are notorious for being overlooked on conventional X-ray, and the threshold for requesting FAST or a chest CT should be low if there are ventilation problems.

If a traumatic *broncho-pleural fistula* is suspected (pneumothorax, increasing mediastinal and surgical emphysema), immediate flexible bronchoscopy is necessary to identify the lesion. Lung separation with a bronchial blocker can be tried at the same time to minimise the air leak. Urgent thoracotomy is necessary to repair the fistula.

Aortic ruptures in children are seen much less frequently than in adults. A widened mediastinum on the chest X-ray after deceleration trauma could indicate such an injury. The diagnosis is confirmed by CT scan or CT angiography. These injuries require management in a paediatric cardiothoracic centre. Thoracotomy and aortic repair is the first choice of treatment in children. Stenting can be an option in the severely compromised patient, but the experience in children is very limited.

Penetrating chest injuries in children are rare but do occur, mainly as stab wounds in the adolescent population. These injuries can present as haemo-pneumothorax, haemopericardium or trans-diaphragmatic injuries. Some patients need immediate thoracotomy for haemorrhage control. The major challenge for the anaesthetist is the high urgency and the massive blood loss these injuries frequently cause. Under exceptional circumstances resuscitative thoracotomy and open cardiac massage can be life-saving.

Anaesthesia for emergency thoracotomy

Emergency thoracotomy in children is mainly undertaken to control intrathoracic haemorrhage. These patients are often under resuscitation conditions and need to be taken to theatres as soon as possible. The anaesthesia principles are outlined in the section on shock, including the need for large-bore venous access, and central venous and arterial access. However, in the exsanguinating patient vascular access can be very difficult and should not delay emergency thoracotomy. Institution of ventilation again bears the high risk of conversion of a pneumothorax into a tension pneumothorax and so any known pneumothorax should be drained. Lung isolation can be helpful in the case of a broncho-pulmonary fistula or intrabronchial haemorrhage to maintain ventilation. This can be either achieved with a bronchus blocker or a double lumen tube. A bronchus blocker needs to be inserted with a flexible fibrescope, which is difficult to use if the patient is bleeding into the lower airway. The first choice therefore would be a double lumen tube (DLT) although these are only available for children above the age of about 10 years.

Abdominal injury and pelvic fracture

Abdominal injuries are the third most frequent injuries after TBI and extremity trauma in children. The solid organs are proportionally larger and therefore not as protected by the thoracic cage as in adults. This exposure leads to a higher incidence of spleen and liver injuries than in adults. Abdominal injuries are the primary cause of circulatory shock, and the abdomen is the most common site of initially unrecognised, fatal injury in traumatised children. FAST is indicated to identify free fluid in the peritoneal cavity. CT scanning is necessary to detect solid organ or retroperitoneal injuries. Fortunately, solid organ injuries rarely require laparotomy, contemporary treatment being primarily conservative or the use of radiological embolisation. This approach requires that the patient remains haemodynamically stable. The success rate for conservative management of splenic injuries is higher than 95%, and 80% of liver injuries can be managed without laparotomy. However, in haemodynamically unstable patients, emergency laparotomy is required.

Fractures of the elastic immature pelvis are relatively rare in children, and generally have a good prognosis. However, if they are associated with other serious injuries (TBI, long bone fractures, intra-abdominal injuries) mortality can increase to 15%. Most pelvic fractures in children can be treated conservatively. In adolescents, fractures of the pelvic ring can lead to severe life-threatening retroperitoneal haemorrhage, which requires external splinting in the emergency department. A C-clamp is used to achieve temporary stabilisation. This approach helps to control haemorrhage and allows surgical access to the abdomen at the same time. Sources of bleeding in pelvic fractures can be arterial, venous, or from bones and ligaments. To control an arterial bleed immediate radiological embolisation should be considered. If the haemorrhage is primarily venous or if there is no immediate access to interventional radiology, temporary retroperitoneal packing can be carried out in theatres or the emergency department.

Anaesthesia for emergency laparotomy

Patients requiring emergency laparotomy usually present hypothermic and in circulatory shock. The anaesthesia principles outlined in the shock section apply. In blunt abdominal trauma the blood loss is always limited by the amount of blood that can be accommodated in the abdominal cavity or retroperitoneal space; eventually the haemorrhage tamponades itself. When opening the peritoneum, tamponade is lost, causing severe hypotension and sometimes exsanguination if the surgeon cannot control the haemorrhage immediately. These patients should be stabilised by transfusion of blood products, with preparation for massive haemorrhage, before the peritoneum is opened. Good communication between surgeon and anaesthetist is essential.

Complex abdominal injuries often require damage control resuscitation before definitive repair can be carried out safely. The goal is to achieve haemostasis and prevent contamination of the peritoneal cavity in case of intestinal perforation. Often intra-abdominal packing is performed as a temporary measure. In these patients the abdominal pressure will increase significantly, leading to high intra-

thoracic pressures. Much higher filling pressures (CVP) are required to achieve normovolaemia. The intra-abdominal pressure needs to be monitored to detect abdominal compartment syndrome early. After damage control surgery, patients are stabilised in the intensive care unit before the definitive repair is carried out.

Limb injuries

The mortality of isolated limb injuries in children and adolescents is low. If associated with injuries to other organ systems the mortality seems to depend on these injuries rather than on the extremity injury.

In the context of damage control resuscitation, definitive repair is postponed until the patient is fully stabilised. However, temporary stabilisation of *long bone fractures* reduces blood loss and the incidence of multiple organ dysfunction syndrome, and is therefore part of the resuscitative efforts. Temporary measures include *external fixation* or casting for more distal fractures.

Crush injuries need early debridement and reconstructive surgery, often staged and tailored to the patient's condition.

Vascular injuries are relatively rare and present with absent pulses and pallor of the affected limb. They are easily overlooked in the polytrauma patient, and they must be actively searched for in order to save the limb.

Minor trauma
Anaesthesia for minor trauma

Most minor trauma in children is managed electively (e.g. forearm fracture, facial laceration). Adequate analgesia is usually achieved with immobilisation and oral paracetamol and ibuprofen, and many of these children are suitable for day-case surgery under general anaesthesia the following day. The exception is supracondylar fracture of the humerus with displacement leading to brachial artery compromise, which requires emergency intervention.

Starvation is of specific concern in these children. Patients in pain have delayed gastric emptying and must be regarded as non-starved even if the accident happened on the day before. Regional anaesthesia is an option in the older child, but often needs to be supplemented with sedation or GA.

Procedural sedation for minor trauma

Children with minor trauma requiring 'procedural intervention' present frequently to emergency departments (EDs). Examples of such presentations include:

- Lacerations requiring suture closure
- Removal of foreign bodies (from ear, nose, soft tissues etc.)
- Reduction of joint dislocation (e.g. shoulder, elbow)
- Repair of crush finger-tip injuries

A lack of understanding, compliance and cooperation on the part of the young patient often makes performing such procedures a challenge, even impossible, and sometimes dangerous. Increasingly in the United Kingdom, EDs are employing IV sedation in children to facilitate these procedures, the benefits to the patient and organisation including:

- A better patient experience – their problem is resolved in 'one-stop';
- Reduced admission rate for day-case procedures;
- Reduction in the number of general anaesthetics given.

While increasingly within the skill set of emergency physicians, the anaesthetist may be called upon to provide support as a 'sedationist' for such procedures, being responsible for administering sedative agents, managing the patient's airway during the procedure and ensuring their recovery from the sedated state. Intravenous ketamine ($1–2\,\mathrm{mg\,kg^{-1}}$) is the drug of choice in this situation.

Intravenous ketamine provides 10–20 minutes of 'surgical' sedation, with children usually returning to a normal sensorium around 40 minutes after administration. Once they have made an adequate recovery they may be discharged home with appropriate written and verbal post-sedation advice.

Key points

- 'Children are not small adults' is a time-honoured paediatric mantra, and while it may hold many truths, it is perhaps least applicable in the context of major trauma. The essence of approach to the injured child follows the same pathway as that for adults, but with some anatomical, physiological and psychological

considerations. The anaesthetist, as an indispensible member of the paediatric trauma team, must be familiar with these differences.
- Trauma care is currently undergoing a paradigm shift with new treatment concepts such as damage control resuscitation, interventional radiology and early full-body CT scanning being introduced. Modern trauma care requires a parallel team approach involving the anaesthetist, as a vital function expert, from the very first minute.
- Early treatment of TIC with substitution of blood products and prevention of hypothermia are life-saving.
- As with the management of adult major trauma, the anaesthetist's success is dependent on competence, meticulous preparation and clear communication, in order to function as a key player in the multidisciplinary team.

Further reading

Bayreuther J, Wagener S, Woodford M *et al*. Paediatric trauma: injury pattern and mortality in the UK. *Arch Dis Child Educ Pract Ed* 2009;**94**:37–41.

Driscoll P, Gwinnutt CL, eds. *European Trauma Course Manual*, 2nd edition. European Resuscitation Council. 2010.

Huber-Wagner S, Lefering R, Qvick LM *et al*. (on behalf of the Working Group on Polytrauma of the German Trauma Society). Effect of whole-body CT during trauma resuscitation on survival: a retrospective, multicentre study. *Lancet* 2009;**373**:1455–61.

Jansen JO, Thomas R, Loudon MA, Brooks A. Damage control resuscitation for patients with major trauma. *Br Med J* 2009;**338**:b1778.

National Confidential Enquiry into Patient Outcome and Death. *Trauma: Who Cares?* NCEPOD. 2007.

Spahn DR, Cerny V, Coats TJ *et al*. Management of bleeding following major trauma: A European guideline. *Crit Care* 2007;**11**:R17.

Acknowledgement

This chapter is partly based, with permission of the editors, on the manual of the European Trauma Course. Please contact the authors for a complete reference list.

Burns in children

40

Bruce Emerson

Introduction

Burns are common throughout the world and are mostly preventable. A moment of inattention by a carer, or an older child playing with fire, can lead to a lifetime of burn care. Children have a higher incidence of burns than adults, although most burns are small. Burns over 10% require formal fluid resuscitation to mitigate the effects of systemic oedema and burn shock. Definitive treatment involves non-operative techniques, such as application of dressings, or for larger or deeper injuries, operations to debride the wound and apply split skin grafts. Each burn generates background, breakthrough and procedural pain that must be managed effectively. Small burns may be complicated by infection, larger burns by multiple organ failure. The outcomes are generally good, and children can survive and thrive even after very large injuries.

Anaesthetists are involved in all aspects of burn care once a child reaches hospital, and they are an essential part of the multidisciplinary burn care team. The aim of this team is to deliver faster healing and better pain control, and to prevent complications. This chapter will describe current burns care for children in the United Kingdom.

Definition and aetiology

A burn is defined as an area of coagulative necrosis of tissue. Burns involve destruction of one or more layers of the skin – the epidermis, dermis and sub-dermis – and may occur by a variety of mechanisms (see Table 40.1). We all experience minor burns and so we can appreciate that the deeper the burn, the longer it will take to heal and the more likely there will be scarring with prolonged recovery.

Table 40.1 Burn depth

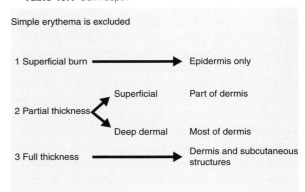

Simple erythema is excluded

1 Superficial burn → Epidermis only

2 Partial thickness → Superficial — Part of dermis
→ Deep dermal — Most of dermis

3 Full thickness → Dermis and subcutaneous structures

Burns are described by their size or percentage of skin loss relative to the body surface area. A minor burn involves less than 10% of the body surface area, a moderate burn 30–60% and a massive burn greater than 60% of the body surface area. The mechanism of the burn injury is important and points to the likely outcome: for example, scalds from hot tea are usually less than 10%, mainly partial thickness, and are generally associated with good recovery. Electrical burns are often smaller and deeper and cause more hidden subcutaneous damage.

A subset of children on burns units have skin loss resulting from desquamating conditions such as staphylococcal scalded skin syndrome, toxic epidermal necrolysis or meningococcal skin loss. They have similar metabolic and wound problems to children with burns.

The six most common causes of burns or skin loss are:

- Thermal burn (scald, flame, contact, cold)
- Electrical burn

- Chemical burn (acid, alkali)
- Radiation
- Friction
- Non-burn skin loss

Burns occur when victims cannot move out of the way of the heat source; babies and those with diseases such as epilepsy are particularly vulnerable. Older children experiment with flammable materials, and young teenage boys will be injured more often than females. Scalds from hot unprotected cooking liquid at ground level are common in developing countries. Wars produce civilian and military casualties and there will be weapon-specific patterns of burns. Children from areas of social deprivation are over-represented because of overcrowding. Children are vulnerable to both non-accidental injury and neglect, so a high level of awareness is needed to prevent further harm. Worrying signs include delayed presentation, physical signs of varying age, or inconsistencies in the history.

The most common type of burn in children in the United Kingdom is a scald. Toddlers learning to walk are particularly vulnerable, for instance by reaching up to a work surface and pulling a hot cup of tea over themselves. Their skin is thin and less resistant to heat damage. Water at 60 °C will burn an infant's skin in 1 second, and a child of five in 5 seconds, yet takes 20 seconds to scald an adult. Five-year surveillance data from St Andrew's Burns Centre (Essex, UK) show 70% of paediatric admissions are scalds, 14% contact burns, 9% flame burns, 2% medical skin loss, 1% chemical burns and 4% mixed other causes. Burn size ranges from less than 1% to 100%, but the majority of burns are small so the median burn size is around 5%.

Rule of tenths for UK burns

There are about 100 000 burns treated in hospital in the United Kingdom per year; half of those are in children under 16. Burns can be described by the rule of tenths:

- One-tenth of children are admitted to hospital.
- One-tenth of these children need formal fluid resuscitation as their burns are over 10%.
- One-tenth of these children will need high-dependency or intensive care.

There are therefore around 50 children each year who may be in hospital for approximately 6 months after suffering a burn injury.

Pathophysiology

The burn wound produces a typical picture described in three concentric zones:

- Coagulative necrosis (central)
- Zone of stasis
- Zone of hyperaemia (peripheral)

If burn wound circulation is optimised the area of stasis can be encouraged to heal rather than convert to a deeper burn.

There are both local and systemic responses to burn injury. Pro-inflammatory molecules are stimulated and the basal metabolic rate can rise by 50%. Mediators include histamine, serotonin, prostaglandins, prostacyclin, bradykinin and catecholamines. There is marked increased microvascular permeability and loss of protein from exudates.

Burn wounds produce large amounts of fluid, and systemic oedema occurs when the burn is over 25%. Oedema formation begins at 4 hours and stops at around 36 hours. This fluid loss causes intravascular volume depletion. Careful fluid replacement is required to avoid under-resuscitation while preventing volume overload. An initial period of myocardial suppression is followed by development of a profoundly hyperdynamic circulation. The hypermetabolic response can last for 18 months in larger burns.

Outcome

Burns of any size may be fatal. The number of children dying in house fires in the United Kingdom remains depressingly static at 50 per year.

Risk factors for mortality are:

- Age of less than 2 years
- Burn larger than 90%
- Smoke inhalation
- More than 1 hour before intravenous fluid replacement is started

There are very few survivors with 90% burns but children have better outcomes for massive burns than adults. Burns as small as 1% can be fatal if complications such as toxic shock syndrome occur. Most patients with small partial thickness burns can be expected to recover within 2 weeks with minimal scarring. Larger burns will take 3 to 6 months; they need long-term burn wound management and often heal with lumpy unstable scars. As a general rule, parents should be advised that their child will need

Table 40.2 St Andrew's Hospital 5 year children's inpatient incidence data

	2004	2005	2006	2007	2008
Number of patients	306	302	303	376	371
Median burn size (%)	3	3	7	5	6
Average length of stay per percent burn	1.1	1	0.7	0.6	0.4

to stay in hospital for 1 or 2 days for each percentage of burn (see Table 40.2).

An experienced multidisciplinary burns team should manage all children with massive burns. Strong family support has a positive benefit on recovery but children will inevitably be left with physical and psychological disabilities. Despite suffering severe injuries, it has been shown that children who survive massive burns can have a quality of life that is comparable to that of non-burned children.

Management of burns

The most important part of burns management in children is prevention. Public education programmes such as encouraging use of smoke alarms, burns prevention advice for parents and the 'Stop, Drop and Roll' campaign for clothing fires have been successful. New standards for equipment may prevent scalds, for instance fitting temperature regulators to all new bathroom appliances.

The practical management of burns can be divided into three phases:

- Emergency care (and referral)
- Acute care
- Reconstructive surgery

Emergency care

Immediate first aid aims to stop the burning process: for instance, flames must be extinguished and clothing contaminated by chemicals must be removed (avoiding danger to the rescuer). The temperature of the wound should be reduced; burns less than 3 hours old should be cooled with cold tap water, but hypothermia must be avoided.

The medical management of burns follows basic ABC principles:

Airway

Assess the patency and safety of the airway and administer supplemental high flow oxygen. There may be an associated cervical spine injury, or other injury, particularly if the child has been involved in an explosion or has jumped or been thrown from a burning building.

Children have narrow airways that may be compromised by oedema. Oedema formation begins in the first 4 hours after a burn injury and may worsen for 36 hours. Early intubation will be necessary if there is concern about airway oedema. Other indications for intubation include respiratory distress, hypoxia, and reduced level of consciousness, or to protect the airway for transfer.

Decisions about intubation for a child with a non-significant facial burn require a pragmatic approach. The aetiology of the burn should be considered and combined with a careful clinical assessment of the child. A facial burn in an enclosed space is more ominous than a flash burn from a garden barbecue. Advice from the burns centre should be sought, but if in doubt, the safer approach is to intubate, especially if transfer is required. The tracheal tube can be placed orally or nasally and should be left uncut, as evolving facial oedema may cause the tube to migrate out of the trachea over the next few hours. It is extremely uncommon to need an emergency tracheostomy.

Breathing

Airway oedema increases the work of breathing; respiratory effort and adequacy of ventilation should be assessed. Smoke, particularly from house fires, may contain toxic particles and poisonous gases that can cause a significant lung injury. Explosions and burns in an enclosed space raise the risk of an inhalation injury.

Routine pulse oximetry may not detect carbon monoxide poisoning. If suspected, carboxyhaemoglobin levels should be measured and high flow oxygen given.

Occasionally full thickness burns to the chest or abdomen will restrict ventilation, and emergency escharotomy may be required. The stiff burn eschar is insensate, but escharotomy should be performed

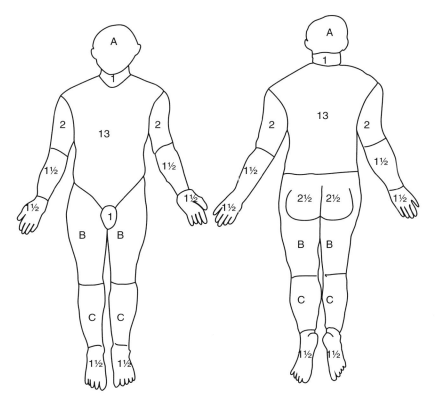

Figure 40.1 Lund and Browder chart for estimating the size of burn. (Redrawn from Lund and Browder 1944; see further reading). The numbers on the figure represent percentage of total body surface area. The letters reflect age-specific areas (see associated table). The Depth of Burn table allows differentiation between superficial and deep burns.

Area	Age					
	<1	1	5	10	15	Adult
A - ½ of head	9½	8½	6½	5½	4½	3½
B - ½ of one thigh	2¾	3¼	4	4½	4½	9¾
C - ½ of one leg	2½	2½	2¾	3	3¼	3½

Depth of burn		
	Superficial	**Deep**
	Shade on figure	*Diagonal lines on figure*
Region	%	%
Head		
Neck		
Anterior Trunk		
Posterior Trunk		
Right Arm		
Left Arm		
Buttocks		
Genitalia		
Right leg		
Left leg		
Total		

under general anaesthesia as the release needs to extend into neighbouring normal tissue that has normal sensation.

Circulation

Fluid is lost from burns, and intravenous access is necessary for all except the most minor injuries.

Circulatory shock is unusual; if present, look for other causes such as long bone fractures or intra-abdominal injury.

Tachycardia, reduced capillary refill and cool peripheries suggest more fluid is needed. Hypotension is a late and ominous sign. A child in circulatory shock requires an initial fluid bolus of 20 ml kg^{-1} of

Table 40.3 Wallace's rule of nines for infants and older children

	Percentage of total body surface area	
	Infant <1 year	Child >10 years
Head/neck	18	9
Each arm	9	9
Anterior thorax	18	18
Posterior thorax	18	18
Each leg	14	18
Perineum	–	1

crystalloid, repeated as necessary. Intraosseous access may be required, but needs to be secure.

Escharotomy may be needed for circumferential burns on arms or legs if the distal circulation is compromised.

Disability

The AVPU score and pupil responses give a rapid description of neurological status. AVPU is scored as the best response of the child: that is, alert (A), responds to voice (V), responds to pain (P), unresponsive (U).

Exposure

Active warming measures are needed as children with burns lose heat quickly. The child should be fully exposed and rolled to document the full extent of injury, then covered to prevent hypothermia. Burns can be covered with non-constricting plastic wrap such as cling film.

The size and depth of the burn should be estimated, excluding soot and erythema, and the burn may need to be washed with warm saline. Burn size is measured using age-specific Lund and Browder Charts (see Further reading), differentiating between superficial and deep burns (see Figure 40.1). This assessment forms the basis for fluid resuscitation, which is required if the burn is over 10%.

The size of the burn can also be estimated using Wallace's rule of nines. Younger children have a relatively larger head and smaller legs, so a modified rule of nines is used for infants (see Table 40.3).

Another way to estimate burn size is that the front of the body represents approximately 50% of the body surface area, and the child's palm and fingers represent 1% body of surface area.

Fluid resuscitation is with Hartmann's solution or Ringer's lactate, using the modified Parkland Formula:

Total volume of Hartmann's in the first 24 hours = % burn × weight × 4 ml

The fluid volume requirement is calculated from the time of burn. Half the volume is given over the first 8 hours (when fluid loss may be greater) and the other half over the next 16 hours.

All formulae are estimates, and the actual fluid rate may need to be increased or decreased according to the child's response. Additional maintenance fluids are no longer recommended.

The end point of resuscitation is when the child is warm and well-perfused and the urine output is $1-2\,ml\,kg^{-1}\,h^{-1}$. Excessive urine output is not desirable, and infusion rates may need to be reduced to avoid fluid overload and respiratory compromise.

Additional fluid may be required if resuscitation is delayed, if there is significant smoke inhalation, electrical injury, or associated injuries, or to prevent renal impairment if haemoglobinuria is present (the urine appears 'dirty' or red coloured).

Parenteral analgesia should be given via the intravenous or intranasal route and titrated to effect for all but the most minor injuries, for example morphine $100-200\,mcg\,kg^{-1}$ IV or intranasal diamorphine $100\,mcg\,kg^{-1}$. Paracetamol should also be given. Non-steroidal anti-inflammatory drugs are relatively contraindicated in larger burns because of concerns about gastric erosion and renal impairment.

If the burn is over 15% a nasogastric tube and a urinary catheter should be inserted. A tetanus booster or tetanus toxoid should be given as indicated. Prophylactic antibiotics are not required. A full history should be taken and documented. A thorough primary and secondary survey will ensure other injuries are not missed.

Referral to a burns unit

Advice and guidelines for referral to a burns unit should be obtained from the local burn service. The nearest paediatric bed may be some distance away. Children with the following conditions should be managed in a specialist burns unit:

- Burn >5% body surface area
- Any burn involving the face, hands, feet, perineum or over a joint
- Circumferential burns

- Burn associated with another injury, or with inhalational injury
- Suspected non-accidental injury
- Electrical burns
- Chemical burns

Anaesthesia for acute burn care

Burns are a surgical problem and need specific burns surgery for successful outcome. Surgical plans may be non-operative, involving dressings only, or operative involving debridement and split skin grafting. The UK National Burn Care Review Committee recommends that the burns theatre is co-located within the burns unit.

Burn care is designed to replicate the functions of the skin, which is to provide the following:

- Physical barrier
- Fluid barrier
- Temperature control
- Sensory
- Psychological
- Immune function
- Metabolic function

Two key functions of the skin are prevention of water loss and protection from bacterial sepsis. The child is susceptible to systemic infection from loss of skin protection, and also immunosuppression from protein loss. A burn injury impairs thermoregulation, and it is difficult to keep the child warm. Pain is reduced if the burn is covered to reduce exposure of sensory nerve endings. Restoration of appearance is vital for children with burns, particularly of the face and hands.

The burn wound heals by re-epithelialisation. It must be allowed to lose exudates but not to dry out. A variety of techniques are used to encourage wound healing: exposure to air, dressings and ointments, as well as operations involving wound debridement and grafts. The endpoint of all treatments is for the patient's own skin to cover the burn.

Dressings cover the wound to protect from bacterial ingress and collect the protein exudates. The classic dressing of paraffin-impregnated gauze covered with crepe and wrapped in bulky cotton wool is imperfect because the dressing needs to be changed and this causes intense (though short-lived) procedural pain. Modern dressings are non-adherent, and dressing changes are less frequent and wound inspection less

painful. Mepitel® is an example of a non-adherent dressing. Another dressing is Biobrane®, which can be closely applied to more superficial partial thickness burns such as scalds and remains in place until the skin is healed. Skin grafts are usually split skin (partial thickness) shaved from the thigh but full thickness grafts are occasionally used. Most skin grafts will be meshed to allow them to stretch like a string vest to cover a larger area. Donor sites temporarily increase the area of injured skin.

Pre-operative care: acute burns

Potential problems will be identified by taking a careful history, examining the child and ordering targeted investigations. The child is at risk of gastric aspiration early in the acute phase of a burn, particularly if the burn is >10%, and our practice is to empty the stomach with a nasogastric tube and to use a rapid sequence induction. Suxamethonium is not used beyond 18 hours after a burn because of the risk of hyperkalaemic cardiac arrest. Routine starvation guidelines are suitable for small scheduled operations.

The burn theatre should be maintained at high ambient temperature and humidity. During surgery, blood loss may be quick, occult and massive, so pre-operative cross-match is necessary for all but the smallest procedures. Our practice is to use normovolaemic haemodilution and replace initial losses with crystalloid, provided the haemoglobin is $\geq 7\,g\,dl^{-1}$, and there are no contraindications to haemodilution such as impaired oxygen delivery due to acute lung injury.

Acute care of small burns

These can be generally managed with a standard anaesthetic. Potential problems include a difficult airway due to oedema, aspiration due to a full stomach, occult blood loss and hypothermia from exposure and cleaning fluids.

Some children require a single general anaesthetic to allow the initial dressing to be applied. Children admitted from a house fire or with flame burns may need to be cleaned under anaesthesia to allow differentiation between smoke discolouration, erythema or burn. One technique is a 'ketamine clean up'. The patient is fully monitored and intermittent bolus doses of ketamine $1\,mg\,kg^{-1}$ IV are titrated to eye nystagmus. The airway is not secured but supplemental facemask oxygen is used. This technique has the advantage of providing analgesia that persists after anaesthesia has worn off.

Typical burn surgery during the acute phase involves preparation of the burn and graft donor site and surrounding areas with iodine-based cleaning solution. Monitoring may be lost during the washing procedure but should be reinstated as soon as possible. Intravenous access needs to be fixed securely. The child often needs to be intubated, but minor procedures away from the face may be undertaken with a laryngeal mask. A single prophylactic dose of antibiotics such as benzylpenicillin 25 mg kg^{-1} IV and gentamicin 2 mg kg^{-1} IV is given to counter the bacteraemia during burn surgery.

Local anaesthesia is useful. Caudal anaesthesia may provide analgesia for both operative and donor sites. Ultrasound-guided blocks under general anaesthesia are possible. Donor site infiltration or topical local anaesthesia onto dressings are useful techniques. The typical donor site is the thigh or buttocks. If there is only a small donor site, a block of the lateral cutaneous nerve of the thigh is simple and effective. Opioid analgesia may be necessary. Addition of clonidine 1–2 mcg kg^{-1} IV is useful.

Post-operative analgesia includes regular paracetamol, NSAIDs and regular opioids with additional rescue doses. Aperients are necessary. The patients will return to theatre at least twice for dressing change and removal of staples from the graft site under general anaesthetic, and hence psychological preparation is crucial.

Acute surgery for large burns

This challenges even experienced anaesthetists and needs as much preparation as a typical adult ruptured aortic aneurysm. There are rapid, occult, massive fluid shifts in patients who are already receiving intensive care and may have multiple organ dysfunction. All patients are hypermetabolic, with high temperature, pulse rate and cardiac output. Starvation must not be prolonged, and patients who have a cuffed tracheal tube and established post-pyloric (nasojejunal) feeding may continue with feeds during the operation.

Early near-total burn wound excision reduces mortality in severely burned children. Full thickness burns may need excision down to fascia whereas partial thickness burns need tangential excision or shaving; paradoxically these wounds bleed more than a deeper injury. Operative blood loss is increased by a factor of three 48 hours after an acute burn owing to increased wound vascularity.

Intubation is often difficult because of airway and facial oedema. Airway loss could be fatal in these patients or necessitate a difficult emergency tracheostomy. An airway exchange catheter such as a Cooks® catheter is useful if the tracheal tube needs to be changed. Pressure controlled ventilation with tidal volume 7 ml kg^{-1} is used to minimise lung injury.

Intravenous access must be secure. Short large-bore IV lines are required for rapid fluid infusion. These lines must be firmly stitched in place with four braided sutures, otherwise they will be dislodged during frequent rolling for cleaning and owing to the presence of emollients. An arterial line may be necessary if there is no limb available for non-invasive measurement. ECG dots will slide off regularly. Fetal scalp electrodes can be fixed into burned or non-burned skin and the wires fixed to standard ECG dots. There may a lack of available digits for pulse oximetry so reflectance probes may be necessary.

It can be difficult to maintain temperature, and surgery may need to be stopped because of hypothermia. It is vital to have a good rapport with the surgical team and to stop surgery if you cannot keep up with blood loss or it is difficult to ventilate the patient. Blood loss may be reduced by the use of tourniquets on limbs, subcutaneous infiltration of 1:100 000 adrenaline prior to excision (maximum dose 10 mcg kg^{-1} i.e. 1 ml kg^{-1}) and topical phenylephrine soaked swabs (20 mg in 1 litre of saline). Systemic absorption of phenylephrine is rarely of clinical significance.

Burns that are older or infected bleed more, and blood transfusion in excess of a blood volume may be required. A useful formula to estimate the blood requirement during surgery is:

$$\text{Blood required during surgery (ml)} = 3 \times \text{weight (kg)} \times \% \text{ burn}$$

Anaesthesia should be maintained with volatile agents and continuation of morphine infusion. Patients are transferred back to the intensive care unit post-operatively with full monitoring.

Anaesthesia for burns reconstructive surgery

Burn scars cause contractures, deformity and dysfunction, especially over mobile areas, and these need release and resurfacing surgery. Normal childhood growth increases tension across burn wounds, and urgent corrective operations may be required to prevent permanent fixed flexion contractures. Burns contractures involving the head and neck may result in difficult intubation from limited mouth opening, reduced neck movement and fixed anterior neck structures. The nasal cavities may be obstructed. Subglottic stenosis may occur if the burn involved the neck or intubation was prolonged. Venous access may still be a problem. Head and neck surgery involves the challenges of the shared airway.

Resurfacing surgery involves excising the burn scar to allow the surrounding skin to spring away from the contracture. This is covered by a split skin graft or artificial skin substitutes such as Integra®. Grafts need to be closely adherent to the wound. For head and neck burns this is achieved using bolster tie-overs that can be bulky and interfere with the airway in recovery or when the child returns to theatre.

Children (and parents) will have fixed views about how they like anaesthesia to be delivered, and these views should be accommodated if possible. Psychological difficulties abound because of the original injury, return to the hospital environment and the need for recurrent operations. Paediatric nurses and play specialists have a pivotal role.

Most reconstructive procedures are painful and require local anaesthetic blocks and infiltration plus opioids. There may still be tolerance to opioids because of long-term exposure.

Airway burns

There are three distinct aspects to consider in airway burns:

- Upper airway obstruction
- The lower airway injury
- Systemic poisoning from smoke inhalation

Upper airway obstruction may be due to the burn or subsequent swelling, but if well managed, rarely leads to fatalities.

Lower airway injury may be due to inhaled soot, oedema, secretions or bronchoconstriction. Chemical pneumonitis occurs when particles in the inhaled smoke adhere to the mucosal surface of the lung. Fortunately, direct thermal injury to the lower airway is rare because of the highly efficient heat exchange mechanisms of the upper airway.

The most serious injuries are from inhalation of toxic gases such as carbon monoxide and hydrogen cyanide, and can be rapidly fatal. Systemic poisoning may complicate hypoxia at the scene of the injury.

Laryngoscopy and bronchoscopy are indicated if a significant upper or lower airway injury is suspected. High concentration oxygen and supportive treatment are usually sufficient.

Electrical injury

Children may be at risk from electrical burns in the home, for instance if toddlers place electrical flexes in their mouths. Electrical injuries cause three distinct problems:

- Electrocution
- Flash burn from explosive arcing as the current jumps from the source to ground
- Injury from being blown away from the explosion.

Electrical current will flow through the line of least resistance, that is, bones, muscles, blood vessels and nerves. Electrocution can produce direct myocardial injury or later rhythm disturbances. If there is a history of loss of consciousness or there are rhythm or ECG changes, the child should be monitored for 24 hours. An electrical burn may cause severe distal ischaemia, and compartment syndrome is a particular risk.

Chemical injury

Young children commonly put things in their mouths and may suffer accidental poisoning from swallowed acids that cause a surface burn, or alkalis that penetrate deeper and cause more prolonged tissue destruction. The management strategy is to reduce the concentration of chemical by dilution. The eyes must be checked as well as the obvious site of burn. Children who have ingested corrosives should be referred for general surgical management.

Use of anaesthetic drugs in burns injuries
Physiological changes affecting anaesthetic drugs

Tissue damage following major burns may result in development of extrajunctional myoneuronal receptors. Fatal increases in serum potassium have occurred owing to depolarisation of these abnormal receptors by suxamethonium. Suxamethonium should therefore be avoided from 18 hours up to 18 months after a major burn.

There are a number of other physiological changes after a burn injury that may affect anaesthetic drugs:

- Plasma albumin is reduced, α_1-acid glycoprotein level is increased.
- Renal blood flow and glomerular filtration rate are increased.
- Hepatic metabolism of drugs is reduced.
- Oedema increases volume of distribution of drugs.
- Basal metabolic rate is increased by up to 50%.

Sensitivity to non-depolarising muscle relaxants is reduced and requires double dosing and boluses at double frequency.

Opioid tolerance occurs easily. Some children develop massive sedation requirements after prolonged intensive care. Changes are unpredictable and vary among individuals.

Management of pain and itch

Burns are painful injuries with background, breakthrough and procedural pain. Early effective pain management is essential to gain the trust and cooperation of the child and their carers. Effective analgesia also modulates the neuroendocrine response to the burn. The link between emotional and physical aspects of pain should not be ignored. Pain must be assessed regularly, recorded, interventions prescribed and the child re-assessed.

The mainstay of pain control in burns is regular oral analgesia using opioids and paracetamol. Extra analgesia must be available to treat breakthrough pain. Patient-controlled analgesia may be used, but burns to the hands and dressings may be a barrier. Switching from morphine to oxycodone or methadone may be useful if tolerance to morphine occurs.

Regular aperients and rescue antiemetics should be given. Adjuncts such as clonidine can be added. Gabapentin is effective in neuropathic pain. Anxiolysis with benzodiazepines may be needed. Non-steroidal anti-inflammatory drugs are effective in small burns but side effects (gastric erosion, renal impairment) preclude their use in the early treatment of larger burns.

Itch from donor sites or regenerating burns can be severe. Gabapentin is helpful with other drugs added using a stepladder approach: cyproheptadine and hydroxyzine then chlorpheniramine.

Procedural pain should be anticipated and treated appropriately. A child may require different levels of anaesthesia, analgesia or sedation, depending on the stage of wound healing. Deep sedation should be carried out in a designated area with full monitoring and by appropriately trained staff. Drugs that have been used for management of procedural pain include:

- Entonox (if child cooperative)
- Fentanyl lozenges (licensed from 16 years)
- Ketamine 7.5 mg kg^{-1} PO, midazolam 0.5 mg kg^{-1} PO
- Remifentanil – profound analgesia, but there is a risk of respiratory depression

Burns critical care

Intensive care for children with burns is a low-volume high-intensity activity that requires close attention to detail, and should be delivered by staff familiar with all aspects of burn care. A 'concertina of care' model works well where facilities and staff can be expanded or contracted to meet the specific needs of the child. A large team is involved including surgeons, intensivists, paediatricians, nurses, theatre teams, physiotherapists, occupational therapists, social workers, psychotherapists, play therapists, dieticians and pharmacists.

Children who require intubation owing to airway oedema or respiratory insufficiency require adequate sedation and ventilation. Tracheal tubes should be fixed securely, which is challenging in the presence of facial burns. Extubation can follow as the oedema resolves.

Management of smoke inhalation is with saline lavage and triple nebulised therapy, which includes alternating bronchodilators, heparin 5000 IU 4 hourly and 20% N-acetylcysteine 3 ml 4 hourly. This reduces microcoagulation, removes toxic soot products, treats bronchoconstriction and stops the formation of bronchial casts, and has been shown to reduce complications following paediatric inhalation injury.

Severe smoke inhalation may be complicated by acute respiratory distress syndrome, and the child may require prolonged respiratory support with protective lung ventilation strategies.

Central venous access is necessary for drug infusions, antibiotic therapy and blood sampling. The use of ultrasound aids line placement as the burn limits potential sites for intravascular lines. A high index of suspicion should be maintained for line-related sepsis, and prompt catheter changes are required. Children with burns are susceptible to serious line-related complications including ischaemic limbs.

Supportive care is required until the burn wound is closed, and this may involve many visits to the operating theatre. There may be worsening of the patient condition during each sequential harvest and skin grafting procedure. The child is susceptible to sepsis originating from the burn itself and to translocation of bacteria from the gut mucosa, or from the lungs or intravascular lines.

The hypermetabolic response to burn injury is minimised by reducing stressful procedures to a minimum, optimal pain control, nursing in a warm environment, effective infection control and provision of additional calories, ideally by early enteral feeding via nasogastric or post-pyloric route. Abdominal complications such as gastric erosions and stress ulceration are common, and were first described in burns patients by the surgeon Thomas Curling in 1842. Antacid prophylaxis is required for all patients.

Fluid requirements and filling are assessed using core–peripheral temperature gradient in conjunction with pulse rate, blood pressure and urine output. Volume status may be difficult to estimate, and daily weight may not be useful because of exudates in dressings. Cardiac output monitoring may be required. Oesophageal Doppler or pulse contour analysis can guide the use of inotropes, although inotropes are rarely required during the resuscitation phase. Norepinephrine may be needed to maintain blood pressure in the face of a hyperdynamic circulation typical of a burns patient. Ongoing fluid and electrolyte requirements including losses through the burn wound need to be assessed and adjusted each day.

Sedation may be difficult because of extreme tolerance to opioids. A combination of IV ketamine and midazolam and oral clonidine is usually used. Additional analgesia is required for dressing changes and showers.

There is inevitable regression of a child's behaviour after a burn. The child may have serious psychological issues, and the parents may be dealing with an enormous burden of guilt about not protecting their child from injury. It is an emotionally exhausting time for the child, family and staff. Psychological support is an essential part of burn care.

Key learning points

- Burns in children are common but massive burns are rare. Outcomes are generally good but require high intensity treatment.
- Start burn treatment early; children with burns over 10% body surface area require fluid resuscitation.
- Complex or large burns should be referred to a burns unit to achieve best outcomes.
- Anaesthetists are an essential part of the large multidisciplinary team involved in achieving the best possible outcomes for children with burns.

Further reading

Education Committee of the Australia and New Zealand Burn Association Ltd. *Emergency Management of Severe Burns Course Manual EMSB* (UK edition). British Burn Association. 2004.

Henry DB, Foster RL. Burn pain management in children. *Ped Clin North Am* 2000;**47**:681–97.

Hettiaratchy S, Papini R, Dziewulski PD, eds. *ABC of Burns*. Blackwell. 2005.

Lund CC, Browder NC. The estimation of areas of burns. *Surg Gyn Obst* 1944;**79**:352–8.

National Burn Care Review Committee. *Standards and Strategy for Burn Care – A Review of Burn Care in the British Isles 2001*. http://

www.britishburnassociation.org/downloads/NBCR2001.pdf (accessed 19 August 2012).

Rabinowitz PM, Siegel MD. Acute inhalation injury. *Clin Chest Med* 2002;**23**:707–15.

Sheridan RL, Hinson M, Liang MH *et al.* Long-term outcome of children surviving massive burns. *J Am Med Assoc* 2000;**283**:69–73.

Chapter

41

Principles of paediatric intensive care

Ian A. Jenkins

Introduction

Critically ill children will continue to require support from anaesthetists, whether these anaesthetists are working in children's hospitals or, just as likely, in a district general hospital (DGH), where they might receive a call to a 'collapsed' infant in the emergency department (ED) for whom their assistance is urgently required. The ED and paediatric staff will probably have already set in motion advanced life support measures, but often they will be looking for additional help. The infant may not be intubated, may look pale, mottled and listless, and may be tachycardic and tachypnoeic. On arrival the differential diagnoses include sepsis and dehydration but could, at this point, still include intussusception, cardiomyopathy, coarctation of the aorta, metabolic disease or even non-accidental injury. Although this may appear to be a bewildering array of differential diagnoses, non-specialist anaesthetists should be able to provide valuable support by understanding key elements of paediatric critical illness.

Anaesthetists will also be required to attend these children in the paediatric ward, the high-dependency unit (HDU), or on a general intensive care unit (ICU), possibly prior to transfer to a specialist centre. Such transfer will generally involve a specialist paediatric intensive care retrieval team, but for certain time-critical conditions the local team may be required to transfer a critically ill child to a tertiary centre. Anaesthetists may also have to provide clinical input to children in a paediatric intensive care unit (PICU), some of whom will need anaesthesia for surgery or imaging, or for their expertise with analgesia and difficult airways.

This chapter will aim to cover some essential aspects of paediatric intensive care that will help the anaesthetist in these situations.

How much paediatric critical care is out there?

Data from the Paediatric Intensive Care Audit Network (PICANet) indicate that there were approximately 47 000 PICU admissions in the UK in the 3 years between 2006 and 2008. Of these approximately 16 000 patients were transported to these PICUs, but nearly a quarter of these were transported by non-PICU teams. From data in southwest England, for every one admission of a child to PICU there are three admissions to DGHs with critical illness; PICU admissions are, therefore, the tip of the iceberg.

Additionally, there is little sign that the number of children admitted to adult ICUs in the United Kingdom is dropping. Children continue to be admitted to DGH emergency departments and paediatric inpatient services because of trauma or critical illness, requiring the services of their local clinicians to resuscitate and stabilise them.

According to data from the UK Intensive Care National Audit and Research Centre (ICNARC), DGH ICUs admit over 800 children per year. Interestingly, data from the southwest region of England for 2006–7 showed that only one-third of these admissions were transferred to a PICU (Figure 41.1), the rest returning mainly to paediatric areas. The reasons for this may include a predicted short ICU admission (e.g. after an operation, a febrile convulsion, or with rapidly resolving croup, asthma or bronchiolitis), or where the child is well known to the local DGH and may have a terminal condition and moving the child may not be in the child's best interests.

Risk adjusted outcomes for the children who were not transferred to PICU and remained in the general

Core Topics in Paediatric Anaesthesia, ed. Ian James and Isabeau Walker. Published by Cambridge University Press. © 2013 Cambridge University Press.

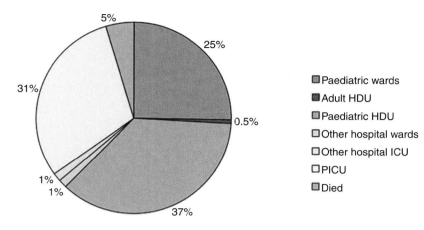

Figure 41.1 Discharge destinations for paediatric admissions to general intensive care units (aggregated data for southwest region 2006–7). See plate section for colour version.

- Paediatric wards
- Adult HDU
- Paediatric HDU
- Other hospital wards
- Other hospital ICU
- PICU
- Died

Total = 217 ICU admissions

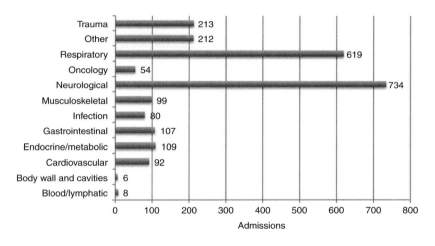

Figure 41.2 Diagnoses in general ICU nationally 2005–7.

ICUs have been shown to be comparable to national PICU outcomes. This would indicate that, where such outcomes are consistently and carefully audited within an active network, not all children admitted to DGH ICUs need to be transferred to the regional PICU.

The type of illness seen in the adult ICU compared with that seen in the PICU is contrasted in Figures 41.2 and 41.3. PICU case mix is affected by its tertiary specialist role and often by a large amount of cardiovascular surgery. Respiratory, neurological and trauma conditions make up the largest groups in children admitted, albeit temporarily, to GICUs.

The age range also differs between adult ICUs and PICUs as seen in Figures 41.4 and 41.5. PICUs see far more young infants, driven to some extent by the

large number of cardiovascular operations in this age group, whereas the age distribution in GICUs is far more evenly distributed.

General principles of paediatric intensive care

Why infants readily develop respiratory inadequacy

- They have small airways; from the Hagen–Poiseuille equation ($Q = \Delta P \pi r^4 / 8\eta l$), any reduction in airway diameter may have a marked effect on airflow and work of breathing.
- They have horizontal and cartilaginous ribs; this causes difficulty in increasing tidal volumes via rib

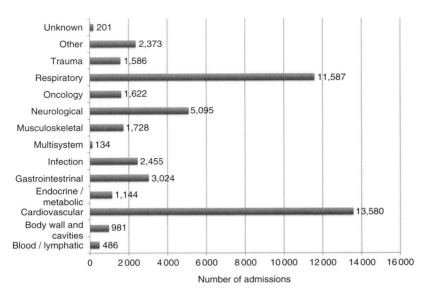

Figure 41.3 Diagnostic groups in PICUs 2006–8.

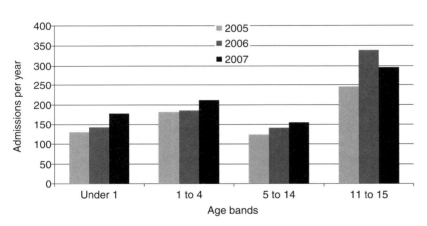

Figure 41.4 Admissions to general ICUs by age.

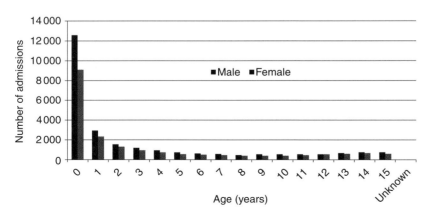

Figure 41.5 Admissions to PICU by age and gender 2006–8.

Table 41.1 Child Glasgow Coma score

	1	2	3	4	5	6
Eyes	No eye opening	Opens eyes to pain	Opens eyes to speech	Opens eyes spontaneously		
Verbal	No verbal response	Inconsolable, agitated	Inconsistently consolable, moaning	Cries but consolable, inappropriate interactions	Smiles, follows objects and sounds, interacts	
Motor	No motor response	Extension to pain (decerebrate)	Flexion to pain (decorticate)	Withdraws from pain	Withdraws from touch	Infant moves spontaneously or purposefully

The lowest score possible is 3; anything below 8 is associated with poor outcomes and is the accepted level for mandatory intubation and ventilation.

movement and a mechanical disadvantage from thoracic cage flexibility. In croup and bronchiolitis, this results in the mechanical inefficiency of subcostal and substernal indrawing and an exacerbation of the work of breathing. In view of the lack of ability to increase tidal volumes, infants must rely on an increased respiratory rate.

Clinical indicators of respiratory inadequacy

- Tachypnoea
- Tachycardia
- Use of accessory muscles
- Subcostal and sternal recession
- Lack of inspiratory reserve
- Stridor – a smaller cricoid ring which may become oedematous in croup or after tracheal intubation
- Deteriorating conscious level
- A rise in $PaCO_2$
- Ultimately, cyanosis

Peculiar to infants and young children with croup is the appearance of expiratory stridor where initially only inspiratory stridor existed. This is a sign that the airway compromise caused by croup is advancing and should precipitate intubation if other measures such as steroids and adrenaline have already been tried (see the 'Croup' section below).

Intubation

Apart from specific respiratory compromise, other indications for intubation include the following:

- Decreased conscious level. Conventionally this becomes definitely indicated with a Glasgow Coma Score of 8 or less (see Table 41.1).
- Smoke inhalation – even when no respiratory effects are present at that time, because respiratory compromise can ensue quickly from airway swelling, pneumonitis or carbon monoxide poisoning.
- Cardiovascular instability. Low cardiac output may be due to intrinsic congenital cardiac problems, myocarditis, cardiomyopathy or dysrhythmias.
- Sepsis. This may be severe, necessitating large volumes of intravenous fluids, e.g. $>60\,\mathrm{ml\,kg^{-1}}$. Pre-emptive support with intubation and ventilation is necessary to offset the development of respiratory compromise due to increased lung water. This path of action, with aggressive fluid resuscitation, control of ventilation and administration of inotropes, is often inadequately managed.

Intubation and ventilatory support also permits easier insertion of central venous and arterial catheters for monitoring and the administration of inotropes, which would be indicated in these circumstances. In all such cases the choice of induction agents can be critical.

Drugs for intubation in the critically ill child

'Which drugs should be used?' is one of the most frequently asked questions when dealing with a seriously ill child. As in any other emergency situation the effects of anaesthetic induction agents on the circulation of a shocked patient still apply. Agents that affect the systemic vascular resistance the least and are less likely to exacerbate any obvious or occult hypovolaemia are the ones to be chosen. Even when children appear normovolaemic, intrinsic cardiovascular compromise still exists in sepsis, metabolic conditions, arrhythmias, cardiomyopathies and cardiac lesions involving left ventricular outflow tract obstruction. Those experienced with critically ill children, particularly those with cardiovascular compromise, find that agents such as ketamine, with *small* doses of fentanyl and/or midazolam, and muscle relaxation with pancuronium cause less instability and have much to commend them. Pancuronium is best avoided in tachydysrhythmias as it increases heart rate, and agents such as vecuronium or rocuronium should be used in preference. Atracurium often releases histamine and is therefore not so useful in cardiovascular compromise. Ketamine has been shown to be safe in head injury.

Respiratory support in children

Continuous positive airways pressure (CPAP) can decrease the work of breathing by decreasing the pressure gradient across the narrowed airways. CPAP is frequently used in infants with less severe forms of croup, bronchiolitis and pneumonias and may obviate the need for intubation and ventilation. In infants under 6 kg this is usually delivered via short nasal prongs connected to a humidified gas supply from a purpose-built 'driver'; small nasal masks are now available. Older children may manage with small (adult) nasal masks. Some conventional ventilators now have software that will allow them to deliver CPAP without alarming continually for the large leaks that inevitably result from the necessary free-flowing gases.

For larger children, purpose-built non-invasive ventilators (NIV) can be used to deliver CPAP or patient-triggered BiPAP via nasal masks or facemasks covering nose and mouth. Even masks covering the whole face can be used successfully, particularly in children whose face shapes do not match conventional masks.

In children up to the age of 5 or so requiring ventilation on the ICU, nasal intubation is better tolerated than oral, with decreased requirements for sedation. Additionally, nasal tubes are more stable, easier to fix and permit easier mouth care.

Pressure-cycled ventilation is very common in paediatric practice because leaks round traditionally used uncuffed tracheal tubes are rendered less significant, although changes in lung or thoracic compliance will alter alveolar ventilation. Volume-cycled ventilation is less vulnerable to compliance changes but is affected by the leaks around non-cuffed tubes. Monitoring of expired tidal volumes is therefore vital. Peripheral oxygen saturations and end-tidal CO_2 where possible, without causing problematic dead space increases, should be continuously monitored.

Cuffed versus uncuffed tracheal tubes in PICU

Cuffed tubes decrease leaks by compensating for tube and larynx size mismatch. For anaesthesia, it has now been shown that they can be used without problem. However, such studies on their use in PICU are still awaited. Cuffed tubes permit greater use of volume-cycled ventilation modes, but there are still unanswered questions regarding the risk of subglottic stenosis or dilation. It is suggested that cuff pressure should remain below 25 cmH$_2$O. However, this may not prevent a leak in conditions requiring high-pressure ventilation, and there is no consensus on the methodology of cuff pressure monitoring in children. In children with prolonged length of stay on the PICU, tracheostomies are less readily employed owing to anatomical difficulties (short necks, short tracheal length), and their use is associated with longer-term problems such as local tracheomalacia or stenosis (even with more modern surgical techniques).

High-frequency oscillatory ventilation (HFOV)

HFOV is a mode of ventilation that delivers minimal tidal volumes into the anatomical dead space at frequencies ranging from 3 to 20 Hz. The faster frequencies are used in neonates. HFOV is used fairly commonly in paediatric practice in diffuse parenchymatous disease where, in order to obtain adequate gas exchange, conventional IPPV ventilator pressures are very high (e.g peaks of $\geq$28 kPa). It is thought that the reduced tidal volumes avoid the shear stresses of pulmonary 'volutrauma' while maintaining a high mean airway pressure (MAP) to maximise alveolar recruitment and minimise atelectasis. While MAP and FIO_2 are dictated by the pressure and composition of the gas flow, CO_2 elimination is dictated by the movement of gas in and out of the airway caused by the action of a piston-driven diaphragm that

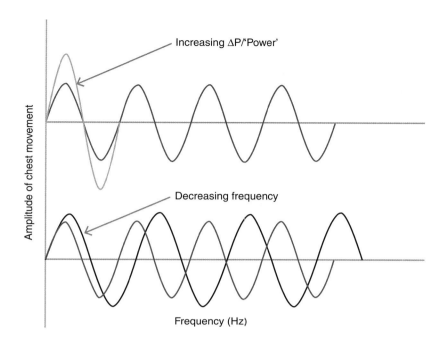

Figure 41.6 Effect of 'power' and frequency on amplitude of oscillation. See plate section for colour version.

oscillates at high frequency. The amplitude of the movement of the gases in and out of the patient is dictated by three variables:

- The patient's total thoracic compliance;
- The 'power' or ΔP driving the ventilator diaphragm; and
- The frequency of the oscillation.

For any given compliance and power, the initial slope of the amplitude of tidal volume against time is also constant. Increasing the 'power' of the driving oscillatory diaphragm in the ventilator will clearly increase the tidal movement of air. However, by decreasing the oscillatory frequency, the wavelength is longer, giving more time for the diaphragm movement to exert an effect. This is shown in Figure 41.6 where the desired elimination of CO_2 may be achieved at lower overall pressure differences by reducing the frequency rather than increasing the 'power' of the diaphragm.

Patient oxygenation will also depend on adequate MAP to exert beneficial effects of alveolar recruitment, but as the pulmonary condition improves this can lead to overinflation with pulmonary capillary compression and decreased gas exchange. Regular chest radiographs are necessary to help assess overinflation.

Transfer to theatre of a patient on HFOV

It may become necessary to move a patient on HFOV to the operating theatres or for a scan. It is possible to perform surgery and insert invasive catheters with a child on an oscillator, but it is technically more difficult, and generally attempts would be made to return them to conventional ventilation. When moving the patient back to a conventional ventilator one has to attempt to replicate the high degree of PEEP and alveolar recruitment that HFOV is achieving. This may mean accepting higher peak pressures than desirable but recognising that this would be only a short-term measure. A trial of conventional ventilation should be attempted to ascertain whether the child will tolerate this. If not, it will be necessary to set up the oscillator in the operating theatre or, in emergency situations, to undertake surgery in the PICU.

Extra-corporeal membrane oxygenation (ECMO)

This comprises an extra-corporeal circuit, draining blood from the venous system and returning it after gas exchange to the arterial system (usually from the internal jugular vein to the carotid artery or, following cardiac surgery, from right atrium to aorta).

The blood is usually pumped by a centrifugal vortex pump round a circuit that contains a heat exchanger and an oxygenator. The circuit must be heparinised and the activated clotting time (ACT) monitored with levels held at 170–200 seconds.

According to the International Extracorporeal Life Support Organisation Registry ('ELSO'), outcomes from ECMO in children appear to be better than in adults. The validity of ECMO in treating neonatal respiratory failure was established after it was subjected to a prospective randomised trial, but evidence for its use in older children and adults has been much less convincing. However, the latest RCT in adults ('CESAR Trial') demonstrated more survivors with ECMO over conventional, non-ECMO treatment. Apart from severe cardiac failure, e.g. cardiomyopathy awaiting transplant or immediately after cardiac surgical operations, the main indication for ECMO is severe respiratory failure. Referral for ECMO should be made when one or more of the following are present:

- Severe hypoxia and/or hypercapnia with lack of response to conventional support measures (this may include high frequency oscillation, inhaled nitric oxide, prone positioning and surfactant). Severe hypoxia in this context is usually defined as:
  - PaO_2 (in mmHg) $\div FiO_2 < 100$; or
  - Oxygenation index (OI) >40, where OI = $FiO_2 \times 100 \times MAP$ (cmH$_2$O) $\div PaO_2$ (mmHg);
- Sustained elevated inflation pressures, e.g. > 24 hours of MAP >20 on conventional ventilation, or MAP >25 on HFOV;
- Persistent air leak or interstitial air;
- Cardiovascular instability with shock (pH <7.25).

ECMO will usually not be offered where there is likely to be irreversible ventilator-induced lung injury, conventionally when mechanical ventilation is longer than 10 days. Early referral is recommended.

Children receiving ECMO occasionally need intercurrent imaging, e.g cardiac catheterisation or CT/MRI scans, or urgent surgery such as re-exploration of a cardiac operation or laparotomy. It is most important that the heparin dosing is kept to a minimum, that all coagulation factors, including fibrinogen and platelets, are optimised and that blood is instantly available. Transferring patients on ECMO is hazardous because of the circuitry and is best avoided if at all possible. A team comprising the perfusionists, ICU nurses and doctors with clearly defined roles should be assembled for any transfer.

Fluids and inotropes in critically ill children

Children, particularly infants, have a large extracellular fluid compartment. This leads to higher maintenance fluid requirements and also, in sepsis, increased capillary leak. Such children will have greater requirements for fluid supplementation on a weight basis than may be anticipated from adult practice. However, children are also more prone to developing inappropriate ADH secretion in respiratory conditions such as bronchiolitis. If given 'normal for age' IV fluid maintenance they can develop severe hyponatraemia. Therefore, in these instances, maintenance fluids are cut back to 80% of normal for that age and fluids containing less than 0.45% saline are not used. If fluid boluses are needed for ongoing deficits then isotonic fluids should be used (0.9% saline or lactated Ringer's solution). See also Chapter 14.

With greater surface area for their body weight, smaller children have higher insensible losses on a volume/weight basis and this is exaggerated in pyrexia. In infants, it is reasonable to allow an extra 10% maintenance fluids for every degree C of pyrexia.

Infants have hearts that differ from older children and adults:

- With less concentration of contractile elements and a relative preponderance of collagen and elastin, cardiac compliance is diminished. Cardiac output is less responsive to volume loading and more dependent on heart rate.
- The Starling curve is flatter with an earlier downward inflection point at shorter fibre lengths (i.e. lower filling pressures).
- After term, myocyte β-receptor populations and response to catecholamines and phosphodiesterase inhibitors are normal. However, the infant heart remains particularly sensitive to and dependent on ionised calcium levels in the ECF; hypocalcaemia is not well tolerated.

Inotrope choice in children is very similar to that in adults, the most common being adrenaline and milrinone. In adult cardiac arrests there may be benefit from using vasopressin 0.2–0.8 units kg^{-1}. There

Table 41.2 Principal clinical features of croup, epiglottitis and bacterial tracheitis

	Croup	Epiglottitis	Bacterial tracheitis
Age range (peak)	6 months to 3 years (1.5 y)	3 months to 5 years (2.5 y)	8 months to 14 years (3.75 y)
Cough	Severe (+++) Barky and non-productive	Minimal	+++ (Productive)
Stridor timing	Early	Late	Early
Stridor onset	Gradual	Sudden (+++)	Sudden mild (+)
Toxic	No, mild pyrexia	Yes	Yes
Dysphagia	Minimal	Pronounced	Minimal
Drooling	No	Yes	No

are no data to support (or refute) its applicability in paediatric practice. The data on its use in PICU in refractory hypotension in sepsis are disappointing.

Specific respiratory conditions

Viral disease accounts for much of the respiratory pathology seen on the PICU. Nasopharyngeal aspirates (NPA) are commonly taken for immunofluorescence and polymerase chain reaction (PCR) to detect viruses. However, where the pathology is in the lower respiratory tract, either endotracheal aspirates (ETA) or broncheoalveolar lavage (BAL) specimens should be obtained.

Croup, epiglottitis, tracheitis

The differing clinical features of these conditions are outlined in Table 41.2.

For croup, dexamethasone, 150 mcg kg^{-1}, is best administered parenterally and can avoid or shorten intubation. Intubation is usually necessary in epiglottitis although it is now an uncommon disease since the introduction of *H. influenzae* vaccination. Conversely the incidence of bacterial tracheitis, which will also usually need tracheal intubation, appears to be on the increase. Severe pseudomembranous bacterial tracheitis has been reported which requires repeated bronchoscopic lavage.

Bronchiolitis

This is an infection of the lower respiratory tract usually involving infants but seen up to 3 years of age. It is characterised by cough, tachypnoea, nasal flaring and subcostal recession. Usually there are widespread crepitations and coarse wheeze. Many patients can be managed conservatively by treating the pyrexia, ensuring

adequate hydration and the use of CPAP delivered by nasal prongs or nasal mask. No benefit from steroids has been demonstrated nor have any sustained effects from bronchodilators been shown, although some temporary improvement in clinical variables may occur.

Intubation and ventilation may be necessary for actual or impending respiratory fatigue, judged on clinical grounds. Pulmonary compliance is often very poor so 'permissive' hypoventilation with modest hypercapnia (6.5–8 kPa), respiratory acidosis (≥7.25) and desaturation (92–95%) should be accepted.

Status asthmaticus

Children present with respiratory distress, cough and wheeze. The factors that suggest that ICU admission is indicated are pleomorphic but might include:

- History of previous ICU admissions
- Rapid deterioration
- Hypoxaemia despite oxygen administration
- Severe distress despite nebulised bronchodilators
- Inability to phonate
- Limited air entry
- Inspiratory as well as expiratory wheezing
- Altered conscious level
- If blood gases are being taken, a rising CO_2 with signs of fatigue

Drug management for severe asthma includes:

Glucocorticoids: these are the key treatment but they may take up to 8 hours to reach full effect so should be given early.

Prednisolone 1–2 mg kg^{-1} orally, or
Hydrocortisone 4 mg kg^{-1} IV if unable to take oral medication.

In the meantime the following should be given by nebulisation, noting that under 2 years β2 agonists may not work and may produce paradoxical bronchoconstriction:

Salbutamol

<5 yrs, 2.5 mg

>5 yrs, 2.5–5 mg

Ipratropium

<5 yrs, 125 mcg

>5 yrs, 250 mcg

If there is inadequate response, *intravenous salbutamol* is given as a bolus over 10 minutes:

<2 yrs, 5 mcg kg^{-1}

>2 yrs, 15 mcg kg^{-1}

In HDU or ICU settings a *continuous infusion of salbutamol* can be started at 1–5 mcg kg^{-1} min^{-1}.

Aminophylline is used in children to supplement β-agonists, bolus 5 mg kg^{-1} over 20 minutes, then infused at 1 mg kg^{-1} h^{-1}, but the evidence for its efficacy has not been established.

The same also applies to IV *magnesium* (25–40 mg kg^{-1} over 20 min) but this is becoming used more frequently after some reports on its use in emergency medicine.

Intubation and ventilation are indicated in the event of life-threatening asthma unresponsive to the above measures. Care needs to be taken on intubation as there may be occult hypovolaemia secondary to a period of decreased fluid intake. Drugs that release histamine, such as morphine and atracurium, should be avoided. Ketamine is useful in preserving blood pressure and in its bronchodilator action. A cuffed tube is useful, given the anticipated high inflation pressures.

Ventilation should adopt the following strategy:

- Modest hypercapnia, accepting an arterial pH of >7.2;
- Slow rates to allow for prolonged expiratory time and avoid air trapping;
- Short inspiratory times to keep an adequate respiratory rate;
- Low PEEP.

Avoidance of PEEP is a mistake as this only encourages small airway closure and exacerbates air trapping. If flow–time curves are available, then the optimal PEEP and expiratory times can be estimated.

Antibiotics are only required where there is evidence of bacterial infection, such as:

- Raised inflammatory markers, such as neutrophil count and C-reactive protein;
- Positive cultures of tracheal aspirates;
- Radiological evidence.

Macroscopically purulent sputum may be misleading as this may contain large amounts of eosinophils.

Sedation for ventilation could include ketamine and fentanyl and possibly a muscle relaxant if it is better to obtund the patient's respiratory activity and coughing in the early stages. It should be remembered that the presence of the tracheal tube may be an ongoing stimulus for bronchospasm and so the tube should be removed at the earliest opportunity, even if there is still some wheeze.

Cardiovascular

Children may present to the emergency department or to PICU in a low cardiac output state in whom the cause may be an undiagnosed cardiac disorder, an acute dysrhythmia, or cardiomyopathy. In a baby who has been discharged from the maternity unit perfectly well but re-presents to the hospital in a collapsed state in the first few days of life, coarctation of the aorta or congenital aortic stenosis should be suspected. The patency of the ductus arteriosus protects them immediately after birth by perfusing the aorta distal to the obstruction. As the duct closes over the next few days, distal systemic flow falls, which can lead to a profound low output state with severe metabolic acidosis and organ dysfunction. This can mimic severe sepsis.

Administering prostaglandins in this situation is essential; this may not reopen the duct fully but may give partial relief to the obstruction and improve distal perfusion to a degree. In aortic stenosis, however, amelioration will depend on re-opening the duct.

Most severe congenital cardiac lesions are identified on antenatal scanning, but occasionally these may be missed. In a newborn presenting with cyanosis, transposition of the great arteries should be considered. Prostaglandin infusion to keep open the ductus will be necessary. The newborn with obstructed total anomalous pulmonary venous drainage will present with cyanosis and a 'hazy' chest X-ray, which can easily be mistaken for meconium aspiration.

Gastrointestinal

Volvulus is a condition caused by malrotation of the gut and is heralded by bilious vomiting or bilious NG aspirates. It is usually seen in the neonate but can occur later. It is a surgical emergency, and it may be faster and therefore more appropriate if the referring team transfers the child to a paediatric surgical centre, rather than waiting for a retrieval team which may double the transfer time and could result in an necrotic intestine with disastrous results.

Intussusception can present rather vaguely with lethargy and intermittent pain rather than the classical vomiting and redcurrant jelly stools, which are seen in only a third of cases. It can develop into a time-critical emergency where the viability of the intestine and of the child itself are at stake with a marked systemic inflammatory response with circulatory failure. Consequently, it is often best that the referring team transfers these patients into the tertiary centre rather than incurring delays caused by retrieval. Local protocols must allow for this.

Diarrhoeal conditions may go on to develop into haemolytic uraemic syndrome, particularly associated with *Escherichia coli* O157-H7 but also with salmonella and campylobacter. It is a condition caused by diffuse small vessel occlusion by thrombotic microangiopathy with a triad of haemolysis, thrombocytopenia and renal failure. Its complications are diffuse and include fits, coma, cardiac failure, pancreatitis and ischaemic colitis where frank necrosis and perforation can occur. The treatment is to support the failing kidney with peritoneal dialysis or haemofiltration and, where possible, avoid platelet transfusion and systemic antibiotics which may fuel the condition. Where CNS involvement occurs, then it more resembles thrombotic thrombocytopenic purpura (TTP) and is often treated with plasmapheresis with replacement of circulating proteins with fresh frozen plasma.

Renal failure and support

The past few years have seen a great refinement in the equipment available for paediatric 'renal replacement therapy' (RRT) in the ICU, and haemofiltration and haemodiafiltration have become relatively commonplace. Mortality is worse if the patients are hypotensive on going onto RRT, particularly if receiving inotropic support, or have secondary renal failure rather than primary single organ renal failure.

RRT is also used as specific therapy in metabolic disease, particularly when there is marked hyperammonaemia, which is only treatable by haemofiltration or haemodialysis. In certain cases, this may have to be used in neonates, which is more of a technical challenge.

The problems seen particularly in smaller patients are:

- Thrombocytopenia due to adsorption of platelets to the filter;
- A tendency to underestimate insensible fluid losses, which can be monitored and corrected for by daily weighing of the child;
- Hypothermia due to the patient's blood travelling through a circuit with a very high relative surface area.

Some manufacturers have started to make proprietary jackets to conserve heat on these parts of the circuit.

Decisions to move the patient for scans or operations need to be considered carefully as each time this occurs the patient will have to be disconnected from the filter and the circuit carefully reprimed with blood when the child is reconnected. Consequently, such procedures are better bunched together to reduce donor exposure.

Neurology
Cerebral blood flow

This accounts for a third of the cardiac output at birth and, at 4 years of age, is still twice that of adults per kilogram. Thus, in cardiovascular compromise, it should be expected that brain function and conscious levels consequently deteriorate and may be demonstrated in the early inconsolable irritability that can develop into the somnolence of the seriously ill child.

Fits and status epilepticus

In a previously well child the differential diagnosis of fits includes infection, trauma and tumours. Meningitis will have to be excluded if the history is suggestive, but the most common causes of seizures in the preschool child (3 months to 5 years old) are so-called 'febrile convulsions'. These appear to be worse where the rise in temperature is fastest (hence occasional lack of prodromal history), may consist of alarming unilateral and prolonged fits, and can be resistant to conventional antiepileptic protocols.

When the fits are unilateral, precautionary CT scanning is essential to exclude more sinister pathology. Generally, after a few hours of ventilation and control of temperature where indicated, these children wake up entirely normally. Further investigation is usually not undertaken unless fits recur.

In status epilepticus, the usual cascade is:

- 2 doses of benzodiazepine,
  - midazolam 500 mcg kg^{-1} buccally or
  - diazepam 500 mcg kg^{-1} rectally; or
  - lorazepam 100 mcg kg^{-1} intravenously, then
- phenytoin 20 mg kg^{-1} IV or
- phenobarbital 20 mg kg^{-1} IV.

At this time paraldehyde 0.4 ml kg^{-1}, dissolved in the same volume of olive oil, can be instilled rectally. If these latter measures do not halt the seizures after 20 minutes, then intubation using intravenous thiopental should be undertaken. It may be necessary to continue a thiopental infusion at 2–6 mg kg^{-1} h^{-1} and proceed to continuous EEG recordings to detect ongoing seizure activity.

Traumatic brain injury (TBI)

Most centres that insert intracranial pressure (ICP) monitoring aim for a minimal cerebral perfusion pressure (CPP) of at least 40 mmHg.

$$CPP = Mean\ arterial\ blood\ pressure - [ICP + CVP]$$

However, in TBI, cerebral blood flow autoregulation is abnormal, and there is recognition that pushing CPP much beyond this risks over-perfusion of the brain and thereby raising ICP. There is no evidence of benefit of hypothermic treatment of paediatric TBI. Jugular venous saturation measurement, although it has been studied in research to a limited extent, has not proved to be consistently useful in practice and may also interfere with jugular venous drainage.

External ventricular drains (EVD) are inserted to decrease ICP by controlled release of cerebrospinal fluid and also for draining obstructed hydrocephalus in haemorrhagic brain injury. When moving patients with EVDs the level of the drain must be controlled carefully. These are usually set 5–10 cm above a zero point at the midpoint between the lateral edge of the orbit and the tragus of the ear. Dropping the drain level may cause precipitous and excessive drainage. If it is raised then there may be some reflux back into the patient leading to a rise in ICP and increasing

danger of infection. Generally it is safer to clamp these drains *briefly* for transfer to scanners or to theatre but, once this is completed, to replicate their setting in ICU and maintain controlled drainage. Above all, it is important to remember to unclamp the drain and then ensure that free drainage has returned. If not, the drain may have blocked and will need attention. These drains should never be laid flat; the porous ventilation holes in the collection chamber will get wet and the drain will no longer function correctly.

Metabolic diseases

Inborn errors of metabolism

These usually declare themselves in early childhood but this may not happen until young adulthood. Many conditions are insidious with 'failure to thrive', but there are a few that can present as medical emergencies, sometimes catastrophically. Some trigger, such as intercurrent infection, precipitates an acute collapse in a previously well child, with variable manifestations: lactic acidosis, hypoglycaemia, and/or hyperammonaemia. The presentation is with 'collapse' with a sick, drowsy, 'shut-down', hypoglycaemic and poorly perfused child. Where doubt exists it is important to measure blood glucose, lactate and ammonia (which must go to the lab *on ice*).

Adequate carbohydrate administration will switch off protein and lipid metabolism, which may be the root cause of the crisis.

- A 10% glucose infusion must be started and run at a minimum of 90 ml kg^{-1} h^{-1} to give about 6 mg kg^{-1} min^{-1}.
- All feeds must be stopped, as they may be substrates for the toxic by-products the child is now failing to clear.

Once this is all accomplished, there will be time to set in motion more detailed metabolic investigations and to start ammonia scavenging medications and co-enzymes. However, very high ammonia levels (>500 mcmol l^{-1}) will require haemofiltration as an emergency to clear this neurotoxic substance.

Diabetic ketoacidosis (DKA)

DKA in children differs significantly from that in adults because of the danger of cerebral oedema. This disastrous complication is thought to be due to the rapidity with which the biochemistry is corrected, such as rapid changes in serum osmolality caused by the fluids used in rehydration, dropping of the high glucose or aggressive correction of the acidosis – particularly in using bicarbonate – or any combination of these.

Consequently, it is managed differently and is subject to widely accepted international guidelines:

- Cautious administration of fluids
- Very gradual correction of the glucose
- No initial insulin bolus, and infusion rates kept to 0.05–0.1 units $kg^{-1} h^{-1}$
- Avoidance of bicarbonate

Shock, caused by dehydration, should be treated with 10 ml kg^{-1} fluid boluses, but even this should be done sparingly and any such fluids should be deducted from the calculation of fluid replacement (in ml) necessary over the next 48 hours (body weight × % dehydration × 10).

If cerebral oedema is suspected, with a deteriorating GCS, then mannitol 10% (1 ml kg^{-1}) or hypertonic saline 3% (5 ml kg^{-1}) should be given, and all IV fluids slowed. If this does not procure a lasting improvement, the child should be intubated and ventilated and nursed head up. Hyperventilation must be avoided owing to worse outcomes although there is some recognition that a low-normal $PaCO_2$ may be physiologically appropriate. A CT scan should be performed to exclude cerebral venous thrombosis, a recognised complication from the profound dehydration.

Sepsis

In severe sepsis, where volumes administered equal or exceed 60 ml kg^{-1}, it is advisable to consider intubation. Not only does this counteract the effects of the pulmonary oedema that often develops to a degree in these situations, but it also presents an opportunity to insert central venous and arterial catheters for more accurate haemodynamic monitoring and to facilitate the use of inotropes. It is a common mistake to underestimate the amount of fluid a child needs to maintain cardiac output in sepsis, and not to intervene early enough with inotropes.

Similar considerations apply as in adults in dealing with 'warm' or 'cold' shock by responding to lack of intravascular volume by administering fluids to ensure the heart is well filled and then using either selective inotropes or adding in agents with

vasoconstrictive effects or even vasodilatory effects (such as with phosphodiesterase inhibitors) depending on the perceived tonicity of the vascular bed.

Limb compromise can be seen in the purpuric septicaemias, owing to either meningococci or pneumococci, and this can be due to either embolic deficits or more global deficits consequent to 'compartment syndromes'. However, compartment involvement can be quite diffuse, involving multiple compartments, even in the same limb. Fasciotomies have been tried in the past but have had disappointing results, perhaps because the vessel compromise has not been as a result of any relievable local pressure and, in turn, the operative wounds also go on to be a source of secondary infection themselves.

Non-accidental injury and child protection ('safeguarding')

Non-accidental injury may present as overt trauma but may 'masquerade' with fits, as 'failure to thrive' or as a 'collapse' in the emergency department. Anaesthetists and general intensivists must be alert to these possibilities, and all now have an obligation to have at least basic training in the recognition of abuse and in knowing what subsequent course of action to take. An ever-present index of suspicion is unfortunately necessary. See Chapter 5.

Managing the potential organ donor

When a child or young person has been subjected to a catastrophic brain injury with incipient brain death, it may not be in the child's (or the family's) best interests to move the child from a DGH to a regional PICU.

When it is apparent the child will not survive the family may be, perhaps should be, approached with a view to organ donation. Historically, the United Kingdom has performed quite poorly in approaching families and securing much needed organs for those on transplant waiting lists (until recently, at half the rate of donors per million population than France and about a third of the rate in Spain) but progress has been made in the past 2 years by the UK Organ Donation Taskforce and rates have increased by about 30%.

Donation after cardiac death (DCD) may also be considered where withdrawal of intensive therapy is being considered owing to the gravity of the underlying condition. These donations may not be suitable for heart and lung transplantation, but liver, kidney and other solid organs and tissues such as corneas and heart valves can be sourced by this method. Provided the best interest principles of the child are upheld, there is no reason why they may not be donors after death, and it has been shown to help families in their grieving. It is mandatory that decisions about withdrawal are made prior to broaching organ donation and it is advisable that the two discussions are carried out by different teams.

In either post-cardiac or post-brain-death situations the advice of the local specialist nurse in organ donation should be sought, particularly before the family are approached in case there is any doubt about the suitability of the donor. In the brain-dead child, they will give important advice about management of the donor, including support of the circulation and consequent optimisation of the donated organs. There are physiological considerations, such as preservation of vasomotor tone and general maintenance of the circulation and biochemistry, sometimes including hormonal therapy with cortisol and thyroxine, that must be attended to if the organs are to be protected. Local protocols should be agreed and easily accessible.

Key points

- It is important that the 'generalist' anaesthetist understands the principles of care of the critically ill child, as they are best placed to provide immediate care to a child presenting to the emergency department, working in conjunction with the paediatricians.
- Ketamine maintains cardiovascular stability in the shocked child.
- Cuffed tracheal tubes should be used in children with reduced lung compliance, but the cuff pressure should be monitored.
- The need for fluid replacement and inotropic support is frequently underestimated in children with shock, with the exception of diabetic ketoacidosis, where fluid boluses should be used with extreme caution.
- Non-accidental injury should be considered in children presenting with trauma.

Further reading

Asthma Guidelines. http://www.brit-thoracic.org.uk/Portals/0/Guidelines/AsthmaGuidelines/sign101%20Jan%202012.pdf

British Society of Paediatric Endocrinology and Diabetes. *DKA Guideline 2009*. http://www.bsped.org.uk/professional/guidelines/docs/DKAGuideline.pdf (accessed 17 June 2011).

Hammer GB, Holzki J, Morton NS. The pediatric airway. *Ped Anes* 2009;**19** (Supp. 1): 1–197.

McKeown DW *et al.* Management of the heartbeating brain-dead organ donor. *BJA* 2012;**108**: i96–i107.

Murphy PJ, Marriage SC, Davis PJ. *Case Studies in Pediatric Critical Care*. Cambridge University Press. 2009.

Nichol DG, ed. *Rogers' Textbook of Pediatric Intensive Care*, 4th edition. Lippincott, Williams & Wilkins. 2008.

Chapter

42
Stabilisation and safe transport of the critically ill child

Daniel Lutman

Introduction

Centralisation of specialist services, such as paediatric critical care, major trauma, cardiac surgery or neurosurgery, improves outcomes. For the critically ill child, accessing specialist services often requires the child to be transported to the appropriate centre, either primarily by ambulance (bypassing non-specialist centres) or secondarily by hospital teams after initial resuscitation and stabilisation in a non-specialist centre.

Children may be particularly vulnerable during transfer. Hospitals that admit children who may be critically ill or injured should be part of a clinical network involving paediatric critical care services and transport teams, with agreed guidelines for referral, immediate care and transport, and appropriate audit and governance arrangements. Transporting a critically ill child carries risks for the patient and requires the involvement of senior clinicians. This chapter describes general principles of secondary transport of critically ill children and specific guidance for the transport of a child with a neurosurgical emergency, which may need to be undertaken by the referring hospital.

Prospective planning

- The secret to efficient stabilisation and transport of critically ill children is anticipation.

It is important to plan for transport in terms of resources, expertise and equipment, before the need arises. This is important for both specialised transport services and for district hospitals who may be required to transport a child, for instance with a time-critical neurosurgical emergency.

The need for transport of critically ill children is relatively predictable. There are common diagnostic categories, and predictable frequency and variations according to time of day and months of the year. Plans should be made for the most commonly encountered scenarios. For example, airway emergencies are common in children, bronchiolitis is most common in the winter months, and children are most commonly involved in trauma out of school hours. Basic support of respiratory and cardiovascular systems is similar for most of the commonly encountered diagnoses.

Guidelines for the following commonly encountered emergencies should be available, ideally via the local retrieval service website (for instance from the Children's Acute Transport Service CATS www.cats.nhs.uk):

- Anaphylaxis
- Asthma
- Bronchiolitis
- Burns
- Coma
- Congenital heart disease
- Diabetic ketoacidosis
- Metabolic emergencies
- Neurosurgical emergencies
- Persistent pulmonary hypertension of the newborn
- Poisoning
- Sepsis
- Status epilepticus
- Upper airway obstruction

Making a referral

- For a critically ill child, the risk of the transport is small compared with the benefit of specialist services.

Core Topics in Paediatric Anaesthesia, ed. Ian James and Isabeau Walker. Published by Cambridge University Press. © 2013 Cambridge University Press.

Most UK centres now have a dedicated transport team for both children and neonates. Establishing the need for transport and the required time frame informs all other decisions. There should be a close dialogue between the referring hospital and the transport team as soon as referral is considered.

Specialist transport teams have dedicated consultant intensivists and are a valuable source of advice for the clinician involved in initial stabilisation of the child. Some referrals may resolve with advice from the intensive care team, and the need for transport will be avoided. Ideally, when a child is referred, the transport team will act as the liaison between the referring hospital and the specialist centre, leaving the referring doctor free to concentrate on the immediate clinical needs of the child.

The most senior clinician available at the referring hospital should assess the balance of risks and direct management once the decision to transport has been made. For instance, an arterial line and a central line may be indicated for a critically ill child, but are they required prior to transport? If central venous access is technically difficult, how long should one persist and at what point should one abandon the attempt? Decisions about urgency of transfer also require an understanding of what will happen in the receiving hospital. Does the patient need emergency neurosurgery, or will they be transferred to the PICU for a period of ventilation and antibiotics?

Information for the transport team should be collated prior to referral. Essential information can be summarised in a referral checklist (Table 42.1).

Acceptance and agreement

- It is vital that a critically ill child is taken to the correct receiving institution and that they are ready to receive the child.

The child may be transported by a specialist transport team, or the local hospital team may be required to transfer the child themselves, depending on the availability of the transport team, the distances involved, and the urgency of the clinical situation.

The transport team must know the name of the accepting consultant and the name of the receiving hospital. As a minimum, a member of the transport team should contact the receiving unit immediately before departure. It is advisable to speak to someone who will be directly involved with the patient,

Table 42.1 Referral checklist

Patient details

Referrer details

Reason for referral

Clinical details. Follow SBAR format:
- Situation
- Background
- Assessment
- Recommendation

Allergies, medications, immunisations

Child protection issues

Trauma: details of injury, including timings

Status at referral:
- Airway
- Breathing
- Circulation
- Disability (AVPU)
- Everything else: blood results, blood gases, imaging, cultures

Planned interventions

Summary of discussion

AVPU stands for Alert, responds to Voice, responds to Pain, Unresponsive

for example the nurse in charge in PICU. Describe the current condition of the child and any immediate needs of the patient, as well as how to get the patient from the ambulance entrance to the receiving ward.

Generic transport rules

There are some rules that are common to all scenarios:
- Before transport, interventions that improve outcomes should be prioritised.
- Recognise the point at which the transport itself becomes the priority.
- For the transporting team, the risk of a transport is small but present. Unnecessary risks should not be taken.

The point at which the transport becomes the priority sometimes occurs surprisingly quickly. It is more easily recognised by someone who is 'hands off' in a leadership role, but the person with most experience is frequently directly involved in clinical procedures.

It is important that the team leader maintains a clear overview of the situation.

Generic goals: ABC

- Physiological support often has to be instituted before a definitive diagnosis has been made.

If paediatric critical care transport is required, only do investigations that change either clinical management or the destination of the child.

Airway

- A clear airway needs to be maintained at all times.

It may be better to intubate a patient electively in the hospital environment rather than risk emergency intubation in the ambulance if the patient deteriorates *en route*. Early intubation is recommended for children with sepsis requiring aggressive fluid resuscitation and cardiovascular support.

Common indications for intubation include:

- Airway protection or to maintain a patent airway
- Respiratory failure
- Cardiovascular support
- Neuroprotection in severe head injury

The expected size and length of tracheal tube should be calculated for every patient, and one size larger and smaller should be carried for the transport. Do not pre-cut the tube, as it may be too short. The aim should be to use a tracheal tube with a snug fit, and if the tube has a large leak it should be changed. Consider a cuffed tracheal tube, particularly in children with respiratory infection or sepsis, as lung compliance may deteriorate. All intubated children should have a nasogastric tube inserted and left on free drainage.

If possible, put together an airway bag specifically for each patient transported. The airway bag should contain the following equipment:

- A functioning laryngoscope
- A replacement tracheal tube
- One larger tracheal tube, one smaller tracheal tube
- Magill's forceps
- Suction catheters
- Tape, scissors
- A facemask

The facemask is commonly forgotten if the patient is intubated prior to departure. Do not overload the bag.

Failed intubation

- The priority is oxygenation; repeated attempts at laryngoscopy should be avoided.

Failed intubation is a particular problem in paediatric patients with respiratory failure. The main group at risk seems to be those under 1 year of age. It is important to consider transport early in any child in whom a difficult intubation is anticipated, before their respiratory status becomes critical. An LMA and Ayre's T-piece may be used to transport patients successfully following failed intubation. This is not ideal as sedation and paralysis are usually required to tolerate an LMA, which places the patient in a precarious position for the journey.

Optical laryngoscopes such as the Glidescope or Airtraq should be considered in children who are difficult to intubate. A technique using an adult fibre-optic scope has been described in situations where a paediatric fibre-optic scope is not available. The scope is used to visualise the larynx, and the suction channel is used to pass a suitable wire into the trachea. A small tracheal tube is then passed over this wire into the larynx.

In some situations, a surgical airway inserted by an ENT surgeon should be considered, particularly if the child has an unstable airway and a long transport time is anticipated.

Breathing

- Respiratory support can become a problem during a transport because the disease process may be evolving, and consumables such as oxygen and power are limited.

A self-inflating bag should be available and in view at all times. A bagging circuit attached to an oxygen outlet should be ready at all phases of the transport.

An adequate supply of oxygen should be carried, and there should always be a back-up supply. Never carry all the oxygen in a single cylinder.

If the patient is intubated, a mechanical ventilator is preferable to ventilation by hand. Hand ventilation uses a high fresh gas flow, and it may not be possible to deliver PEEP or pressure limited ventilation as effectively as via a ventilator, particularly if a self-inflating bag is used.

If a ventilator is used, the consumption of oxygen should be known and a calculation made to ensure that enough oxygen is available for the journey. A calculation can be made using the following formula, always assuming that the patient will require a FiO_2 of 1.0:

$$\text{Oxygen required (litres)} = \text{ventilator consumption}$$
$$(\text{litres minute}^{-1}) \times \text{journey length (minutes)} \times 2$$

Ventilators always consume more gas than the minute volume delivered, so this excess needs to be known to calculate the quantity of gas required.

Some transport ventilators utilise an electrical power source but will have a limited battery life. Always know the battery life of the ventilator that you are using, and plug the ventilator into a suitable power source whenever one is available.

Control and conserve oxygen supplies carefully during a transport. When returning a patient to a ventilator after using a bagging circuit ensure that the supply of oxygen to the bagging circuit is switched off. Monitor oxygen consumption during a transport to make sure it matches the amount calculated.

The transport ventilator and oxygen cylinders need to be restrained so that they do not present a hazard to staff or the patient if the vehicle accelerates, brakes suddenly or is involved in an accident.

Use a filter in the circuit to retain heat and moisture and act as a bacterial and viral filter. If dead space is critical, use filters at the ventilator end of the inspiratory and expiratory limbs to prevent ventilator contamination.

Continuous positive airway pressure

Continuous positive airway pressure (CPAP) is challenging to deliver in a transport environment because the oxygen consumption is very high. Ventilators that contain an air compressor are an option and can deliver CPAP for patients requiring low inspired oxygen, providing that sufficient power is available.

Oxygen failure

The self-inflating bag can provide emergency ventilation in the event of oxygen failure. The ambulance should then be diverted to the nearest emergency department to top up the oxygen supply.

Ventilatory problems during transfer

Significant deterioration may occur during transport, particularly if the child is unstable prior to transport, and children should be monitored carefully. Consider the mnemonic 'DOPES' if ventilatory problems occur after intubation:

- Displaced?
- Obstructed?
- Pneumothorax?
- Equipment?
- Stomach?

Care should be taken to ventilate to normocapnia for the head injured child. Permissive hypercapnia is acceptable in severe lung disease (provided pH >7.2, SpO_2 $>88\%$). Children with acute severe asthma are at risk of dynamic hyperinflation and air-trapping; if this is the case it may be necessary to disconnect the child from the breathing circuit briefly to perform manual decompression.

Circulation

- Two secure IV lines are recommended for transport. A triple lumen central line counts as one site of vascular access.

It is essential to monitor heart rate and non-invasive blood pressure during transport, although measurements do not indicate cardiac output and need to be interpreted in the context of the clinical history, pulse volumes, capillary refill time, urine output, conscious level and response to therapeutic interventions.

An understanding of age-appropriate heart rates and blood pressures is essential. This information is probably best incorporated as an *aide memoire* with the transport documentation. Normal values should be targeted in most clinical situations. Exceptions include:

- Penetrating trauma in the older child, where hypotensive resuscitation may have a role;
- Head injury with raised intracranial pressure, when a higher blood pressure may be required to achieve adequate cerebral perfusion.

Monitoring standards

The monitoring standards defined by the Association of Anaesthetists of Great Britain and Ireland (AAGBI) are appropriate for all ventilated patients. These include:

- Continuous ECG
- Blood pressure
- Pulse oximetry
- Capnography

- Temperature
- Ventilator alarms (minimum disconnect and high pressure alarms)

Capnography is an essential component of respiratory monitoring, and should be used for all transports. It is used to monitor adequacy of ventilation, it identifies correct tracheal tube placement (and displacement) and provides a useful monitor of cardiac output, particularly during cardiopulmonary resuscitation.

Non-invasive blood pressure monitors rapidly deplete the battery power of integrated monitors, and become unreliable if there is a lot of movement. Blood pressure is most efficiently measured using intra-arterial monitoring, but time must not be wasted in failed attempts to insert an arterial line (this applies to any intervention). The time taken must not exceed the benefit of the line, and intermittent non-invasive blood pressure measurements may be the best option.

Documentation

- An anaesthetic record is a good starting point for transport documentation.

A contemporaneous record of the medical decisions and the physiological status should be made. A section summarising medical issues yet to be dealt with or any outstanding investigation results is essential. A copy of relevant documentation, scans and X-rays must be given to the receiving team and a copy returned to the referring hospital.

Ideally, transport documentation should be designed to facilitate decision-making processes by guiding assessment, providing information (drug calculations, tracheal tube sizes, normal physiological variables) and offering therapeutic goals.

Transport team

The skills of the transport team should match the requirements of the patient. A two-person team is the accepted minimum for ventilated patients. Each hospital should develop a contingency plan for emergency paediatric transport, which should identify which personnel will form the transport team.

- *Team Leader.* This should be someone with the ability to lead medical decisions, with the appropriate skills to undertake likely interventions. In practice this is often a physician or advanced nurse practitioner.

- *Assistant.* This should be someone able to assist the team leader in delivering the level of care required. In practice this is often a children's nurse or ODP but could be a paramedic with appropriate skills.
- *Driver/technician.* This should be someone capable of operating the transport ambulance equipment and driving the patient and team to the receiving facility in a safe timely manner. In practice the driver will often be an ambulance driver with experience in emergency response driving. The route to the receiving facility may be unfamiliar so some form of map is essential and a GPS system is helpful.

The local ambulance service should not automatically be asked to supply a paramedic crew for the transport. The main role of the paramedic crew is for primary transport from home or roadside to a hospital facility, and the paramedic crew may be underutilised in a physician-led secondary transport.

Method of transport
Road transport

A 'frontline' NHS ambulance will have some of the equipment required for transport of a critically ill child. The essential requirements include oxygen, suction and a defibrillator suitable for the size of the child. Other equipment such as monitors, syringe pumps and airway/ventilation equipment may have to be sourced from the referring hospital for time critical transfers; specialist children's transport ambulances will be fully equipped.

Power sockets are usually available and there are usually at least three seats, which will permit a parent or carer to accompany the patient, if this is deemed clinically appropriate.

Air transport

- The technical and logistical problems that accompany *ad hoc* secondary aeromedical transfer in the emergency setting are formidable.

The main problem with aeromedical transport using fixed wing aircraft or helicopter transfer is not the physiology of aviation, but coordination of multiple transfers, patient access and monitoring in unfamiliar isolated hazardous environments. Weather and landing site restrictions may reduce any potential time saved. Road ambulances will be required to transport the patient to landing sites, and these will need to be coordinated with the aircraft. The local ambulance service may be able to assist, if this is required.

Helicopter emergency medical service (HEMS) helicopters are limited in capacity and it is likely that only one member of staff will be able to accompany the patient.

A Search and Rescue helicopter can be requested which has the capacity to transfer a medical team with the patient. The team should not expect any medical equipment, power or oxygen to be available. The dual pilot, navigator and winchman crew that accompany a Search and Rescue helicopter are an additional valuable resource for the transporting team.

Altitude

It is important to liaise with the crew if altitude will cause clinical problems. All helicopters are unpressurised and often operate at or below 2000 feet. Fixed wing aircraft may be pressurised or unpressurised. A pressurised fixed wing aircraft will not have a cabin pressure higher than 8000 feet. As a rule of thumb at 8000 feet (2438 m) a healthy individual breathing air would experience a PaO_2 of 7 to 8.5 kPa (SpO_2 of 85 to 91%).

A chartered air ambulance may be able to pressurise the cabin to sea level for the journey – however, there will be a limitation on the aircraft altitude and a fuel penalty.

Because a low ambient pressure causes expansion of trapped gases, the following issues should be considered:

- A pneumothorax will expand at altitude and should be drained pre-departure.
- Air transport is relatively contraindicated if the child has an open head injury or open eye injury.
- Air transport is relatively contraindicated for children with intestinal obstruction, as there is a risk of perforation.
- Tracheal tube cuff pressures should be checked en route.
- Minute volume from ventilators may increase and end-tidal CO_2 monitoring must be used.
- Intravenous fluid bags containing gas may pressurise, increasing infusion rates unexpectedly.
- A vacuum mattress will soften at altitude.

Parents and carers

- A parent or carer should accompany the patient.

Unnecessary separation can add considerably to the distress of parents and carers at a very difficult time. From the perspective of the transport team, parents are an essential source of information, and it is helpful if they are present at the destination hospital when the child arrives. It may be useful to re-examine the medical history with the parent or carer during the journey, if circumstances permit. Parents should be kept fully informed at all times, and ideally, one parent should travel in the transport ambulance.

Health, safety and insurance

- The patient, parent or carer, equipment and staff must be adequately restrained when the vehicle is moving. Seat belts must be used.
- Consider a personal death or injury insurance such as that available to AAGBI, ICS or PICS members.

Some improvisation is usual in an emergency *ad hoc* transport, and inevitably there will be some risk to the team and patient from the transfer. Assessing risks and keeping them to an acceptable level is part of the overall process of transfer, and all members of the team need to participate.

Oxygen cylinders are particularly dangerous unless they are properly restrained when the vehicle is in motion.

All NHS staff are eligible to benefit from the NHS Injury Benefits Scheme via the NHS Litigation Authority. It seems that some form of negligence would need to be demonstrated on behalf of the employer and the benefits are not clear.

As a result the Association of Anaesthetists of Great Britain and Ireland (AAGBI), Intensive Care Society (ICS), Paediatric Intensive Care Society (PICS) and allied organisations have arranged personal accident insurance for members undertaking patient transfers. Those likely to form part of a transport team should consider taking out this kind of insurance.

Death of a patient during transport

If a child has suffered an irrecoverable head injury or major trauma, or brain stem death is inevitable, it is better to spare the family and the child the distress of a futile secondary transfer where no clinical benefit is likely. If a child unfortunately succumbs during transport, it is usual to divert to the nearest hospital able to manage the situation. This is often the nearest hospital with an accident and emergency department. The location of the death will determine which Coroner will investigate the case.

Time-critical neurosurgical emergency

The child requiring urgent neurosurgery, for instance because of extradural haematoma, blocked ventriculo-peritoneal (VP) shunt or bleed into a previously undiagnosed cerebral tumour, should be transferred to a specialist neurosurgical centre as soon as possible. Transfer by the referring hospital team is usually the most appropriate, but decisions should be made in joint consultation with the transport team and neurosurgeons. Transfer by an experienced anaesthetist is usually appropriate.

Useful pointers for urgent transfer

Following trauma

- Rapid loss of consciousness
- Initial lucid interval followed by loss of consciousness
- Unequal pupils
- Cushing's triad – hypertension, bradycardia, abnormal respiration
- Focal neurological deficit e.g. hemiparesis
- Obvious external injury e.g. depressed skull fracture

Non-traumatic

- Suspected blocked VP shunt
- Rapid loss of consciousness in previously well patient
- Unexpected cardiorespiratory arrest in a young infant (consider non-accidental injury)
- Focal neurological deficit, including focal seizures in an older child
- Antecedent severe headache and vomiting

Outcome can be improved by reducing the time to surgery, but basic neuroprotection must be in place prior to transfer. Hypotension and hypoxaemia are associated with poor outcome and must be avoided at all times.

Initial management of acute neurosurgical emergencies is in accordance with APLS guidelines:

Table 42.2 Target values for mean arterial pressure in children with a neurosurgical emergency

Age	Target mean arterial pressure (mmHg)
<2 years	>55
2–6 years	>60
>6 years	>70

- Stabilise airway (and cervical spine), breathing and circulation
- Establish two points of IV access
- Pass a urinary catheter and orogastric tube

Indications for intubation

- GCS ≤8 or rapid decrease in GCS
- Signs of raised ICP: unequal pupils, Cushing's triad
- Loss of airway reflexes
- Ventilatory insufficiency
- Spontaneous hyperventilation ($PaCO_2$ ≤3.5 kPa)

Neuroprotection after intubation

- Secure the tracheal tube and confirm bilateral air entry.
- Continue cervical spine immobilisation if indicated with collar, sandbags and tape.
- Maintain oxygen saturation ≥94%, maintain normocapnia ($PaCO_2$ 4.7–5.3 kPa). Capnography is mandatory.
- Paralyse and sedate with morphine, midazolam and vecuronium infusions. Boluses of fentanyl 5 mcg kg^{-1} may be useful during suction.
- Maintain adequate blood pressure to maintain cerebral perfusion pressure. Target mean arterial pressures according to the age of child are shown in Table 42.2; inotropes may be required:
  - Dopamine 5–10 mcg kg^{-1} min^{-1} IV (peripheral)
  - Noradrenaline 0.02–1 mcg kg^{-1} min^{-1} IV (central)
- If there are concerns about raised ICP or rapid changes in clinical signs (e.g. pupillary changes or Cushing's triad) consider interventions to reduce ICP:
  - Mannitol (0.25 to 0.5 g kg^{-1} IV) and/or
  - Hypertonic saline (3% saline 3 ml kg^{-1} IV over 20 minutes, aim for serum sodium 145 mmol l^{-1}).

- Record pupil signs and vital signs every 15 minutes.
- Maintain central temperature 35–37 °C. Avoid hyperthermia.
- Identify and treat seizures with a loading dose of phenytoin $20\,mg\,kg^{-1}$.
- Fluid restrict to 50% maintenance. Use isotonic fluids only (0.9% saline).
- Maintain normal blood sugar – add dextrose to 0.9% saline:
  - For a child <2 years if blood glucose $\leq 4.4\,mmol\,l^{-1}$
  - For a child ≥2 years if blood glucose $\leq 3.9\,mmol\,l^{-1}$
- Antibiotic prophylaxis is recommended for penetrating head injuries or when there is evidence of CSF leak (co-amoxiclav $20\,mg\,kg^{-1}$ or cefuroxime $20\,mg\,kg^{-1}$ + metronidazole $7.5\,mg\,kg^{-1}$).
- Consider associated injuries if there is hypotension and falling haemoglobin. Ideally associated injuries should be excluded or stabilised prior to transfer.

Urgent CT scan

A CT scan should be done within 30 minutes of suspicion of a mass lesion, but does not take priority over neuroprotection, and should only be carried out once neuroprotection goals are met. If the CT scan indicates that neurosurgery is required, transfer should take place immediately (target maximum <60 minutes from end of scan).

Indications for urgent CT scan in a child are:

- GCS <13 at any time since injury
- GCS equal to 13 to 14 at 2 h after the injury
- Suspected open or basal skull fracture
- Post-traumatic seizure
- Focal neurological deficit
- >1 episode vomiting
- Amnesia >30 minutes of events before impact
- Dangerous mechanism of injury
- Coagulopathy

Although useful, insertion of a central line and arterial line should not delay transport. In this situation inotropes may need to be run peripherally and the non-invasive blood pressure cuff used, such is the importance of timely surgery.

Table 42.3 Checklist for transport of a child from a local hospital to specialist centre

	Tick when completed
Receiving hospital staff spoken to by the responsible consultant	
Ambulance Service request (999 call or via Duty Controller) • State ventilated neurosurgical emergency • Request ASAP response time	
Estimated journey time from Local Ambulance Service	
Call receiving hospital immediately prior to leaving	
Equipment	
Airway (facemask, Ambu bag, tape, tubes, laryngoscope, scissors)	
Drugs (fluid bolus, mannitol, sedation, paralysis, inotropes)	
Ventilator and oxygen calculation	
Infusion pumps	
Mobile phone with appropriate telephone numbers	
Monitoring	
ECG	
SpO_2	
Blood pressure (NIBP or arterial)	
End-tidal CO_2 (mandatory)	
Physiological targets	
$SpO_2 \geq 94\%$	
Blood pressure (NIBP or arterial) – age-appropriate target	
End-tidal CO_2 required to achieve $PaCO_2$ 4.7–5.3	
Full sedation and paralysis	

Time-critical transport checklist (non specialist transport teams)

A checklist suitable for local transport teams such as illustrated in Table 42.3 will reduce critical incidents. It is sensible to prepare equipment in advance.

Penetrating trauma

The majority of blunt trauma can be managed non-operatively and will respond to restoration of circulating volume and attention to coagulation. A specialist transport team can then retrieve the patient.

A child that presents to an adult trauma unit or other non-specialist hospital with penetrating trauma resulting in life-threatening haemodynamic instability requires special consideration.

The decision in this situation hinges on the surgical expertise at the non-specialist hospital at that moment, and damage limitation surgery should be attempted on site if appropriate. If damage limitation surgery cannot be attempted locally, the patient will need to be transported to the nearest Major Trauma Centre or other specialist facility, and the best chance of survival probably lies with an immediate non-specialist team transfer.

The most senior doctor available should accompany the child on the transport. Aggressive fluid resuscitation in this situation may cause exsanguination, and should be limited to achieve low-normal blood pressure.

Key points

- The need for transport of a critically ill or injured child is predictable and should be planned within clinical networks.
- The retrieval team is an invaluable source of advice during initial stabilisation prior to transport.
- The airway should be secured early, prior to transport in critically ill children.
- Time-critical transfers may need to be undertaken by the referring hospital;

appropriate equipment and protocols should be prepared well in advance.
- Completion of a transport checklist reduces critical incidents during transport.

Further reading

AAGBI. *Safety Guideline Interhospital Transfer*. February 2009. www.aagbi.org/sites/default/files/interhospital09.pdf

Advanced Life Support Group (ALSG). *Advanced Paediatric Life Support: The Practical Approach (APLS)*, 5th edition. Wiley-Blackwell. 2011

Advanced Life Support Group (ALSG). In Driscoll, P, ed. *Safe Transfer and Retrieval: The Practical Approach*, 2nd edition. Wiley Blackwell. 2006.

Advanced Life Support Group (ALSG). *Paediatric and Neonatal Safe Transfer and Retrieval: The Practical Approach*. BMJ Books. 2009.

Children's Acute Transport Service (CATS). http://portal.cats.nhs.uk/

Department of Health. *The Acutely or Critically Sick or Injured Child in the District General Hospital. A Team Response.* 2006. Crown Copyright. http://www.dh.gov.uk/prod_consum_dh/groups/dh_digitalassets/@dh/@en/documents/digitalasset/dh_062667.pdf (accessed 2 June 2012).

Martin T. *Aeromedical Transportation: A Clinical Guide*. MPG Books. 2006.

National Health Service Clinical Advisory Group Report. *Management of Children with Major Trauma*. 2011. http://www.ukpics.org.uk/documents/Management%20of%20Children%20wi~dvisory%20Group%20Report%201.pdf (accessed 2 June 2012).

South Thames Retrieval Service (STRS). http://www.strs.nhs.uk

Index